CONSULTATION IN INTERNAL MEDICINE

MEDICAL CONSULTATION® SERIES

Jerome P. Kassirer, M.D.
Consulting Editor

Caplan, Kelly:
    Consultation in Neurology
Harrington:
    Consultation in Internal Medicine
Hedges:
    Consultation in Ophthalmology
Reinhold:
    Consultation in General Surgery
Scott, Scott:
    Consultation in Diagnostic Imaging
Williams:
    Consultation in Chest Medicine

CONSULTATION IN INTERNAL MEDICINE

JOHN T. HARRINGTON, M.D.

Professor of Medicine
Tufts University School of Medicine
Boston, Massachusetts
Chief of Medicine
Newton-Wellesley Hospital
Newton, Massachusetts

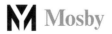 Mosby

St. Louis Baltimore Boston Carlsbad Chicago Naples New York
Philadelphia Portland London Madrid Mexico City Singapore
Sydney Tokyo Toronto Wiesbaden

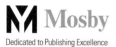
Mosby
Dedicated to Publishing Excellence

A Times Mirror
Company

Printed in the United States of America

Mosby–Year Book, Inc.
11830 Westline Industrial Drive
St. Louis, MO 63146

Library of Congress catalog card number 89–51063

ISBN 1-55664-076-5   10 9 8 7 6 5

CONTRIBUTORS

FREDERICK R. ARONSON, M.D., M.P.H.

Assistant Clinical Professor of Medicine, University of California, San Francisco, School of Medicine; Attending Physician, The Medical Center at the University of California, San Francisco, California

Anemia
Splenomegaly

SANJEEV ARORA, M.D.

Assistant Professor of Medicine, Tufts University School of Medicine; Staff Physician, New England Medical Center, Boston, Massachusetts

Chronic Abdominal Pain
Hepatic Encephalopathy

VINCENT J. CANZANELLO, M.D.

Assistant Professor of Medicine, Nephrology Section, Bowman Gray School of Medicine of Wake Forest University, Winston-Salem, North Carolina

Edema
Recurrent Urinary Tract Infections

JENNIFER DALEY, M.D.

Instructor, Harvard Medical School; Associate Physician, Beth Israel Hospital, Boston, Massachusetts

The Patient with Pain
Diabetes
Hypertension
Medical Noncompliance

N.A. MARK ESTES III, M.D.

Associate Professor of Medicine, Tufts University School of Medicine; Director, Cardiac Electrophysiology and Pacemaker Laboratory, New England Medical Center, Boston, Massachusetts

Syncope
Ventricular Arrhythmias
Pacemaker Therapy: Classification, Indications, and Clinical Considerations

KARIM A. FAWAZ, M.D.

Associate Professor of Medicine, Tufts University School of Medicine; Physician, New England Medical Center, Boston, Massachusetts

Dysphagia
Chronic Abdominal Pain
Upper Gastrointestinal Bleeding
Recurrent Lower Gastrointestinal Bleeding
Acute Diarrhea
Chronic Diarrhea
Elevated Transaminases
Clinical Approach to Jaundice
Hepatic Encephalopathy

NELSON M. GANTZ, M.D.

Professor of Medicine, Microbiology and Molecular Genetics, University of Massachusetts Medical School; Clinical Director of Infectious Diseases, Hospital Epidemiologist, Division of Infectious Disease, Department of Medicine, University of Massachusetts Medical Center, Worcester, Massachusetts

Postoperative Fever
Endocarditis Prophylaxis
Approach to the Patient with Erythema Nodosum
Infections Caused by New Pathogens—Corynebacterium Group JK, Crytosporidium, Capnocytophaga, and Aeromonas

RICHARD A. GLECKMAN, M.D.

Professor of Medicine, University of Massachusetts Medical School; Chief, Infectious Disease, Chief of Medicine, St. Vincent Hospital, Worcester, Massachusetts

Selecting a Parenteral Cephalosporin
Fever of Unknown Origin in the Elderly
Infection in the Diabetic Patient
Fever in the Leukopenic Leukemia Patient

JOHN T. HARRINGTON, M.D.

Professor of Medicine, Tufts University School of Medicine, Boston; Chief of Medicine, Newton-Wellesley Hospital, Newton, Massachusetts

The Patient with Pain
Diabetes
Hypertension
Medical Noncompliance

CHRISTOPHER D. HILLYER, M.D.

Fellow, Division of Hematology/Oncology, New England Medical Center, Boston, Massachusetts
An Approach to the Bleeding Patient

JEFFREY M. ISNER, M.D.

Professor of Medicine and Pathology, Tufts University School of Medicine; Chief, Cardiovascular Research, St. Elizabeth's Hospital, Boston, Massachusetts
Cardiac Consultation in Patients Undergoing Noncardiac Surgery
The Systolic Murmur
Anticoagulation in Cardiac Disorders
Cardiovascular Screening of Competitive and Noncompetitive Athletes

HARRY KIMBALL, M.D.

Professor of Medicine, Tufts University School of Medicine; Chief, Division of General Medicine, New England Medical Center, Boston, Massachusetts
Cancer Screening

MARVIN A. KONSTAM, M.D.

Associate Professor of Medicine and Radiology, Tufts University School of Medicine; Director, Adult Cardiac Catheterization Laboratory, New England Medical Center, Boston, Massachusetts
Congestive Heart Failure

ANDREW S. LEVEY, M.D.

Associate Professor of Medicine, Tufts University School of Medicine; Division of Nephrology, New England Medical Center, Boston, Massachusetts
Hyponatremia and Hypernatremia
Hypokalemia and Hyperkalemia
Acid-Base Disorders
Diagnosis of Renal Insufficiency
Management of Renal Insufficiency
Recurrent Urinary Tract Stones

KENNETH B. MILLER, M.D.

Assistant Professor, Division of Hematology/Oncology, Tufts University School of Medicine; Director of Leukemia Services, New England Medical Center, Boston, Massachusetts
An Approach to the Bleeding Patient
Leukocytosis
Cancer Screening

CHESTER H. MOHR, M.D.

Clinical Fellow in Pulmonary Disease, New England Medical Center, Boston, Massachusetts
Evaluation of Patients With Hemoptysis

LARRY NATHANSON, M.D.

Professor of Medicine, SUNY at Stony Brook; Director, Oncology-Hematology Division, Winthrop-University Hospital, Mineola, New York
Paraneoplastic Syndromes

DOUGLAS T. PHELPS, M.D.

Clinical Fellow, Tufts University School of Medicine; Research Fellow in Pulmonary Disease, New England Medical Center, Boston, Massachusetts
Recurrent Pulmonary Infections

FRANCIS RENNA

Assistant Professor of Dermatology, Tufts University School of Medicine, Boston; Chief of Dermatology, Newton-Wellesley Hospital, Newton, Massachusetts
Pigmented Skin Lesions

JAN ROTHMAN, M.D.

Fellow, Oncology-Hematology Division, Winthrop-University Hospital, Mineola, New York
Paraneoplastic Syndromes

RICHARD A. RUDDERS, M.D.

Professor of Medicine, Tufts University School of Medicine; Physician, New England Medical Center; Director, Lymphoma Service, Boston, Massachusetts
Lymphadenopathy
Adjuvant Treatment of Cancer
Splenomegaly

LEONARD SICILIAN, M.D.

Assistant Professor, Department of Medicine, Tufts University School of Medicine; Director, Medical Intensive Care Unit, New England Medical Center Hospital, Boston, Massachusetts

Evaluation of Patients with Hemoptysis
Management of Acute Asthmatic Attacks
Recurrent Pulmonary Infections
Solitary Pulmonary Nodule
Care of the Intubated and Mechanically Ventilated Patient
Evaluation of the Patient with Suspected Occupational Lung Disease
Acute Inhalation Injury

DAVID R. SNYDMAN, M.D.

Associate Professor of Medicine and Pathology, Tufts University School of Medicine; Pathologist and Physician, Director of Clinical Microbiology and Hospital Epidemiologist, New England Medical Center, Boston, Massachusetts

Evaluation of the Patient with a Positive Tuberculin Skin Test

ANDREW R. WEINTRAUB, M.D.

Fellow in Cardiology, Tufts University School of Medicine; Staff, New England Medical Center, Boston, Massachusetts

Congestive Heart Failure

ALEXANDER WHITE, M.B., M.R.C.P.I.

Clinical Fellow, Tufts University School of Medicine; Clinical Fellow in Pulmonary Disease, New England Medical Center, Boston, Massachusetts

Care of the Intubated and Mechanically Ventilated Patient

PREFACE

The art and science of performing a consultation in internal medicine is often neglected in traditional internal medicine teaching, both in medical schools and in residency programs. In this text, *Consultation in Internal Medicine*, we have provided the systematic approach of a collegial group of clinicians to the clinical problems for which we are most often consulted. All the contributors have (or have had) appointments at the New England Medical Center and/or Tufts University School of Medicine.

In compiling the topics for our text, I asked the contributors to review the specific problems they were asked to address in inpatients. I estimate that more than 90 percent of the problems for which internists or internal medicine subspecialists are called to see patients are covered in this text. The contributors have covered eight topics in cardiovascular medicine, nine topics in infectious disease, gastroenterology, and hematology-oncology, seven topics in nephrology and pulmonary disease, and four topics in general medicine. Endocrinology and rheumatology sections deliberately were omitted because most of these patients currently are cared for as outpatients. Diabetes mellitus is reviewed in the general medicine section, as are other general medicine problems of chronic pain, hypertension, and noncompliance.

Who needs this text? The number of medical texts seems to increase exponentially. We have tried not to be responsible solely for chopping down more trees, but rather to provide a highly focused examination of the diagnosis and treatment of major, common problems. We have aimed the text at the young internist and surgeon who need precise answers to such pragmatic questions as "What do I do with an elderly patient who has fainted once?", "Should I treat every patient with a positive PPD?", "What tests should I order in my patient with dysphagia?", "How should I work up and treat acute bronchospasm? Pigmented skin lesions? Hyponatremia? Chronic pain?"

It is my belief that the thorough, pithy discussion of the problems covered in this handbook provides readily available and invaluable information to young internists and surgeons. I believe that the systematic approach emphasized in this text also will provide sustenance to the seasoned internist in his or her daily practice. The text is designed to be carried in one's pocket for ready consultation at the bedside.

My thanks to our publisher, Brian Decker, for supporting this series; to the editor of the series, Dr. Jerome P. Kassirer, my long-time friend and colleague; and special thanks to Ms. Karen Coyne for her devotion to this task over the last year.

John T. Harrington, M.D.

CONTENTS

GASTROINTESTINAL DISEASE

RENAL DISEASE

PULMONARY DISEASE

HEMATOLOGIC DISEASE AND CANCER

CHRONIC DISEASE

CARDIOVASCULAR DISEASE

1 | SYNCOPE

N.A. MARK ESTES III, M.D.

Syncope, defined as sudden temporary loss of consciousness, results from a variety of pathologic abnormalities or physiologic changes and is a common diagnostic problem. Loss of consciousness generally reflects a transient decrease in cerebral blood flow that is secondary to a fall in systemic arterial blood pressure. The causes of syncope are numerous and can be divided into cardiac and noncardiac etiologies as indicated in Table 1–1. The prognosis of syncope is related to the underlying etiology. With some conditions, such as vasovagal syncope, the prognosis is excellent, whereas with others, such as ventricular tachycardia or aortic stenosis, syncope must be regarded as an ominous event.

Near-syncope, or presyncope, occurs more commonly than true loss of consciousness. Episodes of dizziness or lightheadedness frequently precede episodes of true syncope and differ from loss of consciousness only in degree. The symptoms of near-syncope must be carefully differentiated from vertigo and from functional symptoms.

In up to 50 percent of patients with an episode of syncope, no specific cause is found despite extensive evaluation.[1] However, in recent years, a number of clinical studies have provided clinicians with diagnostic strategies and useful prognostic categories for evaluating patients with syncope. Evaluation usually includes a history, a physical examination, an electrocardiogram (ECG), ambulatory ECG monitoring, and other selected tests. Therapy for syncope is directed by the results of the diagnostic evaluation.

HISTORY

The history elicited from the patient and from observers is essential to proper evaluation of syncope and frequently provides critical diagnostic clues. Vasodepressor syncope (vasovagal syncope), the common "fainting spell", is often experienced by young people under psychological stress. Vasodepressor

TABLE 1-1   Causes of Syncope

Cardiac

Arrhythmias
  Bradyarrhythmia
    Sinus bradycardia
    Sinus arrest, asystole
    High degree AV block
    Atrial fibrillation with slow ventricular response
  Tachyarrhythmia
    Supraventricular tachycardia
    Ventricular tachycardia

Anatomic
  Aortic stenosis
  Hypertrophic cardiomyopathy
  Pulmonary hypertension
  Myocardial infarction
  Atrial myxoma

Noncardiac

Alteration of vasomotor tone
  Vasovagal
  Orthostatic hypotension
  Carotid sinus hypersensitivity
  Cough, micturition, deglutition, defecation

Drug-induced
  Hypotension
  Tachycardia
  Bradycardia
  Overdose

Cerebrovascular disease
  Seizure
  Hemorrhage
  Cerebrovascular insufficiency

syncope is a response enacted through the autonomic nervous system and occurs in patients who have an exaggerated response to stressful circumstances. There is both a vagally-mediated cardioinhibitory component that results in bradycardia and a vasodepressor component that causes hypotension. This syndrome should be suspected when syncope follows a triggering event, such as pain, fear, or other emotional stress. Most commonly, a prodrome of yawning, pallor, sweating, and nausea precede the spell. A trained observer may notice a weak, slow pulse. In elderly patients, vasovagal syncope may occur with a drop in blood pressure (vasodepressor component) that is not accompanied by a decrease in heart rate (cardioinhibitory component). This cause of syncope is usually evident after a careful history is taken.

Vasovagal syncope constitutes the most common cause of syncope in patients presenting to the emergency room after a single episode of loss of consciousness.

Orthostatic hypotension, defined as a drop in systolic blood pressure that is sufficient to cause cerebral hypoperfusion with assumption of an upright posture, is another common cause of syncope. Drugs that cause vasodilation or reduced blood volume or that block the sympathetic nervous system often play a role in precipitating orthostatic hypotension. It may be secondary to other factors, such as impaired vascular regulation by the autonomic nervous system or depletion of circulating blood volume, as with blood loss. One must question the patient in detail regarding changes in posture that precede the episode of loss of consciousness.

Inquiries should also be made regarding cough, micturition, deglutition, and defecation just prior to syncope. Cough syncope is seen most commonly in elderly patients with underlying lung disease and results from impaired cardiac output caused by decreased venous return and increased cerebrospinal fluid pressure associated with vigorous coughing. Similar mechanisms are likely to explain deglutition, micturition, and defecation syncope.

Syncope preceded by exertion should alert the clinician to the possibility of aortic stenosis. Loss of consciousness that develops in association with aortic valve disease was once thought to result from cardiac arrhythmias. However, in patients with aortic stenosis, syncope may also result from a vasodepressor hypotensive reaction of uncertain mechanism. Exertional syncope of a nonarrhythmic nature occurs in patients with hypertrophic cardiomyopathy and in patients with pulmonary vascular disease, especially patients with primary pulmonary hypertension. Less commonly, left atrial myxomas or other large mobile intracardiac masses result in mechanical blockade of the circulation with exertion. Finally, when a history of exertional loss of consciousness is obtained, one must consider the possibility of cardiac ischemia that induces either a low cardiac output or a transient arrhythmia.

Syncope associated with shaving the neck, with application of a tight collar or necktie, or with rotation of the head should raise the possibility of carotid sinus hypersensitivity. With this condition, stimulation of carotid sinus baroreceptors results in bradycardia. Patients with this syndrome often have some degree of intrinsic sinus node disease. A hyperactive reflex may actually be an indicator of hypersensitivity of the sinus node, rather than of excessive activity of the innervation of the sinus node.

A description of the nature, onset, and duration of the spell and any prodrome should be requested from the patient or observer. Abrupt onset of loss of consciousness in which a patient "drops like a stone" suggests sudden loss of cardiac output, as is seen with Stokes-Adams attacks caused by heart block. By contrast, a period of presyncope or dizziness, especially when associated with palpitations, sugests a tachyarrhythmia. Symptoms of near-syncope also may result from bradyarrhythmias, such as sinus bradycardia, sinus arrest, and sinus pauses after the termination of supraventricular tachycardia, or from atrial fibrillation with a slow ventricular response.

Generally, a diagnosis of seizure disorder can be made when loss of consciousness is noted to occur with tonic-clonic movements and postictal confusion. Cerebrovascular disease may predispose to loss of consciousness with transient hypotension causing cerebral ischemic symptoms. Atherosclerosis of both the extracranial arteries, such as the carotids, and the intracerebral vessels can predispose the patient to cardiogenic cerebral hypoperfusion. However, there are rarely any indicators from the history that are helpful in arriving at this diagnosis.

PHYSICAL EXAMINATION

Examination of the patient, an essential component of the initial evaluation, occasionally reveals findings diagnostic of the cause of syncope. A careful check for orthostatic hypotension is mandatory and is done by measuring blood pressure and pulse in the supine and standing positions. Generally, a fall of 25 to 30 mm of mercury in systolic blood pressure is needed to make a diagnosis of orthostatic hypotension. However, some people develop symptoms with a lesser drop, and these individuals still should be classified as having orthostatic hypotension. Any drop in systolic blood pressure that leads to syncope is significant. Some normal elderly patients may have an asymptomatic drop in blood pressure of up to 40 mm of mercury without cerebral hypoperfusion. The diagnosis of orthostatic hyoptension, then, is dependent on replication of symptoms during postural drop in blood pressure, rather than on some arbitrary level of decline in the blood pressure. Many times orthostatic hypotension is transient, such as after the use of vasodilators like nitroglycerin or antihypertensives. Occasionally, a patient with a reduced intravascular volume will have had rehydration by the time the blood pressure is measured, thus eliminating the orthostatic blood pressure drop.

The carotid arteries should be examined in order to detect bruits that would indicate extracranial vascular disease. Although the presence of a bruit raises the possibility of an embolic transient ischemic event, some focal symptoms must be present to make this diagnosis. Furthermore, most experts feel that transient cerebral ischemic attacks rarely, if ever, cause syncope. The presence of a transmitted cardiac murmur raises the possibility of some form of aortic outflow tract obstruction. The classic carotid upstrokes in a patient with significant aortic stenosis are described as "parvus et tardus", thereby indicating a weak and late-peaking carotid upstroke. By contrast, patients with hypertrophic cardiomyopathy generally have bounding carotid upstrokes that are bisferiens in quality.

The distinction between these two murmurs can generally be made with a high degree of confidence based on the cardiac examination (see *The Systolic Murmur*). In summary, patients with significant aortic stenosis frequently have a left ventricular lift at the cardiac apex and occasionally have a palpable thrill at the upper right sternal border. The harsh late-peaking systolic ejection murmur of aortic stenosis is best heard at the upper right sternal border, but radiates to the apex and assumes more of a holosystolic character. With significant aortic stenosis, the aortic closure sound is generally absent. In patients with obstructive cardiomyopathy, one can frequently feel a multi-component apical impulse, the so-called "triple ripple." In addition to a systolic murmur in the aortic listening area, there is commonly a mitral regurgitation holosystolic murmur at the cardiac apex. When the Valsalva maneuver is performed in patients with hypertrophic cardiomyopathy, venous return decreases, the left ventricle gets smaller, and the outflow tract obstruction increases, thereby resulting in intensification of the murmur. In contrast, there is no change in the murmur of aortic stenosis with Valsalva maneuver. Another useful maneuver in patients with suspected hypertrophic obstructive cardiomyopathy is to auscultate when the patient moves from a standing to a squatting position. With obstructive cardiomyopathy, the rapid increase in afterload with squatting results in marked softening of the murmur.

Carotid sinus massage is a diagnostic maneuver that should be performed to detect any abnormal slowing of the heart rhythm. This massage is contraindicated in the presence of a carotid bruit or of other signs of carotid disease because there is a risk of precipitating a neurologic deficit under these circumstances. Both the heart rhythm and blood pressure must be monitored during carotid sinus massage. Gentle massage should be applied to one carotid at the level of the bifurcation for a period of approximately 15 seconds. If this does not result in any diagnostic abnormalities, the other carotid should be massaged in a similar fashion. A normal response consists of a gradual slowing of the sinus rate. Any fall in blood pressure or in heart rate that results in presyncope or syncope is abnormal. Sinus pauses of 3 or more seconds or a fall in systolic blood pressure greater than 40 mm of mercury also is diagnostic of carotid sinus hypersensitivity.

DIAGNOSTIC TESTS

An electrocardiogram is essential in all patients who present with syncope. An ECG not only serves as a screening tool for any bradycardia or tachyarrhythmia, but also as an indicator of any underlying structural heart disease. Abnormalities of conduction systems, such as chronic bifascicular block, raise the possibility of an intermittent progression to a higher degree of block. Occasionally, ventricular preexcitation is noted, with a shortened PR interval accompanied by a delta wave. In patients with Wolff-Parkinson-White syndrome, there is a higher frequency of supraventricular tachycardia and of atrial fibrillation with a rapid ventricular response. Sinus pauses, sinus arrest, blocked atrial premature contractions, and heart block or atrial fibrillation with a slow ventricular reponse suggest bradycardia as the cause of syncope.

Most of the patients in whom a specific cause for the syncopal spell is made have the cause defined on the basis of the history, the physical examination, and an electrocardiogram. However, in the majority of patients one is not able to make a specific diagnosis based on this information alone. Cardiac rhythm disturbances always must be considered in the differential diagnosis of syncope, and 24-hour Holter monitoring should be performed. In most patients, no diagnostic abnormalities are present, and in most patients with episodes of supraventricular tachycardia and ventricular tachycardia, no symptoms are present.[2] Thus, Holter monitoring lacks sufficient sensitivity and specificity to be considered a useful tool in the identification of the cause of syncope. Occasionally the ambulatory electrocardiogram does reveal an abnormality highly suggestive of a diagnosis. Runs of nonsustained ventricular tachycardia are presumptive evidence that a ventricular arrhythmia contributed to the syncope. Generally, this is an adequate indication for institution of antiarrhythmic therapy. Documentation of Mobitz type II block, complete heart block, or sinus pauses over 3 seconds frequently is adequate justification for placement of a permanent pacemaker.

Over the last 6 years, a growing body of data has demonstrated that electrophysiologic testing plays an important role in identifying the cause of syncope and in guiding therapy in carefully selected patients.[3] Patients with recurrent unexplained syncope who have been studied in the electrophysiology lab are selected based on the absence of identifiable causes for their syncope despite a thorough noninvasive evaluation that includes a history and physical examination (including testing for orthostatic hypotension and carotid sinus hypersensitivity), an ECG, and at least 24 hours of continuous ambulatory ECG monitoring. In many instances, exercise tests and echocardiograms also have been nondiagnostic. If there is evidence of structural heart disease, an invasive electrophysiology study may be justified, particularly if the syncope is recurrent. The likelihood of finding a significant abnormality during electrophysiologic testing is directly related to the presence or the absence of heart disease. Between 60 and 90 percent of patients with some form of heart disease and syncope with a nondiagnostic noninvasive evaluation have an abnormality identified in the electrophysiology laboratory. In the absence of structural heart disease, the yield from electrophysiologic testing is considerably lower, only 10 to 50 percent of patients having any abnormality found. Most commonly, ventricular tachycardia is found with programmed ventricular stimulation. Less commonly, supraventricular tachycardia (10 percent of patients), sinus node dysfunction (5 to 15 percent of patients), or His-Purkinje conduction defects (5 to 15 percent of patients) are found. Therapy based on the electrophysiologic abnormalities eliminates recurrent syncope in more than 80 percent of cases. By contrast, recurrent syncope of suspected arrhythmic cause has been reported to cease in only 20 to 70 percent of patients with normal electrophysiologic studies in whom empiric therapy or no therapy has been instituted.

Other specialized diagnostic tests, such as electroencephalograms, skull films, and computed tomography (CT) scans, have extremely low yields as screening tools, particularly if the neurologic examination is normal and if the history is not suggestive of a seizure or of a focal neurologic event.[5,6] Similarly, echocardiography and cardiac catheterization should be reserved for patients with physical findings suggestive of a significant cardiac abnormality, but should not be used as screening tools. In patients with carotid bruits, carotid noninvasive studies can give a reliable indication of the degree of stenosis, but extracranial cerebrovascular disease rarely causes syncope.

THERAPY

The treatment of syncope must be directed by the underlying etiology. The patient with vasodepressor syncope must be advised to avoid the trigger event as much as possible. With an acute episode, the patient should be advised to assume a supine position. Atropine and intravenous fluids may be necessary to treat a severe episode. It is extremely difficult to prevent recurrent episodes. Occasionally, long-term therapy with anticholinergic medication is successful in preventing or in minimizing the severity of these episodes, but these medications must be taken in doses such that side effects (e.g., dry mouth) are common.

Therapy of orthostatic hypotension is directed at the underlying cause of the syndrome. In patients with diabetic or alcoholic neuropathy, improvement in symptoms occasionally occurs with better control of the diabetes or with abstinence from alcohol. In instances where the orthostatic hypotension is caused by the use of drugs, alternate therapy should be instituted. Orthostatic hypotension can result from multiple medications being taken at one time. An alteration in the medication schedule frequently obviates the problem. Volume repletion is the appropriate therapy in patients in whom intravascular volume is depleted by dehydration or blood loss.

Patients with orthostatic hypotension should be instructed to rise gradually from a supine to a sitting position and to spend several minutes in that position before standing slowly. In the event they feel dizzy or presyncopal, they should be instructed to sit down immediately. Elastic stockings or an elastic body garment are sometimes helpful to increase venous return and to minimize symptoms. Occasionally, liberalization of the intake of salt and fluids or treatment with fludrocortisone, a salt-retaining steroid, help when other measures fail.

Somewhat paradoxically, propranolol, a beta-blocker, has been advocated for use of this condition and has been partially successful. In theory, propranolol works because it blocks the peripheral beta receptors that cause vasodilation in patients who have lost the vasoconstrictive alpha-adrenergic response because of some neurologic disease. Pindolol, a beta-blocker with intrinsic sympathomimetic activity, is effective when a peripheral (postganglionic) autonomic defect produces idiopathic orthostatic hypotension. Additionally, clonidine has been reported to be of use in patients who experience postganglionic idiopathic orthostatic hypotension. It is rarely necessary to resort to administration of vasoconstrictors such as phenylephrine or ephedrine. Recent clinical data have indicated that administration of a prostaglandin synthetase inhibitor, such as indomethacin or ibuprofen, results in improvement in orthostatic hypotension by opposing the vasodilatory effects of endogenous prostaglandins. Frequently, many of these measures must be utilized concomitantly to effectively treat this condition.

Pacemaker therapy is frequently necessary when carotid sinus hypersensitivity is documented. Experience with ventricular pacing in patients with carotid sinus hypersensitivity, however, indicates that a significant percentage of patients continue to have syncope. The vasodepressor response (with hypotension) can continue to cause syncope despite protection by the pacemaker against the cardioinhibitory response. An atrioventricular dual-chamber pacemaker is generally needed in patients with carotid sinus hypersensitivity. In refractory cases with severe symptoms, it may be necessary to attempt denervation of the carotid sinus.

Permanent pacemaker therapy is warranted when a clinically significant bradycardia is documented, as discussed in *Pacemaker Therapy: Classification, Indications, and Clinical Considerations*. When supraventricular or ventricular tachycardia is the cause of syncope, initial therapy consists of the selection of appropriate antiarrhythmic agents to suppress the spontaneous arrhythmia (or the arrhythmia induced in the electrophysiology laboratory). Surgical therapy occasionally is necessary for a cardiac arrhythmia because of failure of medical therapy. Rarely, an implantable antitachycardia device, such as an antitachycardia pacemaker or an automatic implantable cardioverter defibrillator, may be required.

When cardiac syncope is caused by aortic stenosis, an echocardiogram and doppler study can estimate the severity of the stenosis and assess left ventricular function. When patients lose consciousness because of aortic stenosis, cardiac catheterization is indicated to measure the gradient between the left ventricle and the aorta, the cardiac output, and the left ventricular function and to define the coronary artery anatomy prior to aortic valve replacement.

An echocardiogram and doppler study provide useful information regarding the magnitude of the outflow tract gradient in patients in whom hypertrophic cardiomyopathy causes syncope. Medical therapy with beta-blockers, calcium-channel blockers, or other negative inotropes such as disopyramide reduces the aortic outflow tract gradient. In an occasional patient, however, repetitive episodes of syncope occur, and surgical therapy with a myotomy or myectomy is mandated. Ventricular arrhythmias frequently occur in patients with hypertrophic cardiomyopathy, and the clinician should diligently search for an arrhythmia as the cause of syncope. Holter monitoring should be liberally performed in this patient population.

Despite major advances in the diagnostic tests that enable the clinician to define the cause of syncope, approximately one-half of all patients who present with syncope have no specific diagnosis found. Prospective studies have shown that the mortality rate is approximately 30 percent over the first year after an episode of syncope in patients with an untreated cardiac etiology of syncope. The mortality rate is considerably less, in the range of 5 to 10 percent per year, for patients who have a noncardiac cause of syncope or who have syncope of unknown origin. Therefore, an individual who presents with an episode of syncope and who has heart disease needs a more extensive evaluation. By contrast, the prognosis is relatively benign in patients who present with syncope, particularly a single episode, and who have no evidence of heart disease on examination or ECG.

References

1. Kapoor WN, Karpf M, Wieand S, et al. A prospective evaluation and follow-up of patients with syncope. N Engl J Med 1983; 309(4):197–204.
2. Gibson TC, Heitzman MR. Diagnostic efficacy of 24-hour Holter electrocardiographic monitoring for syncope. Am J Cardiol 1984; 53:1013–1017.
3. DiMarco JP, Garan H, Harthorne JW, Ruskin J. Intracardiac electrophysiologic techniques in recurrent syncope of unknown cause. Ann Intern Med 1981; 95:542–550.
4. Sharma AD, Klein GL, Millstein S. Diagnostic assessment of recurrent syncope. PACE 1984; 7:749–759.
5. Eagle KA, Black HR, Cook EF, Goldman LE. Evaluation of prognostic classifications for patients with syncope. Am J Med 1985; 79:445–460.

6. Kapoor WN, Karpf M, Maher Y, et al. Syncope of unknown origin: the need for a more cost-effective approach to its diagnostic evaluation. JAMA 1982; 274(19): 2687–2691.

2 | CARDIAC CONSULTATION IN PATIENTS UNDERGOING NONCARDIAC SURGERY

JEFFREY M. ISNER, M.D.

Cardiac disease accounts for a significant proportion of perioperative complications, and mangement of cardiac problems in the perioperative period constitutes one of the most frequent reasons for medical consultations on surgical patients.[1-4] The consultant providing perioperative care for the cardiac patient serves two distinct functions: (1) to assess the degree to which a patient's cardiac disease increases the risk, i.e., the morbidity and mortality, of the surgical procedure and (2) to diagnose and treat cardiac disorders in the perioperative period. I will discuss risk assessment first, then the management of arrhythmias, and conclude by reviewing the management of several known cardiac disorders in the preoperative period.

AGE, TYPE OF SURGERY, AND CHOICE OF ANESTHETIC

Postoperative mortality from cardiac disease is significantly greater in older age groups; the risk becomes striking beyond 70 years of age. There is general agreement on the magnitude of this risk; the combined figure for all series is a mortality of nearly 14 percent for patients over the age of 70. Though few studies have addressed the issue of mortality in patients over 60 but less than 70 years of age, selective analyses of these various series suggest that mortality in patients between 60 and 70 years of age is only about one-half that of patients over 70 (i.e., about 7 percent). Intra-abdominal and thoracic surgery involve greater risk to the patient with cardiac disease than other surgical procedures. Emergency procedures increase fourfold the risk of postoperative myocardial infarction or cardiac death.

Although it has been suggested that the duration of surgery increases the risk in patients with cardiac disease, review of the available data does not support this view. Specifically, the duration of surgery does not influence the risk of perioperative myocardial infarction. Reports of increased risk associated with longer procedures appear to reflect differences in the type of surgical procedure. While there is increased risk of perioperative congestive heart failure and noncardiac death in procedures lasting more than 5 hours, no effect on the incidence of infarction or cardiac death is seen even at this length of procedure.

11

All commonly used general anesthetics given at concentrations that produce surgical anesthesia depress the mechanical performance of isolated heart muscle or decrease the cardiac output of experimental heart-lung preparations. With cyclopropane and ether, the cardiac depressant effect is offset by a simultaneous increase in sympathetic discharge; the net result is that the blood pressure tends to be maintained or even slightly increased. Halothane, enflurane, and methoxyflurane do not cause the same increase in sympathetic tone; the systemic blood pressure, therefore, tends to fall as the level of anesthesia rises. Nitrous oxide may further compromise myocardial contractility in patients with impaired left ventricular function. Spinal and epidural anesthesia do not directly depress myocardial performance, although hypotension may occur as a result of blockade of sympathetic outflow. In general, there is no evidence that the choice of anesthetic agent or the route by which the anesthesia is delivered significantly affects cardiac morbidity or mortality.

Spinal or epidural anesthesia may be advantageous in terms of one cardiac complication: spinal anesthesia rarely results in new or worsened congestive heart failure. In contrast, new congestive heart failure has been reported in 4.3 percent of patients receiving general anesthesia and has worsened in 22 percent of the patients with preoperative failure. This consequence of general anesthesia is probably attributable to its direct myocardial depressant effects, which are not shared by the spinal anesthetics. Thus, although spinal anesthesia carries a risk of intraoperative hypotension and general anesthesia may not significantly alter cardiac mortality or infarction rate, spinal anesthesia is probably preferable to general anesthesia in patients with a history of heart failure.

RELATION OF CARDIAC FACTORS TO PERIOPERATIVE CARDIAC MORBIDITY AND MORTALITY

Congestive Heart Failure

Congestive heart failure (CHF) may have a profound effect on a patient's intraoperative and postoperative course. Careful attention to the etiology, severity, and treatment of CHF is essential.

Preoperative CHF increases surgical risk, and the increment in risk is proportional to the extent of hemodynamic compromise. Multivariate analysis of the signs and symptoms of CHF suggests that only two findings correlate with increased surgical risk: an increased systemic venous pressure (by clinical examination or central venous pressure measurement) and an S_3 (ventricular) gallop sound on auscultatory examination. A past history of CHF without evidence of CHF at the time of surgery is not associated with a statistically significant increase in cardiac mortality.

The incidence of postoperative CHF varies from 0.02 percent to 5.8 percent, and its presence is associated with a mortality of 15 to 20 percent. Postoperative CHF associated with coronary artery disease has a higher mortality (25 to 79 percent) than CHF attributable to other cardiac disease (0 to 17 percent).

Several factors (e.g., chronic obstructive pulmonary disease, emergency surgery, thoracic or major intra-abdominal surgery, and valvular heart disease) have been found to increase the patient's risk of developing postoperative CHF. Significant worsening of preoperative CHF has been commonly found in patients with the preoperative findings of an S_3 gallop heart sound (47 percent) or jugular venous distention (35 percent), or with a history of pulmonary edema (32 percent). This worsening is probably attributable to inappropriate fluid administration in the postoperative period.

Hypotension

The patient with postoperative hypotension presents a challenge to the surgeon, the anesthesiologist, and the internist alike since the etiology may lie in any one of these three bailiwicks. Intraoperative blood loss, postoperative bleeding, gastrointestinal bleeding caused by stress ulceration, or hemorrhage secondary to invasive monitoring devices, such as central venous catheters, arterial lines, or the intra-aortic balloon pump, are common causes of perioperative hypotension. Pneumothorax, particularly in intubated patients ventilated under positive pressure, is another common cause for hypotension in the perioperative period. Reflex mechanisms may play a role in hypotension following intubation, carotid endarterectomy, and thoracic or abdominal procedures in which the vagus nerve is stimulated; excess vagal tone with resultant hypotension may also occur during ocular surgery.

Medications administered intraoperatively and postoperatively must be considered as potential causes of hypotension. These drugs include anesthetic agents, morphine and other analgesics, and antihypertensive or sympatholytic agents. Anaphylactic reactions to drugs, to blood products, or to special substances such as the acrylic cement used in stabilizing orthopaedic prosthetic devices also cause hypotension.

Cardiac disorders that may result in hypotension include arrhythmias, primary depression of left ventricular pump function, and cardiac tamponade. Tamponade is often responsible for hypotension following thoracic procedures, in patients receiving anticoagulant therapy, and in patients with neoplastic disease known to involve the mediastinum. Postoperative hypotension may be attributable to a variety of noncardiac causes, including pulmonary embolism, whether caused by thrombus, fat, or amniotic fluid in the case of the obstetric patient treated by caesarean section. However, only the last cause of embolism is likely to result in hypotension in the immediate postoperative period. Sepsis must always be considered in the differential diagnosis of postoperative hypotension. Although fever and leukocytosis may be clues to the presence of underlying infection, their absence certainly does not exclude septicemia. In the patient with either unrecognized myxedema or Addison's disease, the stress of surgery may precipitate acute crisis with hypotension and/or coma. Hypotension also may occur in patients receiving doses of steroids or in patients who recently have received steroids. Adrenal hemorrhage with acute adrenal insufficiency may produce a similar clinical picture. Patients recently treated with steroids obviously should receive supplemental steroid coverage throughout the perioperative period.

ARRHYTHMIAS IN THE SURGICAL PATIENT

Cardiac arrhythmias are not only the most common of all cardiac disorders, but also potentially the most lethal. The management of these diverse disorders is of paramount importance in caring for the surgical patient.

Supraventricular Arrhythmias

Effect on Risk

Supraventricular tachyarrhythmias are the most frequent type of cardiac rhythm disturbance noted in the surgical patient, even if sinus tachycardia is excluded. Supraventricular tachyarrhythmias in patients with ischemic, myopathic, or valvular heart disease may lead to loss of hemodynamic stability as a result of diminished duration of the diastolic filling period or loss of active atrial contribution to ventricular filling. Furthermore, when atrial arrhythmias are associated with rapid heart rates, otherwise normal patients may experience a significant fall in cardiac output. Supraventricular tachyarrhythmias also may be the initial manifestation of serious medical complications such as myocardial infarction, pulmonary embolism, and sepsis.

Predictably, patients with preoperative supraventricular tachyarrhythmias have a vast increase (up to 13-fold) in similar postoperative arrhythmias. Unfortunately, good data demonstrating a reduction in surgical mortality following treatment of preoperative supraventricular arrhythmias are not available.

Preoperative Evaluation and Management

Careful assessment for other cardiac disease is indicated in the evaluation of the patient with preoperative atrial fibrillation or flutter. Certainly, fixed valvular heart disease should be excluded as well as less common disorders such as atrial septal defect, atrial myxoma, and hypertrophic cardiomyopathy. Echocardiography provides a convenient screening test for these disorders and, in addition, allows accurate measurement of left atrial size. Thyrotoxicosis should also be considered, particularly in the elderly, because its clinical manifestations may be subtle. If atrial fibrillation is of recent onset, more acute problems such as pulmonary embolus, infection, metabolic derangements, myocardial ischemia, and pericarditis should be sought.

Given the high perioperative mortality associated with atrial fibrillation, it is reasonable to question whether patients might benefit from preoperative cardioversion to normal sinus rhythm. Unfortunately, this question has not been well studied. Certainly, normal sinus rhythm following cardioversion is unlikely to persist in a patient with long-standing atrial fibrillation and massive left atrial enlargement. On the other hand, a patient with atrial fibrillation that is acute in onset may benefit from conversion to normal sinus rhythm and, if necessary, from treatment with maintenance drug therapy designed to preserve sinus rhythm. In particular, when a potentially reversible etiology for atrial fibrillation exists, postponement of the planned surgery should be seriously considered. Similar consideration should be given for patients in whom atrial fibrillation can be expected to be poorly tolerated (e.g., patients with aortic stenosis or hypertrophic cardiomyopathy). The decision to proceed with cardioversion becomes more problematic in those patients for whom anticoagulation is indicated prior to conversion in order to prevent systemic embolization. Although the incidence of systemic embolization might be expected to be increased during the perioperative period, available studies fail to document such an increased risk.

Although data are not conclusive, it would seem reasonable to approach anticoagulation in patients with mitral valve disease and atrial fibrillation in the same manner as patients with valvular prostheses (see subsequently). In patients with long-standing atrial fibrillation (caused by other types of disease) who are receiving warfarin therapy, anticoagulation can probably be stopped 3 to 5 days preoperatively and restarted 3 to 5 days postoperatively without adverse effects.

Two groups of patients with atrial fibrillation deserve additional comment. First, in patients with an inappropriately fast (greater than 150 beats per minute) ventricular response, underlying accessory conduction fibers (including Wolff-Parkinson-White) should be suspected. The fast ventricular response results from atrioventricular conduction across the specialized bypass fibers. Hemodynamic decompensation in these patients may occur abruptly. Furthermore, digitalis is contraindicated in such patients because it may enhance conduction across the bypass fibers. Instead, such patients should be treated with electrical cardioversion and subsequently, if necessary, with propranolol. Second, in patients with an inappropriately slow ventricular response (less than 90 beats per minute in the absence of digitalis therapy), underlying atrioventricular node disease should be suspected; this phenomenon may be one manifestation of the so-called sick sinus syndrome. Patients with the sick sinus syndrome present complicated management problems because of their inability to develop appropriate ventricular rates under the stress of surgery or, alternatively, because of associated tachyarrhythmias. Such patients require careful monitoring and, not infrequently, transvenous pacemaker therapy, either temporary or permanent.

Multifocal atrial tachycardia usually occurs in the setting of a compromised pulmonary status and may be associated with life-threatening ventricular ectopy. It is not likely to respond to digitalization; an all-out attack on respiratory tract secretions is often the only effective therapy. The excess surgical risk associated with all these disorders must, of course, be considered when assessing the need for surgical intervention.

Postoperative Evaluation and Management

Atrial arrhythmias are quite common in the postoperative period. Atrial fibrillation and atrial flutter comprise 70 percent of reported postoperative arrhythmias; atrial tachycardia, supraventricular tachycardia, and nodal tachycardia account for another 18 percent. If the type of surgery being performed is a thoracotomy, the risk of developing a postoperative arrhythmia is substantially increased. In addition, a number of other factors appear to be related to an increased incidence of postoperative arrhythmias: age of 70 years or greater, congestive heart failure, chronic obstructive pulmonary disease, nondiagnostic ST-T wave changes, and intra-abdominal, thoracic, or major vascular procedures. There is a definite relationship between the occurrences of these arrhythmias and medical problems such as cardiac disorders, infections, hypotension, anemia, and hypoxia. The mortality of patients with postoperative arrhythmias is not directly attributable to the arrhythmias themselves, but rather to the underlying problem. Most of these arrhythmias revert to normal sinus rhythm without the use of antiarrhythmic agents.

Atrial fibrillation constitutes the most frequently observed postoperative supraventricular tachyarrhythmia. Therefore, preoperative (prophylactic) digitalization is often a consideration in certain high-risk patients. Previous investigations have identified several risk factors for the development of postoperative atrial fibrillation: advanced age, pulmonary resection, congestive heart failure, chronic obstructive pulmonary disease, preoperative pneumonia, or preoperative arrhythmias including atrial premature beats. The risk of a patient with several of these factors developing atrial fibrillation is 10 to 15 percent. Furthermore, a number of studies have demonstrated a reduction in the incidence of postoperative atrial fibrillation in such patients when they are prophylactically digitalized. With respect to overall mortality, however, there appears to be little difference between the digitalized and nondigitalized groups. The decision to prophylactically digitalize such patients must also take into account the fact that many of the same factors that predispose to atrial fibrillation in these patients also predispose to the development of digitalis toxicity.

In summary, I believe that it is justifiable to recommend preoperative digitalization in a metabolically suitable patient who has more than one of the aforementioned risk factors, provided that appropriate precautions are taken to avoid digitalis toxicity. Although it is common practice at many institutions to withhold digitalis on the morning of surgery, there is no evidence to support the efficacy of this approach.

Ventricular Arrhythmias

The majority of ventricular arrhythmias seen in patients undergoing noncardiac surgery fall into the category of isolated ventricular ectopy in asymptomatic patients and do not require therapy. In critically ill patients, patients with underlying cardiac disorders, and patients with various forms of metabolic abnormalities, however, ventricular arrhythmias are much less likely to be benign.

Ventricular Ectopic Activity

Five premature ventricular contractions per minute on any previous ECG increase the cardiac mortality from noncardiac surgery by a factor of 10.

Hypoxia and electrolyte abnormalities are the most common noncardiac causes of reversible ventricular arrhythmias and are generally more common in the postoperative rather than preoperative period. Patients with primary or secondary pulmonary disorders are particularly at risk for hypoxia-related ectopy, while patients with prolonged gastrointestinal disorders are at increased risk for electrolyte abnormalities that may precipitate ventricular ectopic activity. In addition, the use of more potent diuretic agents has greatly increased the incidence of these electrolyte disturbances. Patients with hypokalemia who do not respond to potassium replacement may have associated hypomagnesemia; in these patients, the arrhythmia generally resolves following magnesium replacement.

Often neglected as a source of cardiac ventricular arrhythmias is the displaced intravascular line, whether it be a Swan-Ganz catheter, central venous pressure tubing, a pacemaker electrode, or a sheared indwelling peripheral venous catheter embolism. Ectopic activity resulting from such a foreign body is obviously an indication for immediate removal or repositioning of the mechanical irritant.

Drugs commonly employed during the perioperative period, such as digitalis, adrenergic-stimulating agents, aminophylline, cyclopropane and chloroform anesthetics, psychotropic drugs, or injected radiopaque dyes, need to be ruled out as a basis for ventricular ectopy.

In summary, ventricular arrhythmias may be attributable to a wide variety of etiologies. On the basis of published experience it is not possible to explicitly define which etiologies are specifically responsible for the increased perioperative risk in patients with ventricular ectopy. Nevertheless, on the basis of experience with nonoperative patients, it would appear that high-grade ventricular ectopy, particularly in the patient with underlying ischemic heart disease, increases the risk of perioperative complications of ventricular ectopic activity. I recommend for this group in particular that it would be prudent to use aggressive antiarrhythmic therapy in the perioperative period.

Intraoperative Cardiac Arrest

The incidence of intraoperative cardiac arrest varies from 0.03 to 0.12 percent of all surgical procedures with a resultant mortality of 50 to 93 percent. Fifty percent of cardiac arrests are asystolic, while the remainder are caused by ventricular fibrillation; there is no difference in prognosis between the two groups. Cardiac arrests may occur at any point during the perioperative period; 12 to 24 percent occur during the induction of anesthesia, about 67 percent occur during the surgery itself, and 8 to 22 percent occur during the immediate postoperative period. Approximately 15 to 36 percent of intraoperative arrests are caused by problems with anesthetic management and generally involve patients who were previously healthy. Another 5 to 25 percent of intraoperative arrests are primarily attributable to surgical problems such as excessive blood loss, whereas 13 to 22 percent have been observed in patients classified as poor operative risks for a variety of reasons. The remainder are caused by a combination of these factors. Unfortunately, clearly identifiable risk factors for intraoperative cardiac arrest have not been defined.

Cardiac Conduction Abnormalities

With development of simple, reliable, and safe techniques for the insertion of both temporary and permanent pacemakers, treatment of conduction abnormalities has become an important aspect of the care of the perioperative patient.

First degree heart block is usually a benign abnormality and results in no significant clinical impairment. Second degree heart block of the Wenkebach (Mobitz type I) variety may be seen in otherwise normal hearts and is easily abolished by vagolytic agents such as atropine. Mobitz type II second degree heart block is a more serious disorder, often appearing as a harbinger of complete heart block; pacemaker insertion is routinely recommended.

Acquired third degree (complete) heart block is always an indication for pacemaker insertion. Although patients with bifascicular heart block have been noted to have increased surgical mortality, the excess mortality is attributable to the underlying cardiac disorder, rather than to the conduction abnormality itself.

Patients with an asymptomatic conduction disturbance that otherwise would not be an indication for pacemaker insertion may require such intervention when they develop ventricular irritability requiring antiarrhythmic therapy. Potent antiarrhythmic agents may suppress necessary escape mechanisms and, in addition, may theoretically exacerbate a pre-existing conduction problem, thereby leading to the development of a high degree of atrioventricular block.

In the patient with a conduction disturbance in whom transvenous pacing is not categorically indicated, external stand-by pacing may be a satisfactory contingency. As a final contingent, atropine, epinephrine, and isoproterenol are typically available in the operating room for immediate use for such patients.

Patients with permanent pacemakers pose special problems. Knowledge of the location, type, manufacturer, and age of the pacing unit is important in the management of such patients. Demand pacemakers may be temporarily turned off by the close proximity of use of an electrical cautery, and caution must be taken to keep cauterization units as far as possible from the pacing site. Patients must be monitored carefully while such devices are being used. A magnet for conversion of the pacemaker to fixed mode should be available for use should the demand pacer be suppressed by the cauterization unit. Although present-day pacemakers are said to be protected from the effects of defibrillation currents, initial attempts at defibrillation should be made with the axis of defibrillation perpendicular to the axis of the pacing wire.

SPECIFIC CARDIAC DISORDERS IN THE GENERAL SURGICAL PATIENT

Coronary Heart Disease

The combination of the anesthetic agents and the operative procedure place increased demands on the myocardium through both direct and indiret mechanisms, including pain, anxiety, increased metabolic requirements, catecholamine release, hypoxia, hemorrhage, fever with or without infection, and rapid fluctuations in intravascular volume. Superimposition of these factors on the patient with marginal ability to meet the demand of increased myocardial oxygen consumption, i.e., the patient with coronary heart disease, results in a marked increase in surgical mortality. The magnitude of increased risk for patients with coronary heart disease varies from approximately two to four times that of noncoronary patients in individual series; in the overall compilation of data, surgical mortality is increased more than threefold.

Myocardial Infarction in the Perioperative Period

An ominous prognostic significance is associated with perioperative myocardial infarction: the combined results of 12 different series yield a mortality figure of 51.6 percent for patients with a perioperative myocardial infarction. The peak incidence of perioperative infarcts is on postoperative day 3, while nearly 40 percent of infarctions occur on days 4 to 6.

The diagnosis of myocardial infarction is often limited solely to evaluation of laboratory data because of the high incidence of clinically "silent" infarcts in the perioperative period. In order to interpret elevations of creatine phosphokinase (CK), serum glutamic-oxaloacetic transaminase (SGOT), and lactate dehydrogenase (LDH) caused by tissue trauma during surgery, determination of the isoenzyme fractions of CK and LDH for elevation of the cardiac-specific bands (CK and LDH, respectively) is essential. Postoperative technetium pyrophosphate scanning has also been used to detect postoperative infarctions with some success. Because of the high incidence of perioperative myocardial infarction on postoperative days 3 to 6, serial studies, including ECGs, serum isoenzymes, and radioisotope studies, must be followed for up to 6 days postoperatively in order to document evolution of the majority of postoperative infarcts.

Angina Pectoris

Several studies have evaluated the extent to which a history of angina pectoris affects a patient's surgical risk. The overall surgical mortality in such patients varies from 0 to 16.2 percent, although the only study that segregated out cardiac mortality found the risk to be 4.0 percent. The overall mortality for the combined series is almost 9 percent. Most studies, however, do not comment on the stability of anginal pattern. Nevertheless, given the increased mortality of the operable patient with unstable angina, it would seem prudent to delay noncardiac surgery whenever possible in such patients.

Antianginal medicines should, in general, be continued during the perioperative period in the patient with coronary heart disease. When the patient is unable to take oral medication, either sublingual long-acting nitrates or nitroglycerin ointment may be substituted. In general, propranolol should be continued in the pre- and postoperative periods.

Previous Myocardial Infarction

A history of previous myocardial infarction denotes an increased risk of perioperative myocardial infarction. New perioperative infarction occurs in 6 to 7 percent of patients with evidence of previous myocardial infarction. Furthermore, the interval between a previous infarction and surgery appears to have a dramatic effect on the incidence of new perioperative infarction and mortality. In patients who experience an infarct less than 3 months prior to surgery, the incidence of perioperative infarction is 27 to 54 percent with a cardiac mortality of up to 70 percent. The perioperative infarction rate is reduced by at least 50 percent if the infarct occurred between 3 and 6 months prior to surgery. Most studies indicate that after 6 months the risk of new perioperative infarction and of mortality levels off at approximately 5 percent, a figure that is higher than that of the general population, but comparable to patients with angina pectoris. The risk of noncardiac surgery in the first 3 months following infarction thus is prohibitive for all but life saving surgical procedures.

Electrocardiographic Evidence of Ischemic Heart Disease in the Asymptomatic Patient

The finding of nonspecific ST-T wave changes in a preoperative patient remains problematic. "Nonspecific" or nonclassifiable ST-segment changes and flat or inverted T waves all are associated with an increased postoperative cardiac mortality by univariate, but not multivariate, analysis. In particular, ischemic-appearing ST-segment deviations are not associated with a higher incidence of either postoperative myocardial infarction or cardiac death.

ECG signs of myocardial infarction of indeterminate age in the asymptomatic preoperative patient is another common problem. This may be a critical finding in view of the high risk associated with surgical procedures performed in the first 6 months following a myocardial infarction. Old ECG tracings often yield important information. If no other tracings can be found and if a reasonable likelihood exists that the patient has in fact sustained an unrecognized myocardial infarction at some point in the past, the conservative approach would be to delay elective surgery a minimum of 3 months. If more urgent surgery is indicated, the risks and benefits of early operation must be carefully analyzed. The cardiac risk of early operation under these circumstances, however, must be assumed to be 5 to 10 percent.

Previous Coronary Artery Surgery

Available data suggests that the overall mortality from subsequent noncardiac surgery in patients who have previously undergone coronary artery bypass graft (CABG) appears to be 1 to 2 percent, while the rate of myocardial infarction is about 1 percent and that of serious perioperative arrhythmias about 4 percent. The timing of CABG appears to be critical: 75 percent of the deaths occur in patients undergoing the second procedure within 30 days of bypass surgery.

Aortic Stenosis

The risk of perioperative death in patients with clinically significant valvular heart disease appears to be 6 to 14 percent. This figure is highly dependent, however, on the location of the lesion, the degree of valvular dysfunction, and the extent of associated ventricular dysfunction. In one study, aortic stenosis was the only type of valvular heart disease associated with increased surgical mortality: cardiac mortality in patients with aortic stenosis was 13 percent versus an overall cardiac mortality of only 1.9 percent. Patients with aortic valve disease have a reported surgical mortality of 10 percent. Patients with aortic stenosis who undergo intrathoracic or intra-abdominal surgery have a reported surgical mortality of 20 percent.

Mitral Stenosis

The risk of surgery in patients with mitral stenosis is a function of the presence or absence of (1) atrial fibrillation and (2) pulmonary vascular congestion. The surgical mortality for all patients with mitral stenosis ranges from 5 to 7 percent. When mitral stenosis is complicated by atrial fibrillation, however, there is an 18 percent increase in mortality, as well as a 10 to 18 percent increase in nonfatal complications. The hemodynamic consequences associated with combined loss of diastolic filling time and of active atrial contribution to ventricular filling presumably account for the powerful impact of atrial fibrillation on perioperative mortality.

The relationship between pulmonary vascular congestion and mitral stenosis is similar to that between atrial fibrillation and mitral stenosis: perioperative risk is considerably higher in patients with mitral stenosis and pulmonary vascular congestion and approximates the mortality of patients with cardiac decompensation attributable to other forms of cardiac disease. As well as representing a preoperative risk factor for cardiac mortality in noncardiac surgery, pulmonary vascular congestion is also a frequent postoperative complication of valvular heart disease of all types and occurs in about 20 percent of patients with mitral regurgitation, mitral stenosis, aortic regurgitation, or aortic stenosis.

Mitral Valve Prolapse

Mitral valve prolapse (MVP) usually occurs as an isolated finding, but may occur in association with various cardiac or systemic disorders. MVP is relatively common, occurring in up to 10 percent of patients, male as well as female.

Although supraventricular, ventricular, and bradyarrhythmias have all been described in association with MVP, it is not clear whether arrhythmias associated with mitral valve prolapse syndrome have the same high surgical risk as arrhythmias from other causes. It would seem reasonable to approach both supraventricular and ventricular tachyarrhythmias in these patients at least as aggressively as outlined for the surgical patient in general, thus including perioperative propranolol therapy and continuous ECG monitoring for those patients with high-grade ventricular ectopy. Although the question of endocarditis prophylaxis for patients with MVP remains the subject of debate, evidence of significant mitral regurgitation secondary to MVP is an indication for bacterial endocarditis prophylaxis.

Patients with Valvular Prostheses

Mortality in patients with valvular prostheses is generally related to hemostatic problems: patients in whom anticoagulants are discontinued 1 to 5 days preoperatively have a 5.7 percent mortality and complication rate, whereas patients in whom anticoagulation is continued perioperatively have an 11 percent mortality and a 44 percent complication rate.

It appears that a regimen of anticoagulant therapy maintained in the therapeutic range until 1 to 3 days prior to surgery and resumed 1 to 3 days postoperatively provides reasonable control of thromboembolic complications, but results in an unavoidable incidence of hemorrhagic complications, a fact that must be taken into consideration when calculating the necessity for the planned surgical procedure.

An alternative approach to the problem of perioperative anticoagulation is to discontinue oral anticoagulants 3 to 5 days preoperatively (or reverse anticoagulation with vitamin K), substitute full-dose heparin therapy by continuous infusion up to 6 hours preoperatively, and begin full-dose heparin again 12 to 24 hours postoperatively. Oral anticoagulation can then be reinstituted when the patient is capable of taking medications by mouth; heparin infusion is discontinued when therapeutic prothrombin times have again been achieved by oral anticoagulation. This approach has considerable theoretical merit in terms of providing the fullest possible anticoagulation for the longest period of time while still insuring adequate clotting capabilities during the critical immediate perioperative period.

The preoperative evaluation of the patient with prosthetic valves must also include evaluation of prosthetic dysfunction as well as of the underlying functional status of the myocardium. Routine preoperative blood tests for bilirubin, lactate dehydrogenase, and reticulocyte count are useful in detecting occult hemolysis that might result from prosthetic dysfunction or from a paravalvular leak. Echocardiography and fluoroscopy may be useful for the assessment of prosthetic function. Antibiotic prophylaxis is mandatory in patients with prosthetic valves. Rhythm monitoring and hemodynamic monitoring using a Swan-Ganz catheter during the perioperative period is recommended.

Hypertrophic Cardiomyopathy

Intravascular volume depletion may result in diminution of left ventricular filling and thereby aggravate dynamic left ventricular outflow tract obstruction. Therefore, careful fluid management is probably the single most important aspect of the perioperative care of patients with hypertrophic cardiomyopathy (HC). Preoperative insertion of a Swan-Ganz catheter and an intra-arterial monitoring line allows optimal management of these patients. Care must be used to avoid beta-adrenergic-stimulating agents such as iso-proterenol, dopamine, and epinephrine which may aggravate left ventricular outflow tract obstruction. If hypotension is refractory to treatment with volume replacement, pharmacologic therapy should be limited to alpha-adrenergic-stimulating agents such as Neo-Synephrine. Because of the decreased myocardial compliance in HC, supraventricular tachyarrhythmias may lead to considerable hemodynamic deterioration, and such arrhythmias generally require prompt treatment (including electrical cardioversion). Propranolol is the drug of choice for control of the ventricular response to refractory atrial fibrillation in patients with HC. Although no firm data are available on how atrial fibrillation in the setting of HC influences perioperative mortality in noncardiac surgery, one could reasonably assume that mortality would be at least as high as in those patients with atrial fibrillation attributable to other causes.

SPECIFIC TREATMENT OPTIONS IN PATIENTS WITH CARDIAC DISEASE UNDERGOING GENERAL SURGERY

Digitalis Therapy

The perioperative use of digitalis may be divided into two major categories: (1) continuation of a patient's maintenance regimen of digitalis in the perioperative period and (2) prophylactic digitalization prior to surgery.

Patients already receiving digitalis should continue to receive their medication during the perioperative period. Determination of the serum level of digitalis may be useful as a reference for subsequent perioperative therapy, as well as a screen for subtle digitalis excess. Since absorption of an oral dose of digoxin is less than 100 percent, parenteral maintenance doses should be reduced to 85 percent of the oral dose.

Controversy exists regarding the role of prophylactic digitalization prior to surgery. The greatest potential value of such therapy concerns the group of patients who are at risk for the development of atrial fibrillation, a complication that, as mentioned previously, denotes a high incidence of postoperative complications. The majority of studies demonstrate a reduction in the rate of atrial fibrillation in prophylactically digitalized patients. With respect to overall mortality, however, there is little difference between prophylactically digitalized and nondigitalized groups. Several studies have shown increased incidence of bradyarrhythmias in perioperatively digitalized patients. Although it seems reasonable to prophylactically digitalize patients who appear to be at risk for the development of atrial fibrillation, rigid rules are difficult to support at present.

Beta-blocking Agents

With the widespread use of beta-adrenergic-blocking agents in the management of hypertension, coronary artery disease, cardiac arrhythmias, and hypertrophic cardiomyopathy, increasing attention has been devoted to the proper use of these agents in the perioperative period.

Theoretical concerns have been raised regarding the possible additive myocardial depressant effects of beta-adrenergic-blocking agents and general anesthetics. A number of studies have demonstrated no significant difference in the frequency of perioperative hypotension, congestive heart failure, bradycardia, or mortality when propranol was continued until just prior to surgery. In the only prospective randomized study of this problem, no significant difference in the postoperative incidence of myocardial infarction, hypotension, mortality, or requirement for prolonged intra-aortic balloon support was found when patients whose propranolol was stopped 48 hours prior to surgery were compared with patients who were given propranolol until 1 to 2 hours preoperatively.

With regard to the pharmacokinetics of propranolol withdrawal, it is now fairly clear that neither propranolol nor active metabolites are detectable in the blood or left atrial tissue 24 to 48 hours after discontinuation of propranolol. Although reports based on the use of noninvasive techniques have suggested that some degree of beta-blockade persists for 12 to 24 hours after the last dose of drug, beta-blockade measured in vitro by left atrial sensitivity to norepinephrine or isoprenaline is absent at this time interval.

In summary, both the dangers of continuing propranolol perioperatively and the dangers of abrupt withdrawal probably have been exaggerated. Certainly, there is insufficient evidence to warrant discontinuation of propranolol in a patient receiving the drug for control of arrhythmias or hypertrophic cardiomyopathy. Similarly, in a patient with angina and good left ventricular function, it is probably safer to continue the drug perioperatively. In the patient with severe angina and/or compromised left ventricular function, the decision is more difficult and the approach must be individualized. Should the decision be made to discontinue propranolol preoperatively, discontinuation 48 hours preoperatively should be adequate to avoid the myocardial depressant effect of propranolol at the time of surgery.

References

1. Goldman L, Caldera DL, Nussbaum SR, et al. Multifocal index of cardiac risk in noncardiac surgical procedures. N Engl J Med 1977; 297:845–850.
2. Goldman L, Caldera DL, Southwick FS, et al. Cardiac risk factors and complications in noncardiac surgery. Medicine 1978; 57:357–370.
3. Hills LD, Cohn PF. Noncardiac surgery in patients with coronary artery disease. Arch Intern Med 1978; 138:972–975.
4. Gerson MC, Hurst JM, Hertzberg VS, et al. Cardiac prognosis in non-cardiac geriatric surgery. Ann Intern Med 1985; 103:832–837.

3 | VENTRICULAR ARRHYTHMIAS

N.A. MARK ESTES III, M.D.

The evaluation and treatment of patients with ventricular arrhythmias is one of the most challenging tasks faced by the clinician. In many instances uncertainty exists regarding whom to treat and how to treat; consequently decisions must be made without firm guidelines. Over the last several years, however, insights into the mechanisms and the management of ventricular arrhythmias that have been gained from both basic and clinical investigation have provided a more rational basis for such decisions. The wide-spread existence of electrophysiology laboratories makes possible careful investigation of selected patients with ventricular arrhythmias. Additionally, the recent release of several effective antiarrhythmic agents has improved the pharmacologic treatment of ventricular arrhythmias.

CLASSIFICATION OF VENTRICULAR ARRHYTHMIAS

Multiple classification schemes for ventricular arrhythmias based on mechanism, morphology, frequency, associated clinical features, and prognosis have been proposed. Ventricular premature beats (VPBs) are the most common type of ventricular arrhythmia and occur in individuals with normal hearts. Population surveys that utilize ambulatory electrocardiographic monitoring have demonstrated the presence of VPBs in 20 percent of men aged 35 to 48 years. The incidence increases steadily with aging. By age 65 approximately 70 percent of males have premature ventricular contractions. An association has been noted between frequent premature beats (more than 10 per hour or 10 per 1,000 QRS complexes) and males with some form of structural heart disease, most commonly coronary artery disease. In patients with ischemic heart disease, the frequency of VPBs increases with severity of coronary artery involvement and with impairment of left ventricular function. Ventricular premature beats occur in almost all patients with an acute myocardial infarction and in most patients with cardiomyopathy, myocarditis, valvular heart disease, coronary artery disease, or heart failure.

Ventricular premature beats are classified as uniform, or unifocal, when there is one morphology and multiform, or multifocal, when there is more than one morphology. Repetitive forms include couplets, or two VPBs in a row, and ventricular tachycardia (VT), or three or more consecutive VPBs in a row. By definition, nonsustained ventricular tachycardia (NSVT) occurs when ventricular tachycardia is self-terminating before 30 seconds and 100 beats and does not require intervention with drugs, cardioversion, or pacing techniques. This form of VT becomes more frequent in patients with structural heart disease and advancing age, but does occur in patients with otherwise normal hearts. Sustained VT persists (by definition) for longer than 30 seconds or more than 100 beats, or requires termination because of hemodynamic compromise. Symptoms with sustained VT are variable and depend on tachycardia rate, peripheral vascular resistance, and cardiac output. Sustained VT is usually symptomatic and should be regarded as a life-threatening arrhythmia. When VPBs occur during ventricular repolarization (R-on-T phenomena), repetitive ventricular responses, ventricular tachycardia, or ventricular fibrillation can be initiated. Extrasystoles that occur during this vulnerable period, which corresponds to the peak of the T wave on the surface ECG, cause life-threatening arrhythmias such as ventricular tachycardia or fibrillation most commonly in the setting of acute ischemia, drug toxicity or metabolic derangement.

When VPBs have a constant interval with the preceding QRS complex they are likely caused by reentry within the ventricular myocardium. Parasystolic VPBs, by contrast, demonstrate a fixed interectopic interval to each other, but varying coupling intervals with the preceding beat. This arrhythmia results from the presence of two independently discharging pacemakers, one of which is "protected" from the impulses of the other. VPBs attributable to enhanced automaticity demonstrate a variable relationship to the basic rhythm and to each other. VPBs that occur secondary to slowing of alternate pacemakers are appropriately termed escape beats and typically occur at a constant interval to the last beat of the dominant rhythm.

A classification scheme for ventricular arrhythmias based on the frequency, morphology, and other characteristics was proposed by Lown with the intent of stratifying risk. This classification defines several grades of ventricular arrhythmias as follows:

Grade 0: No ventricular arrhythmias
Grade 1: Uniform ventricular premature beats (fewer than 30 per hour)
Grade 2: Uniform ventricular premature beats (more than 30 per hour)
Grade 3: Multiform ventricular premature beats
Grade 4A: Couplets (2 consecutive ventricular premature beats)
Grade 4B: Ventricular tachycardia (3 or more consecutive premature beats)
Grade 5: R-on-T ventricular premature beats

Limitations of the Lown Classification have restricted its use in recent years. Both couplets and ventricular tachycardia have proven to be more potent indicators of risk than R-on-T beats. It has been demonstrated that, with Grades 4 and 5, the frequency of extrasystoles contributes to an additional risk of sudden cardiac death. However, this classification system does not weigh this impact of VPB frequency on prognosis in patients with Grade 4 or 5 arrhythmias.

Recently, a clinically useful classification scheme has been developed, which considers the nature of the ventricular arrhythmia, any underlying heart disease, and the likely prognosis (Table 3-1). This newer system, evolved from the proposals of Bigger and Morganroth, classifies arrhythmias into "benign", "potentially lethal", and "lethal".[1,2] This classification will likely evolve over the next few years into one based on sound epidemiologic and electrophysiologic data, thereby allowing modification of the somewhat unsatisfactory labels of the classification. Patients with "benign" ventricular arrhythmias generally have no structural heart disease. Population studies indicate that fewer than 5 VPBs per hour or fewer than 100 VPBs per day can be considered normal. Ventricular couplets and nonsustained ventricular tachycardia are rare, but do occur in patients with no evidence of heart disease. Patients may have palpitations with these benign ventricular arrhythmias, but they have no hemodynamic compromise with presyncope or syncope and are at minimal risk for sudden cardiac death.

Patients with ventricular arrhythmias classified as "potentially lethal" usually have some type of structural heart disease, coronary artery disease being the most common. The ventricular arrhythmias range from VPBs to ventricular couplets and nonsustained ventricular tachycardia. Serious hemodynamic consequences from these arrhythmias are usually absent, but

TABLE 3-1 Clinical Classification of Ventricular Arrhythmias

Class	Benign	Potentially Lethal	Lethal
Risk of sudden death	Minimal	Moderate	Highest
Presentation	Palpitations Routine examination	+ Screening	+ Syncope Cardiac arrest
Serious hemodynamic compromise	No	No	Yes
Heart disease	None	Present	Present
Possible type of arrhythmia	VPBs NSVT	VPBs NSVT	VPBs NSVT VT-VF
Treatment objective	Relieve symptoms	+ Possible sudden death prevention	+ Sudden death prevention

symptoms such as palpitations or presyncope may occur. The spectrum of risk for these patients ranges from moderate to high.

The third group in this classification scheme includes patients with "lethal" ventricular arrhythmias. Many have already experienced out-of-hospital cardiac arrest or episodes of sustained ventricular tachycardia. Most commonly, coronary artery disease with left ventricular dysfunction is present. Ventricular arrhythmias seen in these patients include sustained ventricular tachycardia, Torsades de Pointes, nonsustained ventricular tachycardia, and ventricular fibrillation. These patients carry a high risk of sudden cardiac death.

Lethal ventricular arrhythmias occur in 5 to 10 percent of the total population of patients who have ventricular arrhythmias detected. By contrast, approximately one-third of these patients have benign arrhythmias. This leaves approximately 60 percent of these patients with potentially lethal arrhythmias.

EVALUATION OF VENTRICULAR ARRHYTHMIAS

The major goal of evaluation and treatment of ventricular arrhythmias is to minimize the risk of sudden cardiac death. A secondary goal is to eliminate symptoms. The clinician is justified in treating benign ventricular arrhythmias only in the rare patient who has severe symptoms, such as intolerable palpitations. Many patients with mitral valve prolapse have ventricular arrhythmias that are asymptomatic, or minimally symptomatic, and do not require therapy. Accelerated idioventricular rhythm, a type or automatic ventricular arrhythmia characterized by the discharge of a ventricular focus at a rate of 60 to 100 beats per minute, commonly occurs in the settings of acute myocardial ischemia, drug toxicity, particularly digitalis toxicity, or myocarditis. Patients are usually asymptomatic, and the arrhythmia does not degenerate into more malignant arrhythmias. Therefore, this arrhythmia generally does not merit therapy. Although VT was once considered an arrhythmia that unconditionally mandated therapy, under some circumstances there is no need to institute antiarrhythmic agents.

In patients with lethal ventricular arrhythmias, such as prior out-of-hospital cardiac arrest from sustained VT or ventricular fibrillation, prevention of subsequent major arrhythmic events is a major concern. Many studies have shown that there is a recurrence rate of 20 to 30 percent per year in these patients unless they are appropriately evaluated and treated. Prospective studies have demonstrated that the suppression of spontaneous arrhythmias in a highly structured protocol by use of ambulatory monitoring and exercise treadmill testing or the suppression of arrhythmias induced in the electrophysiology laboratory can significantly reduce the risk of sudden cardiac death.[3,4]

However, data showing that suppression of potentially lethal arrhythmias impacts favorably on survival are less compelling. As indicated in Table 3-2, all antiarrhythmic agents have risk, including the potential to cause an arrhythmia, to aggravate heart failure, to cause conduction defects, or to produce other noncardiac toxicity. With impaired left ventricular function (ejection fraction less than 40 percent), the risk of a major life-threatening arrhythmia increases, and thus, the potential benefit of treatment rises. Quantitative information about the frequency of the arrhythmia is essential and can be obtained by ambulatory monitoring and, in many instances, during exercise testing.

However, the decision to institute antiarrhythmic agents in a patient with a ventricular arrhythmia can most rationally be made with additional data regarding the presence or absence of heart disease. Objective assessment of left ventricular function, obtained by an echocardiogram or a gated blood pool scan, is critically important. In selected patients at risk for coronary artery disease, exercise testing is reasonable before a final treatment decision is made.

In the evaluation of a patient with an arrhythmia, quantitative data by Holter monitoring should be obtained to assess, in particular, any correlation of symptoms with the arrhythmia. The risk of the arrhythmia should be defined by establishing the presence, type, and severity of the underlying heart disease by examination, electrocardiogram, and echocardiogram or gated blood pool scan. Initiating factors, such as hypokalemia, hypomagnesemia, disturbances of pH, drug toxicity, or endocrine abnormalities, should be ruled out. Ischemia or left ventricular failure can contribute directly to worsening of acute ventricular arrhythmias and should be considered. Based on this information, ventricular arrhythmias can be classified into the category of "benign", "potentially lethal", or "lethal". The quantitative arrhythmia data and objective information on the presence or absence of any structural heart

TABLE 3-2   Antiarrhythmic Agents for Ventricular Arrhythmia

Benefit

  Sudden death prevention
  Elimination of symptoms

Risks

  Proarrhythmic effects
  Aggravation of heart failure
  Conduction of defects
  Organ toxicity

disease allow the clinician to evaluate the risk versus the benefit of antiarrhythmic therapy. Benign ventricular arrhythmias present no risk of a future major arrhythmic event or sudden death; therefore, the only justification for treatment is intolerable symptoms, such as dizziness or palpitations.

There are few data to support the hypothesis that suppression of spontaneous high-grade ventricular arrhythmias affects survival in patients with potentially lethal arrhythmias. Treatment in this patient population generally is recommended only for symptoms. Patients with potentially lethal cardiac arrhythmias who have survived a recent myocardial infarction are more problematic. Each year in this country there are approximately 750,000 patients hospitalized because of acute myocardial infarction. Of these patients, over 80 percent survive the hospital phase; the average post-hospital mortality rate is 10 percent in the first year and 5 percent each year thereafter. The major mortality risk occurs during the first 6 months after an infarct with an equal distribution of sudden and nonsudden deaths. Based solely on the presence or absence of uniform or complex ventricular premature beats prior to discharge, one can stratify the risk of sudden coronary death in the 5 years after myocardial infarction. Additionally, nonsustained ventricular tachycardia detected on a Holter monitor shortly after the infarct doubles the mortality rate in the first year after a myocardial infarction. The mortality rate of patients with ventricular tachycardia after myocardial infarction rises to as high as 38 percent at 3 years, whereas without ventricular tachycardia, it is one-half that rate.

The presence of both ventricular tachycardia and a depressed left ventricular ejection fraction after myocardial infarction is particularly ominous. If the ejection fraction is greater than 40 percent and if there is no ventricular tachycardia on Holter monitor, the mortality rate is only 2 percent in the first year after an infarct, but rises to 7 percent if ventricular tachycardia is present. Strikingly, however, if the ejection fraction is less than 40 percent, the mortality rate increases from 7 percent in those without ventricular tachycardia to 25 percent in those with ventricular tachycardia. Clearly, noninvasive testing, including ambulatory monitoring and assessment of left ventricular function, can identify a subset of patients at high risk for sudden death after a myocardial infarction. Unfortunately, however, antiarrhythmic agents have not been shown to improve survival in this patient population. Although disagreement still exists, therapy of nonsustained ventricular tachycardia in patients with ejections less than 40 percent frequently is justified by the high mortality. Antiarrhythmic therapy generally is warranted in patients who have had sustained ventricular tachycardia in the in-hospital phase of a myocardial infarction after the initial 72 hours because of the high risk for sudden death. Further studies are currently underway to more accurately identify patients with ventricular arrhythmias after myocardial infarction who are at risk for sudden death. Optimal methods of treatment for these patients are being investigated as well.

By definition, patients with lethal ventricular arrhythmias have a high risk of sudden death. Many of these patients have been resuscitated from out-of-hospital cardiac arrest or have had episodes of sustained ventricular tachycardia with hemodynamic collapse. Therapy of these patients includes initial stabilization of their rhythm with antiarrhythmic agents and treatment of any complications resulting from their arrhythmias. Generally, these patients need cardiac catheterization to define their coronary anatomy and left ventricular function: frequently, therapy for ischemia and congestive heart failure is needed.

One approach to patients with lethal ventricular arrhythmias is to use noninvasive data from ambulatory monitoring to assess drug efficacy. Lown and his colleagues have concluded that antiarrhythmic agents that protect against the recurrence of life-threatening arrhythmias can be identified noninvasively by use of a highly structured protocol with exercise testing as well as with ambulatory monitoring.[3] Their criteria for successful treatment (with 24-hour Holter monitoring and exercise tolerance testing before and after institution of therapy) include total elimination of ventricular tachycardia, a 90 percent reduction in couplets, and a 70 percent reduction in VPBs.

Over the last decade, numerous studies have shown that the incidence of sudden cardiac death is reduced when antiarrhythmic agents prevent the induction of a ventricular arrhythmia in the electrophysiology (EP) laboratory in patients with prior out-of-hospital cardiac arrest or with sustained ventricular arrhythmias.[4] In the EP laboratory, ventricular arrhythmias first are provoked after all drugs with antiarrhythmic effects have been discontinued for five half-lives (usually 2 to 4 days). Serial drug testing is then performed to identify an antiarrhythmic regimen that prevents induction of arrhythmias. The incidence of subsequent arrhythmias is considerably lowered when effective therapy is found by use of such EP testing.[5]

Comparative studies of invasive (EP testing) and noninvasive (Holter monitoring and exercise tolerance testing) testing for the management of life-threatening ventricular tachycardia or fibrillation have been undertaken.[6] The predictive accuracy of invasive testing has been found to be better than noninvasive testing. The primary limitation of the noninvasive approach is a high "false negative" rate, i.e., successful drug treatment is predicted by Holter monitor, yet the arrhythmia recurs. Up to 50 percent of patients with "effective" therapy (defined by Holter monitoring) have had an arrhythmia recur within 18 months. A summary of the factors affecting the difficult choice of noninvasive versus invasive evaluation of ventricular arrhythmias is shown in Table 3–3.

One type of lethal ventricular arrhythmia that is best evaluated non-invasively is Torsades de Pointes because it is not reproducible in the EP laboratory. This term, which literally means "twisting of the points",

TABLE 3-3   Factors Affecting Choice of Noninvasive vs. Invasive Evaluation of Ventricular Arrhythmias

Arrhythmia	Evaluation	
	Noninvasive	Invasive
Nonsustained VT	X	
Exercise-induced VT	X	
Torsades de Pointes	X	
Sustained VT		X
Aborted sudden death		X

describes a rapid, pleomorphic alternation of the electrical axis that occurs in the setting of a long QT interval. Because the arrhythmia usually causes symptoms and can deteriorate to ventricular fibrillation, it merits treatment. The arrhythmia is initiated by a ventricular premature beat that typically occurs as a late-cycle VPB. Prolonged QT interval is a prerequisite for the arrhythmia. The repolarization abnormality resulting in the long QT interval can be either congenital or acquired. When the long QT syndrome occurs in the setting of congenital nerve deafness, it is known as the Jervell and Lange-Nielsen syndrome. When the long QT syndrome is an isolated congenital abnormality, it is known as a Romano-Ward syndrome. Recurrent episodes of Torsades de Pointes are frequently brought on by sudden sympathetic discharge, as in a fear or startle reaction. Beta-blockers are usually effective in suppressing these arrhythmias. A sympathetic imbalance, with the left stellate ganglion being overactive relative to the right, predisposes to Torsades de Pointes by causing a heterogenous repolarization of the myocardium. Permanent pacemaker therapy or ablation of the left stellate ganglion can be used in those individuals who do not respond to beta-blockade.

Type IA antiarrhythmic agent toxicity is a common cause of acquired long QT syndrome. Both hypokalemia and hypomagnesemia predispose to the condition. QT lengthening can occur in association with central nervous problems, such as subarachnoid hemorrhage, head trauma, and cerebral tumors. With acquired long QT syndrome, the life-threatening arrhythmias tend to develop in association with bradycardia. Acutely, treatment to increase the heart rate with isoproterenol or with a temporary pacemaker eliminates the runs of Torsades de Pointes. Chronically, avoidance of the offending agent or, if necessary, treatment of the bradycardia with a permanent pacemaker generally eliminates this life-threatening arrhythmia.

DRUG THERAPY

Once the decision is made to institute an antiarrhythmic agent, the clinician must be familiar with the electrophysiologic and adverse effects of available drugs.[7] Long-term pharmacologic therapy is difficult because of the unfavorable side effect profile of antiarrhythmic agents. With the recent approval by the Food and Drug Administration (FDA) of tocainide, mexiletine, flecainide, encainide, acebutolol, and amiodarone, there has been a dramatic expansion of the drugs available for treatment of ventricular arrhythmias.

Use of the classification scheme of Vaughn Williams for antiarrhythmic agents (Table 3-4) allows for a more systematic approach to therapeutic decisions in the treatment of ventricular arrhythmias. The Class I agents are the membrane-active agents with local anesthetic action. Drugs with anti-sympathetic activity such as beta-blocking agents, are the Class II drugs and include propranolol and acebutolol for treatment of ventricular arrhythmias. The Class III agents include bretylium and amiodarone, which prolong the action potential duration by prolonging the repolarization process, thereby resulting in lengthening of the QT interval. Finally, the Class IV drugs are the calcium-channel blocking agents, such as verapamil, and play no role in the treatment of ventricular arrhythmias. A summary of the pharmacologic properties of currently available antiarrhythmic agents for the treatment of ventricular arrhythmias is presented in Table 3-5.

TABLE 3-4 Classification of Antiarrhythmic Drugs

Class	Effect	Drugs
I	Local anesthetic action	
IA		Quinidine, procainamide, disopyramide
IB		Lidocaine, mexiletine, tocainide
IC		Flecainide, encainide
II	Beta-adrenergic blockade	Propranolol, acebutolol, esmolol*
III	Prolong repolarization	Bretylium, amiodarone
IV	Calcium-channel blockade	Verapamil*

* For supraventricular tachycardia only

TABLE 3-5   Clinical Pharmacology of Antiarrhythmic Agents for Ventricular Arrhythmia

Class	Agent	Oral					Intravenous			Major Side Effects
		Total Daily Dose (mg)	Dosing Interval (hr)	Bioavailability % of Oral Dose	Elimination Half-life (hr)	"Therapeutic" Serum Level Range (μg/ml)	Maximum Loading Dose (mg)	Infusion (mg/min)		
IA	Quinidine	800–1,600	6–8	60–80	5–9	2–6	—	—		GI, fever, thrombocytopenia
	Procainamide	2,000–6,000	4–6	70–85	3–5	3–8	1,000	1–4		Lupus-like syndrome, agranulocytosis
	Disopyramide	400–900	6–8	85	6–9	2–5	—	—		CHF, anticholinergic effects
IB	Lidocaine	—	—	—	1–2	1–5	200	1–4		CNS: confusion, parathesias, seizures
	Mexiletine	300–1,000	6–8	90–100	10–15	1–2	—	—		CNS, GI
	Tocainide	1,200–1,800	6–8	100	10–15	3.5–10	—	—		CNS, GI
IC	Flecainide	200–400	12	>90	12–20	0.2–1.0	—	—		CHF, proarrhythmia
	Encainide	75–200	8	>90	2–3	—	—	—		Proarrhythmia
II	Propranolol	40–360	6–8	20–50	3–6	0.02–0.9	10	0.1–0.3		Bradycardia, fatigue, bronchospasm
	Acebutolol	400–1,200	12	—	8–11	—	—	—		Bradycardia, bronchospasm
III	Bretylium	—	—	—	—	—	30 mg/kg	2		Hypotension
	Amiodarone	200–600	24	50	26–107 days	1–2.5	—	—		All major organ systems

Class IA Agents

Recently, the Class I agents have been divided into three separate groups based on the differences in their electrophysiologic properties.[8] Class IA agents, quinidine, procainamide, and disopyramide, prolong repolarization and slow the conduction velocity in ventricular myocardium. By contrast, Class IB drugs have little effect on conduction velocity or repolarization in normal tissue. Lidocaine is the parenteral preparation available in the Class IB group, while mexiletine and tocainide are the available oral drugs. The Class IC agents, flecainide and encainide, predominantly slow conduction and have minimal effect on repolarization.

Quinidine, the first drug used for the treatment of ventricular arrhythmias, is metabolized by the liver and kidneys and has an elimination half-life of 5 to 9 hours. There is no need to change the loading dose in the presence of renal or hepatic disease, but maintenance doses should be adjusted to maintain therapeutic trough serum levels. Quinidine sulfate is generally given in an initial dose of 200 mg orally every 6 hours, and the effective dose is between 200 and 400 mg every 6 hours.

Quinidine has alpha-adrenergic blocking activity that can cause hypotension, thus severely limiting its intravenous use. Although quinidine gluconate can be injected intravenously at 6 to 10 mg per kilogram given at a rate of 0.3 to 0.5 mg per kilogram per minute, this must be done with careful observation of blood pressure and heart rate. Like other Class IA drugs, the effects of quinidine on the ECG reflect its electrophysiologic actions. The widening of the QRS complex indicates slowing of conduction velocity in the ventricular myocardium, and lengthening of the QT interval occurs because of prolongation of the repolarization process.

The most common adverse effects of quinidine include diarrhea, nausea, and anorexia. Occasionally, central nervous system (CNS) toxicity develops with the syndrome of cinchonism, which includes tinnitus, hearing loss, visual disturbances, confusion, delirium, and in extreme cases, coma. Rashes, fever, immune-mediated thrombocytopenia, anaphylaxis, and hemolytic anemia occur less frequently. Quinidine can predispose to Torsades de Pointes and can predictably raise serum digoxin levels by approximately two-fold.

Procainamide possesses electrophysiologic actions and efficacy that are similar to those of quinidine. Procainamide can be used intravenously for the acute treatment of ventricular arrhythmias or orally for chronic arrhythmias. However, its use as long-term therapy is limited by the frequent development of a positive antinuclear antibody and a lupus-like syndrome. Although the therapeutic blood range is between 3 and 8 μg per milliliter, it is frequently necessary to maintain serum levels higher than this for efficacy. Procainamide is metabolized by the liver to N-acetylprocainamide (NAPA), which also has an antiarrhythmic effect. NAPA is excreted by the kidneys, and therefore accumulates in patients with renal failure. With the short half-life of procainamide, 3 to 4 hours, it is generally necessary to use a sustained release form that can be given every 6 hours.

The most common noncardiac side effects of procainamide are gastrointestinal (GI) disturbances, including anorexia, nausea, and vomiting. Procainamide also can cause fever, rash, and agranulocytosis with the sustained release form. Many patients who take procainamide develop a positive antinuclear antibody and eventually develop a lupus-like syndrome with serositis, arthritis, pleurisy, and pericarditis. However, vasculitis, nephritis, and cerebritis are rare with this drug-induced syndrome.

Disopyramide has electrophysiologic properties and efficacy similar to those of procainamide and quinidine. Absorption of this drug is almost complete with 85 percent oral bioavailability. The half-life is 6 to 9 hours in normal volunteers, but increases to 6 to 15 hours in cardiac patients. Disopyramide is metabolized by both the liver and the kidneys. The side effects of disopyramide include anticholinergic effects such as dry mouth, urinary hesitancy, and difficulty with visual accomodation. Like procainamide and quinidine, it can prolong the QT interval excessively and can cause polymorphic ventricular tachycardia. The drug has a greater myocardial depressant effect than quinidine or procainamide and should be avoided or used with extreme caution in patients with congestive heart failure. In addition to its negative inotropic effects, disopyramide causes an increase in systemic vascular resistance.

Class IB Agents

Lidocaine, the prototype Class IB agent, is used intravenously for the acute treatment of ventricular arrhythmias. It is rapidly metabolized by the liver when taken orally, so its use is limited to parenteral administration. In patients with low cardiac output, hepatic disease, or acute myocardial infarction, the half-life of lidocaine is prolonged and the usual maintenance dose of 2 to 4 mg per minute should be reduced.

Lidocaine, like mexiletine and tocainide, has no significant effects on the QRS complex or the QT interval. Side effects include altered mental status, confusion, seizures, or respiratory arrest. These can be minimized by administering the drug intravenously in divided doses and by reducing the infusion rate in the settings of heart failure, myocardial infarction, liver disease, or infusions of longer than 24-hours duration. The drug can be give intramuscularly in a dose of 4 mg per kilogram and provides therapeutic levels that last for up to 2 hours. This rate of administration has proved useful in emergent, out-of-hospital settings.

Tocainide, developed for oral use in the treatment of ventricular arrhythmias, has a half-life of 10 to 15 hours in normal volunteers. Its oral absorption is complete, and it is metabolized by the kidneys and the liver. The serum therapeutic range of the drug is 3.5 to 10 μg per milliliter. The usual dose is 400 to 600 mg given every 8 hours. The side effects of tocainide include considerable gastrointestinal toxicity with nausea, vomiting, and anorexia. Additionally, neurologic toxicity, such as tremor, dizziness, parasthesias, and confusion, frequently occurs. The drug has to be stopped in approximately 25 percent of patients because of these gastrointestinal or neurologic side effects. Less common side effects include rash, constipation, fever, agranulocytosis, and pulmonary fibrosis. A major advantage of tocainide and mexiletine, another IB agent, is that they have minimal potential for worsening heart failure.

Mexiletine, eliminated by both the kidney and the liver, has a half-life of 10 to 15 hours. The therapeutic range in serum is between 1.0 μg per milliliter and 2.0 μg per milliliter. Epigastric burning and nausea occur commonly with mexiletine. Neurologic side effects are similar to tocainide and include tremor and dizziness. These side effects generally wane following a dose reduction or with administration of the drug after a meal or snack.

Both mexiletine and tocainide have efficacy comparable to that of the IA agents for the treatment of ventricular arrhythmias in patients with good left ventricular function. However, they have limited efficacy in patients with sustained ventricular tachycardia or fibrillation. When used in combination with a IA drug, there is considerable improvement in efficacy, even in patients who had previously failed a Class IA or IB agent alone. The clinical use of combination therapy is gaining wider acceptance and will likely be the major role of the IB agents.

Class IC Agents

Flecainide acetate markedly slows impulse conduction, thereby resulting in lengthening of the PR interval and the QRS complex, but has minimal effect on repolarization in the ventricular myocardium (Table 3–6). The drug is approximately 90 percent bioavailable after oral administration. Peak serum concentrations occur 90 minutes after an oral dose. Flecainide has a half-life of up to 20 hours in normal volunteers and is metabolized by the liver and excreted by the kidney. The efficacy of flecainide and of the other Class IC drug, encainide, is considerably greater in the supression of spontaneous arrhythmias than the IA or the IB drugs. The usual starting dose is 100 mg twice daily with titration to a maximum dose of 200 mg twice daily. The incidence of noncardiac adverse side effects is low, with headache, visual

TABLE 3-6   Effect of Antiarrhythmic Drug Classes on the ECG

Class	PR	QRS	QT	JT*
IA	↑	↑	↑↑	↑↑
IB	–	–	–↓	–↓
IC	↑↑	↑↑	↑	–
II	↑	–	–	–
III	↑	↑	↑↑	↑↑
IV	↑	–	–	–

* JT = QT–QRS

↑ = increase;   ↓ = decrease;   ↑↑ = markedly increase;   – = no effect

changes, constipation, and abdominal cramps occurring in a small percentage of patients. However, there is a greater incidence of cardiac side effects than of noncardiac side effects, particularly in patients with impaired left ventricular function or sustained ventricular arrhythmias. Up to 10 percent of patients with impaired left ventricular function and sustained ventricular tachycardia develop worsening of their arrhythmias, termed a proarrhythmic effect, with this agent. Unlike the proarrhythmic effects of quinidine-like drugs, the characteristic arrhythmias resulting from IC agents are slow wide-complex tachycardias that tend to be resistant to therapy, but that respond to drug withdrawal. Flecainide has negative inotropic effects that are intermediate between quinidine and disopyramide.

Encainide is similar to flecainide in its electrophysiologic effects. The drug is administered in starting doses of 25 mg every 8 hours. It is metabolized by the liver to two metabolites, 3-methoxy-o-demethylencainide (MODE) and O-demethylencainide (ODE), which both have antiarrhythmic effects. Central nervous system and gastrointestinal side effects occur with encainide with a frequency similar to flecainide. Also, the nature and frequency of proarrhythmic effects of encainide are similar to flecainide. However, oral encainide has a minimal negative inotropic effect, and the drug can be used in patients with markedly impaired left ventricular function without worsening of heart failure. A recent study of flecainide and encainide (CAST trial) showed a 2.5- to 3-fold increase in mortality (versus placebo). The Food and Drug Administration accordingly has restricted their use.

Class II Agents

Of the beta-blocking agents, only propranolol and acebutolol have been released for treatment of ventricular arrhythmias. Their efficacy is mainly related to their ability to inhibit the beta-receptor-mediated adrenergic neural activity. These drugs are particularly effective when used for ventricular arrhythmias related to excessive cardiac adrenergic stimulation, such as occurs with exercise, thyrotoxicosis, and pheochromocytoma. Additionally, they are useful in patients with mitral valve prolapse who have ventricular arrhythmias.

The electrophysiologic effects of propranolol include the slowing of conduction through the AV node, thereby prolonging the PR interval. Propranolol has no significant effect on the QRS or the QT interval. The range of serum levels is highly variable with propranolol; the dosage needs to be adjusted in each patient. Generally, the oral dosage ranges from 10 to 80 mg every 6 to 8 hours, although an occasional patient requires considerably higher doses. The usual intravenous dose is 0.05 to 0.10 mg per kilogram which should be given in 1 mg increments approximately every 5 minutes while blood pressure and heart rate are monitored. The onset of action after intravenous administration occurs in 2 to 5 minutes, and the drug exerts its peak effect by 15 minutes. Propranolol is useful in the treatment of digitalis-induced arrhythmias. The mechanism of its control of ventricular arrhythmias in patients with coronary artery disease is likely attributable, in part, to the prevention of ischemia-induced ventricular irritability. The common adverse effects of beta-blockers are congestive heart failure, sinus node dysfunction, slowing of AV conduction, claudication, Raynaud's phenomenon, and bronchospasm.

Recently, acebutolol has been released for the treatment of ventricular arrhythmias. As with propranolol, the predominant electrophysiologic effects of acebutolol are the slowing of conduction and the prolongation of refractoriness in the atrioventricular node. This agent has little effect on intraventricular conduction or ventricular effective refractory periods. Acebutolol is effective in short and long-term management of premature ventricular contractoins in uncontrolled studies. It was found to be superior to propranolol in VPB reduction during exercise. However, there are little or no data on the efficacy of acebutolol in patients with lethal ventricular arrhythmias.

Class III Agents

There are two Class III antiarrhythmic agents available: bretylium and amiodarone. Bretylium's use is limited to acute intravenous administration for arrhythmias refractory to lidocaine or procainamide. The drug is given in doses of 5 mg per kilogram as an intravenous bolus: this can be repeated at intervals of approximately 15 minutes up to a total dose of 30 mg per kilogram. Hypertension and worsening of arrhythmias are frequently seen immediately after the initial bolus because the drug causes the release of catecholamines before exerting its antiarrhythmic effects. Bretylium is effective for the suppression of otherwise refractory acute ventricular arrhythmias, but its use is commonly accompanied by hypotension. Maintenance infusions of 2 mg per minute are standard with this drug.

Amiodarone, a Class III antiarrhythmic agent, is a benzofuran derivative with potent antiarrhythmic effects. This drug prolongs the effective refractory period in all cardiac tissues, including atrium, AV node, His-Purkinje system, ventricle, and bypass tracts in patients with ventricular preexcitation. It has a beta-blocking effect and a relatively minor negative inotropic effect.

The pharmacokinetics of amiodarone are complex and poorly understood. This drug has a very low clearance rate, and the mode of elimination from the body has not been defined. It has a low bioavailability and an extremely large volume of distribution, is highly lipid-soluble, and has a long elimination half-life of 26 to 107 days. A standard maintenance dose of the drug is 400 mg daily after a loading period of 1 to 2 weeks with 1,200 mg daily. The serum level should be kept between 1.0 to 2.5 μg per milliliter.

Side effffects are common with long-term use of amiodarone. Milder side effects include skin reactions with photosensitivity, or deposition of the drug in the skin that causes a peculiar slate-grey pigmentation. Gastrointestinal side effects include nausea and constipation. Corneal microdeposits develop in virtually all patients, but rarely affect visual acuity. However, patients frequently complain of halos and of difficulty with night vision. Neurologic toxicity includes peripheral neuropathy, tremors, ataxia, headaches, and proximal muscle weakness. The drug has a high iodine content, 37 percent by weight, and as a result hyper- or hypothyroidism develops in 3 to 5 percent of patients.

The more serious side effects of amiodarone include pulmonary alveolitis, which occurs in up to 15 percent of patients. Frequently, this manifests with subtle complaints of dyspnea or nonproductive cough. The chest roentgenogram shows diffuse interstitial or alveolar infiltrates. Routine screening of pulmonary function tests is the most sensitive indicator of amiodarone pulmonary toxicity. A reduction in diffusion capacity for carbon monoxide of 15 percent compared to a predrug study indicates probable amiodarone pulmonary toxicity. Amiodarone increases the serum digoxin level and can unpredictably potentiate the hypoprothrombinemic effects of Coumadin. Although an extremely effective drug in the suppression of spontaneous arrhythmias, amiodarone use should be limited to patients with lethal ventricular arrhythmias, which are not controlled by alternate antiarrhythmic agents.

TREATMENT OF VENTRICULAR ARRHYTHMIAS

Once the decision has been made to treat, the clinician is faced with the difficult task of selection of an antiarrhythmic agent, taking into account its pharmacokinetics, electrophysiologic effects, efficacy, and toxicity.[9] An approach to pharmacologic therapy initially proposed by Morganroth is summarized in Table 3-7. It is reasonable to treat patients who have symptomatic benign or potentially lethal ventricular arrhythmias with a beta-blocker. If this fails, owing to either lack of efficacy or toxicity, a IA agent should be used next. The third step includes the addition of a IB drug to the IA drug. Amiodarone therapy is inappropriate in this patient population, given its toxicity. A reasonable approach for patients with lethal ventricular arrhythmias is to start with a IA agent. IC agents have a less favorable side effect profile in this patient population, and Class II agents have lower efficacy. The addition of a IB agent, if necessary, to the IA drug initially started, is a reasonable second step. If this fails, a IC agent can next be tried. The use of amiodarone would be justified only in patients with lethal arrhythmias who fail other available agents. A nonpharmocologic approach to arrhythmia control, such as surgical resection of the site of the tachycardia, or implantation of an automatic implantable cardioverter-defibrillator, should be considered for any patient prior to amiodarone use, given its toxicity profile.

NONPHARMACOLOGIC APPROACHES TO VENTRICULAR ARRHYTHMIAS

Surgical techniques for the management of ventricular tachycardia are being used with increased frequency in selected patients.[10] In 1959 it was discovered that removal of a left ventricular aneurysm resulted in elimination of ventricular tachycardia. Since that time a number of surgical procedures have been developed in an effort to cure ventricular arrhythmias. These procedures include a simple ablative operation, a simple ventriculotomy, the use of cryosurgery, and an exclusion technique called an "encircling endocardial ventriculotomy." However, the most commonly used technique is a resection using an "endocardial peel." This is done in selected patients with lethal ventricular arrhythmias after an evaluation in the electrophysiology

TABLE 3-7   Proposed Algorithm for Antiarrhythmic Drug
Treatment for Ventricular Arrhythmias

Benign or Potentially Lethal

    II   → IA → IA or IB → IA + IB —X→ NEVER III*

Lethal

    IA   → IA + IB → IC → III

* Amiodarone not appropriate for benign or potentially lethal arrhythmias

laboratory that includes induction of the tachycardia and localization of the site of origin by "mapping" the ventricles. This mapping process is repeated in the operating room to confirm the site of earliest activation during the ventricular tachycardia; the site is then surgically removed. The efficacy of this technique is approximately 75 percent with surgical mortality in the range of 10 to 15 percent.

Implantable devices for the treatment of ventricular arrhythmias are gaining more widespread acceptance as their technology improves. Antitachycardia pacemakers have the ability to monitor the ventricular rhythm; with sustained ventricular tachycardia the pacemaker uses pacing techniques to automatically terminate the dysrhythmia. Although this is effective in selected patients, its use is limited by the potential for arrhythmia acceleration. The capacity to provide an antitachycardia pacemaker with a backup automatic defibrillator capability is currently being developed.

Over the last decade the technology of the automatic implantable defibrillator has evolved rapidly.[11] This device consists of sensing electrodes that are placed on the epicardial surface or in the apex of the right ventricle and that monitor the heart rhythm on a beat-to-beat basis. In addition, electrodes are placed on the surface of the heart or in the superior vena cava and epicardial surface and serve as the anode and cathode for defibrillation. In the event ventricular tachycardia or fibrillation develops, a 25 joule shock is delivered to convert the patient back to sinus rhythm. If this fails, subsequent rescue shocks at 30 joules are delivered. The device has been put in several thousand patients and has resulted in a marked improvement in survival. The incidence of sudden death is approximately 3 percent per year in a group of patients in whom the expected incidence would be many times higher. There is little doubt that this and other devices currently being developed will play a major role in the therapy of patients with lethal ventricular arrhythmias.

References

1. Bigger JT. Definition of benign versus malignant ventricular arrhythmias: targets for treatment. Am J Cardiol 1983; 52(6):47–55.
2. Morganroth J. Premature ventricular complexes: diagnosis and indications for therapy. J Am Coll Cardiol 1984: 252:673–676.
3. Graboys TB, Lown B, Podrid PJ, DeSilva R. Long-term survival of patients with malignant ventricular arrhythmia treated with antiarrhythmic drugs. Am J Cardiol 1982; 50:437–443.
4. Ruskin JN, Schoenfeld MH, Garan H. Role of electrophysiologic techniques in the selection of antiarrhythmic drug regimes for ventricular arrhythmias. Am J Cardiol 1983; 52(6):41–47.

5. Cameron J, Isner J, Salem D, Estes NAM. Cardiac electrophysiologic testing: its role in the selection of antiarrhythmic drug regimes for supraventricular and ventricular arrhythmias. Pharmacotherapy 1985; 5(2):95–108.
6. Platia EV, Reid PR. Comparison of programmed electrical stimulation in ambulatory electrocardiographic (Holter) monitoring in the management of ventricular tachycardia and fibrillation. J Am Coll Cardiol 1984; 4(3):493–500.
7. Morganroth J. Differential utility of antiarrhythmic agents. Cardiology 1987; 57(Suppl 2):57–66.
8. Estes NAM, Garan H, McGovern B, Ruskin J. Class I antiarrhythmic agents: classification, electrophysiologic considerations and clinical effects. In: Reiser HJ, Horowitz LN, eds. Mechanisms in treatment of cardiac arrhythmias: relevance of basic studies to clinical management. Baltimore/Munich: Urban and Schwarzenberg 1985:183.
9. Surawicaz B. Pharmacologic treatment of cardiac arrhythmias: 25 years of progress. J Am Coll Cardiol 1983; 1:365–381.
10. Boineau JP, Cox JL. Rationale for a direct surgical approach to control ventricular arrhythmias. Am J Cardiol 1982; 49:381–396.
11. Mirowski M. The automatic implantable cardioverter-defibrillator: an overview. J Am Coll Cardiol 1985; 6(2):461–466.

4 | THE SYSTOLIC MURMUR

JEFFREY M. ISNER, M.D.

Auscultation of a previously undescribed systolic murmur in an adult being seen by an internist for the first time or being evaluated for a noncardiac surgical procedure is one of the most common bases for cardiac consultation. The history, physical examination, and a variety of noninvasive diagnostic tests may be used to good advantage in most cases to avoid invasive evaluation of such a murmur. On the other hand, in occasional patients, the necessity for performing invasive evaluation is unequivocal. Therapeutic responses to the finding of a new systolic murmur are dependent on the results of the diagnostic work-up.

DIAGNOSIS

History

Certain elements of the patient's personal medical history are essential to proper evaluation of the systolic murmur, and include the age of the murmur, the age and sex of the patient, the presence or absence of syncope, chest pain, and/or dyspnea, and the family history. The first element is establishing whether the murmur is old or new. If the patient has been previously healthy and has not been followed regularly by a physician, no information may be available in this regard. A childhood history of a heart murmur is notoriously unreliable; a positive history often reflects a so-called "innocent murmur," unrelated to organic heart disease; a negative history may be the result of limited examinations and/or limited information transmitted from the pediatrician to the mother to the patient. Two sources of routine examination that merit inquiry are examination for life insurance and examination on entry into or discharge from the armed forces. In these cases, a positive history is generally more reliable than a negative history.

If the history is known to be reliable, the absence of a previous history of a murmur virtually excludes the possibility that the systolic murmur is being generated across the right ventricular outflow tract and/or pulmonic valve.[1] In the adult patient in whom the murmur is caused by left ventricular outflow tract obstruction, a history of a previous murmur is consistent with both a congenitally bicuspid aortic valve and a hypertrophic cardio-myopathy.[2] In cases in which the systolic murmur is believed to be related to the mitral apparatus, a positive history most commonly indicates a preexisting floppy mitral valve, whereas a negative history indicates the likelihood of papillary muscle dysfunction and/or spontaneous rupture of a mitral valve chordae tendineae.[3,4]

The patient's sex and age are often overlooked in assessing the basis for a systolic murmur. In general, valvular aortic stenosis is much more common in men than in women.[5] Mitral regurgitation caused by mitral valve prolapse appears to be more common in women than in men. In the adult between 21 and 45 years of age, principal differential diagnostic considerations include a congenitally bicuspid aortic valve, mitral valve prolapse, and hypertrophic cardiomyopathy. In patients over 45 years of age, the principal considerations become aortic stenosis attributable to a calcified, congenitally normal, tricuspid aortic valve; mitral regurgitation caused by papillary muscle dysfunction; and mitral regurgitation caused by a calcified mitral annulus.

A history of syncope is likewise contributory as it generally indicates that the source of the systolic murmur is the left ventricular outflow tract. Syncope represents one of the classic manifestations of critical aortic stenosis, and as such, represents an ominous finding that is generally considered to be an indication for prompt, definitive therapy. On the other hand, when syncope complicates hypertrophic cardiomyopathy it is not uncommon for the patient to complain of multiple syncopal episodes; in this setting syncope does *not* have the same ominous prognostic significance as in patients with critical aortic stenosis. Syncope is an unusual feature of a systolic murmur associated with the mitral valve apparatus unless it is due to associated conduction disturbances and/or tachyarrhythmias.

Complaints of angina-type chest discomfort are most often associated with a systolic murmur generated in the left ventricular outflow tract. Chest discomfort that may be indistinguishable from angina is common in both critical aortic stenosis and hypertrophic cardiomyopathy. When angina-type chest discomfort is associated with a systolic murmur that represents mitral regurgitation, the angina generally indicates that the systolic murmur is secondary to the basis for angina; a typical example is the patient with papillary muscle dysfunction attributable to ischemic heart disease. Angina is much less common in cases of primary mitral valve dysfunction, although patients with substantial mitral regurgitation may often complain of an anginal-equivalent pain resulting from severe pulmonary vascular congestion.

A complaint of dyspnea on exertion is less helpful in discriminating the source of the systolic murmur. Dyspnea on exertion is typically the first symptom that results from aortic stenosis, but may occur in patients with hypertrophic cardiomyopathy and mitral regurgitation as well, because of pulmonary vascular congestion.

Although the patient's personal history may offer clues to the basis for the systolic murmur, the patient's family history is helpful in essentially only one situation, hypertrophic cardiomyopathy. In more than 50 percent of the cases hypertrophic cardiomyopathy is a familial disease; accordingly, a family history of premature sudden unexpected death, syncope, or heart murmur may constitute useful clues towards this diagnosis.

Physical Examination

While the physical examination may leave undecided the magnitude of physiologic dysfunction represented by a systolic murmur, it may nevertheless be adequate to identify the source of the murmur.

Examination of the carotid pulses is extremely helpful: The classic "parvus et tardus," bilaterally symmetrical carotid upstroke, is typical of critical aortic stenosis. In the elderly patient, the contour of the pulse is more useful than auscultation of the pulse, inasmuch as the latter may be more unduly influenced by local carotid vascular disease. A "spike-and-dome" contour to the carotid pulse is the classic physical finding of hypertrophic cardiomyopathy. Mitral regurgitation classically produces a bounding pulse with a fast descent. In a younger patient, particularly if carotid disease is excluded, the finding of a bruit in association with an abnormal carotid examination is a clue that the systolic murmur is due to left ventricular outflow tract obstruction.

Examination of the jugular venous pulse is more useful in the evaluation of systolic murmurs generated on the right side of the heart than on the left side of the heart. The finding of large v waves in the jugular venous pulse is typical of tricuspid regurgitation. The finding of a well-defined, double-impulse ("a" and "v" wave) jugular venous contour is more typical of pulmonary outflow tract obstruction.

Palpation of the precordium is an often neglected examination that is crucial to the evaluation of the systolic murmur. Palpation of a systolic thrill (best performed using the portion of the palm at the base of the digits, with the patient lying in either the left lateral decubitus position or sitting upright) may indicate that the murmur is due to left ventricular outflow tract obstruction when the thrill is palpated along the upper sternal border. In contrast, when the thrill is palpated at the left ventricular apex, the murmur is more likely due to mitral regurgitation. The exception to this is the patient with a recent myocardial infarction in whom a systolic thrill caused by a ruptured ventricular septum may be palpable at any site between the lower left sternal border and the left ventricular apex, although the lower left sternal border is the classic location for this murmur. The finding of a so-called "triple ripple," i.e., three distinct precordial palpatory impulses, is typical of hypertrophic cardiomyopathy. A well-localized, protracted precordial impulse generally represents left ventricular outflow tract obstruction; a diffuse, fleeting precordial impulse is more typical of a volume overload lesion such as mitral regurgitation.

While the auscultatory features of S_1 are generally not helpful, detection of two clear components to the S_2 may be extremely helpful: Absence of an aortic component of the second heart sound indicates the presence of valvular aortic stenosis. Prolonged splitting of the second heart sound may be due to pulmonic stenosis. The finding of gallop sounds are nonspecific, although the finding of gallop sounds that augment with inspiration may indicate that the associated systolic murmur is right-sided.

Discreet sounds between S_1 and S_2 may be specific for the anatomic basis of the systolic murmur. An ejection sound is typical of a noncalcified, congenitally bicuspid aortic valve. The finding of a systolic click, particularly when it occurs during the latter two-thirds of systole, is typical of mitral valve prolapse. In the rare adult who escapes detection of a congenital right-sided murmur during childhood, an ejection click may be associated with valvular pulmonic stenosis.

Careful attention to the auscultatory features of the systolic murmur are critical in determining its origin and importance. A holosystolic blowing murmur almost always is due to mitral regurgitation, and is heard best at the left ventricular apex, radiating well to the left anterior axillary line. A harsh, diamond-shaped murmur is generally due to valvular aortic stenosis; *it is important to note that in the elderly patient the murmur of valvular aortic stenosis may be heard better at the left ventricular apex than along the left upper sternal border.* The murmurs of hypertrophic cardiomyopathy, mitral valve prolapse, and papillary muscle dysfunction are highly variable in configuration, intensity, and quality. As a result, the performance of several maneuvers is mandatory in the evaluation of the undefined systolic murmur. The most useful of these maneuvers, provided the patient is physically able to cooperate, is the standing-squatting maneuver. An increase in the intensity of the murmur going from the squatting to the standing position is typical of patients with hypertrophic cardiomyopathy and mitral valve prolapse. A similar response to the Valsalva maneuver occurs in these two entities; however, the Valsalva maneuver is less reliable than standing-squatting for two reasons. First, it is difficult for many patients to perform the maneuver correctly, particularly if they are told to "bear down as if you are having a bowel movement." It is generally more useful to ask the patient either to purse his lips around his index finger and "blow on your finger as if you are blowing up a balloon," or to ask him to "press your belly against my hand." Second, if the outflow tract obstruction caused by hypertrophic cardiomyopathy is particularly severe, the Valsalva maneuver may result in total obstruction to left ventricular outflow, causing a paradoxical diminution in the intensity of the murmur.

One "maneuver" that does not require any active participation on behalf of the patient is evaluation of the systolic murmur in response to a premature beat, or a short cycle followed by a long cycle in patients with atrial fibrillation. The murmur of valvular aortic stenosis typically increases during the long cycle, while the murmur of mitral regurgitation typically remains unchanged.

Whether or not the systolic murmur is accompanied by a diastolic murmur provides an important clue to the site at which the systolic murmur is being generated, and to the morphology of the responsible valve. The diastolic "blowing" murmur of aortic insufficiency, best heard at the lower left sternal border, is common with either rheumatic aortic stenosis and/or valvular aortic stenosis attributable to a congenitally bicuspid aortic valve. On the other hand, aortic insufficiency present in more than "trace" amounts is rare in patients with a calcified, congenitally normal, tricuspid aortic valve. The presence of a diastolic murmur is rare in patients with dynamic subaortic left ventricular outflow tract obstruction, although common in patients in whom left ventricular outflow tract obstruction is due to a subvalvular discrete membrane. The finding of an opening snap and a diastolic low-frequency rumbling murmur at the left ventricular apex suggests that the systolic murmur of mitral regurgitation is rheumatic in origin. Diastolic rumbles in the absence of an opening snap may be due to torrential mitral regurgitation and/or severe mitral valve annular calcification.

Electrocardiography

Until recently the electrocardiogram was more important in the evaluation of the systolic murmur than it is now with the currently available noninvasive imaging techniques. The absence of any electrocardiographic abnormalities is consistent with a nonorganic basis for the systolic murmur, such as anemia, an alternative high-output state, or innocuous valvular calcification. The most useful positive finding is left ventricular hypertrophy, which favors a diagnosis of left ventricular outflow tract obstruction. It is important to note that in elderly individuals, due to changes in chest wall configuration, voltage criteria for left ventricular hypertrophy may be fulfilled less often than other criteria, such as ST–T wave changes. While the finding of left atrial enlargement is generally a clue to the presence of mitral valve disease, left atrial enlargement may occur in patients with left ventricular outflow tract obstruction caused by a hypertrophied noncompliant left ventricle. Electrocardiographic evidence of myocardial infarction may suggest that papillary muscle dysfunction due to ischemic heart disease is the basis for the systolic murmur. Finally, in any patient with a systolic murmur and a "bizarre" electrocardiogram, the patient should be considered to have hypertrophic cardiomyopathy until proven otherwise.

Echocardiography

Cardiac ultrasonography has proved invaluable in the evaluation of the systolic murmur. Characterization of hypertrophic cardiomyopathy, for example, has paralleled the development of increasingly sophisticated ultrasound capabilities. The principal findings of an asymmetrically hypertrophied ventricular septum and systolic anterior motion of the mitral valve are the classic sine qua non findings for hypertrophic cardiomyopathy on M-mode echocardiography. Evaluation of such patients by two-dimensional echocardiography has indicated that the site of asymmetric hypertrophy may be occasionally located outside the M-mode beam; thus two-dimensional echocardiographic examination is recommended for thorough evaluation of this entity. Moreover, left ventricular outflow tract obstruction has been documented in a small number of patients with symmetric ventricular hypertrophy, so that even the finding of asymmetry may not be required in order to establish this diagnosis.

Likewise, the clinical description of the "floppy mitral valve" or "mitral valve prolapse" syndrome was fueled by the advent of M-mode echocardiography. An echocardiogram that is diagnostic of mitral valve prolapse, whether by M-mode or two-dimensional examination, is obviously helpful in establishing that mitral valve as the source of a systolic murmur. On the other hand, it must be noted that echocardiographic patterns of mitral valve prolapse are highly variable and are extremely subject to viewer interpretation. Therefore, the isolated finding of atypical mitral valve prolapse by cardiac ultrasonography particularly if unaccompanied by typical clinical ausculatatory findings, must be regarded with caution.

Evaluation of aortic stenosis perhaps is most valuable when the aortic valve is clearly seen, when opening can be recognized to be totally normal, and when there is no increased echo intensity of the aortic valve to indicate fibrosis or calcification; in such a case, the diagnosis of hemodynamically significant aortic stenosis can be confidently excluded. On the other hand, when the aortic valve leaflets are heavily calcified, when no opening can be recognized, and when no discernible movement can be observed, then a diagnosis of calcific aortic stenosis can be established with certainty. In intermediate cases, the echocardiogram may be useful in establishing that the aortic valve is the likely source of the systolic murmur, but may not be adequate for defining the presence or absence of a hemodynamic deficit.

The recent addition of Doppler echocardiography to the ultrasound examination promises to be helpful in grading more accurately the severity of the deficit associated with the systolic murmur. Preliminary use of this modality has indicated a relatively close correspondence between gradients measured at the time of cardiac catheterization and gradients estimated on the basis of Doppler-derived algorithms. The use of color-coded Doppler recently has been suggested as a promising means of quantifying the extent of mitral regurgitation, but further confirmatory studies are required to establish the accuracy of this technique.

Radioisotope Ventriculography

Radioisotope ventriculography perhaps is most useful in the evaluation of mitral regurgitation. In such patients, the finding of a left ventricular stroke volume that is more than twice the right ventricular stroke volume indicates that the systolic murmur likely is due to mitral regurgitation, provided a ventricular septal defect has been excluded. The finding of segmental wall motion abnormalities, whether by radioisotope ventriculography or two-dimensional echocardiography, may suggest that papillary muscle dysfunction related to ischemic heart disease is the basis for the systolic murmur.

Fluoroscopy

The importance of fluoroscopy in detecting aortic valve calcification is frequently overlooked. Hemodynamically significant aortic stenosis in patients over 55 years of age is rare in the absence of detectable valvular calcium. The converse, however, is not true: Valvular calcification may exist and may cause a murmur to be heard without resulting in a hemodynamic deficit.

Invasive Evaluation

A decision regarding the necessity for additional invasive examination is made following a synthesis of data gathered from the history, physical examination, and noninvasive tests.

Of the possible etiologies for a systolic murmur, the one that most often mandates invasive examination is valvular aortic stenosis. When two-dimensional echocardiography and/or cardiac fluoroscopy demonstrate a normal aortic valve, the need for invasive evaluation is obviated. If one of these evaluations is abnormal, however, determination of the hemodynamic severity of aortic stenosis becomes increasingly difficult as the appearance of the valve, determined noninvasively, becomes progressively more abnormal. Virtually every noninvasive evaluation that has been proposed at one time or another to be capable of discriminating hemodynamically significant from insignificant aortic stenosis has ultimately failed. The additional fact that so often dictates invasive evaluation for the question of aortic stenosis is the well-documented propensity for this lesion to cause sudden unexpected death. The 10-year follow-up of patients with asymptomatic aortic stenosis in whom the calculated valve area is less than 0.5 cm^2 is poor enough that surgery is considered mandatory for all such patients. Thus the imperfect nature of noninvasive tests designed to evaluate aortic stenosis, combined with the frequently fatal nature of this lesion, most often lead to cardiac catheterization.

In contrast, the noninvasive diagnosis of hypertrophic cardiomyopathy in a patient who has not been previously treated for that condition does not require further invasive evaluation. Likewise, in most patients in whom mitral regurgitation is the basis for the systolic murmur, further invasive evaluation is unnecessary, provided that the patient is asymptomatic or only mildly symptomatic, and that ventricular function is still intact (left ventricular ejection fraction greater than 55 percent). A possible exception to this rule is mitral regurgitation caused by papillary muscle dysfunction; in this case, the decision to proceed to invasive evaluation is based principally on considerations related to ischemic heart disease. For systolic murmurs originating on the right side of the heart, invasive evaluation is mandated only if the patient is symptomatic enough to be considered a candidate for operative intervention.

TREATMENT

Treatment of the various lesions responsible for a systolic murmur differs markedly, depending on the anatomic basis for the murmur. In the case of a patient with mitral valve prolapse, for example, the only "treatment" required is antibiotic prophylaxis for bacterial endocarditis. Although recommendations have varied to some extent as to which patients with mitral valve prolapse require prophylaxis, my opinion is that all patients with this diagnosis should receive prophylaxis, provided there is no demonstrated allergy to the particular antibiotic to be used. The bases for this recommendation are as follows:

1) Patients with isolated systolic clicks, in the absence of a murmur, have been documented to develop endocarditis.
2) The auscultatory findings in this syndrome, even in a given patient, are so

variable that it is common for a patient to have a murmur heard on one occasion and then on another occasion to demonstrate only a click.

3) If the echocardiographic pattern is absolutely diagnostic of mitral valve prolapse, it is possible that an associated murmur may be heard on some occasions but not on others; thus this group of patients should not be excluded from prophylaxis.

4) In patients with isolated clicks, the murmur may at times be provoked by various maneuvers, while at other times, in part because of poor patient cooperation, it may not be possible to provoke; the presence or absence of a provokable murmur is thus an inadequate criterion on which to base the decision for prophylaxis.

5) The risk:benefit ratio of prophylaxis versus endocarditis justifies liberal use of prophylaxis in this syndrome.

At the other extreme is the treatment of the patient with hemodynamically significant aortic stenosis. Because of the well-documented propensity of this lesion to cause sudden unexpected death,[6] surgical intervention is recommended for any symptomatic patient with hemodynamically significant aortic stenosis. While controversy exists regarding the advisability of surgical versus medical therapy in asymptomatic patients, the scant data that exist in this regard suggest that in the younger patient surgical intervention is advised. In the elderly patient, particularly the "oldest old," the natural history of hemodynamically significant aortic stenosis is unknown. Therefore in this age group, particularly when other confounding medical illnesses exist, the decision to recommend surgery may not be straightforward.

In the patient with hypertrophic cardiomyopathy, the first line of treatment is medical therapy consisting of adrenergic beta-blockade or calcium-channel blockers. Available evidence would suggest that beta-blockers are interchangeable for the treatment of this disorder. Among the calcium-channel blockers, verapamil has been used most extensively in the treatment of this disorder; nifedipine has been used successfully, but less widely. Few data exist regarding the treatment of hypertrophic cardiomyopathy with diltiazem. Finally, Norpace has been used successfully in selected patients. The decision to recommend surgical intervention for the patient with hypertrophic cardiomyopathy can only be made, with rare exception, after failure of the patient to respond to medical therapy.

In the patient with mitral regurgitation caused by primary valve dysfunction, no surgical intervention is required provided that the patient is asymptomatic or mildly symptomatic with intact ventricular function. In the patient with class III or class IV congestive heart failure symptoms who has failed to respond to conventional medical treatment, and in whom ventricular function remains intact, surgical therapy is advised. The difficult decision concerns patients who, according to symptoms alone or in combination with the results of medical therapy, do not require surgical intervention, but in whom there is evidence of progressive deterioration of left ventricular function. The decision to operate in these patients is strictly a matter of attempting to intervene at a time when further deterioration of left ventricular function may be prevented. Unfortunately, experience has been less than perfect with both noninvasive and invasive tests designed to predict the progression of left ventricular dysfunction. Thus a decision to operate in such patients must rest on the practitioner's preferred means of predicting the integrity of left ventricular function.

As mentioned previously, the decision for surgical intervention in the patient in whom a systolic murmur is due to papillary muscle dysfunction rests principally on considerations related to ischemic heart disease. In particular, however, it should be noted that ejection-phase indices or other tests of left ventricular function do not have the same meaning in the patient with mitral regurgitation due to ischemic heart disease that they may have in patients with primary mitral valve dysfunction. Specifically, the patient with impaired left ventricular function and secondary mitral regurgitation is more likely to improve following surgery, as the result of revascularization combined with mitral valve replacement and/or left ventricular aneurysmectomy.

Finally, surgery is rarely required in the adult patient with a systolic murmur caused by pulmonary outflow tract obstruction. The same is true for isolated tricuspid regurgitation. One significant exception to the latter statement, however, is the patient with isolated tricuspid regurgitation due to infective endocarditis, in whom simple excision without valve replacement is generally successful.

References

1. Johnson LW, Grossman W, Dalen JE, Dexter L. Pulmonic stenosis in the adult: long-term follow-up results. N Engl J Med 1972; 287:1159–1163.
2. Epstein SE, Henry WL, Clarke CE, et al. Asymmetric septal hypertrophy. Ann Intern Med 1974; 81:650–671.
3. Roberts WC, Perloff JK. Mitral valvular disease: a clinicopathologic survey of the conditions causing the mitral valve to function abnormally. Ann Intern Med 1972; 77:939–956.
4. O'Rourke RA, Crawford MH. The systolic click-murmur syndrome: clinical recognition and management. Curr Probl Cardiol 1976; 1:1–60.
5. Roberts WC, Perloff JK, Constantino T. Severe valvular aortic stenosis in patients over 65 years of age: a clinicopathologic study. Am J Cardiol 1971; 27:487–496.
6. Frank S, Johnson A, Ross J Jr. Natural history of valvular aortic stenosis. Br Heart J 1973; 35:41–45.

5 | ANTICOAGULATION IN CARDIAC DISORDERS

JEFFREY M. ISNER, M.D.

Internists frequently are called upon for an opinion regarding the use of anticoagulation in the treatment of certain forms of heart disease. In most cases the opinion rendered is just that, i.e., an opinion. Uncertainty exists because of a paucity of data relating the *risks* of anticoagulation in an individual patient with a particular cardiac disorder and the *benefits* of anticoagulation. Such risk-benefit analyses are further confounded by the fact that the level of anticoagulation that represents the optimum compromise between efficacy and toxicity (bleeding) remains a matter of controversy. The conventional teaching states that the prothrombin time should be maintained at 1.5 to 2.5 times control. More recent data suggest that much lower levels of anticoagulation (1.2 to 1.5 times normal) may be effective and less likely to provoke bleeding, at least for treatment of recurrent venous thromboembolism. Furthermore, while there exists a consensus regarding the need, or the lack of need, for anticoagulation for several cardiovascular disorders, data are inadequate to allow definite recommendations for the large majority of situations in which the internist is consulted. This caveat must be kept in mind when seeing patients with these conditions. I will focus on the situations in which the issue of anticoagulation is most often raised.

RHEUMATIC MITRAL VALVE DISEASE

The subset of patients with documented mitral stenosis and atrial fibrillation with no contraindications to anticoagulant therapy represents the group of patients in whom there is least debate regarding the necessity for chronic anticoagulation. This consensus in favor of therapy exists even in the absence of a history of systemic emboli. I would recommend that all patients in this subgroup be prophylactically anticoagulated because of the high risk of peripheral embolic phenomena. Previous investigators have concluded that a patient with rheumatic valve disease has at least one chance in five of having a clinically detectable systemic embolus during the course of his or her disease. The incidence of such systemic emboli increases by a factor of seven when mitral valve disease is complicated by atrial fibrillation. In the setting of mitral stenosis associated with atrial fibrillation, a correlation between systemic emboli and certain associated findings—such as atrial size, sex, mitral calcification, or age—is too weak to rely on. Consequently, anticoagulation is recommended for all patients at least up to the age of 80 with mitral stenosis and atrial fibrillation.

Treatment of mitral stenosis in patients with atrial fibrillation—whether by operative commissurotomy, percutaneous valvuloplasty, or prosthetic valve replacement—does not eliminate the need for chronic anticoagulation. Some degree of mitral stenosis persists after all of these procedures, including prosthetic valve replacement. The potential for systemic embolization thus persists, and as a consequence, anticoagulation must be continued. Remember that the use of tissue valve prostheses in patients with mitral stenosis and atrial fibrillation does not obviate the need for chronic anticoagulation. The advantage of using a tissue valve is limited to those patients who subsequently develop an absolute contraindication to continued anticoagulation. Discontinuation of anticoagulation with warfarin is theoretically more acceptable in a patient with a tissue valve than in a patient with a mechanical valve; in this setting, the efficacy of antiplatelet therapy as a substitute for warfarin therapy remains unproven.

The decision to anticoagulate patients with mitral stenosis who have not had a systemic embolus and who are in normal sinus rhythm is difficult. Some investigators have recommended that left atrial diameter greater than 55 mm in these patients serves as a good guideline for institution of anticoagulant therapy. Other physicians have strongly recommended that these patients be prophylactically treated with anticoagulant therapy (regardless of left atrial size) because atrial fibrillation and/or systemic embolization may represent the presenting manifestation of mitral stenosis. I believe therapy probably is indicated in individuals with no contraindications to anticoagulation, particularly in patients who can be expected to scrupulously adhere to the plan of management.

Rheumatic mitral valve disease that consists of mild mitral stenosis with predominant mitral regurgitation does not, in my opinion, change the indications for chronic anticoagulation. Although previous studies had suggested that emboli are more common in mitral stenosis than in mitral regurgitation of rheumatic etiology, the fact that at least mild mitral stenosis complicates most cases of rheumatic mitral valve disease argues for anticoagulant therapy even in the patient with predominant mitral insufficiency.

ATRIAL FIBRILLATION UNASSOCIATED WITH VALVULAR HEART DISEASE

Patients with atrial fibrillation unaccompanied by valvular heart disease constitute a more controversial group of patients with regard to anticoagulant therapy than those in whom mitral stenosis co-exists. There is no question that the risk of peripheral embolic events is increased in patients with chronic atrial fibrillation as oposed to individuals with normal sinus rhythm. What remains unclear is the magnitude of this risk and its relation to the poorly defined risk of bleeding from warfarin in such patients. Some evidence suggests that the likelihood of peripheral embolic events in patients with atrial fibrillation is increased by the association of organic heart disease, such as left ventricular dilatation or hypertrophy. Certainly in patients with atrial fibrillation and a history of a previous embolic event, I would recommend chronic anticoagulation. I also recommend such therapy for patients in whom two-dimensional echocardiography or other noninvasive tests disclosed evidence of atrial thrombus. Unfortunately, two-dimensional echocardiography is not optimally sensitive or specific for the detection of such clots. Consequently, in the absence of a history of peripheral embolic events or noninvasive evidence of left atrial thrombus, I currently do not recommend anticoagulant therapy for isolated atrial fibrillation unassociated with organic heart disease. When chronic atrial fibrillation is complicated by co-existent organic heart disease, assessment of the relative risk of bleeding from warfarin must dictate the decision whether or not to anticoagulate such patients.

Paroxysmal atrial fibrillation previously had been suggested to constitute a more compelling basis for chronic anticoagulation than chronic atrial fibrillation. The rationale for this conclusion was based on the assumption that thrombus was likely to develop in the left atrial appendage during periods of atrial fibrillation, and that such a thrombus then could be dislodged when the patient spontaneously reverted to normal sinus rhythm with the onset of coordinated left atrial contractions. We have reviewed a large series of patients with paroxysmal atrial fibrillation at our institution. We have found that, in the absence of associated organic heart disease, there is an exceptionally low incidence of peripheral embolic events and that this incidence of peripheral emboli does not exceed even the lowest estimates of complications from anticoagulation. Therefore, I do not recommend chronic anticoagulant therapy for patients with paroxysmal atrial fibrillation unassociated with organic heart disease. However, because we have observed systemic emboli in patients with paroxysmal atrial fibrillation in the *presence* of organic heart disease, I do recommend anticoagulant therapy for these patients.

CARDIOMYOPATHY

A number of studies have suggested that the incidence of ventricular and atrial thrombus in patients with dilated cardiomyopathy is sufficiently high, when examined at autopsy, to constitute a sound basis for chronic anticoagulation. Clinical studies have shown a variable risk of peripheral embolic events in patients with dilated cardiomyopathy. Thus, it is our policy to recommend chronic anticoagulation to such patients, provided that the basis for their dilated cardiomyopathy is not chronic ethanol use. Such therapy obviously is contraindicated when a dilated cardiomyopathy is associated with secondary hepatic insufficiency.

The basis for cerebrovascular accidents in patients with hypertrophic cardiomyopathy remains incompletely defined. Some investigations have suggested that such strokes are related to peripheral embolic events with a cardiac origin. Other studies have suggested, however, that the incidence of left atrial thrombus at autopsy is increasingly rare and that cerebrovascular accidents are more likely to be attributable to paroxysmal arrhythmias, intermittent outflow tract obstruction, or extracranial vascular disease. Left atrial size has been suggested as a useful guide for predicting the likelihood of cerebrovascular accidents, i.e., anticoagulation is warranted, when the left atrial size exceeds 55 mm in diameter by echocardiography. I recommend anticoagulation to patients with hypertrophic cardiomyopathy and associated atrial fibrillation. At least some of these patients have mitral annular calcium deposits that may be associated with a transvalvular gradient in the absence of rheumatic mitral valve disease. Even without associated mitral annular calcium deposits, the marked decrease in left ventricular compliance characteristic of such patients might be expected to produce variable degrees of left atrial stasis in association with atrial fibrillation. Such a combination of factors might constitute a basis for chronic anticoagulation. When hypertrophic cardiomyopathy is not accompanied by atrial fibrillation, I do not recommend chronic anticoagulation unless there is a well-documented history of a focal cerebrovascular accident.

In general, the diagnosis of a restrictive cardiomyopathy does not constitute an indication for chronic anticoagulation. The exception to this rule is the patient with the hypereosinophilia syndrome in whom there is a higher likelihood of left atrial thrombus formation and in whom chronic anticoagulation may actually diminish the chronic deposition of ventricular cavity thrombus.

DILEMMAS

Pregnancy in a patient with a preexisting indication for chronic anticoagulation constitutes a moderately difficult clinical problem. A more difficult dilemma exists with regard to a patient in whom infective endocarditis has been complicated by a cerebrovascular accident believed caused by a septic embolism. In both of these situations, hard data on which to base a firm clinical recommendation are not available. I believe that the best recommendations for these two situations are those recommended by the recent ACCP-NHLBI National Conference on Antithrombotic Therapy.*

With regard to pregnancy, the Conference recommended the following.

> It is recommended that pregnant patients...should be treated with adjusted-dose subcutaneous heparin (subcutaneous heparin q 12 hours with a PTT 1.5 to 2 times control 6 hours after injection) from the time pregnancy is diagnosed until delivery. This recommendation is based on a study demonstrating a very high incidence of cerebral embolism when antiplatelet agents alone were used and a high frequency of embryopathy and fetal death in mothers treated with warfarin.

With regard to infective endocarditis, the recommendations of the same Conference were as follows:

1. It is strongly recommended that antithrombotic therapy is not indicated in patients with uncomplicated infective endocarditis involving a native valve or a bioprosthetic valve in patients with normal sinus rhythm. This...recommendation is based on the increased incidence of hemorrhage in these patients and the lack of demonstrated efficacy of antithrombotic therapy in this setting.
2. It is recommended that long-term warfarin therapy be continued in patients with endocarditis involving a prosthetic valve unless there are specific contraindications. This...recommendation is based on the high frequency of systemic embolism in these patients. However, it is to be noted that the risk of intracranial hemorrhage in this circumstance is substantial.
3. The indications for anticoagulant therapy when systemic embolism occurs during the course of infective endocarditis involving a native or bioprosthetic heart valve are uncertain. The therapeutic decision should consider comorbid factors, including atrial fibrillation, evidence of left atrial thrombus, evidence and size of valvular vegetations, and the distribution and severity of embolism.

*Recommendations regarding the use of anticoagulation obviously must be individualized. The reader is referred to the excellent consensus report of the ACCP-NHLBI National Conference on Antithrombotic Therapy published in Chest 1986; 89(Suppl):IS–99S.

6 | CONGESTIVE HEART FAILURE

MARVIN A. KONSTAM, M.D.
ANDREW R. WEINTRAUB, M.D.

Heart failure is generally defined in terms of the effects of myocardial or valvular dysfunction on end-organ perfusion or on venous hydrostatic pressure. Heart failure is present if systemic blood flow is inadequate to satisfy the aerobic metabolic needs of end-organs, either at rest or during usual stress such as exercise. Alternatively, heart failure is present if pulmonary venous (left heart failure) or systemic venous (right heart failure) pressure rises to abnormal levels. Hydrostatic forces may then be sufficient to induce pulmonary edema (left heart failure) or peripheral and systemic organ edema (right heart failure).

Therapy for heart failure must be aimed at both the underlying cardiac functional disorder and the systemic manifestations of heart failure. Some modes of therapy may be directed toward a given manifestation of heart failure, regardless of etiology. For example, diuretics are used to reduce elevated venous pressure, regardless of cause. Other therapies are directed toward the cardiac disorder and may benefit all of the manifestations of that disorder. An example is inotropic therapy, which may reduce all of the consequences of myocardial systolic dysfunction. Still other forms of therapy act at multiple sites and may therefore benefit a given manifestation of heart failure, but may be more effective in the presence of some functional disorders than in others. For example, calcium-channel antagonists, through peripheral arterial dilatation, reduce systolic load and may, therefore, augment systemic perfusion, regardless of the functional disorder. The myocardial actions of calcium antagonists include reduction of contractility, but accelerated relaxation. Therefore, these drugs tend to be more effective in the presence of myocardial diastolic dysfunction and less effective, or possibly detrimental, when systolic dysfunction predominates.

"Conventional wisdom" regarding therapy for heart failure has been changing rapidly as newer diagnostic techniques become perfected, as newer modes of treatment become available, and as the effects of these various therapeutic modalities undergo more intensive and extensive investigation. In addition to being a debilitating illness, heart failure carries a poor prognosis for survival, with 50 percent mortality within 6 months to 3 years, depending on the primary diagnosis and the severity of hemodynamic and clinical derangement. Despite the poor prognosis, therapy has been directed primarily to relief of symptoms, with little expectation that survival can be prolonged. This approach now has begun to change, as we seek and begin to identify treatment modalities that are able to alter the natural history of disease.

This chapter is divided into two sections. In the first section, we will discuss the physiologic factors that influence cardiac performance, categorize disorders that lead to heart failure accordingly, and discuss therapeutic approaches in these specific disorders. In the second section, we will discuss treatment strategies and modalities, with attention to (1) the changing view of indication for treatment, (2) an approach to treatment, and (3) a review of available modes of therapy, with emphasis on matching treatment to both cardiac functional disorders and peripheral manifestations. We have placed a heavy emphasis on the basic pathophysiology because this knowledge is mandatory in order to manage patients with this all-too-common condition.

FACTORS INFLUENCING CARDIAC PERFORMANCE

Preload

Preload can be defined as the extent of myocardial fiber stretch immediately preceding contraction. It may be gauged experimentally as the length of an isolated muscle strip, or clinically as ventricular end-diastolic dimension, end-diastolic volume, or end-diastolic pressure. A commonly employed clinical index of left ventricular preload is mean pulmonary artery wedge pressure, which generally reflects pulmonary venous pressure and, in the absence of mitral stenosis, parallels changes in left ventricular end-diastolic pressure. Because it reflects pulmonary venous pressure, the pulmonary artery wedge pressure is not only an indicator of left ventricular preload but also a gauge of the effectiveness of therapy directed against pulmonary interstitial and alveolar edema. Similarly, right atrial or central venous pressure, measured clinically as jugular venous pressure, is both an indicator of right ventricular preload and a gauge of effectiveness of therapy for right heart failure.

The relation between ventricular preload and systolic performance is described by the Starling relation, which, in its clinical format, plots stroke volume, stroke work, or cardiac output against one of the aforementioned indicators of preload. At relatively low levels of preload, systolic performance rises with preload until a relative plateau is reached. Beyond this point, with additional increases in preload, ventricular systolic performance increases only modestly, and may even decline. In managing heart failure, it is often appropriate to maintain intravenous volume at a level that places preload near the start of this plateau. Further reduction in preload, as with diuretics or venodilators may reduce the manifestations of elevated pulmonary or central venous pressure, but may also reduce cardiac output. Further increases in preload, as with intravascular volume loading, tend to worsen pulmonary edema and systemic venous congestion without substantial gain in cardiac output.

In the setting of reduced peripheral perfusion caused by myocardial infarction and in the absence of antecedent cardiac disease, preload is optimized when pulmonary artery wedge pressure is in the range of 15 to 18 mm Hg. Further increases may result in pulmonary edema, whereas further decreases may reduce cardiac output. When there is no clinical evidence of low cardiac output, there is no reason to maintain pulmonary artery wedge pressure at this level, which exceeds the normal range of 5 to 12 mm Hg. On the other hand, patients with chronic elevation in ventricular filling pressure and/or with noncompliant ventricles, e.g., with severe left ventricular hypertrophy, may have an "optimal" pulmonary artery wedge pressure that exceeds 18 mm Hg. Under such circumstances either greater ventricular filling pressure is needed to achieve the same myocardial fiber stretch (due to diminished compliance), or the slope of the Starling curve is altered such that increases in pulmonary artery wedge pressure above 18 mm Hg may be accompanied by further increases in cardiac output. Furthermore, when pulmonary venous pressure is chronically elevated, mechanisms develop to diminish pulmonary interstitial or alveolar edema at any given pulmonary venous pressure. These include an increase in pulmonary lymphatic flow and thickening of the alveolar-capillary membrane. For these reasons, in the management of heart failure the target ventricular filling pressures must be geared to the needs of the individual patient.

Treatment in Conditions of Primary Ventricular Volume Overload

Heart failure may be primarily the result of increased preload, i.e., ventricular volume overload. The most common etiologies of left ventricular volume overload are mitral regurgitation, aortic regurgitation, and ventricular septal defect with left-to-right shunt. Right ventricular volume overload most commonly results from tricuspid regurgitation (although tricuspid regurgitation usually is functional, secondary to pressure overload), atrial-level left-to-right shunt, or, less commonly pulmonic regurgitation. In all of these circumstances, the involved ventricle receives a diastolic volume that exceeds forward stroke volume, thereby causing increased preload. As a result, conditions of ventricular volume overload may directly cause manifestations of left or right heart failure because of excessive pulmonary or systemic venous pressure, respectively. Furthermore, chronic ventricular volume overload may cause progressive depression of myocardial contractility, thereby producing or exacerbating heart failure.

In conditions causing ventricular volume overload, therapy should be directed primarily toward reducing the excessive preload. Under these circumstances, the most rational medical regimen includes diuretics, venous dilators, and/or systemic arterial dilators.[1] Both diuretics and venodilators directly reduce ventricular preload, whereas arterial dilators augment systolic ejection performance, thereby secondarily reducing preload. Arterial dilators, by reducing aortic pressure and impedance to forward flow, are particularly efficacious in reducing diastolic load and augmenting cardiac output in settings of aortic regurgitation and ventricular-level left-to-right shunt. In the setting of mitral regurgitation, regurgitant flow is more closely related to systolic mitral orifice size than to left ventricular systolic pressure. Therefore, therapy is best implemented by direct reduction in preload, using diuretics and venodilators, with resulting reduction in systolic mitral orifice size.

As in other causes of heart failure, therapy for patients with primary left ventricular volume overload is directed toward improving symptoms. In addition, since chronic ventricular volume overload leads to progressive myocardial dysfunction, it is a reasonable conjecture that early institution of therapy directed toward reducing the diastolic load will improve the natural history and prolong survival. However, at present, data are not available to confirm this hypothesis.

In aortic regurgitation, symptoms of congestive heart failure indicate left ventricular systolic dysfunction and therefore mandate aortic valve replacement, even if symptoms are manageable with medical therapy. Delay of valve replacement may lead to irreversible loss of ventricular contractile function. In the absence of symptoms, noninvasive assessment of left ventricular systolic performance is employed to identify subclinical degrees of contractile dysfunction, thereby aiding in the optimum timing of valve replacement. In the presence of mitral regurgitation, since the left ventricle is ejecting directly into the left atrium and pulmonary veins, symptoms of heart failure may develop in the absence of substantial ventricular contractile dysfunction. Therefore, mitral valve replacement need only be performed for mitral regurgitation if symptoms persist despite medical therapy or if early left ventricular systolic dysfunction is evident (by radionuclide ventriculography, echocardiography, or contrast ventriculography). More severe degrees of left ventricular systolic dysfunction (ejection fraction less than 40 percent) are associated with a poorer prognosis following aortic or mitral valve replacement for regurgitant lesions.

Afterload

In preparations of isolated myocardial tissue, afterload may be defined as the systolic tension developed. Clinically, afterload may be defined as ventricular systolic stress. Systolic wall stress is related directly to intracavitary pressure and radius and inversely to ventricular myocardial thickness. In most clinical circumstances acute changes in left and right ventricular afterload may be approximated by changes in systemic arterial and pulmonary arterial end-systolic pressure, respectively, as measured at the dicrotic notch. Acute changes in left ventricular afterload roughly parallel, but frequently exceed, acute changes in systolic blood pressure.

Increases in afterload reduce the effectiveness of ventricular systolic contraction. Conversely, systolic performance may be augmented in patients with heart failure by interventions designed to reduce afterload, notably administration of agents that directly or indirectly decrease systemic arteriolar resistance.[2-12] In isolated muscle preparations, the interaction between afterload and contractile function may be described by the relation between velocity of fiber shortening and systolic tension. With increasing levels of systolic load, myocardial fiber shortening slows progressively. Clinically, this interaction may be described by the relation of ventricular pressure or wall stress versus ventricular volume or dimension at end-systole. As end-systolic pressure is reduced, a linear decrease in end-systolic volume is achieved. Herein lies the basis for afterload reduction therapy in patients with heart failure and inadequate systemic perfusion. Arteriolar dilatation causes reduction in systemic vascular resistance, thereby decreasing ventricular systolic pressure and myocardial stress, and in turn reducing end-systolic volume and augmenting stroke volume and cardiac output.

Decreases in systemic perfusion pressure limit the extent to which afterload reduction may be employed in the treatment of heart failure. When direct or indirect systemic arteriolar dilators are administered, care must be taken to maintain blood pressure in an acceptable range. Furthermore, it is unusual in the clinical setting to reduce afterload without altering preload. Although combining these two effects may be desirable in the management of the various manifestations of heart failure, concomitant preload reduction may diminish the degree to which afterload reduction augments cardiac output.

Treatment in Conditions of Primary Ventricular Pressure Overload

An abnormal increase in afterload may be the cause of left ventricular failure in settings of aortic stenosis, hypertrophic cardiomyopathy with left ventricular outflow obstruction, and severe systemic hypertension. Likewise, abnormal afterload is the cause of right ventricular failure in patients with left heart failure, mitral valve disease, pulmonary emboli, obstructive lung disease, primary pulmonary hypertension, and with stenosis of pulmonary arteries, pulmonic valve, or right ventricular infundibulum. In patients with left heart failure of other causes, afterload may be inappropriately high because of stimulation of the sympathetic nervous system and the renin-angiotensin axis, and may contribute to a vicious cycle of increasing heart failure.

Patients with severe systemic hypertension may develop manifestations of heart failure related to acute increases in systolic load in the absence of significant myocardial contractile impairment. Alternatively, patients with chronic severe hypertension may develop chronic heart failure secondary to myocardial hypertrophy, with resulting reduction in systolic performance or, more commonly, diastolic performance. Treatment is best directed toward reduction in blood pressure through direct or indirect arteriolar dilators.

Ventricular systolic performance is generally adequate in patients with aortic stenosis if systolic wall stress has been normalized by an increase in myocardial thickness. In such cases, heart failure may still occur as a consequence of myocardial diastolic dysfunction (see subsequently). In the absence of adequate myocardial thickening, afterload is excessive, resulting in heart failure due to reduced systolic performance. Although symptoms of heart failure may be improved in aortic stenosis through use of a variety of pharmacologic agents, such interventions may be fraught with greater risk than is usual. For example, drugs that reduce preload, such as diuretics or nitrates, may diminish symptoms of pulmonary venous hypertension, but carry the risk of markedly reducing stroke volume and cardiac output, which are highly preload-dependent in the hypertrophied left ventricle of aortic stenosis. In addition, prognosis is poor in uncorrected aortic stenosis once symptoms of heart failure, syncope, or angina occur. Therefore, the treatment of choice is correction of the primary abnormality, through aortic valve replacement or aortic valvuloplasty. Once symptoms have appeared, corrective surgery or valvuloplasty should *not* be delayed by a trial of medical therapy.

Heart failure in hypertrophic cardiomyopathy with subaortic stenosis may result from dynamic obstruction of the left ventricular outflow tract and/or from abnormal myocardial relaxation and compliance. Treatment should be initiated with a calcium-channel antagonist and/or beta-adrenergic blocker.[13] Although these drugs may be relatively contraindicated in patients with heart failure related to ventricular systolic dysfunction, systolic function is usually normal in patients with hypertrophic myopathy. Both beta-blockers and calcium-channel blockers may diminish dynamic outflow obstruction through reduction in contractility. Both classes of drugs also may improve ventricular filling through reduction in heart rate.

Calcium-channel blockers have the additional action of augmenting relaxation (see subsequently), which has been shown to be impaired in patients with hypertrophic myopathy. Both agents may reduce the incidence of supraventricular arrhythmias, which often are poorly tolerated in the preload-dependent hypertrophic ventricle. Beta-blockers may additionally reduce the incidence of ventricular arrhythmias, which are frequently responsible for sudden death in patients with hypertrophic myopathy. However, neither calcium-channel blockers nor beta-blockers have been demonstrated to improve survival in this disease. Inotropic drugs are contraindicated, since these may augment the degree of outflow obstruction. Although venodilators and diuretics may directly reduce pulmonary venous hypertension, they must be employed with caution for two reasons: (1) reduction in left ventricular end-diastolic volume may exacerbate outflow obstruction; (2) the hypertrophied ventricle is highly dependent on adequate preload to maintain forward flow. Cautious use of arteriolar dilators may have benefit, particularly if there is superimposed systemic hypertension. Patients who are significantly symptomatic despite medical treatment may benefit from surgery directed at relieving the outflow obstruction through septal myotomy and/or myectomy.

Contractility

Contractility, or inotropic state, may be defined as the effectiveness of myocardial contractile performance, independent of preload and afterload. In an isolated myocardial preparation, under isometric conditions, inotropic state may be gauged by the maximum tension developed or by the rate of tension development at a given end-diastolic fiber length. In a contracting preparation, inotropic state may be gauged as velocity of shortening for a given end-diastolic length and a given systolic tension. In an intact ventricle, inotropic state may be judged prior to ejection or during ejection. Prior to ejection (during isovolumic systole), contractility may be estimated by the peak rate of ventricular pressure rise (dP/dt_{max}) at a given level of preload. During ejection, contractility may be estimated by examining the relation of the velocity of contraction to the maximum contractile tension at a given level of preload. With increased contractility, velocity of shortening is increased for any given level of systolic load. During ejection, contractility also may be judged by the relation of ventricular end-systolic pressure or wall stress to the end-systolic dimension or volume. With increased contractility, the volume to which the ventricle contracts (end-systolic volume) is reduced for any given level of systolic load (end-systolic pressure or wall stress). Increases in inotropic state also are accompanied by increases in the slope of the ventricular end-systolic pressure (wall stress)–volume (dimension) relation. In the assessment of contractility, this relation has the advantage of being independent of preload.

Treatment in Conditions Where Myocardial Contractility is Reduced

Decreased ventricular contractile function may result either from reduction in the mass of functional myocardium, as with ischemic heart disease, or from global reduction in myocardial contractility, as in dilated cardiomyopathy. These two conditions are the most common causes of heart failure in adults. In addition, the hypertrophied myocardium associated with chronically abnormal ventricular loads may manifest altered contractile properties. Reduction in myocardial contractility frequently contributes to the development of heart failure in the setting of chronic volume overload (as with aortic or mitral insufficiency) and occasionally in the setting of chronic pressure overload (as with aortic stenosis or long-standing hypertension).

Primary contractile abnormalities are frequently associated with secondarily altered ventricular loading conditions. Preload is increased because of an inability of the failing heart to eject its diastolic load. This effect may be viewed as serving to maintain cardiac output via the Starling mechanism. Afterload often is relatively high as a consequence of inappropriate "compensatory" mechanisms that serve to maintain blood pressure at the expense of cardiac output. These include vasoconstriction through activation of the sympathetic nervous system and of the renin-angiotensin system.

Therapies for patients with heart failure attributable to reduced contractile performance have been directed toward reduction in preload and in afterload, as well as toward augmentation of contractility. Therapy generally is designed initially to reduce preload through sodium restriction, diuretics, and venodilators. These agents are particularly effective against manifestations of increased pulmonary and systemic venous pressure. Reduction in afterload, through use of direct arteriolar dilators, alpha-adrenergic blockers, beta-adrenergic agonists, or angiotensin converting enzyme inhibitors, is particularly directed toward augmenting cardiac output. Inotropic agents may benefit manifestations of both "forward" and "backward" failure, although the long-term clinical usefulness of these agents is presently in dispute (see subsequently). Drugs that augment contractility of the failing heart, such as beta-adrenergic agents, often have several concomitant effects. These may include direct chronotropic effect and direct vascular effects: i.e., vasoconstriction or vasodilatation. These effects may be desirable or undesirable, depending on the clinical circumstance. Additionally, since contractility is one of the major determinants of myocardial oxygen demand (others being wall stress and heart rate), beneficial effects of inotropic augmentation may be countered by an increase in myocardial oxygen requirement. Where active myocardial ischemia is contributing to reduction of contractile performance, attempts should be made to reverse this process by medical or surgical means (see subsequently).

Relaxation, Compliance, and Ventricular Filling

The diastolic behavior of myocardium may be divided into the active process of relaxation during which calcium is actively transported from the sarcolemma, and the passive process of stretch (compliance) during ventricular filling. Relaxation properties are judged by examination of the rate of ventricular pressure decay during isovolumic relaxation. Compliance is judged by the relation between ventricular pressure and volume during filling. Alterations of either relaxation or compliance may produce manifestations of heart failure, since either may increase ventricular end-diastolic pressure and therefore increase pulmonary and/or systemic venous pressure. Alternatively, decreased compliance (increased slope of the ventricular diastolic pressure–volume relation) may reduce forward flow since normal end-diastolic pressure is associated with lesser end-diastolic volume or fiber stretch. Cardiac output may therefore suffer because of reduced preload.

In addition to abnormalities of myocardial compliance or relaxation, ventricular filling may be mechanically impaired due to pericardial constriction, infiltrative processes that restrict filling (restrictive cardiomyopathy), or lesions that directly limit venous or atrial emptying into the right or left ventricle. Examples of the latter include mitral or tricuspid stenosis, atrial myxoma obstructing the atrioventricular valve, and pulmonary venous occlusive disease.

Treatment in Conditions of Altered Diastolic Function or Ventricular Filling

Clinically relevant reduction in ventricular compliance and/or relaxation may occur as a result of acute myocardial ischemia, in which case therapy is best directed toward medical or surgical relief of ischemia. Alternatively, abnormalities of diastolic performance result from severe ventricular hypertrophy. The latter may be physiologic, as a consequence of systemic hypertension, aortic stenosis (inducing left ventricular hypertrophy), pulmonary hypertension, or pulmonic stenosis (inducing right ventricular hypertrophy). Ventricular hypertrophy also may be nonphysiologic in the case of hypertrophic cardiomyopathy. In addition to relieving the stimulus to hypertrophy (see the section Treatment in Conditions of Primary Ventricular Pressure Overload), therapy may be instituted to directly improve myocardial relaxation. Calcium-channel antagonists improve relaxation in the setting of hypertrophic cardiomyopathy and may have a similar action in hypertensive hypertrophic cardiac disease. Calcium-channel antagonists generally should be avoided in patients with aortic stenosis because any benefit afforded by improving relaxation is likely to be offset by the negative inotropic action of these agents.

Patients with restrictive cardiomyopathy may present with manifestations of pulmonary and systemic venous hypertension, although the latter generally predominate. Therapy consists primarily of sodium restriction and diuretic administration, with dosage limited by manifestations of low cardiac output. This condition must be distinguished from pericardial constriction, in which the treatment of choice is surgical pericardial stripping.

Therapy for patients with mitral stenosis consists of sodium restriction, diuretics, and reduction in heart rate to minimize ventricular filling time. The latter may be achieved with digitalis (in the presence of atrial fibrillation), beta-blockers, or calcium-channel antagonists. When these measures fail to achieve adequate symptomatic benefit, surgical correction should be undertaken.

TREATMENT STRATEGIES AND MODALITIES

Indications for Treatment

Therapy for patients with left ventricular systolic dysfunction has been directed primarily toward relief of symptoms. Until recently, no data have existed to indicate that any medical treatment affected the progression of ventricular dysfunction or altered the natural history of disease. For this reason, a rationale has not existed previously to justify initiating therapy in asymptomatic patients with depression of left ventricular systolic function attributable to dilated cardiomyopathy or to prior myocardial infarction. However, trials have emerged that suggest that long-term afterload reduction prolongs survival in such patients, perhaps by chronic reduction in left ventricular myocardial stress. In patients with symptomatic heart failure, the combination of hydralazine and nitrates has been found to improve survival slightly, compared with placebo.[14] In severely symptomatic patients, angiotensin converting enzyme inhibition with enalapril likewise has been found to prolong survival.[15] These findings, as well as others that substantiate the symptomatic benefit derived from certain vasodilator agents, have caused many clinicians to employ vasodilator agents, particularly angiotensin converting enzyme inhibitors, earlier in the course of heart failure management. Studies are underway to determine whether such agents alter natural history in patients with asymptomatic depression of left ventricular systolic function.

Approaches to Therapy

Concepts in the management of patients with congestive heart failure are undergoing continuous evolution. A search for one of the remediable causes mentioned herein always is indicated. The advent of powerful noninvasive diagnostic tools, particularly echocardiography, has markedly improved the ease and accuracy with which such remediable disorders may be recognized. These techniques also have permitted more precise categorization of functional myocardial disorders (e.g., systolic dysfunction, altered compliance, restrictive disorder), thereby facilitating the tailoring of therapy to the underlying pathophysiology.

Acute Therapy

During acute exacerbation of congestive heart failure or when heart failure is severe at onset, as in the presence of a major myocardial infarction, therapy must be instituted quickly and aggressively and it must carefully be directed toward the specific hemodynamic derangement present. Simultaneously, efforts should be initiated to identify a remediable etiology.

When heart failure is accompanied by symptomatic hypotension or inadequate systemic perfusion, as evidenced by altered mentation or reduced renal function, therapy must be guided carefully by monitoring pulmonary arterial wedge pressure, cardiac output, and blood pressure. Under these circumstances, measures first must be taken to maintain adequate blood pressure. If overt pulmonary edema is absent and if pulmonary arterial wedge pressure is low enough to be safely raised, then initial therapy should consist of volume administration to augment ventricular preload. Guidelines for optimizing pulmonary arterial wedge pressure are described in the section Preload. If hypotension cannot be safely corrected with intravascular volume expansion, then pressors should be administered. Dopamine is a good pressor-of-choice in heart failure due to its pharmacologic actions (described subsequently). When hypotension is accompanied by pulmonary edema, dopamine and a diuretic should be administered concomitantly. In the presence of symptomatic hypotension, drugs with predominant vasodilator action are contraindicated.

If pulmonary edema is present without hypotension or manifestations of low cardiac output, treatment may be instituted with diuretics alone. If diuresis cannot be readily achieved or if inadequate cardiac output becomes evident, then vasodilators and/or inotropic agents should be added. Vasodilators such as intravenous nitroprusside or nitroglycerin may be employed only if blood pressure is adequate; however, under these circumstances they may dramatically reduce ventricular filling pressures while augmenting cardiac output. Similar results may be achieved by administering a nonpressor inotropic vasodilator such as dobutamine or amrinone. Various combinations of inotropic and vasodilator agents may be employed when adequate improvement is not otherwise achieved.

When heart failure occurs in the setting of acute myocardial infarction, several additional considerations must be stressed. First, drugs with inotropic, and particularly chronotropic, action should be used less readily, since these agents may increase myocardial oxygen consumption, thereby potentially worsening ischemia and increasing infarct size. Secondly, as long as blood pressure is adequate, nitrates should be used more readily, since these agents have been found in some studies to reduce infarct size. Third, during the first 6 hours following onset of symptoms, consideration should be given to halting the progression of the infarction through thrombolysis and/or emergent coronary angioplasty. Finally, specific remediable etiologies of heart failure and cardiogenic shock, namely papillary muscle dysfunction or rupture or acute ventricular septal defect, should be considered and investigated.

When medical measures are inadequate to remedy acute severe heart failure, intra-aortic balloon counterpulsation should be considered. This maneuver reduces ventricular preload and augments cardiac output through reduction in systemic arterial impedance. Intra-aortic balloon placement is most rational when a definable acute event is responsible for the abrupt deterioration, and when correction or recovery reasonably may be expected. In acute myocardial infarction or severe ischemia, balloon counterpulsation serves the additional function of reducing ischemia, in part by augmenting diastolic coronary perfusion pressure. Counterpulsation is specifically indicated in the settings of severe acute mitral regurgitation or acute ventricular septal defect, where considerable benefit may be derived from reduction in aortic impedance. It is contraindicated in the presence of significant aortic regurgitation because of increases in aortic diastolic pressure.

Chronic Therapy

Until recently, standard medical treatment of chronic heart failure began with the onset of symptoms and was initiated with restriction of physical activity, sodium restriction, and digitalis administration. If symptoms persisted, diuretics were added in increasing doses (Table 6-1). More recently, data have indicated that vasodilator therapy, particularly with angiotensin converting enzyme (ACE) inhibitors, provides objective symptomatic improvement and alters the natural history of disease. These findings have

TABLE 6-1 Drug Therapy in Chronic Congestive Heart Failure

Drug Class	Actions	Indications	Examples
Diuretics	Preload reduction by diuresis	Systemic and pulmonary venous congestion	Hydrochlorothiazide 25–100 mg daily Lasix 20–400 mg daily
ACE inhibitors	Inhibition of angiotensin II production Vasodilation	Pulmonary congestion or low output; prolongs survival in at least some patient groups	Captopril 6.25–50 mg qid Enalapril 2.5–10 mg bid
Nitrates	Direct systemic venous and arterial vasodilation Epicardial coronary artery vasodilation	Pulmonary congestion, particularly associated with cardiac ischemia Shown to prolong survival in combination with hydralazine	Isosorbide dinitrate 10–40 mg bid or tid Topical nitroglycerin
Calcium channel antagonists	Systemic, coronary, and pulmonary arterial dilation Augmentation of myocardial relaxation Decrease in heart rate	Ischemia-induced pulmonary congestion Hypertrophic cardiomyopathy Diastolic ventricular dysfunction	Verapamil 80–160 mg tid Diltiazem 30–120 mg tid Nifedipine 10–40 mg tid
Alpha-blockers	Systemic arterial vasodilation	Chronic low output states	Prazosin 1–8 mg tid
Other vasodilators	Systemic arterial vasodilation	Chronic low output states Increased patient survival (hydralazine and nitrates)	Hydralazine 10–100 mg qid
Digitalis	Direct increase in cardiac inotropy	Chronic low output or pulmonary congestion Reduction of heart rate in atrial fibrillation	Digoxin 0.125–0.375 mg daily
Phosphodiesterase inhibitors	Increase in cyclic AMP Augmentation of cardiac inotropy Additional vasodilator effects	Documented to improve exercise capacity Exact indications to be determined	Milrinone* 5–12.5 mg qid Enoximone* 50–150 mg tid

*Not FDA approved as of this writing. ACE = angiotension converting enzyme.

caused vasodilator therapy to be employed earlier in the course of symptom development. A variety of orally active inotropic agents have recently come under investigation; however the role of these agents in the scheme of heart failure management is yet to be clearly defined. At the same time, the clinical role of digitalis as an inotropic agent has come into question. Some investigators even have advocated a place for beta-adrenergic blockade as a means for improving the natural history of disease in selected patients with severe ventricular systolic dysfunction. At present, this concept is not accepted broadly and requires additional investigation.

Sodium Restriction and Diuretics

These measures are traditionally the first lines of intervention following the advent of symptoms of heart failure and are primarily effective for symptoms of pulmonary venous hypertension (exertional dyspnea and orthopnea) and elevated systemic venous pressure (edema and ascites). As previously discussed, diuresis may augment or reduce systemic perfusion, depending on the relation between preload and forward output in the individual patient. Diuresis is most likely to be accompanied by increase, or at least maintenance, of cardiac output in the presence of functional mitral and/or tricuspid regurgitation, which may be diminished by reduction in ventricular volumes. In addition, when edema and/or ascites is present, considerable diuresis often may be achieved without significant reduction in cardiac output, since fluid may be mobilized from extravascular spaces without substantial reduction in intravascular volume. When diuresis is induced, the patient must be monitored for manifestations of reduced systemic perfusion, particularly for worsening renal function, for potassium depletion, and for hyponatremia. The last may be avoided by free water restriction.

Vasodilators

Vasodilator agents may be classified as predominantly arteriolar, such as hydralazine, predominantly venous, such as nitrates, and mixed arteriolar-venous, such as prazosin. Vasodilators also may be classified according to mechanism of action: direct vascular smooth muscle relaxation (including calcium-channel antagonism), angiotensin converting enzyme inhibition, or alpha-adrenergic blockade. In addition, the beta-adrenergic agents and phosphodiesterase inhibitors, described in the section Inotropic Agents, also function as vasodilators.

In theory, predominant venodilators, such as nitrates, are most effective at reducing symptoms of systemic venous and pulmonary venous pressure, whereas predominant arteriolar dilators, such as hydralazine, are most effective at augmenting forward cardiac output. In practice, considerable overlap exists among the clinical benefits of these various drug classes. This overlap is partly due to the multiple sites of drug action; for example, nitrates reduce systemic vascular resistance as well as increase systemic venous capacitance. In addition, drugs that directly reduce systemic vascular resistance secondarily reduce ventricular preload by augmenting ventricular systolic emptying. The need to maintain adequate systemic arterial pressure is always a limiting factor for vasodilator drug dosage. Vasodilator therapy tends to effect the greatest hemodynamic and symptomatic benefit in patients with relatively large left ventricular end-diastolic volumes and in patients with valvular regurgitation, including those with functional mitral regurgitation.[16,17] Earlier institution of therapy in patients with less severely dilated left ventricles may yield less evidence of acute benefit, but may limit the progression of left ventricular dilatation and systolic dysfunction. Further studies are needed to confirm these possibilities.

Angiotensin Converting Enzyme Inhibitors

Patients with heart failure tend to have elevated plasma renin levels, thereby resulting in increased systemic vascular resistance secondary to angiotensin effect. This response augments systemic arterial pressure at the expense of forward flow. The angiotensin converting enzyme inhibitors, captopril and enalapril, inhibit the conversion of angiotensin I to the active angiotensin II and, in patients with heart failure, reduce ventricular filling pressure and augment cardiac output. Although angiotensin converting enzyme inhibitor administration may augment renal perfusion, azotemia also may emerge or worsen with initiation of therapy. Azotemia has been described especially in patients with significant renal vascular disease, but may occur in its absence. Azotemia may result from reduced glomerular filtration pressure related to a fall in efferent arteriolar blood pressure. For this reason, and because of the potential for inducing symptomatic hypotension, administration of angiotensin converting enzyme inhibitors always should be initiated with small doses, and increased as tolerated. Hyponatremia in patients with heart failure tends to be a marker not only for severity of illness but also for increased plasma renin levels, a finding that has several implications for therapy with angiotensin converting enzyme inhibitors. Such patients may be more dependent on angiotensin levels for maintaining systemic arterial pressure and may be more prone to develop hypotension upon institution of therapy. However, if the drug is administered cautiously in gradually increasing doses, thereby avoiding hypotension, greater hemodynamic and symptomatic benefit may be expected. Institution of combined therapy with diuretics and an angiotensin converting enzyme inhibitor has been reported to correct hyponatremia in patients with heart failure.

At present, this class of agents most clearly has been demonstrated to chronically augment exercise capacity during placebo-controlled trials in patients with heart failure secondary to reduced left ventricular systolic function. The improvement in exercise capacity is not directly linked with the observed acute hemodynamic benefits, and may require chronic drug administration to take effect. In addition, at least one study performed to date has found an improved survival induced by angiotensin converting enzyme inhibition in patients with severely symptomatic left ventricular systolic dysfunction.[15] Studies are under way to investigate whether similar benefit may be derived in less severely symptomatic patients.

Nitrates

These agents are direct vasodilators that have greater effect on venous capacitance than on systemic arteriolar resistance, and therefore may be particularly effective in reducing symptoms of systemic venous and pulmonary venous hypertension. However, they tend to reduce blood pressure and increase cardiac output. Chronic placebo-controlled trials have documented slightly improved exercise capacity as a result of nitrate administration in patients with symptomatic left ventricular systolic dysfunction. Nitrate therapy has the additional benefit of reducing the frequency and severity of active myocardial ischemia in patients in whom ischemia contributes to symptoms of heart failure. Nitrates reduce myocardial ischemia through at least two mechanisms: (1) by reducing myocardial oxygen demand and (2) by reducing epicardial coronary arterial tone. The latter effect may be particularly important in patients in whom increased coronary tone augments the resistance to coronary flow imposed by fixed vascular occlusive disease. Evidence is accumulating to indicate that nitrate therapy should not be administered continuously, either intravenously in management of acute heart failure, or topically in the management of chronic heart failure. Drug tolerance occurs under these circumstances and may be avoided by intermittent oral therapy.

Calcium-Channel Antagonists

These agents have several sites of action where they may help patients with heart failure. As systemic and pulmonary arteriolar dilators, they may reduce left and right ventricular systolic stress, thereby augmenting cardiac output and reducing pulmonary and systemic venous pressures. As dilators of both small and large coronary arteries, they may reduce any contribution of myocardial ischemia to altered ventricular systolic and diastolic performance. They may directly improve myocardial relaxation, thereby further reducing ventricular filling pressures. This effect is particularly beneficial in circumstances where altered relaxation is a primary pathophysiologic mechanism for development of heart failure, such as in patients with hypertrophic cardiomyopathy. Calcium-channel antagonists tend to variably reduce heart rate, an effect that has particular benefit where myocardial compliance is reduced, such as in patients with hypertrophic cardiomyopathy or where ventricular filling is directly impeded, as in mitral stenosis. Reduced heart rate also diminishes myocardial ischemia by reducing myocardial oxygen demand. Of presently available agents, verapamil has the greatest negative chronotropic effect, and nifedipine the least, with diltiazem intermediate.

A potentially deleterious action of the calcium-channel antagonists is their variable negative inotropic action. In patients in whom heart failure results from depressed ventricular systolic performance, the risk of further reducing systolic function must be individually weighed against the potential beneficial effects. In such patients, therapy must be instituted cautiously. In contrast, the negative inotropic effect of the calcium-channel antagonists may be beneficial in patients with dynamic obstructive hypertrophic cardiomyopathy in whom reduced contractility may be accompanied by reduction in the degree of dynamic aortic outflow obstruction. Of the presently available agents, verapamil has the greatest negative inotropic effect, diltiazem probably the least, with nifedipine probably being intermediate.

Inotropic Agents

Several drugs possessing positive inotropic action have been employed both acutely and chronically for management of congestive heart failure due to depressed left ventricular systolic function. At present, the role of many of these agents in treating symptoms of heart failure remains uncertain. Controversy surrounds the use of inotropic drug therapy in several respects. First, to what extent does chronic administration of inotropic drug therapy establish and maintain hemodynamic and clinical benefit? It may be argued that the failed ventricle is intrinsically exposed to near-maximal inotropic stimulation because of elevated levels of circulating catecholamines, and the degree to which long-term clinical benefit may be derived from additional inotropic stimulation may be questioned. Short-term hemodynamic benefit has been well documented, and trials are under way to investigate the chronic clinical efficacy of a number of newer orally-active drugs with inotropic action. The second controversy surrounds the degree to which acute and chronic hemodynamic and symptomatic benefit of any inotropic agent results from augmented contractility or from the concomitant vasodilator action possessed by many of these agents. Finally, since contractility is a determinant of myocardial oxygen requirement, concern must be voiced that inotropic drug therapy may increase this requirement, resulting in increased potential for ischemic and arrhythmic events. Most studies to date have failed to indicate consistent increases in myocardial oxygen consumption following administration of inotropically active drugs in patients with ventricular systolic failure. These findings are presumed to be related to reduction in systolic stress, which may offset any increase in myocardial contractility in the determination of oxygen demand. Nevertheless, the potential for increased myocardial oxygen requirement in individual patients must be considered whenever drugs possessing inotropic effect are administered.

Inotropic agents exert greatest direct benefit on symptoms of low cardiac output, but also are likely to reduce ventricular filling pressures by augmenting systolic emptying and/or by exerting concomitant direct or indirect vasodilator effect. Inotropic augmentation has no role in the management of heart failure caused by altered diastolic performance and is specifically contraindicated in patients with obstructive hypertrophic cardiomyopathy, where enhanced contractility may result in increased dynamic left ventricular outflow obstruction.

Digitalis

The digitalis glycosides were the first effective pharmacologic agents available for treating congestive heart failure, with clinical effects described by William Withering in the eighteenth century. The inotropic action of this class of drugs is presumed to be related to its inhibition of myocardial sodium–potassium adenosinetriphosphatase (ATPase) and may result from slight increases in intracellular sodium, leading to augmented sodium–calcium exchange. Digitalis has long been employed as an early intervention following development of symptoms of reduced cardiac output and/or pulmonary or systemic venous hypertension due to ventricular systolic dysfunction. The validity of this approach recently has been questioned by some investigators, and several placebo-controlled trials have failed to demonstrate effectiveness of digoxin in reducing the clinical manifestations of heart failure. However, other studies indicate that digoxin therapy does improve symptoms, and most clinicians continue to employ this drug for treating heart failure. With the growing body of evidence demonstrating the clinical benefit of certain vasodilator agents, and the narrow toxic–therapeutic margin of digoxin, the use of digoxin early in the course of symptom development may be questioned. Rather, it may be argued that therapy should be initiated with diuretics and/or vasodilators, and an inotropic agent such as digoxin should be added only if symptoms persist. This issue remains controversial.

In addition to its inotropic effect, digitalis is an important agent in the control of supraventricular arrhythmias and in the regulation of ventricular response to atrial fibrillation. In contrast with digitalis, other classes of agents with similar effects on atrioventricular conduction, namely beta-adrenergic blockers and calcium-channel antagonists, exert hypotensive and negative inotropic effects. Digoxin is therefore central in the management of patients in whom heart failure is complicated and/or exacerbated by supraventricular arrhythmias.

Beta-Adrenergic Agents

These agents exert their cellular effects after binding to cytoplasmic receptors of either the beta-1 class, with a preponderance in myocardium, or the beta-2 class, with a preponderance in vascular and bronchial smooth muscle. Cardiac beta-1 stimulation causes augmented inotropy and chronotropy, whereas smooth muscle beta-2 stimulation causes vasodilatation and bronchodilatation. These effects are mediated by increased intracellular concentrations of adenosine 3':5'-cyclic phosphate (cyclic AMP) resulting from augmented adenyl cyclase activity. Although various pharmacologic agents are said to be relatively beta-1 or beta-2 selective, in clinical practice this selectivity is relatively unimportant, and most beta-adrenergic agents exert chronotropic, inotropic, vasodilator, and bronchodilator actions. These actions, particularly the last three, have potential benefit in the acute management of severe congestive heart failure.

Dopamine and dobutamine are intravenously administered drugs with beta-adrenergic activity and have a role in the management of patients with acute exacerbations of congestive heart failure, particularly when reduced cardiac output is a prominent feature.[18,19] In low to moderate doses, dopamine exerts beta-adrenergic as well as dopaminergic action. The former results in inotropic, chronotropic, and systemic vasodilator actions, whereas the latter results in renal vasodilation, causing preferential increases in renal blood flow. In higher doses, dopamine exerts greater alpha-adrenergic action, resulting in systemic vasoconstriction, an effect that is undesirable in heart failure management unless blood pressure cannot otherwise be maintained. Used in moderate doses, dopamine tends to increase blood pressure, while augmenting cardiac output and renal blood flow, with variable reduction in ventricular filling pressures. Its chronotropic action is less evident in the presence of heart failure where this action tends to be balanced by partial withdrawal of intrinsic catecholamines as cardiac output is improved.

Dobutamine possesses less alpha-adrenergic action and less dopaminergic action than dopamine. Because it is more exclusively beta-adrenergic, it tends to effect greater degrees of systemic vasodilatation. It is not a pressor agent, and should not be employed as primary treatment in the setting of systemic hypotension. In patients with severe acute heart failure, it may be extremely effective at both augmenting cardiac output and reducing ventricular filling pressures. Some evidence exists to suggest that several days of dobutamine infusion achieve a more protracted improvement in hemodynamics and clinical status in patients with severe heart failure.[20-22]

Continued administration of a beta-adrenergic agent inevitably leads to tachyphylaxis because of reduction in beta-receptor density. Drug tolerance limits the usefulness of orally-active beta-adrenergic agents in the management of chronic heart failure. Pulse therapy with either orally-active agents or intravenous agents may serve some role in selected patients with intractable symptoms, but this possibility has not been adequately investigated.

Phosphodiesterase Inhibitors

A series of nondigitalis, nonadrenergic, orally-active agents with inotropic effect recently has been investigated for both acute and chronic therapy in heart failure. These include amrinone, milrinone, and enoximone. The mechanism of their inotropic action may be related to their phosphodiesterase inhibitory effect, resulting in increased intracellular concentrations of cyclic AMP and augmented transmembrane calcium transport.[23] They exert bronchodilator and systemic and pulmonary vasodilator effects as well as inotropic action, and some investigators have contended that hemodynamic benefit is more closely related to vasodilator than to inotropic action. However, clinical inotropic action has been demonstrated by increases in isovolumic phase indices of contractility and by the fact that ventricular systolic performance is increased beyond that which may be explained by the degree of afterload-reduction that occurs.[24-26]

Acute administration of intravenous amrinone in patients with severe left ventricular systolic dysfunction predictably augments cardiac output and variably reduces ventricular filling pressures. Blood pressure tends to be reduced slightly. Although this class of agents possesses chronotropic action, heart rate remains unchanged or increases only slightly in patients with heart failure, presumably because of concomitant withdrawal of endogenous circulating catecholamines. At least one study has indicated that amrinone augments renal perfusion, although data on this matter are conflicting. Intravenous amrinone is an effective agent in the management of patients with acute exacerbations of heart failure with reduced cardiac output and in the maintenance of acceptable hemodynamics during and following surgical procedures in patients with left ventricular systolic dysfunction.[27-30]

Unlike the beta-adrenergic agents, the phosphodiesterase inhibitory inotropic agents have not been found to manifest tachyphylaxis. For this reason and because they are orally active, they have been attractive drugs to investigate in the chronic management of heart failure. Investigations presently are being conducted to determine whether long-term administration of these agents achieves persistent improvement in functional capacity.[31-33]

Beta-Blockade

Patients with symptomatic heart failure are characterized by increases in circulating endogenous catecholamines, presumably in response to depressed systemic perfusion. Administration of beta-blocking agents to patients with heart failure due to ventricular systolic dysfunction is potentially hazardous, since endogenous catecholamines may be responsible for maintaining adequate blood pressure and cardiac output. Therefore, these agents have long been considered contraindicated in this setting. A cautious trial of beta-blockade is occasionally indicated for patients in whom heart failure is related to active myocardial ischemia. In addition, it has been speculated that chronic catecholamine stimulation may, in part, be responsible for progressive myocardial dysfunction, and blockade of this stimulation may therefore limit the progression of disease. Several clinical trials of beta-blocking agents have been carried out in patients with severe left ventricular systolic dysfunction, with varied results. Beta-blockade, instituted cautiously in selected patients, possibly may effect long-term benefit. However, at present such therapy must be considered investigational.

Beta-blocking agents are effective in patients with hypertrophic cardiomyopathy by augmenting ventricular filling through reduction in heart rate and by decreasing dynamic outflow obstruction through reduction in contractility. Likewise, in mitral stenosis, heart rate reduction by beta-blockade is effective in improving ventricular filling and reducing left atrial pressure, particularly in the presence of atrial fibrillation.

Surgical Approaches

Valvular Disease

The aggressiveness with which a surgical approach should be taken in patients with congestive heart failure secondary to valvular disease depends on the lesion that is primarily responsible for symptoms. In both aortic stenosis and aortic regurgitation, valve replacement or repair should be undertaken at the onset of symptoms. In the case of aortic stenosis, the advent of symptoms signifies a poor prognosis in the absence of surgical correction. Reduced left ventricular systolic function in the face of hemodynamically relevant aortic stenosis should not deter surgical intervention, since ventricular performance is likely to improve with relief of abnormal afterload. In aortic regurgitation, symptoms of heart failure indicate at least moderate left ventricular systolic depression and represent a signal that further delay in surgical repair may lead to irreversible ventricular dysfunction. A somewhat more conservative approach may be taken in the presence of mitral valve disease. In mitral regurgitation, a surgical approach need only be taken if symptoms cannot be readily controlled medically or if left ventricular function has begun to deteriorate. As in aortic regurgitation, long-term prognosis is poor in patients who undergo mitral valve replacement for mitral regurgitation following development of severe left ventricular systolic dysfunction. In congestive heart failure due to mitral stenosis, surgery is indicated primarily for relief of symptoms.

Ischemic Heart Disease

A subset of patients with heart failure related to ischemic heart disease have active myocardial ischemia, in addition to healed myocardial infarction, as the cause of left ventricular systolic dysfunction. Such patients may manifest improvement in systolic function, with relief of heart failure, following revascularization by either coronary bypass surgery or angioplasty. Identification of such patients represents a challenge. Evidence of active ischemia clinically or by thallium imaging should trigger consideration of coronary revascularization. Selected patients with heart failure benefit from resection of a left ventricular aneurysm, which is generally performed in conjunction with coronary bypass surgery. In patients with severe heart failure following acute myocardial infarction, consideration should be given to the diagnoses of papillary muscle infarction (with or without rupture) or ventricular septal defect, which generally should be emergently surgically corrected.

Cardiac Transplantation

In the last several years, cardiac transplantation has progressed from an experimental procedure to one of proven clinical benefit to selected patients with severe congestive heart failure. The two advances that most markedly have improved survival following transplantation are (1) the use of endomyocardial biopsy to diagnose rejection and guide therapy and (2) the development and use of cyclosporin as a component of the immunosuppressive regimen. At present, 3-year survival following cardiac transplantation is approximately 75 percent. When this is compared with the 50 percent 6-month survival in patients with New York Heart Association functional class IV due to congestive heart failure, it is evident that cardiac transplantation offers greater hope for improved survival in such patients than any other presently available form of therapy. Unfortunately, lack of donor availability markedly limits the application of this therapeutic modality. Approximately 1,650 cardiac transplants were performed in the United States in 1988, whereas it is estimated that 15 times that number of patients could have benefited from transplantation. At present, transplantation is indicated in patients with less than 1-year expected survival in the absence of other significant disease processes.

References

1. Chatterjee K, Parmley WW, Swan HJC, Berman G, Forrester J, Marcus HS. Beneficial effects of vasodilator agents in severe mitral regurgitation due to dysfunction of subvalvular apparatus. Circulation 1973; 48:684–690.
2. Cohn JN, Franciosa JA. Drug therapy: vasodilator therapy of cardiac failure. N Engl J Med 1977; 297:27–31, 254–258.
3. Franciosa JA, Cohn JN. Hemodynamic responsiveness to short- and long-acting vasodilators in left ventricular failure. Am J Med 1978; 65:126–133.
4. Cohn JN. Physiologic basis of vasodilator therapy for heart failure. Am J Med 1981; 71:135–139.
5. Franciosa JA, Dunkman WB, Leddy CL. Hemodynamic effects of vasodilators and long-term response in heart failure. J Am Coll Cardiol 1984; 3:1521–1530.
6. Chatterjee K, Parmley WW, Cohn JN, et al. A cooperative multicenter study of captopril in congestive heart failure: hemodynamic effects and long-term response. Am Heart J 1985; 110:439–447.
7. Captopril multicenter research group. A placebo-controlled trial of captopril in refractory chronic congestive heart failure. J Am Coll Cardiol 1983; 2:755–763.
8. Kramer BL, Masie BM, Topic N. Controlled trial of captopril in chronic heart failure: a rest and exercise hemodynamic study. Circulation 1983; 67:807–816.
9. Cleland JGF, Dargie HJ, Hodsman GP, et al. Captopril in heart failure; a double bind controlled trial. Br Heart J 1984; 52:530–535.
10. Cleland JGF, Dargie HJ, Ball SG, et al. Effects of enalapril in heart failure: a double blind study of effects on exercise performance, renal function, hormones, and metabolic state. Br Heart J 1985; 54:305–312.
11. McGrath BP, Arnolda L, Matthews P, et al. Controlled trial of enalapril in congestive heart failure. Br Heart J 1985; 54:405–414.
12. Konstam MA, Weiland DS, Conlon TP, et al. Hemodynamic correlates of left ventricular versus right ventricular radionuclide volumetric responses to vasodilator therapy in congestive heart failure secondary to ischemic or dilated cardiomyopathy. Am J Cardiol 1987; 53:1131–1137.

13. Bonow RO, Ostrow HG, Rosing DR, et al. Verapamil effects of left ventricular systolic and diastolic function in patients with hypertrophic cardiomyopathy: pressure-volume analysis with a non-imaging scintillation probe. Circulation 1983; 25:1062–1073.

14. Cohn JN, Archibald DG, Phil M, et al. Effect of vasodilator therapy on mortality in chronic congestive heart failure. N Engl J Med 1986; 314:1547–1552.

15. The CONSENSUS Trial Study Group. Effects of enalapril on mortality in severe congestive heart failure: Results of the Cooperative North Scandinavian Enalapril Survival Study (CONSENSUS). N Engl J Med 1987; 316:1429–1435.

16. Packer M, Meller J, Medina N, Gorlin R, Herman MV. Importance of left ventricular chamber size in determining the response to hydralazine in severe chronic heart failure. N Engl J Med 1980; 303:250–255.

17. Weiland DS, Konstam MA, Salem DN, et al. Contribution of reduced mitral regurgitant volume to vasodilator effect in severe left ventricular failure. Am J Cardiol 1986; 58:1046–1050.

18. Leier CV, Heban PT, Huss P, Bush CA, Lewis RP. Comparative systemic and regional hemodynamic effects of dopamine and dobutamine in patients with cardiomyopathic heart failure. Circulation 1978; 58:466–475.

19. Stoner JD, Bolen JL, Harrison DC. Comparison of dobutamine and dopamine in treatment of severe heart failure. Br Heart J 1977; 39:536–539.

20. Akhtar N, Mikulic E, Cohn JN, Chaudhry MH. Hemodynamic effect of dobutamine in patients with severe heart failure. Am J Cardiol 1975; 36:202–205.

21. Tuttle RR, Mills J. Dobutamine: development of a new catecholamine to selectively increase cardiac contractility. Circ Res 1975; 36:185–196.

22. Sonnenblick EH, Frishman WH, LeJemtel TH. Dobutamine: a new synthetic cardioactive sympathetic amine. N Engl J Med 1979; 300:17–22.

23. Lejemtel TH, Keung E, Sonnenblick EH, et al. Amrinone: a new non-glycoside, non-adrenergic cardiotonic agent effective in the treatment of intractable myocardial failure in man. Circulation 1979; 59:1098–1104.

24. Millard RW, Dube G, Grupp I, Alousi A, Schwartz A. Direct vasodilator and positive inotropic actions of amrinone. J Mol Cell Cardiol 1980; 12:647–652.

25. Konstam MA, Cohen SR, Weiland DS, Martin TT, Das D, Isner JI, Salem DN. Relative contribution of inotropic and vasodilator effects to amrinone-induced hemodynamic improvement in congestive heart failure. Am J Cardiol 1986; 57:242–248.

26. Firth BG, Ratner AV, Grassman ED, Winniford MD, Nicod P, Hillis LD. Assessment of the inotropic and vasodilator effects of amrinone versus isoproterenol. Am J Cardiol 1984; 43:1331–1336.

27. Benotti JR, Grossman W, Braunwald E, Davolos DD, Alousi AA. Hemodynamic assessment of amrinone. N Engl J Med 1978; 299:1373–1377.

28. Wilmshurst PT, Thompson DS, Jenkins BS, Coltart DJ, Webb-Peploe MM. Haemodynamic effects of intravenous amrinone in patients with impaired left ventricular function. Br Heart J 1983; 49:77–82.

29. Klein NA, Siskind SJ, Frishman WH, Sonnenblick EH, Lejemtel TH. Hemodynamic comparison of intravenous amrinone and dobutamine in patients with chronic congestive heart failure. Am J Cardiol 1981; 48:170–175.

30. Gage J, Rutman H, Lucido D, LeJemtel TH. Additive effects of dobutamine and amrinone on myocardial contractility and ventricular performance in patients with severe heart failure. Circulation 1986; 74:367–373.
31. Baim DS, McDowell AV, Cherniles J, et al. Evaluation of a new bipyridine inotropic agent — -milrinone — -in patients with severe congestive heart failure. N Engl J Med 1983; 309:748–756.
32. Borow KM, Come PC, Neumann A, Baim DS, Braunwald E, Grossman W. Physiologic assessment of the inotropic, vasodilator and afterload reducing effects of milrinone in subjects without cardiac disease. Am J Cardiol 1985; 55:1204–1209.
33. Ludmer PL, Wright RF, Arnold MO, Ganz P, Braunwald E, Colucci WS. Separation of the direct myocardial and vasodilator actions of milrinone administered by an intracoronary infusion technique. Circulation 1986; 73:130–137.

7 | PACEMAKER THERAPY: CLASSIFICATION, INDICATIONS, AND CLINICAL CONSIDERATIONS

N.A. MARK ESTES III, M.D.

Since the initial reports of implantation of an artificial cardiac pacemaker for treatment of classic Stokes-Adams attacks 2½ decades ago, there has been a revolution in the technology and the clinical applications of this electronic device. The pacemaker has three essential parts—the battery, which serves as a power source; the circuitry, which regulates the timing, sensing, and energy output of the pacemaker; and the lead. The lead has an insulated portion for conducting the impulses from the pulse generator (battery and circuitry) and an uninsulated portion, the electrode, in contact with the atrial or ventricular myocardium at the site of stimulation. With "dual-chamber" devices, it is possible to stimulate and sense contractions of the atrium or ventricle. Most present-day systems have a range on noninvasively programmable stimulation and sensing parameters. In many instances, information regarding the function of the pacemaker can be transmitted noninvasively by telemetry from the pacemaker to an external programmer.

An international code based on a five-letter reference system has been developed to provide a standard reference system. The complexity of current pacemakers has underscored the need for uniform terminology for the description of various pacing modalities. Table 7-1 shows the five-position pacemaker code developed by the Inter-Society Commission on Heart Disease as modified by the North American Society of Pacing and Electrophysiology. This code assigns one position to each of the five major characteristics of a permanent pacemaker, thereby including the chamber paced (position 1), the chamber sensed (position 2), the mode of response to sensed events (position 3), programmable functions (position 4), and special tachyarrhythmia functions (position 5). Thus, the commonly-used ventricular demand pacemaker would be referred to as "VVIOO" and a dual-chamber device as "DDDOO". These are commonly abbreviated as "VVI" and "DDD", respectively.

TABLE 7-1   Five-Position Pacemaker Codes

I Chamber Paced	II Chamber Sensed	III Response To Sensing	IV Programmability	V Tachyarrhythmia Functions
V = ventricle	V = ventricle	I = inhibited	P = program- mable and/ or output	P = pacing
A = atrium	A = atrium	T = triggered	M = multi- program- mable	S = shock
D = atrium and ventricle	D = atrium and ventricle	D = atrial- triggered and ventricular- inhibited	C = communi- cating	D = dual (pacing and shock)
	O = none	O = none	R = rate- modulated	O = none
			O = none	

INDICATIONS

The indications for insertion of permanent and temporary cardiac pacemakers have evolved from the initial use of asynchronous single-chamber devices for the treatment of life-threatening bradycardia to the use of sophisticated dual-chamber devices for a variety of cardiac dysrhythmias.[1] Indications for permanent pacemakers recently have been grouped into three major operational classifications by the American College of Cardiology and the American Heart Association:[2]

Class I indications for pacing are those in which there is general agreement that a permanent pacemaker should be implanted.

Class II indications are those indications for which permanent pacemakers are frequently used, but among experts there is a divergence of opinion regarding the necessity of their insertion.

Class III indications are conditions for which there is general agreement that pacemakers are unnecessary.

The decision to implant a pacemaker is based not only on the patient's rhythm disturbance, but on such factors as symptoms, underlying cardiac disease that may be adversely affected by a bradycardia, the need to operate a motor vehicle, and the time required for the patient to reach medical care. The overall physical and mental status of the patient also is appropriately weighed when the clinician considers pacemaker implantation.

PACING IN ACQUIRED AV BLOCK IN ADULTS

Clinically, atrioventricular (AV) block can be classified as first degree with prolongation of the PR interval beyond 200 msec, second degree, or third degree (complete heart block). Second degree heart block includes delayed conduction within the atrioventricular node with progressive prolongation of the PR interval before a blocked ventricular response (Wenckebach phenomenon). Block within or below the bundle of His, represented on the surface ECG by a nonconducted P wave without a preceding prolongation of the PR interval, is Mobitz type II block. As indicated in Table 7–2, neither first degree AV block nor asymptomatic Wenckebach-type block are indications for pacemaker placement.[3] Symptomatic Wenckebach and Mobitz type II block are well-accepted (Class I) indications for placement of a permanent pacemaker. There remains controversy regarding the necessity of pacing patients with asymptomatic Mobitz type II block (Class II indication), although there is a considerable incidence of progression to a higher degree of AV block. Complete heart block (CHB) that is associated with symptomatic bradycardia or congestive heart failure, or ventricular arrhythmias that require antiarrhythmic agents that might suppress the escape focus are clear indications for permanent pacemaker placement. Additionally, a permanent pacemaker is indicated in the presence of complete heart block if there are documented periods of asystole of 3 seconds or longer, or of an escape rate of less than 40 beats per minute (bpm), even in patients free of symptoms. Finally, a permanent pacemaker is indicated in any patient who has an acute confusional state related to a bradyarrhythmia in whom it has been documented that there is improvement with temporary pacing. Abnormalities of AV conduction, in adults, for which permanent pacemakers are frequently used, but for which there is a divergence of opinion with respect to the necessity of their insertion (Class II), include asymptomatic complete heart block with an escape rate of 40 bpm or faster.

PACING IN BIFASCICULAR AND TRIFASCICULAR BLOCK

Complete heart block usually is preceded by a variable period of bifascicular block. However, the rate of progression of asymptomatic chronic bifascicular block to complete heart block generally is low. There are currently

TABLE 7-2 Indications for Permanent Pacemaker Therapy

Dysrhythmia	Class I (Indicated)	Class II (Sometimes Indicated)	Class III (Not Indicated)
First degree AV block			X
Second degree AV block			
Type I (Wenckebach)			
Asymptomatic			X
Symptomatic	X		
Type II (Mobitz II)			
Asymptomatic		X	
Symptomatic	X		
Complete AV block			
Congenital			
Asymptomatic			X
Symptomatic	X		
Acquired			
Asymptomatic		X	
Symptomatic	X		
Chronic bifascicular and trifascicular block			
Intermittent CHB			
with symptoms	X		
Intermittent Mobitz type II			
with symptoms	X		
Intermittent Mobitz type II			
without symptoms		X	
With syncope not proven to			
be due to CHB, but other			
causes not identifiable		X	
No AV block or symptoms			X
With first degree AV block			
without symptoms			X
AV block associated with myocardial infarction			
CHB	X		
First degree AV block with			
new BBB		X	
Transient advanced AV block			
and BBB		X	
Transient AV block			
without BBB			X
Transient AV block			
with LAHB			X
Acquired LAHB			
without AV block			X
Acquired bifascicular BBB			X

TABLE 7-2 Continued

Dysrhythmia	Class I (Indicated)	Class II (Sometimes Indicated)	Class III (Not Indicated)
Sinus node dysfunction (sick sinus syndrome)			
Symptomatic bradycardia	X		
With heart rates <40 bpm without documented symptomatic bradycardia		X	
Asymptomatic			X
Hypersensitive carotid sinus syndrome			
Recurrent syncope associated with carotid sinus stimulation and with >3 second pauses with carotid sinus massage	X		
Recurrent syncope without clear provocative event and with a hyperactive cardioinhibitory response		X	
Asymptomatic			X
Syncope from vasodepressor responses			X
Atrial fibrillation or flutter with slow ventricular response			
Asymptomatic			X
Symptomatic	X		
Tachycardia prevention			
Associated with bradycardia	X		
Associated with long QT syndrome—Torsades de Pointes		X	
Tachycardia termination			
Atrial flutter	X		
Atrial fibrillation			X
AV nodal re-entry	X		
Reciprocating tachycardia in WPW	X		
Ventricular tachycardia	X		

BBB = bundle branch block; CHB = complete heart block; LAHB = left anterior hemiblock

no clinical variables that identify asymptomatic patients at high risk for progression to complete heart block. The conduction time from the bundle of His to the ventricle (HV interval), an invasive measurement of conduction through the His-Purkinje system, is not a reliable indicator of risk in patients with asymptomatic bifascicular block. In symptomatic patients, however, such as those with recurrent syncope and bifascicular block in whom no cause can be found by noninvasive means, one can quantitate the risk of progression to complete heart block based on the HV interval. It is generally accepted that a permanent pacemaker is warranted if atrial pacing with rates of less than 125 bpm produces block below the bundle of His.

Accepted (Class I) indications for permanent pacing of bifascicular block include Mobitz type II or complete heart block associated with symptomatic bradycardia. Class II indications include bifascicular or trifascicular block with intermittent type II second degree AV block without symptoms. Another Class II indication is bifascicular or trifascicular block with syncope that is not proven to be caused by complete heart block, but with no other identifiable cause for the syncope. Finally, if atrial pacing induces block within or below the bundle of His, many experts consider this to be an indication for permanent pacing. Patients with fascicular blocks without AV block who are asymptomatic and patients with fascicular blocks and first-degree AV blocks who are asymptomatic are not candidates for permanent pacemakers (Class III).

PACING WITH AV BLOCK ASSOCIATED WITH MYOCARDIAL INFARCTION

The indications for permanent pacing after myocardial infarction in patients experiencing AV block include persistent, advanced second degree AV block with two or more nonconducted P waves or with complete heart block.[4,5] Class II indications include patients with persistent first degree AV block in the presence of a new bundle branch block and patients with transient advanced AV block with an associated bundle branch block. Permanent pacing is not needed in patients in whom AV conduction disturbances are transient in the absence of ventricular conduction defects. Unlike indications for patients with chronic structural heart disease, the criteria for permanent pacing in patients with an acute myocardial infarction and AV block are independent of the presence or absence of symptoms; the long-term survival of patients with acute myocardial infarctions with AV block is related primarily to the extent of the myocardial injury, rather than to the AV block per se. Patients with transient AV block in the presence of isolated left anterior hemiblock and those with left anterior hemiblock in the absence of AV block do not have adequate indications for pacing.

PACING FOR SINUS NODE DYSFUNCTION

Sick sinus syndrome remains the most common indication for pacing in the United States. The spectrum of sinus node dysfunction includes sinus bradycardia, sinus arrest, sinus exit block, and sinus pauses at the termination of tachycardias. Common accompaniments of these bradyarrhythmias are periods of atrial fibrillation or of other supraventricular arrhythmias that require drugs to prevent the arrhythmia or to control the ventricular response. Documented symptomatic bradycardia represents an accepted (Class I) indication for permanent pacing in patients with sinus node dysfunction. Patients in whom drug therapy exacerbates the bradycardia, but is essential, also require a permanent pacemaker. Arguable (Class II) indications for pacing with sick sinus syndrome include sinus node dysfunction that occurs spontaneously or as a result of necessary drug therapy with heart rates below 40 bpm and without a clear association between symptoms and the bradycardia. Pacing is not indicated for asymptomatic patients with sinus node dysfunction, including those in whom there are sinus rates less than 40 bpm as a consequence of drug therapy. Additionally, pacing is not indicated in patients whose symptoms suggestive of bradycardia are clearly documented not to be associated with bradycardia.

HYPERSENSITIVE CAROTID SINUS SYNDROME

The syndrome of hypersensitive carotid sinus results from a marked cardioinhibitory and vasodepressor response to carotid sinus stimulation, as discussed in detail in *Syncope*. The cardioinhibitory response results from increased parasympathetic tone and is demonstrated by slowing of the sinus rate and prolongation of the PR interval, occasionally with AV block. The vasodepressor component, secondary to reduction in sympathetic activity, results in vasodilatation and hypotension. It is essential to have some estimation of the relative contribution of the two components of the abnormal carotid sinus response prior to deciding about pacing. A hyperactive response to carotid sinus syndrome is defined as asystole, from sinus arrest or AV block, lasting 3 seconds with symptomatic hypotension. Approximately 15 to 20 percent of patients with carotid sinus hypersensitivity have a significant vasodepressor component. These patients frequently have persistent symptoms if they are paced with ventricular inhibited (VVI) pacing. Accepted (Class I) indications for permanent pacemaker implantation with this syndrome include recurrent syncope that is associated with spontaneous events and provoked by carotid sinus stimulation, and asystole of 3 seconds or greater with minimal carotid sinus pressure. Class II indications for pacing with this syndrome include patients with recurrent syncope without clear provocative events and with hypersensitive cardioinhibitory responses. Finally, pacemakers are not indicated (Class III) in asymptomatic patients with hyperactive cardioinhibitory responses to carotid sinus stimulation. Pacing also is not indicated in patients with vague symptoms, such as dizziness or lightheadedness, or in those with recurrent syncope, lightheadedness, or dizziness in whom the vasodepressor component of the carotid sinus response is the primary cause for symptoms.

PACING WITH ATRIAL FIBRILLATION

A permanent pacemaker is warranted in patients with atrial fibrillation or flutter with advanced degrees of AV block and with resulting symptomatic bradycardia. Drugs that are known to impair AV conduction, such as digitalis or verapamil, should be discontinued, and if the slowed ventricular response persists, placement of a pacemaker is justified.

PACING FOR TACHYARRHYTHMIAS

Increasingly, pacemaker therapy is being used as an alternative to drugs for the prevention or the termination of supraventricular or ventricular arrhythmias. The decision to use pacing for control of tachycardias should be made only after detailed cardiac electrophysiologic evaluation. It is generally accepted that selected patients with symptomatic supraventricular tachycardias who have failed multiple drug trials should be treated with antitachycardia pacemakers. At the time of a detailed electrophysiology study, an external form of the device to be implanted should be available to document its efficacy prior to permanent placement. Antitachycardia pacemakers are contraindicated in patients with ventricular preexcitation (Wolff-Parkinson-White syndrome [WPW]) in whom atrial fibrillation with rapid response has occurred spontaneously or during electrophysiology testing.

TEMPORARY VENTRICULAR PACING

Temporary ventricular pacing, using an endocardial electrode, was initially described by Furman in 1958. Since that time, a variety of new access techniques, lead systems, and pulse generators have made the technique safer and more effective. Generally accepted indications for temporary pacing include acute treatment of sinus bradycardia, sinus arrest, or heart block (Table 7–3). Frequently, temporary pacing is used in the settings of acute myocardial infarction, metabolic disturbances, or drug toxicities, or is justified in patients with atrial fibrillation with a slow ventricular response. Finally, a prophylactic temporary pacemaker is justified in any patient with an anterior wall myocardial infarction and subsequent development of Mobitz type II block, new bundle branch block with transient complete heart block, new bifascicular block, or complete AV block. Some experts feel that a temporary pacemaker is justified in patients with a new right bundle branch block in the setting of an acute myocardial infarction.

TABLE 7-3   Indications for Temporary Ventricular
Pacing

With symptoms

Sinus bradycardia
Hypersensitive carotid sinus syndrome
Type I second degree AV block
Type II second degree AV block
Complete heart block
Atrial fibrillation with slow ventricular response

With acute myocardial infarction (anterior or inferior)

Any pharmacologically unresponsive symptomatic
bradycardia

With acute anterior myocardial infarction

New bifascicular bundle branch block
New bundle branch block with transient complete heart
block
Type II second degree AV block
Complete AV block

CLINICAL APPLICATIONS OF VARIOUS PACING MODALITIES

The choice of an optimal pacing mode for a particular patient has become more difficult with the evolution of pacing technology and the multiplicity of options. Dual-chamber cardiac pacemakers, capable of pacing and sensing the atrium and ventricle, coordinate the events occurring in one chamber with those occurring in the other. These devices can be programmed noninvasively to pace or to sense a single chamber, e.g., atrial-inhibited (AAIOO) or ventricular-inhibited (VVIOO) pacers. Generally more expensive than single-chamber pacemakers, the added expense is justified in many patients. A dual-chamber pacemaker is indicated in patients with intact sinus node function and high-grade persistent or intermittent AV block. Additionally, DDD pacemakers are indicated when there is a particular need for maximum hemodynamic advantage or when there are situations in which there is danger of hemodynamic deterioration, i.e., a patient with aortic stenosis, hypertrophic cardiomyopathy, or congestive heart failure in whom there is a significant contribution of atrial priming to cardiac output. Dual-chamber pacing also is indicated in patients with symptomatic sinus node dysfunction with questionable or inadequate AV conduction. Basically, DDD pacing is indicated in patients in whom restoration of AV synchrony can be expected or shown to cause an improvement in hemodynamics. In questionable cases, cardiac output can be determined during both temporary ventricular and temporary AV sequential pacing, either before or during implantation of the pacemaker.

Patients in whom the "pacemaker syndrome" can be anticipated or in whom the syndrome has previously occurred during ventricular pacing also are candidates for DDD pacemakers. The pacemaker syndrome consists of a spectrum of symptoms resulting from loss of AV synchrony with ventricular pacing. Elevation of the right and left atrial pressure results in shortness of breath and fatigue with signs of left or right heart failure. Approximately 10 percent of patients with single-chamber fixed-rate ventricular pacemakers develop pacemaker syndrome.

There may be some disagreement on the indications for dual-chamber pacing (Class II indications) in patients with symptomatic carotid sinus hypersensitivity and related vagally-mediated bradyarrhythmias. Another Class II indication would be symptomatic sinus bradycardia with intact AV conduction in which single-chamber atrial pacing may be considered an option. Sinus node dysfunction in the setting of the brady-tachycardia syndrome is considered a Class II indication. DDD pacemakers are contraindicated in patients with persistent or chronic atrial flutter or fibrillation or other supraventricular tachycardias. DDD pacemakers also are contraindicated in patients with silent atria or in patients who have a short life expectancy.

Although ventricular-inhibited (VVI) and dual-chamber synchronous (DDD) are the most widely utilized pacing modes, single-chamber rate-adaptive pacing (VVIRO, AAIRO) has been introduced recently. In the United States, rate-adaptive pacing has been limited to an "activity-sensing" device. Other sensors, such as temperature, QT interval, respiration, and pH, are under clinical evaluation. The principle of these single-chamber devices is to respond with a change in paced rate to a physiologic variable detected by a sensor. Currently, the experiences with these devices is limited, but there are several clinical situations where they would be of theoretical benefit. These situations include atrial fibrillation and a slowed ventricular response, sinus bradycardia with inability to exceed 70 percent of maximum predicted heart rate during exercise (chronotropic incompetence), and technical inability to pace the atrim. A proposed algorithm for choice of pacing modalities is shown in Figure 7-1.

EXTERNAL CARDIAC PACEMAKERS

Recently, temporary cardiac pacing has become possible with the use of a pacemaker that stimulates the ventricle via electrodes applied to the chest wall.

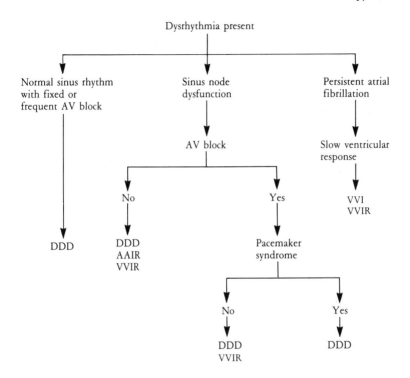

Figure 7-1 Clinical algorithm for choice of optimal pacing modalities

The ease of application of adhesive pads allows the physician to rapidly begin pacing in emergency situations. These devices can be used for temporary bradycardia therapy in any acute setting and can be applied prophylactically for patients at high risk for bradycardia. Use of this device is generally limited by patient discomfort to a period of several hours, but does allow for placement of a standard endocardial temporary pacemaker.

References

1. Harthorne J. Indications for pacemaker insertion: types and modes of pacing. Prog Cardiovasc Dis 1981; 23(6):393–400.

2. Joint American College of Cardiology/American Heart Association Task Force on Assessment of Cardiovascular Procedures (Subcommittee on Pacemaker Implantation, May, 1984). Guidelines for permanent pacemaker implanation. J Am Coll Cardiol 1984; 4(2):434–442.
3. Zipes DP, Duffin EG. Cardiac pacemakers in heart disease. In: Braunwald E, ed. A textbook of cardiovascular medicine. Philadelphia:WB Saunders, 1984:744.
4. Hindman MC, Wagner GS, Jaro M, Atkins J, Scheinman M, DeSanctis R, Hutter A, Rubenfire M, Yeatman L, Pujura C, Rubin M, Mars J. The clinical significance of bundle branch block complicating acute myocardial infarction I: clinical characteristics, hospital mortality, and one year follow-up. Circulation 1978; 58:679–688.
5. Hindman MC, Wagner GS, Jaro M, Atkins J, DeSanctis R, Hutter A, Morris J, Rubenfire M, Scheinman M, Yeatman L. The clinical significance of bundle branch block complicating acute myocardial infarction II: indications for temporary and permanent pacing. Circulation 1978; 58:689–699.

8 | CARDIOVASCULAR SCREENING OF COMPETITIVE AND NONCOMPETITIVE ATHLETES

JEFFREY M. ISNER, M.D.

Exercise training is becoming a way of life not only for athletes but also for millions of men and women seeking its potential cardiovascular and recreational benefits. This phenomenon has drastically increased the number of individuals who may need medical screening prior to participation in vigorous exercise programs. In addition to the problem of a major increase in the number of individuals participating in regular exercise, there has also been a wider spectrum of basal physical fitness and cardiac status among participants varying from that of an elite long-distance runner to that of an elderly person with a history of multiple myocardial infarctions.

Permission to participate in competitive or noncompetitive athletic opportunities constitutes a frequent basis for consultation. With regard to athletes under 35 years of age, the results of the physical examination, electrocardiography, chest roentgenography, and echocardiography must be interpreted in the framework of what constitutes a "normal" examination for this highly select subset of individuals. I will discuss this group in some detail and finish by briefly summarizing my approach to the individual over age 35.

PHYSICAL EXAMINATION

The evaluation of a systolic heart murmur is a frequent problem in the cardiac examination of a young athlete. Approximately 85 percent of young athletes have audible ejection type murmurs. These traumas are caused by forward flow of blood across the normal right or left ventricular outflow tract. Since most of the cardiac stroke volume is ejected during the first half of systole, one would anticipate that such flow murmurs would peak early in the systolic cycle. The velocity of blood flow at this phase of the systolic cycle may cause turbulence, thereby producing the systolic murmur. Since the major determinant of the intensity of such murmurs is the velocity of blood flow, it is no surprise that conditions that increase peak flow, such as exercise, anxiety, or fever, increase the intensity of these murmurs.

The vibratory systolic murmur (Still's murmur) is most often detected in individuals between the ages of three and seven, with a diminishing incidence toward adolescence. This murmur is usually heard best along the left sternal border in the third and fourth interspaces or just medial to the left ventricular apical region. The quality of this murmur is quite distinctive; it is a buzzing or vibrating sound best heard with the bell of the stethoscope. Still's murmur, short in duration, occurs in the first half of systole. The "supraventricular systolic murmur" is often heard in children and young adults. This murmur, heard best above the clavicles, tends to be louder on the right side than on the left, but often is heard bilaterally. The flow through the supraventricular vessels may even cause a palpable thrill. Shoulder maneuvers should be performed when evaluating this murmur since the murmur diminishes or disappears when the shoulders are hyperextended. A third, and by far the most common, innocent murmur in adolescents and young adults is the "innocent pulmonic systolic murmur" (pulmonary flow murmur). This murmur is usually best heard in the second left interspace, but may be transmitted along the left sternal border and even toward the cardiac apex. It is usually Grade 1 to 2 in intensity, but may be as loud as Grade 3. As do all innocent murmurs, this murmur may change with position and typically increases with exercise and anxiety and decreases with standing.

Apparently innocent flow murmurs must be distinguished from murmurs that result from outflow tract obstructions or other organic valvular disease. The murmur of aortic stenosis, for example, may be associated with an ejection sound in the case of a bicuspid aortic valve or with a diastolic murmur of aortic regurgitation attributable to either a congenitally malformed valve or rheumatic aortic valvular disease. Dynamic outflow tract obstruction (idiopathic hypertrophic subaortic stenosis) characteristically causes a systolic murmur that increases with the Valsalva maneuver and increases with standing from a squatting position. The same observations can be found in patients with the systolic murmur of mitral valve prolapse, another common murmur in young patients. This murmur frequently is heard in association with a midsystolic click. Finally, the murmur of an atrial septal defect also may be confused with an "innocent" flow murmur, but can be identified by abnormal (fixed) splitting of the second heart sound.

Physical examination of trained athletes frequently discloses a forceful left ventricular impulse, diastolic filling sounds (S_3 or S_4 gallops), and vascular bruits because of increased stroke volume.

ELECTROCARDIOGRAPHY

The ECG of elite distance runners typically demonstrates routine physiologic responses to training, including bradycardia, increased precordial R wave voltage, and increased PR intervals; significant ST segment depression and T wave inversion are not uncommon. First degree atrioventricular block, junctional rhythms, and premature ventricular contractions have all been described frequently. An incompete right bundle branch block pattern, an S_1-S_2-S_3 pattern, or a slurred contour to the QRS and a Wolff-Parkinson-White pattern on the electrocardiogram seem to occur in conditioned athletes more often than in the general population. Arrhythmias found at rest are almost always reduced or abolished by exercise. These arrhythmias include sinus arrhythmias, junctional rhythms, coronary sinus rhythms, a Wenckebach type of second degree atrioventricular block, and ventricular premature contractions. An increase in the height of P waves and ST-T changes ranging from J-point to elevation to frank ST elevation also are commonly seen in well-conditioned athletes.

NONINVASIVE STUDIES

Echocardiography constitutes a useful adjunct for the noninvasive evaluation of the so-called "athlete's heart." A number of studies have now documented by echocardiography what had been previously recognized at necropsy, that left ventricular mass is substantially increased in a conditioned, competitive athlete. What had not been previously appreciated is that the increase in ventricular mass may result from increased wall thickness or from increased cavity size, depending on the nature of the athletic endeavor. Echocardiograms performed on athletes who specialize in isometric exercise (such as wrestling or shotput) versus those who specialize in isotonic activities (such as swimming or running) have demonstrated an increase in left ventricular mass in both groups. In the isometric exercise group, however, increase in ventricular mass is primarily caused by an increase in left ventricular wall thickness (maximum 14 mm), while the left ventricular volume tends to remain normal. In contrast, maximum left ventricular free wall thickness seldom exceeds 12 mm in any of the isotonic exercise subjects, whereas left ventricular volume is considerably increased (maximum 60 mm), thereby accounting for the increase in left ventricular mass. These findings have been interpreted as demonstrating a chronic volume overload "lesion" for the isotonic activity, which requires a prolonged increases in stroke volume, as opposed to a pressure overload "lesion" for isometric activities. Isometric exercise demands episodic bursts of energy typically associated with increased mean arterial pressure.

Subclassification of competitive runners into sprinters versus endurance runners discloses left ventricular enlargement in both groups, but more left ventricular hypertrophy in the endurance runner as opposed to the sprinter. The endurance runners also have higher ejection fractions and left atrial enlargement.

DISORDERS RESPONSIBLE FOR
EXERCISE-RELATED DEATHS

In order to prospectively identify the athlete who is at high risk for adverse consequences of vigorous physical activity, it is necessary to know which disorders are responsible for exercise-related deaths in such individuals. The results of several necropsy studies of sudden death in athletes provide this information. Reports of sudden death associated with exertion make the important observation that in few of the cases is "death . . . due to the effects of extreme exertion in a previously healthy heart." Thus, a thorough evaluation of the cardiovascular system should be a mandatory part of the screening examination of prospective athletes.

Anomalous origin of both the right and left main coronary arteries from the anterior sinus of Valsalva is a cause of sudden unexpected death associated with exertion.[1] These patients often may be identified by a history of exertion-related syncope; unfortunately, electrocardiographic or radioisotopic response to an exercise stress test usually is normal. The mechanism of death in these patients is thought to be exercise-related encroachment on the acute angle of the left coronary artery as it arises from the aorta.

Hypertrophic cardiomyopathy (idiopathic hypertrophic subaortic stenosis) has been frequently described as the basis for sudden death in athletes.[2] A history of syncope, familial premature sudden death, or auscultatory evidence of hypertrophic cardiomyopathy are all clues to this diagnosis. Two-dimensional echocardiography may frequently establish the diagnosis noninvasively.

Coronary heart disease, contrary to previous speculation, is a cause of sudden death in athletes, including those capable of running a 26-mile, 385-yard marathon.[3] The so-called Bassler hypothesis, which alleged that the ability to finish a marathon conferred "virtual immunity from fatal heart attacks," has now been debunked by at least three separate necropsy studies. Autopsy-proven cases of fatal coronary atherosclerosis have been documented in several marathon runners. Necropsy findings in patients who have died during or shortly after running (including one accomplished distance runner who ran 23 miles the day before his death) typically disclose evidence of coronary heart disease.

The results of these necropsy studies suggest that the screening of individuals for participation in sports should, at the very least, be directed at excluding the presence of anomalous origin of the left main coronary artery, hypertrophic cardiomyopathy, Marfan's syndrome, and coronary heart disease. Anomalous origin of the left main coronary artery, as previously stated, may be suggested by a history of syncope. Unfortunately, however, this anomaly may be otherwise unsuspected by noninvasive cardiac examination.

The diagnosis of hypertrophic cardiomyopathy may be at least suspected, if not clearly documented, by M-mode echocardiography. Furthermore, M-mode echocardiography should be a reliable means of identifying those individuals with concentric left ventricular hypertrophy that is excessive even for well-conditioned athletes. The echocardiogram also is useful in delineating the size of the aortic root in patients with Marfan's syndrome; in many individuals, particularly basketball players, the distinction between a tall, attenuated body habitus and the classic features of Marfan's syndrome is not necessarily obvious. Finally, although electrocardiographic and/or radiographic exercise testing are widely employed as noninvasive screening tests for coronary heart disease, both are clearly imperfect. In fact both become more imperfect in a population of individuals with a low prevalence of coronary disease. Accordingly, in rare instances cardiac catheterization with coronary angiography may be necessary to definitely rule out obstructive coronary disease.

OLDER ATHLETES

With respect to the management of patients with known heart disease or of untrained individuals starting exercise programs above the age of 35, the role of the physician does not end with screening procedures, but becomes one of continuous guidance and periodic evaluation. Exercise stress testing should be performed in all such individuals, not only for diagnostic purposes but, more importantly, to help set limits on the amount of exercise that can be safely tolerated. Patients with no history of cardiac disease and with negative stress tests usually can embark on a loosely supervised self-training program after becoming acquainted with the general principles of slowly increasing the level of training. Patients with known coronary artery disease can show dramatic improvement in exercise training. Such training, however, should be done under close medical or paramedical supervision. Whether cardiac exercise rehabilitation will increase the longevity of these patients is yet to be proved.

Cardiac disorders such as congenital heart disease, cardiomyopathies, and valvular heart disease may respond adversely to exercise training. Such training, if attempted at all, should be done only under close and expert supervision. If syncope is a clinical feature of one of these disorders in a given individual, water sports activities generally should be discouraged.

References

1. Cheitlin MD, DeCastro CM, McAllister HA. Sudden death as a complication of anomalous left coronary origin from the anterior sinus of Valsalva. A not-so-minor congenital anomaly. Circulation 1974; 50:780–787.

INFECTIOUS DISEASE

9 | POSTOPERATIVE FEVER

NELSON M. GANTZ, M.D., F.A.C.P.

Fever occurs frequently after surgery. The origin of the fever may be occult or it may be obvious, such as when a surgical wound dehisces and pus is extruded. The fever may have an infectious or a noninfectious cause. Atelectasis, the most frequent cause of postoperative fever, does not have an infectious basis. Any major surgical procedure can produce a fever for approximately 1 to 3 days after the operation. The fever is usually low grade (99° to 100°F; 37.2° to 37.8°C) and self-limited with no cause determined. However, a localized or a systemic infectious disease is always a consideration, especially when the patient's postoperative temperature exceeds 101°F (38.6°C) in magnitude, when the elevation persists for 72 hours duration, or when the temperature becomes elevated after an initial afebrile interval. If antibiotic therapy has been continued after surgery, the fever may be low grade and the only clue may be the presence of leukocytosis with an increase in immature granulocytes (left shift). In the elevation of a febrile postoperative patient, it is important to note the type of surgery, the anesthetic used, the transfusions administered, and the medication record, as well as to perform a meticulous physical examination to obtain clues to the source of fever.

Certain causes of postoperative fever, such as atelectasis or wound or urinary tract infection, are associated with a variety of surgical procedures. Other causes, such as mediastinitis or a prosthetic graft infection following the insertion of a heart valve, are specific for a particular type of operation. Occasionally, the fever represents an infectious disease problem unrelated to the surgical procedure, such as acute cholecystitis after a hernia repair.

FEVER DURING THE FIRST 24 POSTOPERATIVE HOURS

In the evaluation of a patient with postoperative fever, it is helpful to note the temporal relation of the fever to the operation. Causes of fever during the procedure or within the first 24 hours include malignant hyperthermia, transfusion reactions, atelectasis, aspiration pneumonia, wound infection, drug reactions, or endocrine disorders such as acute adrenal insufficiency, thyroid storm, or pheochromocytoma. Malignant hyperthermia is a rare, but life-threatening, cause in which high fever (105° to 106° F; 40.6° to 41.6° C) and severe metabolic acidosis occur immediately after the introduction of the anesthesia.[1] The disease occurs in approximately one of every 40,000 adults having surgery. A family history of fatal reactions, such as anaphylactic shock associated with anesthesia, may be the only clue present. The disease is inherited as an autosomal dominant trait. Anesthetic agents that commonly trigger the reaction include halothane, enflurane, isoflurane, and succinyl-choline. The susceptibility to malignant hyperthermia can be determined by obtaining a muscle biopsy and performing an in vitro contracture test on the muscle specimen. All patients with a family history of suspected malignant hyperthermia should undergo diagnostic muscle testing. Measurements of serum creatine kinase (CK) levels as a screening test for this disease should be abandoned, since false positive and false negative results occur frequently.[1]

Fever occurs commonly with blood transfusions. Although these reactions are usually self-limited, they may represent red cell or granulocyte incompatibility or contamination of the blood with microorganisms. Atelectasis is the most frequent cause identified for fever during the first 24 hours postoperatively. The aspiration of a foreign body, such as a denture, should be excluded. Although wound infections are usually not detected until after several days, those caused by group A streptococci or by clostridia may present during the first 24 hours after surgery.

FEVER THAT OCCURS 24 TO 72 HOURS POSTOPERATIVELY

The possible causes of fever that begins after the initial 24 to 48 post-operative hours are numerous. The most frequent causes, however, are infection at an intravenous or an arterial line site, infection of the wound, infection of the urinary tract, deep venous thrombosis, or a pulmonary problem.[2,3] "Third-day surgical fever" denotes fever that occurs on the third postoperative day as a result of an infection at the intravenous site.[4] Such fevers are not limited to the third day and may result from contaminated intravenous fluid as well as from infection at the catheter insertion site. Inflammation may be absent from the intravenous site, thereby making the diagnosis more difficult. Arterial, pulmonary artery, and central venous pressure catheters are important sources of nosocomial bacteremias in patients hospitalized in intensive care units. This source of bacteremia can be decreased by removal of central lines when they are no longer medically indicated. Therapy consists of removal of the catheters, culture of the tips, and collection of several blood cultures. Never obtain a single set of blood cultures. Instead, draw two or three sets, using both aerobic and anaerobic bottles, before starting antibiotics.

WOUND SEPSIS

Most wound infections are seen 4 to 10 days after an operation. Increased warmth, redness, pain, and tenderness, along with purulent drainage, may be detected. A gram stain and culture of the discharge should identify the causative agent. Adequate drainage and antibiotics are usually required. Toxic shock syndrome (TSS) can develop as a complication of a surgical wound infection.[5] The syndrome usually develops within 2 days of surgery with a range of 1 to 7 days after the operation. The local signs of surgical wound infection may be unimpressive. *Staphylococcus aureus* is isolated from the wound culture. The diagnosis should be considered in a postoperative patient with fever, diffuse erythroderma that resembles a sunburn-like rash, watery diarrhea, and hypotension. Other findings that may be present include pyuria, an elevated CK level, abnormal liver function tests, a reduced serum calcium level, and a decreased platelet count. Treatment of TSS consists of fluid replacement, use of pressor agents, drainage of the local wound, and antistaphylococcal antibiotics.

URINARY TRACT INFECTION

A urinary tract infection should be suspected in any patient with an indwelling catheter or who has had any urinary tract instrumentation.[6] Although infrequent, the source of the fever may be in the prostate; thus, a rectal examination should be done. Fever that develops 5 to 7 days or more after an operation should always raise the possibility of deep venous thrombosis, which can present with fever as its only clinical manifestation. The lungs are the other common site of infection. Atelectasis, aspiration, bacterial pneumonia, or pulmonary embolism are the most likely possibilities.[7,8] Atelectasis with or without pleural effusion may be a clue to an intra-abdominal abscess beneath the diaphragm.

NOSOCOMIAL SINUSITIS

Nosocomial acute maxillary sinusitis is a frequently overlooked cause of fever in a postoperative patient with a nasogastric tube, nasotracheal tube, or other foreign body that causes mechanical obstruction of the sinus ostia.[9,10] A history of extensive facial or cranial fracture is often present. Purulent nasal discharge may provide a clue, but its absence does not exclude the diagnosis. Purulent discharge was present in only 25 percent of patients with sinusitis in one report.[9] Many of the patients are obtunded and unable to complain of facial pain. A leukocytosis is usually present, and x-ray films of the maxillary sinuses or a computed tomography scan of the sinuses confirms the diagnosis. Unlike community acquired acute maxillary sinusitis in otherwise healthy adults where the causative organisms are usually *Streptococcus pneumoniae* or *Haemophilus influenzae*, nosocomial sinusitis is most commonly caused by gram-negative aerobic bacilli, such as *Escherichia coli*, *Klebsiella* species, *Enterobacter* species, or *Pseudomonas aeruginosa*. Polymicrobic infections occur in 40 percent of patients.[9] Since it is difficult to predict the causative organisms in patients with nosocomial sinusitis, antibiotic therapy should be guided by the gram stain and culture results of material obtained by sinus aspiration. Definitive therapy consists of removal of the nasal tube responsible for obstructing the sinus ostia and administration of appropriate antibiotics based on the results of the gram stain and culture.

PSEUDOMEMBRANOUS COLITIS

Fever, abdominal tenderness, and profuse watery diarrhea that occurs following surgery should raise the possibility that the patient has pseudomembranous colitis[11] caused by a gram-negative anaerobe, *Clostridium difficile*. The disorder is more common and severe in the elderly patient who has undergone abdominal surgery and received antibiotics. The syndrome is highly variable, and some patients have fever and abdominal tenderness without diarrhea.[11] Fecal leukocytes are detected in about half of the patients. Symptoms occur as early as a few days after the start of an antibiotic to as long as 6 weeks after antibiotics have been discontinued. The diagnosis can be established by the visualization of pseudomembranes by proctosigmoidoscopy and by the detection of *C. difficile* cytotoxin in the stool. The extent of elevation of the cytotoxin titer does not correlate well with the disease severity, nor should it be used to follow response to therapy. Almost every antibiotic has been implicated as a cause of *C. difficile* colitis, with the exception of vancomycin. Therapy consists of fluid and electrolyte replacement and administration of oral vancomycin or oral metronidazole. When postoperative patients have an ileus, vancomycin should be given intravenously as well as by enema and nasogastric tube. The offending antibiotic should be discontinued, although no firm data exist regarding the efficacy of this measure. Patients with pseudomembranous colitis should be placed on stool precautions.

OTHER CAUSES OF DELAYED POSTOPERATIVE FEVER

Additional causes of fever with an onset at least 24 hours after an operation include the complications associated with anesthesia (e.g., halothane hepatitis), viral hepatitis (particularly non-A, non-B type), cytomegalovirus (CMV), Epstein-Barr virus, *Babesia microti* (malaria transmitted through transfused blood), sterile or infected hematomas, drug fever, and infections unrelated to the operation (e.g., acute cholecystitis). Halothane and methoxyflurane may cause postoperative fever, although this is infrequent. The features observed in a patient with halothane hepatitis are fever during the second postoperative week, malaise, anorexia, right upper quadrant pain, an increase in serum glutamic-oxaloacetic transaminase (SGOT) levels, and occasionally, a rash or jaundice. Multiple exposures to halothane may be associated with a shorter postoperative incubation period. Risk factors associated with halothane hepatitis include middle age, previous closely-spaced administrations of halothane, obesity, female sex, and genetic predisposition.[12] Chemical and bacterial meningitis are other reported causes of fever that may occur with spinal anesthesia. Transmission of CMV is not restricted to patients after open heart surgery; CMV can develop after any blood transfusion. Fever that develops 2 to 4 weeks after an operation and that is accompanied by atypical lymphocytes is a clue to a mononucleosis syndrome caused by CMV or by Epstein-Barr virus.

The spectrum of disease associated with *B. microti* infection ranges from an asymptomatic disorder to an illness characterized by fever, myalgias, fatigue, and hemolytic anemia. Microscopic examination of Giemsa-stained blood smear reveals the intraerythrocytic protozoan. Patients who are seriously ill should receive treatment with clindamycin and quinine sulfate.

Non-A, non-B hepatitis is the major cause of transfusion hepatitis, but fever is usually absent. Drug fever is an important noninfectious cause of persistent postoperative fever, especially in patients taking antibiotics, quinidine, phenytoin, methyldopa, procainamide, allopurinol, or sleeping medications. Drug fever may be caused by any drug, however, and the associated rash and eosinophilia may be absent. Finally, there is always the possibility of an infection unrelated to an operation, such as cholecystitis, hospital-acquired influenza, or Legionnaire's disease.

Acute cholecystitis can occur after operative procedures unrelated to the biliary tract. This infection often develops in patients with no prior history of biliary tract disease. Symptoms include right upper quadrant pain, nausea, vomiting, and fever. At times, fever is the only feature. Right upper quadrant tenderness is a helpful finding. The inability to detect biliary stones by radiologic techniques does not exclude the diagnosis of acute cholecystitis, since the patient may have acalculous cholecystitis. Postoperative cholecystitis often results in gangrene, perforation, or empyema of the gall bladder. Other complications include intrahepatic abscesses, cholangitis, and intra-abdominal abscesses. Organisms recovered most often from patients with postoperative cholecystitis include *E. coli, Klebsiella* species, enterococci, *Bacteroides fragilis,* and *Pseudomonas aeruginosa.*[13] Difficulties in establishing the diagnosis and in initiating appropriate therapy are reflected in high mortality rates ranging from 10 to 50 percent. The mortality rate in patients with acalculous cholecystitis is usually twice that of patients who have calculi and acute cholecystitis.[13] Once the disease is recognized, early operative intervention and appropriate antibiotics are indicated.

Disseminated candidiasis is a consideration in patients who have had operations of the gastrointestinal tract.[14] Risk factors that predispose patients to systemic candidiasis include exposure to multiple broad-spectrum antibiotics, impaired host defenses caused by the patient's underlying illness, corticosteroids, parenteral catheters, and total parenteral nutrition. Fever, leukocytosis, and hypotension in a patient who has had abdominal surgery and who has received broad-spectrum antibiotics should raise the suspicion of disseminated candidiasis. Diagnosis depends on isolation of the yeast from the blood and/or detection of the typical focal chorioretinal lesions. Blood cultures are frequently negative, and serologic tests have not been helpful in establishing the diagnosis.

As previously mentioned, in addition to the complications that occur with various surgical procedures, the cause of the fever may be closely related to the particular kind of operation performed. An intra-abdominal, subphrenic, hepatic abscess or pancreatitis may develop after abdominal surgery. A foreign body, such as a surgical sponge retained following abdominal surgery, may be responsible for postoperative fever. A pelvic operation may be complicated by septic pelvic thrombophlebitis, pelvic abscess, or cellulitis. Diagnostic considerations after cardiovascular surgery are sternal osteomyelitis, endocarditis, mediastinitis, venous graft-site infections, or the postcardiotomy syndrome. Similarly, in neurosurgical, orthopaedic, and other specialist-performed operations, the causes of fever may be unique to the procedure. The cause of fever may become apparent only after an analysis of the fever onset and its relation to surgery in general or to the particular operation, the patient's complaints, and the physical and laboratory findings. As I have tried to stress, in the evaluation of a patient with postoperative fever, it is important to perform a careful history and physical examination and to obtain focused laboratory tests based on the likely source of the fever, rather than to order a routine battery of tests as part of a "fever work-up".[15,16]

References

1. Paasuke RT, Brownell AK. Serum creatine kinase level as a screening test for susceptibility to malignant hyperthermia. JAMA 1986; 255:769–771.
2. Maki DG. Epidemic nosocomial bacteremias. In: Wenzel RP, ed. Handbook of hospital acquired infections. Boca Raton, FL: CRC, 1981:371–512.
3. Polk HC Jr, Simpson CJ, Simmons BP, et al. Guidelines for prevention of surgical wound infection. Arch Surg 1983; 188:1213–1217.
4. Altemeier WA, McDonough JJ, Fuller WD. Third day surgical fever. Arch Surg 1971; 103:158–166.
5. Bartlett P, Reingold AL, Graham DR, et al. Toxic shock syndrome associated with surgical wound infections. JAMA 1982; 247:1448–1450.
6. Warren JW. Infections associated with urological devices. In: Sugarman B, Young EJ, eds. Infections associated with prosthetic devices. Boca Raton, FL: CRC, 1984:219.
7. Bartlett JG, Gorbach SL, Finegold SM. The bacteriology of aspiration pneumonia. Am J Med 1974; 56:202–207.
8. Wynne JW, Modell JH. Respiratory aspiration of stomach contents. Ann Intern Med 1977; 87:466–474.
9. Caplan ES, Hoyt NJ. Nosocomial sinusitis. JAMA 1982; 247:639–641.
10. Deutschman CS, et al. Paranasal sinusitis: a common complication of nasotracheal intubation in neurosurgical patients. Neurosurgery 1985; 17:296–299.
11. Fekety R. Recent advances in management of bacterial diarrhea. Rev Infect Dis 1983; 5:246–257.
12. Farrell G, Prendergast D, Murray M. Halothane hepatitis. N Engl J Med 1985; 313:1310–1314.
13. Devine RM, Farnell MB, Mucha P Jr. Acute cholecystitis as a complication in surgical patients. Arch Surg 1984; 119:1389–1393.
14. Solomkin JS, Flohr A, Simmons RL. Candida infections in surgical patients. Ann Surg 1982; 195:177–185.
15. Freischlag J, Busuttil RW. The value of postoperative fever evaluation. Surgery 1983; 94:358–363.
16. Stone HH. Infection in postoperative patients. Am J Med 1986; 81:39–44.

10 | EVALUATION OF THE PATIENT WITH A POSITIVE TUBERCULIN SKIN TEST

DAVID R. SNYDMAN, M.D.

The presence of a positive tuberculin skin test (purified protein derivative [PPD]) has implications for the patient's lifetime risk of tuberculous disease. Therefore, it is incumbent upon the internist or the consultant who is seeing a patient with a positive PPD to assess this finding accurately in order to provide appropriate prophylaxis or therapy. The clinical history, physical examination, and a limited number of laboratory studies can be used in most cases to determine whether the patient has active disease.

DIAGNOSIS

The presence of a positive tuberculin skin test indicates that the patient has had infection with tuberculosis and requires further evaluation. A positive PPD may be the first clue to the physician that tuberculosis is present and has important clinical and epidemiologic implications. For example, some studies have shown that the degree of PPD positivity correlates with the subsequent risk of developing active disease. These findings are especially true for patients with very large reactions (usually greater than 15 mm).

The tuberculin skin test is the traditional method of diagnosing tuberculous infection.[1] The intradermal (Mantoux) test, using a 5-tuberculin unit (TU) Tween-stabilized preparation, is the standard method. However, it is important to note that this test is not totally specific and that atypical mycobacterial disease may cause a falsely positive PPD. In addition, the reaction to tuberculin is dose-related; use of a larger strength test, such as with 250 TU, increases the rate of a nonspecific reaction.

A positive skin test is classified as greater than or equal to 10 mm of induration 48 hours after the application of the skin test. If a patient has 5 to 9 mm of reactivity, the reaction is considered intermediate. A reaction of less than 5 mm is considered negative. The PPD may be negative in as many as 20 percent of patients with tuberculosis because of errors in administration or in interpretation of the test, or because of immunosuppression, protein malnutrition, or anergy in the subject being tested.

Application of the tuberculin test will not sensitize an uninfected individual; however, the test may stimulate hypersensitivity that has waned. This so-called "booster effect" may be problematic in individuals given yearly testing, such as hospital employees. This phenomenon is also more commonly seen in older individuals. Therefore, when the reaction to tuberculin is assessed, it is important to determine the latest test date. If the most recent testing period was more than a year ago, then a positive PPD is unlikely to be caused by the booster phenomenon.

Once a diagnosis of a positive PPD is made, completion of the evaluation is important in order to determine whether there is active disease and whether the patient qualifies for preventive therapy. The history and the physical examination can be helpful in making the appropriate medical decisions in this consultation.

CLINICAL HISTORY

In an individual with a positive PPD, it is important to determine whether the patient has had a positive PPD, whether there is a family history of tuberculosis, which might indicate that the patient has a longstanding positive PPD, or whether the patient has recently emigrated to the United States from a country where tuberculosis is endemic. For example, Indo-Chinese refugees have extraordinarily high rates of active tuberculosis and PPD positivity. Furthermore, it is important to determine whether the patient has received bacille Calmette-Guérin (BCG) vaccination in the past. BCG vaccine is used in many countries and can be associated with a false-positive PPD. If the patient has received BCG vaccination more than 10 years ago, one should generally consider that the positive PPD is attributable to tuberculous infection and not attributable to the vaccine. In addition, any strongly-positive PPD (i.e., 15 mm) in a BCG recipient should be considered evidence of infection, not vaccination.

Once the possible length of time during which the individual may have been PPD-positive is determined, it is important to assess the patient for the absence or presence of symptoms that might indicate active disease. One should inquire about fever, night sweats, weight loss, cough, sputum production, malaise, fatigue, or any systemic symptom that might indicate active disease. An absence of symptoms generally indicates that the patient does not have active tuberculosis; however, physical examination and laboratory determinations are necessary for the total analysis.

PHYSICAL EXAMINATION

As a general rule, the physical findings in a patient with tuberculosis are not specific and therefore may lead to underestimation of the extent of disease. A complete physical examination is always required, although there are certain aspects of the examination upon which to focus. It is important to examine the eye grounds for retinal lesions that might be indicative of disseminated tuberculosis. A scar on the arm may be apparent in a patient with a history of BCG vaccination. It is also useful to examine for the presence of lymphadenopathy and to provide a complete chest examination. The presence of rales may indicate that a cavitary lesion is present. Occasionally, rales may be heard only when the patient breathes in after a short cough (post-tussive rales). Larger lesions may present more obvious signs of consolidation (e.g., whispered pectoriloquy, tubular breath sounds).

The examination should also include the abdomen and the genitourinary tract. Occasionally, individuals with a positive PPD have genitourinary tuberculosis, the only manifestation of which may be an epididymal nodule.

LABORATORY EVALUATION

A complete blood count with differential is useful. Disseminated tuberculosis or active tuberculosis is frequently associated with anemia, monocytosis, or thrombocytopenia. Rarely, neutropenia may also be seen. Hypoalbuminemia is common in advanced disease. The sedimentation rate may also be an indication of disease activity and may be useful to follow.

RADIOLOGIC EVALUATION

A chest roentgenogram is essential to the evaluation of a patient with a positive PPD. Apical scarring, contraction of the upper lobes, and a Ghon complex or a Simon's focus are indications of old tuberculosis and signify that the positive PPD may be longstanding. The presence of any lung lesion in a symptomatic patient requires isolation of the patient and sputum screening for acid-fast bacilli and culture positivity. Furthermore, a positive chest film in a PPD-positive individual may require more extensive radiologic evaluation by the use of apical lordotics, tomography, or computed tomography (CT) scan.

If disease activity is questioned, the physician must obtain multiple sputum samples for acid-fast smear and culture. The urinalysis also may be helpful, since sterile pyuria may indicate that the genitourinary tract is involved. Furthermore, it has been documented that, in 10 percent of patients with active pulmonary tuberculosis, the organism may be cultured from the urine. Therefore, if active disease is highly suspected, a urine culture may be a useful adjunct to making a diagnosis.

PREVENTIVE THERAPY

The vast majority of cases of tuberculosis in the United States arise from individuals who have a positive PPD. Therefore, the prevention of reactivation disease is extremely important in the elimination or the reduction of the risk of tuberculosis in the infected individual.[2] Preventive therapy is generally achieved with isoniazid (INH), 300 mg per day for 6 months. Clinical trials have demonstrated a 60 percent to a 90 percent reduction in subsequent tuberculous disease in INH-treated subjects compared with those who were given placebo.[3] Furthermore, 6 months of INH may actually reconvert a positive PPD to a negative one if given early after the establishment of infection, i.e., 3 to 6 months postexposure. It must be emphasized, however, that a single drug, such as INH, must not be used in someone with active disease.

The risk-benefit ratio is an additional consideration in evaluating the use of preventive therapy. The major risk of INH is hepatic dysfunction and, therefore, patients receiving INH preventive therapy should be evaluated for the presence of liver disease. Hepatitis caused by INH is rare in individuals below the age of 20 years. Epidemiologic studies have shown that the rate of INH hepatotoxicity is 0.3 for individuals between 20 and 35 years of age, 1.2 for individuals between 35 and 45 years of age, and 2.3 for individuals between the ages of 50 and 64 years. The yearly, or lifetime, risk of tuberculosis, the rate of hepatotoxicity, and the efficacy of INH must all be taken into consideration in the evaluation of the risk-benefit ratio.[4]

The benefits of preventive therapy far outweigh the risk of hepatitis for the following groups:

1. Household members and other close contacts of infectious cases
2. Positive tuberculin reactors with chest x-rays suggestive of inactive tuberculosis
3. Recent skin test converters
4. Tuberculin reactors with medical conditions that increase the risk of development of active disease, such as immunosuppressive illnesses, chronic renal failure, silicosis, gastrectomy, or jejunoileal bypass for morbid obesity
5. Any skin test reactor who is younger than 35 years of age.

The risk-benefit ratio of preventive therapy becomes 1:1 at the age of 45 years for a skin test reactor with an uncertain history of duration. Therefore, I think that individuals between the ages of 35 to 45 years need to be considered on an individual basis. Factors to weigh when INH prophylaxis is considered should include the size of the tuberculin test and the reliability of the patient.

I am of the opinion that a reliable individual between 35 and 45 years of age who does not have other risk factors for hepatitis may benefit from INH preventive therapy and should be seriously considered for such prophylaxis.

A somewhat more controversial subject is the use of INH prophylaxis in older individuals.[5] In general, the risk-benefit ratio has been assumed to favor no prophylaxis in the PPD-positive older individual. However, recent studies in nursing home populations in Arkansas have demonstrated the need for screening and prophylaxis in this population. Not only was INH effective in preventing active tuberculosis in this population, but its use was not associated with marked untoward reactions. Therefore, when epidemiologic circumstances warrant, INH prophylaxis for the PPD-positive elderly may be prudent.

There are certain contraindications to INH preventive therapy. These include the presence of progressive tuberculous disease, in which case more than one drug is necessary. This situation should have already been ruled out by the steps outlined earlier. Documentation of completion of an adequate course of INH or of a previous severe reaction to INH would be contraindications to therapy. Furthermore, acute liver disease of any etiology represents a major contraindication to INH therapy.

Special attention must be paid to the concurrent use of other medications that may result in drug interactions, the daily use of alcohol, or chronic liver disease. In the latter two circumstances, there may be difficulty in the evaluation of change in hepatic function. The pregnant patient with a positive PPD must also be handled with special attention; to defer prophylaxis until after delivery may be prudent, unless there are urgent indications.

When evaluating preventive therapy, consideration must be given to the risk of INH drug resistance. INH alone may be insufficient in populations such as Indo-Chinese refugees where INH resistance is extremely common. It may be necessary to monitor these patients more carefully or even to consider two-drug prophylactic regimens after active disease has been ruled out.

Occasional patients may not be able to tolerate INH because of hepatitis, central nervous system reactions, or allergic reactions. Rifampin is an acceptable alternative agent in such patients; the dose is 600 mg daily.

Monitoring in INH Therapy

I generally monitor patients at monthly intervals and check them for symptoms of hepatic dysfunction. Although the role of routine monitoring of liver function is considered controversial, there are published studies that support its use. As many as 20 percent of individuals taking INH may have serum transaminase elevations at some time during INH preventive therapy. In some studies, the liver function indicators were elevated in some patients without any symptoms being present. For this reason, I favor routine liver function testing. The drug should not be discontinued unless the liver function tests, such as the serum glutamic-oxaloacetic transaminase (SGOT) or the serum glutamic-pyruvic transaminase (SGPT), exceed by five-fold the upper limit of normal or unless the patient develops overt symptoms. In general, I do not prescribe pyridoxine with INH as long as the nutritional status of the patient is satisfactory.

References

1. Glassroth J, Robins AG, Snider DE Jr. Tuberculosis in the 1980s. N Engl J Med 1980; 302:1441–1450.
2. Johnston RF, Wildrick KH. State of the art review. The impact of chemotherapy on the care of patients with tuberculosis. Am Rev Respir Dis 1974; 109:636–664.
3. Hsu KHK. Thirty years after isoniazid. Its impact on tuberculosis in children and adolescents. JAMA 1984; 251:1283–1285.
4. Comstock GW, Edwards PQ. The competing risks of tuberculosis and hepatitis for adult tuberculin reactors. Am Rev Respir Dis 1975; 111:573–577.
5. Ferebee SH. Controlled chemoprophylaxis trials in tuberculosis. A general review. Adv Tuberc Res 1970; 17:28–106.

11 | ENDOCARDITIS PROPHYLAXIS

NELSON M. GANTZ, M.D., F.A.C.P.

The subject of endocarditis prophylaxis continues to stir controversy. Recommendations for prevention of endocarditis from committees of The American Heart Association (AHA),[1] the Working Party of the British Society for Antimicrobial Chemotherapy,[2] and the Medical Letter[3] are not based on controlled clinical studies. No such studies have been published or are likely to be forthcoming. A number of questions regarding prophylaxis remain unanswered, such as: Can endocarditis be prevented by giving prophylactic antibiotics? What is the risk of endocarditis following procedures, such as dental extraction, associated with transient bacteremia? Which antibiotic regimens for prophylaxis are the best? Are parenteral antibiotics more effective than oral drugs? Is it necessary to use a bactericidal drug for prophylaxis? Are the data derived from the animal models of experimental endocarditis relevant to prophylaxis in humans? Which procedures merit the use of prophylactic antibiotics to prevent endocarditis? How should patients with mitral valve prolapse who are to undergo various diagnostic or therapeutic manipulations be managed? Should patients with arterial grafts or orthopedic devices (e.g., prosthetic hip) receive prophylactic antibiotics for special clinical situations associated with a transient bacteremia?

This is only a partial list of questions that the clinician faces daily when caring for patients at risk for endocarditis. Despite the widespread availability of antibiotics, the incidence of endocarditis has not declined in recent years.[4]

Infective endocarditis has major morbidity and mortality, despite the availability of antimicrobial agents. Patients who have underlying valvular heart disease are at risk for the development of infective endocarditis when organisms invade the bloodstream. A key factor in the pathogenesis of infective endocarditis is the occurrence of a transient bacteremia.[5] The AHA recommends that patients with rheumatic, congenital, or other cardiovascular diseases, as well as those with a prosthetic heart valve, receive prophylactic antibiotics when they have a procedure associated with a transient bacteremia.[1,6,7]

In this chapter I shall discuss the procedures associated with transient bacteremia, the types of underlying cardiovascular diseases that predispose a patient to infective endocarditis, and the antibiotic regimens recommended for prevention of endocarditis in predisposed patients.

Most cases of endocarditis are not preventable by the administration of prophylactic antibiotics. Only half of the patients who develop endocarditis have a recognized cardiac lesion for which prophylaxis would be a consideration. Furthermore, less than 25 percent of patients with endocarditis caused by viridans streptococci and about 40 percent of patients with endocarditis caused by enterococci have an identified portal of entry for which prophylaxis could be given. In addition, the usually recommended antibiotics are likely to be effective in only 67 percent of cases of endocarditis. Therefore, it is estimated that only 8 to 10 percent of cases of endocarditis are potentially preventable.

TRANSIENT BACTEREMIA

Transient bacteremias occur commonly.[5] They may occur spontaneously, such as with chewing food or with defecation. They may result from many procedures that traumatize mucous membranes with an indigenous microbial flora, such as with a dental extraction or a urethral catheterization. Bacteremias that follow procedures resulting in mucosal trauma are asymptomatic, usually occur about 1 to 5 minutes following the procedures, and generally last less than 15 minutes. Blood cultures are usually sterile 30 minutes after the procedures. Quantitative blood cultures usually reveal colony counts of less than 10 organisms per milliliter of blood. Transient bacteremias also occur with local infections, such as those that occur with incision and drainage of an abscess or with manipulation of the urinary tract in a patient with asymptomatic bacteriuria. The organisms associated with these bacteremias reflect either the normal flora at the manipulated site or the pathogen causing the local infection.

A history of a predisposing event can at times be elicited from patients with endocarditis. A preceding dental procedure has been noted in 15 to 20 percent of patients with nonenterococcal streptococcal endocarditis. A preceding genitourinary tract procedure has been reported in 40 percent of patients with enterococcal endocarditis. A preceding infection of the skin or soft tissue has been noted in 35 percent of patients with staphylococcal endocarditis.[8]

The oropharynx is a frequent portal of entry for organisms into the bloodstream. Blood cultures are positive in 18 to 85 percent of patients after a dental extraction.[5] The frequency of bacteremia correlates with the severity of gingival infection and the extent of tissue trauma. The organisms isolated reflect the normal mouth flora. Viridans streptococci are isolated most frequently, but anaerobic streptococci, coagulase-negative staphylococci, diphtheroids, and fusobacteria are also seen. Strains of viridans streptococci account for 50 to 75 percent of cases of endocarditis and are usually penicillin-sensitive. Streptococci that are relatively resistant to penicillin are found in patients receiving prophylactic penicillin for rheumatic fever and in those starting antibiotic prophylaxis 1 to 2 days before a procedure.[9]

Prophylaxis should begin 1 to 2 hours prior to a procedure so that serum levels of the antibiotic are adequate at the time of anticipated bacteremia. Penicillin given just prior to a dental extraction decreases the incidence of positive blood cultures after the procedure. Gingival degerming agents (compared with placebo), such as povidone-iodine mouthwash, also reduce the incidence of bacteremia associated with dental procedures. Topical antiseptic agents, however, should never be given without concomitant systemic antibiotic therapy.

Other dental procedures that may result in a transient bacteremia include periodontal operations, such as gingivectomy, root canal surgery, and dental cleaning. Blood cultures are positive in up to 88 percent of patients, depending on the severity of gum disease.[5] The predominant organisms are the same as those found following dental extraction. Positive blood cultures are also seen after tooth brushing (0 to 26 percent), after the use of oral irrigation devices (7 to 50 percent), after the use of dental floss (20 percent), and after gum cleaning or eating hard candy (0 to 22 percent). Antibiotic prophylaxis obviously is impractical for prevention of transient bacteremias secondary to these common daily activities. The cumulative risk of transient bacteremia is far greater for the usual daily events of living, such as eating, brushing the teeth, or defecation, compared with the risk from an occasional surgical procedure.[10] Maintenance of good oral hygiene decreases the amount of gum disease, which is a key determinant of the frequency of transient bacteremia following any dental manipulation.

Other procedures involving the oropharynx and the respiratory tract may result in bacteremia; these include tonsillectomy, nasotracheal intubation, and rigid-tube bronchoscopy. Positive blood cultures, however, rarely occur in association with flexible fiberoptic bronchoscopy and lung biopsy. This contrasts with the 15 percent rate of bacteremia that is associated with the use of a rigid bronchoscope.[5]

Diagnostic procedures that involve the gastrointestinal tract are another source of transient bacteremias.[5,11] Positive blood cultures are found in 0 to 10 percent (4 percent overall) of patients having fiberoptic gastrointestinal endoscopy, in 0 to 9.5 percent (5 percent overall) of patients undergoing rigid sigmoidoscopy, in 3 to 14 percent of patients undergoing liver biopsy, in 11 percent of patients having a barium enema, and in 0 to 27 percent (5 percent overall) of patients undergoing colonoscopy.[11] The predominant organisms isolated with these procedures are enterococci, which are frequent causes of endocarditis, and gram-negative bacilli, organisms rarely involved in endocarditis.

Transient bacteremia and infective endocarditis can occur following urinary tract, obstetric, and gynecologic procedures.[5] The urinary tract is the portal of entry in 20 to 50 percent of patients with enterococcal endocarditis, while 20 percent of cases caused by this organism are related to obstetric and gynecologic procedures. A genitourinary tract source is implicated in about 15 percent of all patients with endocarditis. A transient bacteremia occurs in 8 percent of patients undergoing urethral catheterization, in 24 percent of patients undergoing urethral dilation, in 17 percent of patients having cystoscopy, and in 12 to 31 percent of patients having transurethral prosthetic resection. The frequency of positive blood cultures increases several-fold in patients with infection at the instrumented site.[12] One example of such an infection is that of the urinary tract.

Transient bacteremia also occurs in 0 to 5 percent of patients after vaginal delivery, cesarean section, and dilation and curettage of the uterus and during insertion or removal of an intrauterine contraceptive device.[5]

Manipulation of an infected focus, such as massage of an infected prostate or incision and drainage of an abscess, is associated with bacteremia and the risk of endocarditis. Transient bacteremia, however, is rare with cardiac catheterization and angiographic procedures.

Table 11–1 lists the procedures associated with transient bacteremia and the indications for antibiotic prophylaxis.

CARDIAC LESIONS PREDISPOSING TO ENDOCARDITIS

Prevention of endocarditis requires a knowledge of the events likely to produce bacteremia, as well as the patients with predisposing cardiac lesions. Unfortunately, half the patients with endocarditis have no recognized underlying heart disease, thus making antibiotic prophylaxis impossible for this group.[8] Rheumatic valvular disease still remains the most common form of underlying cardiac disease in patients in whom endocarditis develops. The frequency has declined in recent years, however, because of the decreasing incidence of rheumatic fever. Patients with a bicuspid aortic valve are predisposed to endocarditis, as are patients with calcific or atherosclerotic changes in the aortic and mitral valve or anulus.

Patients with mitral valve prolapse—click murmur syndrome—have been reported to be at increased risk of endocarditis. In a case-controlled study, the risk of endocarditis in patients with mitral valve prolapse was approximately 8 times higher than that for the matched controls.[13] In a study of endocarditis prophylaxis failures, mitral valve prolapse was the most frequent cardiac abnormality identified and accounted for 33 percent of the cases of endocarditis.[14] Bor and Himmelstein estimated the risks and benefits of antibiotic

TABLE 11-1 Indications for Antibiotic Prophylaxis in Procedures Associated with Transient Bacteremia

Antibiotic prophylaxis recommended for all patients with valvular heart disease

  Dental procedures with gingival bleeding
    Dental extraction
    Dental cleaning
    Periodontal surgery (e.g., gingivectomy)

  Procedures involving the airways
    Tonsillectomy or adenoidectomy
    Bronchoscopy with a rigid bronchoscope

  Genitourinary manipulations
    Cystoscopy
    Transurethral prostatic resection
    Urethral dilation

  Gastrointestinal tract
    Cholecystectomy
    Intestinal surgery

  Gynecologic and obstetric conditions
    Dilation and curettage of uterus
    Vaginal hysterectomy
    Vaginal delivery (complicated)
    Cesarean section

  Manipulation of septic foci
    Incision and drainage of abscesses

Antibiotic prophylaxis recommended only for patients at high risk, i.e., presence of prosthetic or bioprosthetic heart valves

  All procedures listed previously

  Procedures involving the airway
    Nasotracheal intubation
    Fiberoptic bronchoscopy (?)

  Gastrointestinal procedures
    Sigmoidoscopy
    Barium enema
    Colonoscopy
    Liver biopsy
    Upper gastrointestinal endoscopy with biopsy
    Endoscopic retrograde cholangiopancreatography

Procedures for which antibiotic prophylaxis is not indicated for patients with valvular heart disease

  Procedures involving the airway
    Orotracheal intubation
    Nasotracheal suctioning

TABLE 11-1   Continued

Gynecologic procedures
Insertion or removal of intrauterine device
Vaginal delivery (uncomplicated)

Other procedures
Cardiac catheterization and angiographic procedures
Pacemaker insertion
Peritoneal dialysis

prophylaxis for patients with mitral valve prolapse who are undergoing a dental procedure. For such patients, their analysis suggested that the risk of fatal outcomes to penicillin reactions far outweighed the benefits of endocarditis prevention.[15] They suggested either no prophylaxis or prophylaxis with erythromycin, rather than prophylaxis with penicillin. This is only a theoretical analysis, however, and not a controlled clinical trial. Prophylaxis in all such patients would be difficult because of the high incidence of mitral valve prolapse; 5 to 6 percent of the American population is affected. I therefore recommend that antibiotic prophylaxis should only be given to those patients with associated mitral insufficiency documented by a holosystolic murmur, and not to those who have only a systolic click.

Patients with a previous episode of endocarditis should receive prophylaxis for predisposing events. Patients with prosthetic or bioprosthetic heart valves are also predisposed to endocarditis. Because infection of a prosthesis is often difficult to eradicate and carries a high mortality, antibiotic prophylaxis is recommended both for the usual predisposing events and for additional procedures that are associated with a transient bacteremia, but with a lower risk of infection, such as sigmoidoscopy (see Table 1).[1,5]

Although there are no controlled studies to establish the effectiveness of prophylactic antibiotics in patients with predisposing cardiac lesions, prophylaxis is generally recommended. The value of prophylaxis for procedures that may be associated with a transient bacteremia is unclear in patients with transvenous pacemakers, arteriovenous shunts for hemodialysis, and ventriculoatrial shunts. The risk in the last situation is probably low, and the majority of experts do not recommend prophylaxis in such cases.

RISK OF ENDOCARDITIS

Only rough estimates are available for the incidence of endocarditis in susceptible persons after exposure to an event associated with transient bacteremia. The incidence is clearly low, because bacteremias often occur after operative procedures, and resultant endocarditis is relatively rare. One report noted no instance of endocarditis after 403 tooth extractions among 98 patients with rheumatic heart disease.[16] In another report, there were four cases of endocarditis among 350 children with rheumatic heart disease who had a recent tooth extraction without antibiotic prophylaxis.[17]

Similarly, the effectiveness of antibiotic prophylaxis for infective endocarditis remains undetermined. Because a carefully controlled study with a large number of patients would be required to answer some of the questions surrounding this issue, animals have been used to study the pathogenesis and efficacy of antibiotic prophylaxis on infective endocarditis.

In the rabbit model of Garrison and Freedman, a polyethylene catheter is inserted across the tricuspid or aortic valve, thereby resulting in sterile vegetations.[18] A suitable organism is injected intravenously 24 to 48 hours later, thus causing endocarditis. The efficacy of various antibiotic regimens is tested by administration of the drugs 30 minutes before the injection of the bacteria. The animal is later sacrificed, and cultures of the vegetations are obtained. A major criticism of this model is the high inoculum (e.g., 10^5) of organisms per milliliter used to produce infection, compared with 100 organisms per milliliter in the blood after a dental extraction. Therefore, the animal models tend to overestimate the margin of safety of any antimicrobial regimen.

PRINCIPLES OF ANTIBIOTIC PROPHYLAXIS

Effective use of prophylactic antibiotics requires that adequate drug levels be present at the appropriate site at the time of the event posing the risk of transient bacteremia. According to data from the rabbit model of experimental endocarditis, it is necessary to have bactericidal activity in the serum for 9 hours after the bacterial challenge.[19] The 3-g amoxicillin prophylactic regimen advocated by the British provides 10 hours of serum inhibitory activity.[2, 20] To accomplish this goal, the antimicrobial should initially be given 1 to 2 hours prior to the procedure and continued for 12 to 24 hours. An increase in the duration of treatment beyond one dose after the initial loading dose only raises the cost and increases the possibility of an adverse drug reaction.

The antibiotic selected for dental procedures and other procedures involving the airway should be directed against viridans streptococci. Genitourinary manipulations and gastrointestinal, gynecologic, and obstetric procedures require that the antibiotic prophylaxis be adequate for enterococci. Antibiotics should be directed against penicillinase-producing staphylococci in a predisposed person having incision and drainage of an abscess. A urine culture should be obtained prior to a genitourinary procedure so that any infection can be identified and treated before the instrumentation. Bactericidal antibiotics should be used, if possible, because all the bacteriostatic agents tested were ineffective in the animal model.

Table 11-2 lists the regimens of antibiotic prophylaxis preceding dental and surgical procedures.[1]

TABLE 11-2   Antibiotic Prophylactic Regimens*

Situation	Antibiotic
Dental procedures and upper respiratory tract surgical procedures	Penicillin V 2 g PO 1 hr prior to procedure, then 1 g 6 h later *or* Aqueous crystalline penicillin G 2 million units IM or IV ½ to 1 hr before procedure, then 1 million units 6 hr later *or* Ampicillin 1 to 2 g IV or IM plus gentamicin 1.5 mg/kg IM or IV, not to exceed 80 mg, ½ to 1 hr before procedure. Repeat once 8 hr later *or* Amoxicillin 3 g PO 1 hr prior to procedure, then amoxicillin 1.5 g PO 6 hr later
If patient allergic to penicillin or receiving continuous oral penicillin for prevention of rheumatic fever	Erythromycin 1 g PO 1½ hr prior to procedure, then 500 mg PO 6 h later *or* Vancomycin 1 g IV given over 30 min. Start infusion ½ to 1 hr prior to procedure. Then give erythromycin 500 mg PO 6 hr after instrumentation
Urinary, gynecologic, and gastrointestinal procedures	Ampicillin 2 g IV or IM plus gentamicin 1.5 mg/kg IM or IV, not to exceed 80 mg. Give the two drugs ½ to 1 hr prior to procedure, then repeat in 8 hr as one additional dose *or* Amoxicillin 3 g PO 1 hr prior to procedure, then amoxicillin 1.5 g PO 6 hr later
If patient allergic to penicillin	Vancomycin 1 g IV over 30 min, plus gentamicin 1.5 mg/kg IM or IV, not to exceed 80 mg. Give drugs 1 hr prior to procedure and repeat in 8 hr as one additional dose.
Incision and drainage of skin abscesses caused by coagulase-positive staphylococci†	Nafcillin or oxacillin 2 g IV ½ to 1 hr prior to procedure, then 2 g IV q4h *or* Dicloxacillin 500 mg PO 1 hr prior to procedure, then 500 mg q6h

Table continues on following page

TABLE 11-2   Continued

If patient allergic to penicillin	Cephalothin 2 g IV ½ to 1 hr prior to procedure, then 2 g IV q4h
	or
	Cefazolin 1 g IM 1 hr prior to procedure, then 500 mg IM q6h
	or
	Vancomycin 1 g IV over 30 min. Start infusion ½ to 1 hr prior to procedure, then give 500 mg IV q6h.

* Parenteral regimens are recommended for patients with prosthetic or biosynthetic heart valves.[2]
† Route and duration of therapy depend on the severity of the infection and whether or not the predisposed person is at high risk (e.g., prosthetic heart valve). Results of Gram's stains and cultures should also guide antibiotic selection.

The recommendations for prophylaxis for the various procedures are empiric. It is useful to classify procedures into those that are low risk, such as barium enema, and those that are higher risk, such as dental extraction.[21] The classification of the various procedures into risk groups is arbitrary. Similarly, one can categorize patients into risk groups based on the underlying cardiac lesion. Patients with a prosthetic heart valve or an arterial graft would be at high risk and those with rheumatic valve disease at lower risk. The consequences of infection of a prosthetic heart valve and the difficulty in erradicating this infection are far greater than those of a native heart valve. If both procedural and patient risks are high, then prophylaxis is indicated: for example, endoscopy with biopsy in a patient with a prosthetic heart valve. If a patient has underlying rheumatic valvular heart disease, then prophylaxis would be indicated for a dental extraction, but not for a low-risk procedure, such as a barium enema. If neither risk is high, then prophylaxis is optional. I do not recommend prophylaxis for patients with prosthetic joints who are to undergo various diagnostic or therapeutic manipulations, although this is controversial.

References

1. Shulman ST, Amren DP, Bisno AL, et al. Prevention of bacterial endocarditis. Circulation 1984; 70:1123A–1127A.
2. Working Party of the British Society for Antimicrobial Chemotherapy. The antibiotic prophylaxis of infective endocarditis. Lancet 1982; 2:1323–1326.
3. Prevention of bacterial endocarditis. Med Lett Drugs Ther 1987; 29:109–110.
4. Bayliss R, Clarke C, Oakley C, et al. The teeth and infective endocarditis. Br Heart J 1983; 50:506–512.
5. Everett ED, Hirschmann JV. Transient bacteremia and endocarditis prophylaxis. A review. Medicine 1977; 56:61–76.
6. Sipes JN, Thompson RL, Hook EW. Prophylaxis of infective endocarditis: A re-evaluation. Annu Rev Med 1977; 28:371–391.

7. Lowy F, Steigbigel NH. Infective endocarditis. Part III. Prevention of bacterial endocarditis. Am Heart J 1978; 96:689–695.

8. Kaye D. Prophylaxis against bacterial endocarditis: A dilemma in infective endocarditis. In: Kaplan EL, Taranta AV, eds. Infective endocarditis. American Heart Association Monograph Series, No. 52. Dallas: American Heart Association, 1977:67.

9. Garrod LP, Waterworth PM. The risks of dental extraction during penicillin therapy. Br Heart J 1962; 24:39–46.

10. Guntheroth WG. How important are dental procedures as a cause of infective endocarditis? Am J Cardiol 1984; 54:797–801.

11. Shorvan PJ, Eykyn SJ, Cotton PB. Gastrointestinal instrumentation, bacteremia, and endocarditis. Gut 1983; 24:1078–1093.

12. Sullivan NM, Sutter VL, Mims MM, et al. Clinical aspects of bacteremia after manipulation of the genitourinary tract. J Infect Dis 1973; 127:49–55.

13. Clemens JD, Horowitz RI, Jaffe CC, et al. A controlled evaluation of the risk of bacterial endocarditis in persons with mitral-valve prolapse. N Engl J Med 1982; 307:776–781.

14. Durack DT, Bisno AL, Kaplan EL. Apparent failures of endocarditis prophylaxis. Analysis of 52 cases submitted to a national registry. JAMA 1983; 250:2318–2322.

15. Bor DH, Himmelstein DU. Endocarditis prophylaxis for patients with mitral valve prolapse. A quantitative analysis. Am J Med 1984; 76:711–717.

16. Schwartz SP, Salman I. The effect of oral surgery on the course of patients with disease of the heart. Am J Orthod 1942; 28:331–345.

17. Taran LM. Rheumatic fever in relation to dental disease. NY J Dent 1944; 14: 107–113.

18. Garrison PK, Freedman LR, Experimental endocarditis I: Staphylococcal endocarditis resulting from placement of a polyethylene catheter in the right side of the heart. Yale J Biol Med 1970; 42:394–410.

19. Durack DT, Petersdorf RG. Chemotherapy of experimental streptococcal endocarditis: I. Comparison of commonly recommended prophylactic regimens. J Clin Invest 1973; 52:592–598.

20. Kaye D. Prophylaxis for infective endocarditis: An update. Ann Intern Med 1986; 104:419–423.

21. Durack DT. Current issues in prevention of infective endocarditis. Am J Med 1985; 78 Suppl 6B:149–156.

12 | APPROACH TO THE PATIENT WITH ERYTHEMA NODOSUM

NELSON M. GANTZ, M.D., F.A.C.P.

Erythema nodosum is the most common cause of inflammatory cutaneous nodules of the legs and is associated with a number of different underlying disorders.[1-3] While the mechanism responsible for the inflammation remains unknown, it is probably an immunologically-mediated host reaction to a number of unrelated infectious, inflammatory, or hormonal disorders. The initial classic description by Willan in 1798 of "discrete, tender erythematous, indurated protuberances, one to five cm in diameter with a bruised appearance occurring predominately in the pretibial areas and lasting three to six weeks" is still accurate. Variations on this theme occur occasionally. Adjacent nodules can coalesce into larger lesions. Lesions can evolve without the bruised appearance, and rarely, the lesions persist for months to years. Although much less common, erythema nodosum can occur on the buttocks, soles, and extensor surface of the arm.[3] Patients commonly have chills, fever, and malaise in addition to the cutaneous lesions. There may be an associated edema of the legs, and in one report, 60 percent of patients had arthralgias that usually involved the ankles or knees.[3] Polyarthritis may be present. Laboratory abnormalities frequently include an elevated sedimentation rate, leukocytosis, mild anemia, and an increase in gamma globulin. Hilar lymphadenopathy may be seen on chest roentgenogram. Other laboratory abnormalities may provide a clue to the specific disorder associated with erythema nodosum.

EPIDEMIOLOGY

The disease occurs predominantly in women. During its peak incidence in the third and fourth decades of life, women account for 90 percent of cases. The sex ratio is nearly equal in other age groups. The disease is uncommon in children younger than 15 years old. The female predominance occurs also in patients with associated fungal diseases. In one outbreak of histoplasmosis, 90 percent of the cases of erythema nodosum were found in women, even though only half of the patients with histoplasmosis were female.[4] Erythema nodosum occurs four to five times more often in women than in men with coccidioidomycosis, even though the disease occurs more commonly in males.[5] The epidemiology of disorders associated with erythema nodosum also has changed in recent years. Before the 1950s, tuberculosis was a common cause associated with erythema nodosum, while today this is an infrequent cause. In Europe, infection with *Yersinia* species is a common cause of erythema nodosum.

DIAGNOSIS

Usually the diagnosis of erythema nodosum is made by the clinical appearance of the lesions. The diagnosis is best confirmed by a skin biopsy, however, since the differential diagnosis of tender nodules on the legs includes erythema induratum, nodular vasculitis, panniculitis secondary to pancreatitis or pancreatic carcinoma, polyarthritis nodosa, leukemic infiltrates, superficial thrombophlebitis, cryptococcal cellulitis, Sweet's syndrome, and factitial disease. The pathologic changes that occur primarily in the subcutaneous tissue consist of lymphocytic and neutrophilic cell infiltration around the small vessels. The findings vary within each nodule, so an ellipse biopsy that contains subcutaneous fat is essential to supply a specimen large enough to ensure an adequate diagnosis. The smaller punch biopsy is reported to be adequate in only 20 percent of cases.[6]

Once a diagnosis of erythema nodosum is made, a search for an underlying disorder must begin. In approximately one-third to one-half of the patients, no precipitating disorder can be identified. The most common disorders associated with erythema nodosum, in order of decreasing frequency, are infections, sarcoidosis, inflammatory bowel disease, drug reactions, and hormonal disturbances (Table 12–1).[1-3]

ASSOCIATED DISORDERS

Streptococcal infections probably account for the majority (50 percent) of cases of erythema nodosum in the United States. Typically, lesions occur about 2 weeks after streptococcal pharyngitis or, less commonly, after cellulitis. Especially in children, but also in adults, erythema nodosum may develop with primary tuberculosis at the time of or slightly prior to the conversion of the purified protein derivative (PPD) skin test. Geographic considerations are important when pursuing the etiology. There are areas of the world where certain endemic diseases commonly precipitate erythema nodosum. For example, coccidioidomycosis frequently causes erythema nodosum in the San Joaquin Valley of California. Histoplasmosis is a common cause of erythema nodosum in the Mississippi and Missouri Valleys.[7] When erythema nodosum is associated with coccidioidomycosis and histoplasmosis, the coccidioidin and

TABLE 12-1   Disorders Associated with Erythema
Nodosum

Infections/Agent
    Group A beta-hemolytic streptococci
    Yersinosis
    Salmonellosis
    Chlamydial
    Campylobacter
    Mycobacterial
    Histoplasmosis
    Coccidioidomycosis
    Syphilis

Drugs
    Estrogens
    Oral contraceptives
    Sulfonamides
    Iodides
    Bromides

Miscellaneous
    Inflammatory bowel disease—Ulcerative colitis
    Sarcoidosis
    Behçet's disease

histoplasmin skin tests are usually positive, and there is a decreased incidence of disseminated disease. In Scandinavian countries, *Yersinia enterocolitica*, which may produce symptoms of gastroenteritis and mesenteric arteritis, has been associated frequently with erythema nodosum. Lymphogranuloma venereum and psittacosis have been associated with erythema nodosum. Other infectious diseases less commonly reported with erythema nodosum include infectious mononucleosis, toxoplasmosis, *Salmonella* gastroenteritis, leptospirosis, hepatitis B, syphilis, and, recently, *Campylobacter* gastroenteritis. The erythema nodosum-like lesions that occur with leprosy are unique in that the mycobacterial organisms are found in the lesions.

After infectious disorders, the next most common cause of erythema nodosum is sarcoidosis. Erythema nodosum, an early manifestation of sarcoidosis, occurs in approximately 20 percent of patients. The typical patient has erythema nodosum, bilateral hilar adenopathy, arthralgias, and a low-grade fever. However, the hilar adenopathy is not specific for sarcoidosis, since it may occur with streptococcal, as well as idiopathic, erythema nodosum. In general, sarcoidosis, associated with erythema nodosum has a benign self-limited course, but some patients have progressive pulmonary involvement.[1,3]

Approximately 10 percent of patients with ulcerative colitis and, less often, with regional enteritis have erythema nodosum. Early in the course of inflammatory bowel disease, the activity of erythema nodosum parallels the activity of the gastrointestinal disease. After approximately 2 years, however, this no longer holds. In one study, erythema nodosum heralded the onset of Behçet's disease, preceding it by up to 2 years.[2] Reiter's disease has also been associated with erythema nodosum.

With the exception of oral contraceptives, drugs very seldom cause erythema nodosum. Those drugs that infrequently have been implicated are sulfonamides, iodides, and bromides.[3]

There is an interesting relationship between erythema nodosum and estrogens. As previously stated, the incidence of erythema nodosum between the sexes in prepuberty is similar, but during the childbearing years the disease occurs much more frequently in women. There are several reports of women developing erythema nodosum in the first and second trimesters of pregnancy with resolution of the lesions in the third trimester. In one woman, this pattern recurred in four successive pregnancies and was reproduced when she was given birth control pills.[8]

PATHOGENESIS

The pathogenesis of erythema nodosum remains an enigma. Some of the evidence points toward a cell-mediated type of reaction. Erythema nodosum usually occurs at the time of conversion of delayed hypersensitivity skin tests, such as the PPD, coccidioidin, or histoplasmin. Furthermore, patients who have erythema nodosum seldom develop disseminated fungal disease. Evidence also implicates humoral reaction because circulating immune complexes have been reported in patients with sarcoidosis and erythema nodosum.[9] Finally, a 10-fold rise in IgE in some children has been noted with poststreptococcal erythema nodosum.[10]

EVALUATION

The evaluation of erythema nodosum should include a detailed study of antecedant illnesses, a complete physical examination, a complete blood count, a sedimentation rate, an intermediate PPD skin test, a chest x-ray, and possibly a skin biopsy. The work-up should begin without delay, since it is important to detect early the various treatable associated disorders. With the appropriate geographical history, complement fixation titers for histoplasmosis or coccidioidomycosis should be obtained. An antistreptolysin O titer or streptozyme test may be helpful to establish a streptococcal etiology. If gastrointestinal complaints are present, the patient should have stool cultures for *Salmonella*,

Campylobacter, and *Yersinia* species. Barium studies are indicated for possible inflammatory bowel disease. A scalene node biopsy is helpful to distinguish patients with sarcoidosis who have bilateral hilar adenopathy from those with idiopathic erythema nodosum.[9]

THERAPY

No established treatment for erythema nodosum exists at the present time. The skin lesions are usually self-limited and resolve without therapy within 3 to 6 weeks. Bruise-like lesions may persist for months, but recurrences are rare. Specific therapy, if available, should be directed at the underlying disorder. Some patients may benefit from rest and salicylates for pain. Corticosteroids are only marginally effective and may worsen the underlying illness. Corticosteroids are contraindicated if the underlying illness is unknown. Administration of potassium iodide for 1 month seems to have helped selected patients, but its effectiveness has not been proven.[11] The role of the nonsteroidal anti-inflammatory agents, such as indomethacin or naproxen, remains unclear. Colchicine may be efficacious.

References

1. Weinstein L. Erythema nodosum. Disease-a-month. Chicago: Year Book 1969.
2. Bullock WE. The clinical significance of erythema nodosum. Hosp Pract 1986; 21:102E–102X.
3. White JW Jr. Hypersensitivity and miscellaneous inflammatory disorder. In: Moscella SL, Hurley HJ, eds. Dermatology. Philadelphia: WB Saunders 1985: 464–467.
4. Ozols II, Wheat LJ. Erythema nodosum in an epidemic of histoplasmosis in Indianapolis. Arch Dermatol 1981; 117:709–712.
5. Smith CE. Epidemiology of acute coccidioidomycosis with erythema nodosum ("San Joaquin" or "Valley Fever"). Am J Public Health 1940; 30:600–611.
6. Winkelmann RK. New observations in the histopathology of erythema nodosum. J Invest Dermatol 1975; 65:441–446.
7. Medeiros AA, Marty SD, Tosh FE, et al. Erythema nodosum and erythema multiforme as clinical manifestations of histoplasmosis in a community outbreak. N Engl J Med 1966; 274:415–420.
8. Bombardieri S, DiMunno O, DiPunzio C, Pasero G. Erythema nodosum associated with pregnancy and oral contraceptives. Br Med J 1977; 1:1509–1510.
9. Jones J, Cumming R, Asplin C. Evidence for circulating immune complexes in erythema nodosum and early sarcoidosis. Ann NY Acad Sci 1976; 278:212–219.
10. Mandalenaki-Lambrou C, Thomaidis TH, Benetos S, Ladis B, Matsaniotis N. Immunoglobulin E in erythema nodosum. Arch Dis Child 1976; 51:391–393.
11. Horio T, Imamura K, Danno S, Ofuji S. Potassium iodide in the treatment of erythema nodosum and nodular vasculitis. Arch Dermatol 1981; 117:29–31.

13 | SELECTING A PARENTERAL CEPHALOSPORIN

RICHARD A. GLECKMAN, M.D.

The cephalosporins are the most commonly prescribed parenteral antibiotics in the United States. This statement is particularly ironic when one realizes that the original source fungus, known as *Cephalosporium acremonium*, was isolated from sewer water effluent by Professor Guiseppe Brotsu on the island of Sardinia in 1945. The first parenteral cephalosporin, cephalothin sodium, became clinically available in the United States in 1964. Between that historic event and the present, sixteen additional parenteral cephalosporins have been released by the Food and Drug Administration.

I believe there are a number of reasons why the cephalosporin family of compounds has been so popular with physicians. When used appropriately, these agents have performed extremely well in the clinical arena. They have provided effective treatment for a wide range of infections, including skin and soft tissue infections, pneumonia, bacteremia, urinary tract sepsis, biliary tract infections, peritonitis, meningitis, and endocarditis. As importantly, the cephalosporins, as a class of antibiotics, have been remarkably safe drugs, particularly when compared to the aminoglycosides. With rare exceptions, cephalosporins have not produced serious or irreversible neurologic, hematologic, hepatic, renal, cardiac, or pulmonary toxicity.[1,2] In addition, in contrast to aminoglycosides, clinicians do not need to monitor serum drug concentrations when cephalosporins are administered.

A real concern with the administration of cephalosporins, particularly in penicillin-allergic patients, is their ability to produce immediate hypersensitivity events, namely laryngeal edema and anaphylaxis. These adverse life-threatening events result from the presence of preformed IgE antibody directed against the antigenic determinants of the antibiotic. The reactions appear to be mediated by potent vasoactive mediators released from tissue mast cells and blood eosinophils.[3] Cephalosporins are well-tolerated by most patients with IgE antibody to penicillin. However, until a specific immunologic test is available to predict hypersensitivity in a patient with a history of type 1 allergy to penicillin, it is best to avoid the use of cephalosporins in patients who have experienced laryngeal edema or anaphylaxis.

As clinicians, we refer to the members of the cephalosporin family of drugs as if they comprise a homogeneous group of antibiotics. In fact, this group of agents is heterogeneous and consists of (1) members derived from cephalosporin C, the cephalosporins, (2) members derived from cephamycin C (such as cefoxitin), known as cephamycins, and (3) a totally synthetic agent, called oxabeta-lactam or moxalactam, in which an oxygen atom is substituted for the sulfur atom in the cephem nucleus.

The cephalosporins are bactericidal antibiotics. Their antibacterial effects (as well as those of the penicillins, monobactams, and carbapenems) are dependent on their ability to inhibit enzymes, known as penicillin-binding proteins, that are located in the bacterial plasma membrane.[4] The penicillin-binding proteins catalyze the terminal stages involved in the assembly of the peptidoglycan network that forms the bacteria's inner cell wall. In order for the cephalosporin to bind, complex, and inhibit the penicillin-binding proteins, the antibiotic must be able to penetrate the bacteria's cell wall membrane, as well as to resist destruction by beta-lactamase enzymes located in the periplasmic space.

Cephalosporins have traditionally been described as first, second, and third generation compounds. The classification according to generation has most frequently been determined by the drug's spectrum of inhibitory activity for gram-negative aerobic bacilli. The first generation parenteral compounds (Table 13-1) (cephalothin, cephapirin, cefazolin, and cephradine) are active against the majority of strains of *Escherichia coli, Klebsiella pneumoniae,* and *Proteus mirabilis* that cause community-associated infections, such as pneumonia, cholangitis, and pyelonephritis. A second generation cephalosporin (see Table 13-1), such as cefamandole, may possess some inhibitory activity for additional organisms, including *Citrobacter* species and *Providencia* species. Another second generation drug, namely cefoxitin, extends its spectrum of activity to some strains of *E. coli, Klebsiella, Citrobacter,* and *Serratia* that are resistant to the first generation cephalosporins. The third generation cephalosporins (see Table 13-1) further augment the spectrum of activity, and these compounds often possess inhibitory activity for additional gram-negative aerobic bacilli, including *Enterobacter* species, *Proteus* species (indole positive), and *Serratia marcescens.*

FIRST GENERATION

For more than 20 years, the first generation parenteral cephalosporins have enjoyed wide popularity for empiric in-hospital therapy of patients with the following community-acquired infections: skin and bone infections caused by susceptible strains of streptococci and *Staphylococcus aureus*; pneumonia

TABLE 13-1 Available Cephalosporins

First Generation Cephalosporins
  Cephalothin (Keflin)
  Cephapirin (Cefadyl)
  Cephradine (Velosef)
  Cefazolin (Ancef, Kefzol)

Second Generation Cephalosporins
  Cefamandole (Mandol)
  Cefuroxime (Zinacef, Kefurox)
  Cefonicid (Monocid)
  Cefoxitin (Mefoxin)
  Cefotetan (Cefotan)

Third Generation Cephalosporins
  Cefotaxime (Claforan)
  Moxalactam (Moxam)
  Cefoperazone (Cefobid)
  Ceftizoxime (Cefizox)
  Ceftriaxone (Rocephin)
  Ceftazidime (Fortaz, Tazidime, Tazicef)

caused by susceptible strains of *Streptococcus pneumoniae, Staphylococcus aureus*, and *Klebsiella pneumoniae*, as well as pyelonephritis caused by susceptible strains of *E. coli, Proteus mirabilis,* and *Klebsiella pneumoniae*. In addition, these compounds have emerged as the agents of choice for perioperative prophylaxis for selective, elective surgical procedures.[5] These procedures include orthopaedic operations (total hip replacement, hip fracture repair), cardiovascular operations, femoral artery surgery, abdominal aorta surgery), and obstetric and gynecologic operations (vaginal hysterectomy, caesarean section for the high-risk patient). No convincing evidence exists to show that second or third generation cephalosporins are more effective prophylactic agents for these procedures. However, limited data show that, for patients experiencing elective colorectal surgery, the addition of preoperative cefoxitin, as compared to cefazolin, to the standard neomycin-erythromycin bowel preparation results in fewer postoperative incisional and intraperitoneal infections.

I believe cefazolin is the preferred agent among the first generation cephalosporins. It has a longer half-life and therefore requires fewer intramuscular injections or intravenous infusions when prescribed in the hospital or when administered at home or in an outpatient setting. Cefazolin achieves the highest and most prolonged serum concentrations and, in contrast to some of the other parenteral first generation cephalosporins, appears to be free of nephrotoxicity.

SECOND GENERATION

Soon after its introduction, cefamandole, a second generation cephalosporin, gained wide acceptance as empiric treatment for elderly patients (excluding leukopenic patients and nursing home residents) with community-acquired bacterial pneumonia. The reason for the appeal of this compound was that it possessed inhibitory activity for *Streptococcus pneumoniae, Staphylococcus aureus,* and *Klebsiella pneumoniae,* respiratory pathogens that contribute to these bacterial pneumonias. In addition, in contrast to the first generation cephalosporins, cefamandole extended the spectrum of activity to include *Hemophilus influenzae,* including many beta-lactamase-producing strains. This broader activity represented an important advantage for this compound, because the bacterial cause of community-acquired pneumonia in the elderly is often difficult to identify. As importantly, *Hemophilus influenzae* probably is the second most common cause of this infection in this age group.

In the late 1970's, some clinical investigators endorsed the use of cefamandole to treat endometritis and secondary peritonitis. Universal agreement now exists, however, that these infections are caused by a complex microflora consisting of aerobes and anaerobes, and that cefamandole does not constitute appropriate therapy. Finally, cefamandole's potential to cause hypoprothrombinemia and, on occasion, clinically significant bleeding, has placed a further restraint on enthusiasm for this antibiotic.[6]

Cefuroxime possesses a spectrum of activity similar to that of cefamandole, but there are some important differences between these compounds. In contrast to the experience with cefamandole, the development of hypoprothrombinemia with an increased bleeding tendency has not been observed with the administration of cefuroxime. Additionally, cefuroxime penetrates the leptomeninges in therapeutic concentrations. Cefuroxime has a proven track record for the therapy of community-acquired pneumonia caused by *Streptococcus pneumoniae* and *Hemophilus influenzae.* Cefuroxime can be considered appropriate onset therapy for the patient with pneumonia caused by *Hemophilus influenzae* while the clinician awaits susceptibility and beta-lactamase testing of the isolate.

Limited clinical studies indicate that cefuroxime is an effective antibiotic to treat adults with community-acquired bacterial meningitis caused by *Streptococcus pneumoniae, Neisseria meningitidis,* and *Hemophilus influenzae,* including beta-lactamase-producing strains.[7] However, penicillin remains the agent of first choice to manage life-threatening disease caused by *Streptococcus pneumoniae* and the meningococci. The third generation cephalosporins, specifically cefotaxime and ceftriaxone, which possess more potent antimicrobial activity and enhanced penetration into the leptomeninges, appear to be preferred therapy for patients with meningitis caused by beta-lactamase and non-beta-lactamase-producing strains of *Hemophilus influenzae*.

Cefonicid is distinguished by its relatively long half-life and inhibitory activity for *Hemophilus influenzae*, including beta-lactamase-producing strains. The compound can be administered as infrequently as once daily (1 to 2 g per day), thereby making cefonicid a cost-effective parenteral form of treatment of community-acquired pneumonia caused by *Streptococcus pneumoniae* or *Hemophilus influenzae*.[8] Cefonicid can be delivered by either the intramuscular or intravenous route, thus rendering the agent invaluable for therapy administered in the hospital, the nursing home, or the community. Hypoprothrombinemia with bleeding has not been associated with cefonicid. Cefonicid should not be prescribed for patients with pneumonia complicated by meningitis. Limited data exist to confirm the efficacy of cefonicid or cefuroxime for the treatment of staphylococcal pneumonia or gram-negative pneumonias caused by *E. coli* or *Klebsiella pneumoniae*. Alternative agents should be prescribed until additional studies have been published.

Cefoxitin has enjoyed a reputation as a safe and effective antibiotic to serve as monotherapy for a wide range of polymicrobic infections. Convincing data support the administration of cefoxitin to patients with community-associated peritonitis that results from appendicitis, trauma, and diverticulitis, as well as to diabetic patients with foot infections.[9] The therapeutic success of cefoxitin in these and in additional infections, such as endometritis and pelvic inflammatory disease, can be attributed to the compound's broad spectrum of activity, particularly the drug's unique ability to inhibit the growth of approximately 80 percent of strains of the anaerobe, *Bacteroides fragilis*.

Cefotetan was specifically developed to compete with cefoxitin and to dislodge the latter compound from its preeminent status as the most frequently prescribed parenteral cephalosporin in the United States. When compared to cefoxitin, cefotetan offers two major advantages: (1) cefotetan can be prescribed less frequently (two times a day in contrast to four to six times a day for cefoxitin) to treat community-acquired secondary peritonitis, and (2) this dosing schedule can result in considerable cost savings. A number of concerns should be resolved, however, before clinicians elect to prescribe cefotetan, rather than cefoxitin.

Few American investigators have published their experience with cefotetan. However, this newer second generation cephalosporin does appear to be comparable in clinical efficacy when compared to a predecessor, cefloxitin. In addition, cefotetan possesses less inhibitory activity for some strains of *Bacteroides fragilis* that are non-subspecies fragilis, as well as *B. bivius* and *B. disiens.* The clinical importance of this latter observation is unknown, although the latter organisms have been implicated in tubo-ovarian abscesses and postpartum endometritis. Of additional concern is the fact that cefotetan contains the N-methyl-thio-tetrazole side chain, which is considered by some researchers as a possible mechanism for antibiotic-associated hypoprothrombinemia and clinical bleeding.[10] Antibiotic-associated hypoprothrombinemia occurs particularly in elderly postoperative patients who have renal failure and who have been deprived of oral intake. Prophylactic administration of vitamin K_1 prevents the coagulation defect. The limited data available suggest that clinical bleeding will not prove to be a problem with cefotetan.

THIRD GENERATION

Third generation cephalosporins offer considerable appeal for the treatment of specific life-threatening infections (nosocomial pneumonia, meningitis, urosepsis) when the disorders are caused by susceptible aerobic gram-negative bacilli. Their broad spectrum of inhibitory activity for gram-negative aerobic bacilli rivals that of the aminoglycosides, and they often provide synergistic inhibitory activity when combined with an aminoglycoside. The third generation cephalosporins appear to be preferable treatment when compared with the aminoglycosides, particularly for those patients with renal insufficiency, vestibular damage, or hearing loss. Third generation cephalosporins have successfully cured serious infections caused by strains of *Enterobacteriaceae* resistant to the aminoglycosides. In addition, the third generation cephalosporins have not only been safe compounds, but they penetrate the leptomeninges in therapeutic concentrations, thereby establishing these compounds (other than cefoperazone) as the agents of choice to treat a meningitis caused by susceptible aerobic gram-negative bacilli.[11]

A number of important differences exist among the third generation cephalosporins. These are outlined in Table 13-2. The clinician who prescribes these compounds should be aware of their limitations.[12] The third generation cephalosporins are extremely expensive drugs, and they should not be prescribed to patients with infections caused by anaerobes or by gram-positive cocci.

The third generation cephalosporins should not be used as monotherapy to treat serious abdominal or pelvic infections in which *Bacteroides fragilis* and other anaerobes are contributing, and they are not appropriate treatment for life-threatening infections caused by *Staphylococcus aureus, Staphylococcus epidermidis,* streptococci (including enterococci), *Streptococcus pneumoniae,* or *Listeria monocytogenes.* No third generation cephalosporin should be pre-

TABLE 13-2 Unique Features of the Third
Generation Cephalosporins

Drug	Feature
Cefotaxime	Established track record from gram-negative meningitis
Moxalactam	Clinical bleeding may result
Cefoperazone	No dosage adjustment needed in renal failure
Ceftizoxime	Similar to cefotaxime, but less frequent dosing
Ceftazidime	Preferred compound for disease caused by *Pseudomonas aeruginosa*
Ceftriaxone	Dosing as infrequent as every 12 to 24 hours

scribed as exclusive onset therapy for the febrile leukopenic patient with presumed bacteremia. In addition, when ceftazidime is prescribed for the treatment of a serious infection caused by *Pseudomonas aeruginosa,* the clinician should also administer an aminoglycoside.

The third generation cephalosporins should not be used for perioperative prophylaxis. Disulfiram-like reactions can occur when patients receive moxalactam or cefoperazone with either alcohol or alcohol-containing medications. These reactions consist of flushing, nausea, vomiting, headache, and hypotension. Patients should not ingest alcohol until at least 3 days after these drugs have been discontinued. The third generation cephalosporins can cause pseudomembranous colitis, and they have been associated with superinfection caused most often by enterococci, *Pseudomonas aeruginosa,* and *Candida* species.

Bleeding has resulted from the administration of moxalactam and cefoperazone. Moxalactam can produce clinical bleeding by inhibiting platelet aggregation and by inducing hypoprothrombinemia.[13] At least two mechanisms may explain the compound's capacity to cause hypoprothrombinemia. It has been suggested that the moxalactam destroys menaquinone-producing gut flora. Alternatively, the development of hypoprothrombinemia has been attributed to the ability of the drug's N-methyl-thio-tetrazole side chain to interfere with prothrombin synthesis, or to moxalactam's inhibition of vitamin K-dependent carboxylation.

A major concern with the third generation cephalosporins is the emergence of resistance during therapy, particularly by *Enterobacter* species, *Citrobacter freundii, Serratia* species, and *Providencia* species. The antibiotics appear to cause a depression of beta-lactamases in these organisms.[14] Routine laboratory testing does not detect this phenomenon. These inducible beta-lactamase enzymes seem to prevent access of the cephalosporins to their binding proteins in the inner membranes of the bacteria.

I would consider ceftazidime the preferred third generation cephalosporin for initial treatment of a life-threatening gram-negative bacillary infection, pending identification and susceptibility testing. This compound can be administered as infrequently as every 8 hours, it has not been associated with bleeding, it has successfully treated meningitis, and, among all the third generation cephalosporins, it possesses the greatest inhibitory activity for *Pseudomonas aeruginosa.* I regard ceftriaxone, because of its extended serum half-life, the ideal cost-effective third generation cephalosporin.[15] This compound can be administered intravenously in the hospital, or at home following discharge, as infrequently as once or twice a day. Ceftriaxone possesses excellent inhibitory activity for many *Enterobacteriaceae* and *Hemophilus influenzae*, but has inadequate activity for *B. fragilis* or *Pseudomonas aeruginosa.* Ceftriaxone is also an effective therapy for pharyngeal and rectal gonorrhea when caused by beta-lactamase negative or positive *Neisseria gonorrhea* and appears as a promising drug to treat syphilitic meningitis and the neurologic manifestations of Lyme disease. When profound renal insufficiency exists, ceftizoxime becomes a highly cost-effective third generation compound. Dosing can be reduced to every 36 to 48 hours for patients with a creatinine clearance of 10 to 49 ml per minute.

References

1. Snavely SR, Hodges GR. The neurotoxicity of antibacterial agents. Ann Intern Med 1984; 101:92–104.
2. Barza M. The nephrotoxicity of cephalosporins: an overview. J Infect Dis 1978; 137 Suppl:S60–S73.
3. Saxon A. Immediate hypersensitivity reactions to beta-lactam antibiotics. Rev Infect Dis 1983; 5 Suppl 2:S368.
4. Tomasz A. Penicillin-binding proteins and the antibacterial effectiveness of beta-lactam antibiotics. Rev Infect Dis 1986; 8 Suppl 3:S260–S278.
5. DiPiro JT, Bowder TA, Hooks VH III. Prophylactic parenteral cephalosporins in surgery. JAMA 1984; 252:3277–3279.
6. Bertino JS, Kozak AJ, Reese RE, Chiarella LA. Hypoprothrombinemia associated with cefamandole use in a rural teaching hospital. Arch Intern Med 1986; 146:1125–1128.
7. Swedish Study Group. Cefuroxime versus ampicillin and chloramphenicol for the treatment of bacterial meningitis. Lancet 1982; 1:295–298.
8. Wallace RJ Jr, Neifield SL, Waters S, Waters B, Awe RJ, Wiss K, Martin RR, Greenberg SB. Comparative trial of cefonicid and cefamandole in the therapy of community-acquired pneumonia. Antimicrob Agents Chemother 1982; 21:231–235.
9. Malangoni MA, Condon RE, Spiegel CA. Treatment of intra-abdominal infections

is appropriate with single-agent or combination antibiotic therapy. Surgery 1985; 98:648–655.

10. Lipsky JJ. N-methyl-thio-tetrazole inhibition of the gamma carboxylation of glutamic acid: possible mechanism for antibiotic-associated hypoprothrombinaemia. Lancet 1983; 2:192–193.

11. Landesman SH, Corrado ML, Shah PM, Armengaud M, Barza M, Cherubin CE. Past and current roles for cephalosporin antibiotics in treatment of meningitis. Am J Med 1981; 71:693–703.

12. Gleckman R, Gantz NM. The third-generation cephalosporins: a plea for restraint. Arch Intern Med 1982; 142:1267–1268.

13. Weitekamp MR, Aber RC. Prolonged bleeding times and bleeding diathesis associated with moxalactam administration. JAMA 1983; 249:69–71.

14. Sanders CC, Sanders WE Jr. Emergence of resistance during therapy with the newer beta-lactam antibiotics: role of inducible beta-lactamases and implications for the future. Rev Infect Dis 1983; 5:639–648.

15. Baumgartner JD, Glauser MP. Single daily dose treatment of severe refractory infections with ceftriaxone. Arch Intern Med 1983; 143:1868–1873.

14 | FEVER OF UNKNOWN ORIGIN IN THE ELDERLY

RICHARD A. GLECKMAN, M.D.

Classically, fever of unknown origin (FUO) has been defined as a fever that persists for at least 3 weeks, that is accompanied by documented temperatures of 101°F or greater, and that remains unexplained despite at least a week of intensive diagnostic evaluation. Researchers studying patients with febrile disorders have uncovered a number of descriptive and distinctive fever patterns, such as the remittent, intermittent, hectic, and sustained fever patterns. Unfortunately, however, identification of these fever patterns fails to provide useful clinical information since these patterns do not have specific diagnostic value. Of greater importance to the physician evaluating the febrile geriatric patient is the recognition of a relapsing fever or the detection of a reversal of the normal diurnal temperature curve. The former abnormality would suggest the presence of lymphoma, and the latter observation should evoke a concern for miliary tuberculosis or polyarteritis nodosa.

CAUSES

The most common causes of FUO in elderly patients include neoplasms (particularly lymphoma, nephroma, and carcinoma of the pancreas or gastrointestinal tract, the latter often associated with liver metastases), infections (specifically occult abdominal and retroperitoneal abscesses, infections following prosthesis and graft insertions, miliary tuberculosis, and subacute bacterial endocarditis), and collagen vascular diseases (such as giant cell arteritis).[1] Additional causes of FUO to be considered in the geriatric patient include preleukemia, polyarteritis nodosa, recurrent pulmonary emboli, dissecting aortic aneurysm, adverse drug reactions, and two viral disorders (transfusion-related cytomegalovirus, and infectious mononucleosis).[2] Some well-recognized causes of FUO in younger adults (inflammatory bowel disease, sarcoidosis, rheumatic fever, granulomatous hepatitis, Still's disease, systemic lupus erythematosus, and "factitious" fever) rarely cause FUO in aged patients.

A clinician assessing an elderly patient for FUO should not yield to the temptation to turn to a checklist and simply order a battery of sophisticated, expensive, and sometimes, invasive tests. The individual patient must remain the centerpiece of the diagnostic evaluation. A thorough history is indispensable. Knowledge that the patient has travelled to an endemic area raises the suspicion of malaria, amebic liver abscess, tuberculosis, brucellosis, trypanosomiasis, leishmaniasis, salmonellosis, and schistosomiasis. The patient who participates in camping or hunting and who is at risk of exposure by handling or by consuming infectious material is a candidate for borreliosis, trichinosis, and leptospirosis.

Medications

A review of the list of medications that the patient is receiving is essential.[3] Patients with drug-induced fever can appear otherwise well or can experience concomitant symptoms (headache, myalgia, rigors) and appear severely ill. The height of the fever is not a distinguishing feature of drug-related fever, and patients can develop drug-related fever months after the onset of therapy. In my experience, the most common drugs to produce prolonged fever in the aged include dilantin, quinidine, cimetidine, and antimicrobial agents, particularly trimethoprim-sulfamethoxazole. Prolonged unexplained fever in the elderly has also been attributed to intramuscular injections of the antihistamine hydroxyzine (Atarax). As a general rule, drug-induced fever disappears 12 to 96 hours after discontinuation of the medication.

Neoplasms

Contemporary reviews indicate that neoplasms are the most common disorders causing FUO in elderly patients.[1] Hodgkin's disease and non-Hodgkin's lymphoma represent less than 5 percent of all new cancers in the United States, but these two malignancies account for an inordinately large percent of cases of FUO that are ultimately found to be caused by tumors. Hodgkin's disease and nonHodgkin's lymphoma present as prolonged unexplained fever when there are no remarkable peripheral nodes and when the disease exclusively involves subdiaphragmatic structures, such as the liver, spleen, and retroperitoneal nodes.

Renal cancer is occasionally heralded by a combination of flank pain, palpable mass, and hematuria. However, FUO can be the initial and exclusive manifestation of a hypernephroma, with fever occurring independently of concomitant metastases or renal infection. Carcinoma of the liver or a metastatic tumor of the liver can be signaled by protracted fevers accompanied by sweats and impressive leukocytosis, thus conveying the impression of an infection.

Protracted fever can serve as the presenting and dominant feature of preleukemia in elderly patients. The symptoms and physical findings lack specificity, but the typical abnormalities detected in the blood (anemia, granulocytopenia, poikilocytosis) and bone marrow (megakaryocytosis, erythroidhyperplasia) suggest the diagnosis of this myeloproliferative disorder.

The presence of fatigue, fever, weight loss, shortness of breath, and pedal edema raises an awareness of cardiac myxoma. Recognition of this cause of FUO in the elderly patient may avoid disabling complications or even death from congestive heart failure or from tumor embolization.[4]

Occult Infections

Abdominal abscesses are a frequent, important, and often overlooked source of FUO in the aged patient. These infections usually arise from contiguous inflammatory or neoplastic disease of the hepatobiliary system, gastrointestinal tract, and kidneys. Such infections have a predilection for the liver, as well as for the subphrenic, pelvic, paracolonic, and retroperitoneal spaces.

The clinician may not immediately consider the possibility of a liver abscess to explain FUO, particularly when the patient does not manifest jaundice, right upper quadrant pain, or hepatomegaly. Further challenging the clinician's diagnostic capability is the fact that elderly patients can have what has been termed 'cryptogenic' liver abscesses. These abscesses have no readily identifiable precipitating event, such as prior trauma, biliary tract disease, or disease of the colon.

A number of factors contribute to the delay in detection or the inability to detect abdominal abscesses in older individuals. There may be neither localized tenderness nor palpable abdominal mass. Patients may fail to demonstrate a ''hectic'' fever pattern or to muster an impressive leukocytosis. In addition, clinicians may not appreciate the limitations of the newer imaging procedures, such as [67] gallium citrate scanning, ultrasonography, and even computed tomography, to detect abdominal and pelvic abscesses.[5]

Infections following insertion of a prosthesis or a graft are often associated with minimal symptoms, and the surgical site is not suspected as the cause of the FUO. To detect these localized infections, it is usually necessary to perform computed tomography of the abdomen (if the prior surgery was abdominal) or bone scanning with gallium scanning (if the prior surgery involved the extremities).

Localized tuberculosis that involves bones, joints, lymph nodes, bladder, or kidneys rarely causes FUO.[6] Fever of unknown origin produced by tuberculosis occurs in those elderly patients with miliary disease. Alcoholism, diabetes mellitus, malignancies, and immunosuppressive therapy are often associated factors in these patients. The diagnosis of miliary tuberculosis is difficult and often delayed because these patients have nonspecific clinical features, such as fever, weight loss, cough, abnormal mental status, abdominal pain, hepatomegaly, and/or splenomegaly, as well as normal chest roentgenograms, at least initially. Physicians often consider these abnormalities an indication of an occult neoplasm.

There are a number of reasons why clinicians may fail to consider the diagnosis of subacute bacterial endocarditis when elderly patients experience FUO. The manifestations of the disease, such as myalgias or backache, may be vague or subtle. There may be no murmur, or the physician may consider the murmur to be insignificant. The symptoms of the disease, including fever, chills, headache, sweats, anorexia, and weight loss, can resemble a flu-like viral syndrome. Alternatively, neurologic abnormalities resulting from subacute bacterial endocarditis, such as hemiplegia, ataxia, or seizures, direct the physician's attention towards a primary central nervous system disease. When blood cultures become a routine component of the diagnostic assessment of the febrile aged patient, subacute bacterial endocarditis will virtually disappear from diagnostic consideration in the elderly with FUO.

Although considered a disease of young adults, infectious mononucleosis does occur in the elderly.[7] Aged patients experience fever, malaise, and fatigue without the presence of localizing findings, such as pharyngitis, lymphadeno-pathy, or splenomegaly. The detection of an absolute lymphocytosis, atypical lymphocytes, and abnormal liver enzymes suggest the possibility of infectious mononucleosis, and these findings should encourage the performance of the more specific antibody determinations.

Transfusion-related cytomegalovirus infection manifests as prolonged, unexplained fever that develops 2 to 6 weeks after a blood transfusion. Usually, but not invariably, atypical lymphocytes are detected in the peripheral blood and the serum glutamic-oxaloacetic transaminase (SGOT) concentration becomes elevated. Although no effective antiviral chemotherapy exists to hasten the rate of clinical resolution, recognition of this disorder is important to reduce patient anxiety, to obviate unnecessary antibiotic administration, and to curtail extensive and expensive diagnostic testing. The diagnosis of transfusion-related cytomegalovirus can be most readily achieved by the identification of the IgM-specific antibody in serum.

Vasculitis

Giant cell arteritis, the most common collagen vascular disease to cause FUO in aged patients, can masquerade as a malignancy or as an infection. This vasculitis is characterized by prolonged unexplained fever, weakness, weight loss, anemia, and an elevated sedimentation rate. Patients can experience shaking chills, drenching sweats, and fever that can exceed 103°F. The full spectrum of giant cell arteritis is continuing to evolve as new manifestations, including cough, are being recognized.[8] Absence of symptoms such as headache, jaw claudication, change in vision, or tenderness of the temporal artery should not dismiss giant cell arteritis from diagnostic consideration.

Polyarteritis nodosa can present as FUO in the elderly. Constitutional symptoms such as weight loss, anorexia, myalgia, and articular abnormalities, as well as nausea, vomiting, and abdominal pain, are common early manifestations of this systemic vasculitis. There is no specific laboratory test for the diagnosis of polyarteritis nodosa, but many patients demonstrate anemia, leukocytosis, an elevated sedimentation rate, hepatitis B surface antigen, proteinuria, hematuria, pyuria, and azotemia. The absence of hypertension, renal abnormalities, and dermal lesions does not exclude the diagnosis. Arteriographic findings of aneurysms and sharply segmental narrowing of medium-sized arteries of the renal, hepatic, and visceral vasculature is virtually pathognomonic of polyarteritis nodosa.

Miscellaneous

On occasion, recurrent pulmonary emboli may be signaled by FUO in the bedridden elderly patient.[9] These patients often have coexistent chronic obstructive lung disease or chronic congestive heart failure, disorders that reduce the specificity of the perfusion lung scan and make accurate diagnosis more difficult.

Rarely, a dissecting aneurysm of the aorta can cause FUO in an elderly patient. This disease usually occurs in hypertensive patients in the sixth and seventh decades of life. The combination of constitutional symptoms (including drenching night sweats), anemia, and an elevated sedimentation rate usually suggest an alternative systemic disorder.

EVALUATION

The initial FUO evaluation consists of a complete medical history and a meticulous physical examination. If the cause of the FUO is not promptly discovered, both of these elements should be periodically repeated and supplemented by essential laboratory and radiographic studies. Those procedures that form the foundation of the FUO work-up include the following: complete blood count with differential; sedimentation rate; stool guaiac; urinalysis with sediment examination and urine culture; liver enzymes; serum uric acid; rheumatoid factor; serum creatinine; chest X-ray; tuberculin skin testing with purified protein derivative (PPD-S); and storage of 5 to 10 ml of serum (the 'acute phase' serum).[2] Three sets of blood cultures should be performed on two consecutive days. Each set must include a bottle that enhances the yield of aerobes and a bottle that permits the growth of anaerobes.

Neither arterial blood cultures nor blood cultures inoculated into hypertonic culture media have proven helpful to assess patients with FUO. The physician should also resist the temptation to request the "febrile agglutinin battery", unless there is epidemiologic information to suggest the possibility of exposure to *Brucella* species.[10] The "febrile agglutinin battery" assesses the Widal reaction (*Salmonella* antibodies), Weil-Felix reaction (*Proteus* OX-cross-reacting antibodies to *Rickettsia* species), and agglutinin titers for *Brucellosis* species.

In the absence of clinical or laboratory clues to the cause of the FUO, the clinician should proceed to noninvasive radiographic techniques, including two-dimensional echocardiography to detect valvular vegetations in patients with blood culture-negative endocarditis as well as left atrial myxoma, and computed tomography of the abdomen. Culture-negative endocarditis usually results from indiscriminate administration of antibiotics prior to the performance of the blood cultures. Computed tomography of the abdomen is performed to detect abdominal and perinephric abscesses, to identify retroperitoneal tumor, carcinoma of the pancreas, and nephroma, and to delineate hepatic and splenic masses.[11] Although computed tomography is not infallible, this imaging technique often permits an early diagnosis when patients have nonspecific physical and laboratory findings. Computed tomography has virtually replaced excretory urography (IVP) in the detection of renal masses and perinephric abscesses, and it has proven to be superior to lymphangiographic examination in revealing lymphomatous masses involving the mesenteric, periportal, and perirenal lymph node groups.

At this stage in the evaluation, the physician should consider sigmoidoscopy and barium enema, even if the stool is negative for occult blood, in order to discover a 'silent' colon cancer.

More invasive procedures become indicated when the noninvasive tests, coupled with history, physical, and radiographic studies, fail to identify the cause of the FUO in patients who remain ill or who seem to be deteriorating.

Bone marrow trephine biopsy may provide invaluable information by detecting nonHodgkin's lymphoma, the lymphocyte depletion type of Hodgkin's disease, metastatic carcinoma, or miliary tuberculosis. Although liver biopsy appears to provide a higher diagnostic yield for miliary tuberculosis, bone marrow biopsy is a more benign procedure and, on occasion, confirms the diagnosis of miliary tuberculosis when liver biopsy proves negative.

Temporal artery biopsy should be performed to diagnose giant cell arteritis before the patient is offered a therapeutic trial of corticosteroid. It is essential to attempt to secure a definitive diagnosis because chronic steroid therapy can result in serious sequelae, particularly symptomatic vertebral fractures. Temporal arteriography is not a satisfactory alternative to biopsy. For patients with giant cell arteritis, corticosteroid therapy usually results in a resolution of fever and weakness within a few days and, most importantly, prevents blindness.

Elderly patients who have been subjected to a thorough investigation and who still have no identifiable cause of FUO should not be relentlessly evaluated with expensive, uncomfortable, invasive, and potentially harmful tests if there is no evidence of deterioration, such as significant weight loss or incapacitation.[9] These patients should be discharged, advised to maintain a diary of daily temperatures and weight, and instructed to return for a follow-up outpatient visit in 2 weeks.

For the patient who does appear to be deteriorating a liver biopsy is indicated.[12] This procedure may reveal evidence of miliary tuberculosis, alcoholic cirrhosis, hepatoma, or metastatic tumor to explain the patient's FUO. If this study is contraindicated or is not diagnostically helpful, the clinician should elect to either perform an exploratory laparotomy or initiate a diagnostic and/or therapeutic drug trial. The need for exploratory laparotomy has been largely obviated by computed abdominal tomography. On occasion, however, when the patient is deteriorating, the computed tomography is indecisive, or when some data indicate that the abdomen is the source of the disease process, exploration may identify a disorder amenable to therapy, such as an abscess, miliary tuberculosis, or polyarteritis nodosa.[13] A decision to perform a laparotomy should not be made out of frustration, but only after a careful review of the patient's medications, physical examination, x-ray films, laboratory studies, and prior biopsies.

The physician may elect to initiate a therapeutic drug trial if the patient refuses abdominal exploration or if no data indicate that the cause of the FUO is a disease in the abdomen. Therapeutic and/or diagnostic drug trials for the aged patient with FUO would include the following; heparin for recurrent pulmonary emboli; ampicillin with an aminoglycoside antibiotic to treat subacute bacterial endocarditis; isoniazid with rifampin as therapy of miliary tuberculosis; a corticosteroid for giant cell arteritis; and a nonsteroidal anti-inflammatory agent to suppress the fever caused by hepatic metastases.[2]

These drug trials must not be used to circumvent a meticulous diagnostic assessment, especially since they occasionally provide misleading information. Some patients with lymphoma have defervesced when receiving antituberculous medication. Also, a decline in temperature following corticosteroid therapy cannot be used to differentiate fever of an infectious disease from fever caused by collagen vascular diseases.[14]

Nonsteroidal anti-inflammatory agents have been known for more than 15 years to be able to eliminate fever associated with malignancies when aspirin and corticosteroids had previously failed. Recently, it has been observed that naproxen, prescribed as 250 mg orally every 12 hours, selectively causes lysis of neoplastic-induced fever, but fails to cause resolution of fever when infection complicates the malignancy.[15] This important observation requires confirmation.

References

1. Larson EB, Featherstone HJ, Petersdorf RG. Fever of undetermined origin: diagnosis and follow-up of 105 cases, 1970–1980. Medicine 1982; 61:269.
2. Gleckman RA, Esposito AL. Fever of unknown origin in the elderly: diagnosis and treatment. Geriatrics 1986; 41:45.
3. Young EJ, Fainstein V, Musher DM. Drug-induced fever: cases seen in the evaluation of unexplained fever in a general hospital population. Rev Infect Dis 1982; 4:69.
4. Davison ET, Mumford D, Zaman Q, Horowitz R. Left atrial myxoma in the elderly. J Am Geriatr Soc 1986; 34:229–233.
5. Pitcher WD, Musher DM. Critical importance of early diagnosis and treatment of intra-abdominal infection. Arch Surg 1982; 117:328.
6. Alvarez S, McCabe WR. Extrapulmonary tuberculosis revisited: a review of experience at Boston City and other hospitals. Medicine 1984; 63:25.
7. Horwitz CA, Henle G. Schapiro R, Borken S, Bundtzen R. Infectious mononucleosis in patients aged 40 to 72 years: report of 27 cases, including 3 without heterophil-antibody responses. Medicine 1983; 62:256.
8. Larson TS, Hall S, Hepper NGG, Hunder GG. Respiratory tract symptoms as a clue to giant cell arteritis. Ann Intern Med 1984; 101:594.
9. Gleckman R, Crowley M, Esposito A. Fever of unknown origin: a view from the community hospital. Am J Med Sci 1977; 274:21.
10. Zuerlein TJ, Smith PW. The diagnostic utility of the febrile agglutinin tests. JAMA 1985; 254:1121.
11. Quinn MJ, Sheedy PF, Stephens DH, Hattery RR. Computed tomography of the abdomen in evaluation of patients with fever of unknown origin. Radiology 1980; 136:407.
12. Masana L, Guardia J, Clotet B, Cuxart A, Vilaseca J, Bacardi R. Liver biopsy in fever of unknown origin. Gastroenterol Clin Biol 1980; 4:215.
13. Greenall MJ, Gough MH, Kettlewell MG. Laparotomy in the investigation of patients with pyrexia of unknown origin. Br J Surg 1983; 70:356.
14. Flatauer FE, Ballou SP, Wolinsky E. Comparative response of fever to corticosteroids in tuberculous and in connective tissue disease. Am J Med 1981; 281:111.
15. Chang JC, Gross HM. Utility of naproxen in the differential diagnosis of fever of undetermined origin in patients with cancer. Am J Med 1984; 76:597.

15 | INFECTION IN THE DIABETIC PATIENT

RICHARD A. GLECKMAN, M.D.

Infection is an important precipitant of both ketoacidosis and hyperosmolar nonketotic coma for the approximately 5 million diabetics in the United States, and often necessitates hospitalization. Most infection-related hospitalizations in diabetics are caused by pneumonia, urinary tract infections, and infections of the feet.

The diabetic patient, a compromised host, is susceptible to a number of unusual infections and is less able to confine those infections that do develop. The precise biochemical defect that predisposes diabetics to unusual and unique infections remains unknown. Some diabetics manifest altered cell-mediated immunity. Others display abnormalities of polymorphonuclear leukocytic function, including impairment of adherence, chemotaxis, phagocytosis, and intracellular killing.

Contrary to general belief, the data are not convincing that gram-negative bacteremia, staphylococcal furuncles, or staphylococcal bacteremia are more prevalent in the diabetic patient. Of interest, however, is the observation that, if staphylococcal bacteremia should develop in a diabetic patient who has a primary focus of infection, such as a foot infection, the bacteremia is more likely to result in bacterial endocarditis than it would in a nondiabetic host.[1] A consensus exists that the following infections are more prevalent in the diabetic: erythrasma, emphysematous cholecystitis, emphysematous pyelonephritis, papillary necrosis associated with pyelonephritis, rhinocerebral mucormycosis, invasive ('malignant') external otitis, necrotizing and/or crepitant soft tissue infections (phycomycotic gangrenous cellulitis, necrotizing fasciitis, synergistic necrotizing cellulitis, nonclostridial gas gangrene), and foot infections. Some researchers suggest that infections caused by group B streptococci are also more prevalent in the diabetic.

ERYTHRASMA

Erythrasma is a chronic bacterial infection of the stratum corneum caused by the organism *Corynebacterium minutissimum*.[2] This skin infection, consisting of well-defined brown to red-brown patches, has a predilection for the groin, axillae, toe webs, and breast folds. Skin lesions can be asymptomatic or pruritic. A distinctive feature of these lesions is the coral-red fluorescence seen under a Wood's light. A groin eruption caused by erythrasma must be differentiated from candidiasis and tinea cruris. Characteristically, erythrasma has no raised borders, is not associated with satellite lesions, and gives a negative potassium hydroxide (KOH) preparation. Oral erythromycin is one of the preferred treatments for erythrasma.

EMPHYSEMATOUS CHOLECYSTITIS

Emphysematous cholecystitis, an unusual form of acute cholecystitis, appears to be more common among diabetics. Presumably, ischemia is an important pathogenetic component, as contrasted with conventional acute cholecystitis. A number of features distinguish emphysematous cholecystitis: the disease is more common in men; often there is no concomitant cholelithiasis; the predominant causative organisms are anaerobes, particularly clostridia; there are usually advanced stages of gallbladder pathology (gangrene, perforation) by the time the disease is recognized; and there is a rather diagnostic roentgenographic appearance. The x-ray film demonstrates air in the gallbladder wall and the pericholecystic area in the absence of an abnormal communication with the gastrointestinal tract. On occasion, however, the initial x-ray film is normal.

The signs and symptoms of acute cholecystitis and acute emphysematous cholecystitis are similar. Patients with acute emphysematous cholecystitis do not appear any more severely ill than do those with conventional acute cholecystitis, nor do they experience fevers of greater magnitude or exhibit more impressive peritoneal signs, even though acute emphysematous cholecystitis is more commonly lethal. Treatment of acute emphysematous cholecystitis consists of fluid and electrolyte support, the administration of broad-spectrum antibiotics, including at least one agent that inhibits the growth of *Clostridium* species (e.g., penicillin or ampicillin), and emergent cholecystectomy.

RENAL PAPILLARY NECROSIS

Renal papillary necrosis with pyelonephritis occurs in patients who have sickle cell trait, urinary tract obstruction, a history of prolonged analgesic consumption, and diabetes mellitus. In the diabetic, the disease, also known as necrotizing pyelonephritis, is often bilateral. Papillary necrosis can appear as an acute fulminating disorder, or it can manifest as a subacute process. The disease can also be entirely asymptomatic and be discovered incidentally at autopsy. This diagnosis should be considered when the diabetic patient manifests florid pyelonephritis, hematuria, renal colic, or ketoacidosis. On urographic examination, papillary necrosis has a distinctive appearance. Ultrasound is a valuable technique to diagnose obstructive uropathy caused by papillary necrosis. Therapy of the seriously ill diabetic patient consists of supportive measures, antibiotic treatment, regulation of concomitant ketoacidosis, and relief of obstruction.

EMPHYSEMATOUS PYELONEPHRITIS

Emphysematous pyelonephritis is a necrotizing, potentially life-threatening bacterial infection caused by aerobic gram-negative bacilli, particularly *Escherichia coli*.[3] This rare suppurative kidney infection is characterized by the presence of gas formation in renal tissue. Most patients who have emphysematous pyelonephritis are diabetics, and some have coexistant papillary necrosis. These patients appear critically ill and experience fever, vomiting, and flank pain. On occasion, the infection can be indolent and can be caused by fungi. Antibiotic therapy usually has been unsuccessful. Most experts suggest that these patients require nephrectomy in addition to antibiotics.

RHINOCEREBRAL MUCORMYCOSIS

Rhinocerebral mucormycosis, a rapidly-spreading invasive fungal infection caused by Mucor species, is usually accompanied by ketoacidosis in the diabetic.[4] The disease presumably begins in nasal tissue or palate and extends to the paranasal sinuses (maxillary, ethmoid) where it threatens the orbit and brain. Rarely, the disease pursues an indolent course unassociated with ketoacidosis. The fungus that causes this potentially life-threatening infection has the unique predisposition to invade blood vessels, both arteries and veins, thereby producing thrombosis, infarction, and necrosis.

Initial manifestations consist of facial or ocular pain and a characteristic blood-tinged nasal discharge. The latter material, which exudes from black necrotic crusts in the nasal septum and turbinates, resembles dried blood. Additional features include fever, lethargy, headache, proptosis, periorbital edema, visual blurring, increased lacrimation, tenderness over the maxillary sinus, and facial cellulitis. Rhinocerebral mucormycosis requires differentiation from acute bacterial sinusitis, cavernous sinus thrombosis, and carcinoma of the sinus. X-ray films of the maxillary sinus reveal nodular thickening of the lining and spotty destruction of the bony walls. In contrast to acute purulent bacterial sinusitis, air-fluid levels do not develop.

The diagnosis should be confirmed by biopsies of infected tissues, which are submitted for histologic examination and culture. Precise identification of the infecting organism is imperative, because other fungi (*Aspergillus* species, *Pseudoallescheria boydii*), as well as bacteria (*Pseudomonas aeruginosa, Haemophilus* species), can cause progressive invasive sinusitis in diabetic patients, and the latter three organisms require alternative therapies. Treatment consists of control of the ketoacidosis, administration of amphotericin B, and debridement of necrotic tissue. Patients who survive have often sustained orbital or maxillary destruction, and these patients are candidates for orbital and facial prosthesis.

INVASIVE EXTERNAL OTITIS

Invasive external otitis, formerly known as malignant external otitis, occurs in patients with longstanding diabetes mellitus. In contrast to rhinocerebral mucormycosis, invasive external otitis does not develop in the setting of ketoacidosis.[5] Invasive external otitis, usually a unilateral disease, begins in the external ear canal and spreads to the pinna, as well as to the temporal bone. The infection can advance along the base of the skull, infect the opposite side, and cause cranial nerve palsy, thrombosis of the sigmoid sinus, and death. Impaired cellular immunity has been identified in some diabetic patients with invasive external otitis. Otalgia and otorrhea are the dominant presenting features. The external auditory canal is inflamed and contains granulation tissue. Patients do not appear toxic, are usually afebrile, and fail to muster a leukocytosis. The disease must be differentiated from squamous cell carcinoma.

The cause of this infection is almost always *Pseudomonas aeruginosa*. The pathogenesis of this life-threatening illness is, perhaps, best understood in terms of characteristics attributable to the organism and to the diabetic host. *Pseudomonas aeruginosa* elaborates a number of extracellular factors, including exotoxin A, various proteases, and phospholipase and has the predisposition to invade blood vessels. In addition, the diabetic host presumably has a microangiopathy with thickening of the subepithelial capillary basement membrane.

Technetium and gallium scintigraphy are more sensitive than conventional x-rays, thin section tomography, and computerized tomography for the early detection of the temporal bone osteomyelitis. In fact, [67]gallium citrate scanning, but not Tc 99 m scanning, can be used to assess radiographic resolution following successful antimicrobial therapy.[6]

Two-antibiotic combination therapy has been the standard treatment to manage invasive external otitis caused by *Pseudomonas aeruginosa*. Therapy has consisted of an aminoglycoside (gentamicin, tobramycin, amikacin) plus an antipseudomonal penicillin (ticarcillin, mezlocillin, azlocillin, piperacillin). I recommend combination treatment for the following reasons: susceptibility patterns for *Pseudomonas aeruginosa* are not predictable; synergistic activity is achieved; the emergence of resistant organisms is prevented; and relapse is prevented. Limited data suggest that monotherapy with selective third genera-tion cephalosporins, such as ceftazidime and cefsulodin, is also effective. Antibiotics should be prescribed for 6 weeks to prevent relapse, and even then some patients relapse. Surgery plays an ancillary role to antibiotic treatment. Isolated reports published in the medical literature suggest that cure of inva-sive external otitis was attributed to adjunctive hyperbaric oxygen therapy. However, no controlled studies have defined the role of this modality.

PHYCOMYCOTIC GANGRENOUS CELLULITIS

Phycomycotic gangrenous cellulitis, known as cutaneous mucormycosis, is a rare, progressive, invasive, necrotizing fungal infection caused by members of the *Mucoraceae* family. This soft tissue infection develops at a site of prior tissue injury and is characterized by a central black necrotic area with a margin of red to purple edematous cellulitis. The disease consists of fungal invasion of the vasculature, thus resulting in thrombosis and tissue necrosis. The disease can assume a subacute course or can be rapidly progressive, thereby resembling necrotizing fasciitis or synergistic necrotizing cellulitis.

The definitive diagnosis requires isolation of the organism and/or demon-stration of the fungus in tissue. The distinguishing characteristic of the fungus is the wide, nonseptate, irregularly-branching hyphae. Treatment consists of metabolic control of the diabetes, surgical debridement, and administration of amphotericin B.[7] On occasion, there is a coexistant bacterial infection that necessitates antibiotic therapy.

NECROTIZING FASCIITIS

Diabetics who experience trauma to the extremities, colon, or perineum are predisposed to the development of necrotizing fasciitis.[8] This rapidly progressive bacterial infection of the fascia and subcutaneous tissue causes obliterative arterial thrombosis and vasculitis, which results in dermal gan-grene. Originally considered a disease caused exclusively by group A beta-hemolytic streptococci, it is now appreciated that this soft tissue infection is caused by a complex microflora consisting of streptococci (group A, non-group A beta-hemolytic strains), anaerobes (*Bacteroides* species, peptostrepto-cocci) and Enterobacteriaceae. These patients appear ill, are febrile, and some experience bacteremia. Initially, the skin appears somewhat edematous, but it is not noticeably abnormal; it thus conceals both the severity and the extent of the infection of the superficial fascia and deep dermis. Later, the skin becomes warm, tender, painful, and red. The disease resembles acute cellulitis and erysipelas, but necrotizing fasciitis does not yield to antibiotic treatment. As the infection spreads, the skin's blood supply becomes compromised, thereby resulting in crepitus, cyanosis, vesicle formation, and gangrene. The lesion exudes a dark-brown turbid fluid, not frank pus.

The diagnosis of necrotizing fasciitis is established by frozen section examination of an incisional biopsy or by detailed exploration of the fascia.[9] Treatment consists of hemodynamic support, wide debridement, drainage and excision of all necrotic soft tissue, and combination antibiotics that possess inhibitory activity for those pathogens most commonly recovered from this life-threatening infection. The patient should be reexamined in the operating room within 12 hours of the initial debridement in order to excise residual necrotic and/or infected soft tissue.

SYNERGISTIC NECROTIZING CELLULITIS

Synergistic necrotizing cellulitis, a life-threatening soft tissue infection that primarily involves fascia and muscle, secondarily affects the subcutaneous tissue and skin. This infection most often occurs in the perineum or the legs and is caused by a complex microflora consisting of anaerobes and gram-negative aerobic bacilli. Patients appear toxic, are usually febrile, and experience marked local tenderness. On occasion, the skin exudes a characteristic reddish-brown, foul-smelling, thin exudate that has been termed "dishwater pus." Synergistic necrotizing cellulitis can be accompanied by bacteremia and gas in tissues and resembles necrotizing fasciitis. Therapy consists of the intravenous administration of antibiotics, fluids, and electrolytes, correction of concomitant ketoacidosis, and excision of infected and/or necrotic ischemic tissue.

NONCLOSTRIDIAL GAS GANGRENE

Nonclostridial gas gangrene, also known as infected vascular gangrene, is a polymicrobic infection that usually consists of gram-negative aerobic bacilli and streptococci that commonly involves the muscles of the legs. Most patients appear toxic and manifest gas in the subcutaneous tissue. The intensity of the pain varies, presumably because the concomitant diabetic neuropathy often renders patients somewhat insensitive to painful stimuli. Treatment consists of antibiotics and excisional surgery, usually an amputation.

FOOT INFECTIONS

Foot infections are the most common reason for hospitalizing the diabetic patient, and more in-hospital days are spent treating diabetic foot infections than any other complication of diabetes. Of all nontrauma-related amputations of the lower extremities performed in the United States, 50 percent or more involve diabetics. Prevention is superior to treatment, and active podiatric care must be carried out in all diabetics. A number of factors contribute to the predisposition of the diabetic to foot infections: functional abnormalities of neutrophils; foot deformities; trauma; peripheral neuropathies; and occlusive vascular disease. These foot infections consist of cellulitis, extensive deep soft tissue infections, and osteomyelitis. There are no precise guidelines to determine when the diabetic patient requires hospitalization for the treatment of an infected foot, but there is a concensus that in-hospital therapy is appropriate when the patient cannot comply with home care, when outpatient management has been unsuccessful, when toxicity or fever exist, when significant soft tissue swelling has developed, and when gangrene or crepitus have been identified.[10]

It is important to try to distinguish a cellulitis from a concomitant osteomyelitis because the latter infection requires more prolonged antibiotic therapy and extensive debridement. Pain, swelling, erythema, indolent ulcers, and a combination of these abnormalities occur in both disorders. Conventional x-ray films usually identify chronic osteomyelitis if the process has been present for more than 6 weeks. Radionuclide scanning permits earlier detection of osteomyelitis than do conventional x-ray films. Coexistent cellulitis, however, hinders the interpretation of a bone scan. This problem can be remedied somewhat if the radiologist analyzes both early ("blood pool") and late ("uptake") imaging phases of the bone scan because with osteomyelitis, in contrast to cellulitis, radioactive uptake increases over time. However, it would be accurate to state that both x-ray films and bone scans are fallible in the identification of chronic osteomyelitis in infected feet of diabetic patients.

Cellulitis involving the foot of the diabetic is caused by a complex microflora involving both aerobic and anaerobic bacteria. The organisms most commonly isolated from the deep tissue of diabetics with infected feet are enterococci, *Proteus mirabilis, Staphylococcus aureus, Peptococcus magnus,* and *Bacteroides* species. In febrile patients with foul-smelling lesions, anaerobes are invariably recovered. When these soft tissue infections are accompanied by bacteremia, the organisms most frequently isolated from the blood are *Staphylococcus aureus* and *Bacteroides fragilis.* Precise identification of the microbiology of soft tissue infection of the diabetic patient's foot is difficult to achieve. A swab of the ulcer provides no valid bacteriologic information. To obtain meaningful information, the physician should obtain either a needle aspiration or a biopsy specimen of the deep tissue.

Treatment consists of antibiotics, metabolic control of the diabetes, and local care (such as debridement, application of warm moist compresses, modest elevation, and protection of the wound). No antibiotic therapy has emerged as the preferred treatment. I suggest the following antibiotic programs: clindamycin plus an aminoglycoside; cefoxitin (if *Staphylococcus aureus* and *Pseudomonas aeruginosa* are not contributing to the infection); the ticarcillin and clavulanic acid combination; and perhaps the imipenem and cilastatin combination. If the patient has previously experienced an immediate or accelerated hypersensitivity reaction from a penicillin or a cephalosporin, I employ tobramycin (1.5 mg per kilogram every 8 hours intravenously after an initial dose of 1.75 mg per kilogram). When an aminoglycoside antibiotic is prescribed, however, it is necessary to obtain peak and trough serum assays to ensure precise dosing, to achieve therapeutic drug concentrations, and to avoid toxicity. I use tobramycin, rather than the less expensive gentamicin, because *Pseudomonas aeruginosa* often contributes to these infections, and the former antibiotic has been associated with decreased nephrotoxicity, an important consideration for elderly diabetic patients who often have marginal or reduced renal function.

Chronic osteomyelitis in the diabetic initially involves the toes. Radiologically, there is periosteal elevation and mottled, lytic lesions. On occasion, cultures taken from sinus tracts provide invalid microbiologic information and, therefore, cannot be relied on as a guide to antibiotic therapy. Therapy consists of removal of all sequestra, devitalized tissue, and sinus tracts and protracted, specific antibiotic administration.

The most accurate technique to identify the pathogen(s) responsible for chronic osteomyelitis is the performance of a bone biopsy. However, trauma can result in bone necrosis, the histology of chronic osteomyelitis can resemble the pathology caused by diabetic osteopathy, and cultures obtained through an area of soft tissue infection may not be reliable.[11] Unfortunately, chronic osteomyelitis is often recalcitrant to the therapy outlined, and it is necessary to amputate the foot to arrest the destructive process. The type of operation performed depends on the extent of the tissue damage and the status of the vasculature.

Some studies suggest that soft tissue infections, endometritis, and pneumonia caused by group B streptococcus, also known as *Streptococcus agalactiae*, occur more commonly in diabetics. Penicillin is the drug of choice to treat these infections. On occasion, strains are "tolerant" to penicillin (inhibited by the usual concentrations of the antibiotic, but requiring concentrations greater than 16 to 32 times the minimum inhibitory concentration to achieve 'killing'). When life-threatening infections are caused by these tolerant strains of group B streptococci, I recommend a combination of penicillin plus an aminoglycoside to achieve a synergistic effect, a situation analogous to the therapy of enterococcal endocarditis.

References

1. Cooper G, Platt R. Staphylococcus aureus bacteremia in diabetic patients. Am J Med 1982; 73:658.
2. Sarkany I, Taplin D, Blank H. The etiology and treatment of erythrasma. J Invest Dermatol 1986; 37:283.
3. Klein FA, Smith JV, Vick CW III, Schneider V. Emphysematous pyelonephritis: diagnosis and treatment. South Med J 1986; 79:41.
4. Meyers BR, Wormser G, Hirschman SZ, Blitzer A. Rhinocerebral mucormycosis: premortem diagnosis and therapy. Arch Intern Med 1979; 139:557.
5. Salit IE, McNulty DJ, Chait G. Invasive external otitis: review of 12 cases. Can Med Assoc J 1985; 132:381.
6. Parisier SC, Lucente FE, Som PM, Hirschman SZ, Arnold LM, Roffman JD. Nuclear scanning in necrotizing progressive malignant external otitis. Laryngoscope 1982; 92:1016.
7. Parfrey NA. Improved diagnosis and prognosis of mucormycosis: a clinicopathologic study of 33 cases. Medicine 1986; 65:113.
8. Miller JD. The importance of early diagnosis and surgical treatment of necrotizing fasciitis. Surg Gynecol Obstet 1983; 157:197.
9. Stamenkovic I, Lew PD. Early recognition of potentially fatal necrotizing fasciitis. N Engl J Med 1984; 310:1689.
10. Gleckman RA, Roth RM. Diabetic foot infections—prevention and treatment. West J Med 1985; 142:263.
11. Wheat J. Diagnostic strategies in osteomyelitis. Am J Med 1985; 78 Suppl 6B:218.

16 | FEVER IN THE LEUKOPENIC LEUKEMIA PATIENT

RICHARD A. GLECKMAN, M.D.

Fever, an inevitable development in the course of a patient with leukemia and leukopenia, can be caused by the leukemic process itself, by the chemotherapy, by a hematoma, by a superimposed inflammatory disorder (aspiration chemical pneumonitis, deep venous thrombosis of the legs, pulmonary embolism, phlebitis related to an intravascular device), by a transfusion reaction, or, most frequently, by an infection. The most common identifiable infections are bacterial and consist of pneumonia, cellulitis, pharyngitis, sinusitis, urinary tract infections, perirectal cellulitis, and bacteremia. Often no source for the bacteremia is discovered. Presumably, these bloodstream infections arise from disease-induced ulcerations of the pharynx, esophagus, or colon (Table 16–1). Less frequently, fever can be attributed to pseudomembranous colitis or to disease produced by viral agents (transfusion-related cytomegalovirus, cytomegalovirus pneumonia, and herpes simplex esophagitis or pneumonia), by parasites (*Pneumocystis carinii* pneumonia and *Toxoplasma gondii*-related encephalitis or pneumonitis), by *Nocardia* species, or by fungi (fungemia, esophagitis, meningitis, pneumonia, or occult abdominal dissemination).

In the leukopenic leukemic patient the risk of infection varies directly with the duration of the granulocytopenia and inversely with the quantity of granulocytes. Infections, the most common cause of death in the leukemic patient, occur more often when the leukemia is in relapse rather than in remission. Most fatal infections are caused by bacteria and, less commonly, by fungi, particularly *Candida* species and *Aspergillus* species. The most impor-

TABLE 16–1 Most Common Bacteria Recovered from the Blood of Febrile, Leukopenic Leukemic Patients

Gram-negative Rods
E. coli
Pseudomonas aeruginosa
Klebsiella species
Gram-positive Cocci
Staphylococcus epidermidis
Staphylococcus aureus
Streptococcus pyogenes
Streptococcus pneumoniae
Streptococcus faecalis

tant determinant for a favorable outcome in patients with profound granulo-cytopenia and gram-negative sepsis is the recovery of the patient's granulo-cytes during antibiotic therapy.[1]

The diagnosis of infection in the febrile leukopenic leukemic patient is difficult because of the subtleness of the signs and symptoms. The anticipated host responses are blunted. Patients with pharyngitis have pain and erythema, but no exudate. Skin and anorectal infections manifest as erythema and local pain, usually without prominent local heat, swelling, exudation, fluctuation, or regional adenopathy. Urinary tract infections occur in the absence of irritative voiding symptoms (dysuria, frequency, urgency) and pyuria. Patients with pneumonia may not experience cough or sputum production, and there may be no rales or evidence of consolidation.

As a general clinical guide, fever caused by the leukemia is usually not associated with rigors, sweats, or hypotension, whereas the presence of shaking chills or a toxic appearance suggests that a bacteremia exists.[2] However, these guides are not infallible since the leukemic patient can experience bacteremia unassociated with shaking chills or a toxic appearance.

A detailed history and physical examination are essential to assess the febrile leukemic patient. No clinical or laboratory feature reliably distinguishes an infection caused by gram-negative bacilli from one caused by gram-positive cocci or one of polymicrobic origin.[3] The major exception to this dictum is the presence of ecthyma gangrenosum, a skin lesion that consists of a central necrotic area surrounded by an erythematous base and that is most often recognized in *Pseudomonas aeruginosa* bacteremia.

The patient's history can provide invaluable diagnostic information. A sore throat in association with fever and ulceration of the pharynx caused by antineoplastic compounds can be an early sign of bacteremia caused by *Pseudomonas aeruginosa* or *Capnocytophagia*. Pain on swallowing accompanied by substernal burning suggests esophagitis caused by *Candida* species, herpes simplex, bacteria, and, less commonly, cytomegalovirus, *Aspergillus*, or *Mucor* species.[4] Pain on defecation or recent development of hemorrhoids can alert the physician to the possibility of perirectal cellulitis or abscess, life-threatening lesions usually caused by *Pseudomonas aeruginosa* and anaerobes. Fever, vomiting, abdominal pain, and abdominal tenderness in the leukemic patient who has received antineoplastic therapy or antibiotics may be symptoms of cytosine arabinoside-induced toxicity, pseudomembranous colitis, candidal hepatitis, or typhlitis (an inflammation of the cecum).[5]

On physical examination, attention should be directed to the detection of painful or erythematous skin and anorectal lesions, pharyngeal edema, perio-dontal inflammation, sinus tenderness, and rales. Periodontal infection is mani-fested by local tenderness and fever accompanied by minimal signs and symp-toms of inflammation.[6] The presence of a Hickman catheter necessitates careful inspection of the insertion site and tunnel and raises the possibility of an intravascular device-related bloodstream infection. Normal repetitive physical examinations do not exclude an infectious disorder as a cause of the patient's fever, however.

A chest X-ray, a urine culture, and blood cultures are essential components of the laboratory assessment of the febrile, leukopenic leukemic patient. Serial chest X-rays are indicated because pneumonia is one of the most common infections in the leukemic patient. Pneumonia can exist in granulocytopenic leukemic patients who do not cough, produce sputum, or demonstrate rales or evidence of consolidation on physical examination. Multiple sets of blood cultures should be obtained with the use of media that support the growth of aerobes, anaerobes, and fungi. There should be no reluctance to perform a series of blood cultures over several days, even if the patient is receiving antibiotics. If the antimicrobial removal device (ARD blood-culture system) is available, some, but not all, of the blood cultures should be processed with this technique.

If the patient has an altered mental status or meningeal signs or symptoms, X-rays are indicated to exclude mass lesions. Examination of the cerebrospinal fluid should be performed when localized mass effect has been excluded by contrast-enhanced CT. Two groups of organisms account for the majority of infections in this setting: gram-negative bacilli (*Pseudomonas aeruginosa* and *Enterobacteriaceae*) and fungi (particularly hematogenously born *Candida* species and *Aspergillus* species). Sugical wedge biopsies performed on skin lesions can provide invaluable diagnostic information.[7] The tissue removed should be subjected to culture and special stains to demonstrate bacteria and fungi.

X-rays of the sinuses, including a Caldwell view, an upright Water's view, and a lateral view for evaluation of the sphenoid sinus, should be performed when facial pain or pressure exists or when the patient has nasal congestion or a discharge. Transillumination is difficult to perform correctly, can only assess the maxillary and frontal sinuses, and is too unreliable to be used as the exclusive means of examining the sinuses. Abnormalities identified by conventional X-rays can be further evaluated by computed tomography (CT). Fiberoptic esophagoscopy, with appropriate biopsies (if the procedure is not precluded by thrombocytopenia that is recalcitrant to platelet transfusions), cultures, and cytologic studies, is a useful procedure for the patient with dysphagia or odynophagia.

The detection of one or both *Clostridium difficile* toxins in the stool provides strong support that fever and diarrhea are symptoms of cancer chemotherapy-related or antibiotic-related pseudomembranous colitis. These test can prove particularly valuable when there is reluctance to perform endoscopy on neutropenic, thrombocytopenic leukemic patients.

After the history and physical examination have been performed and appropriate cultures obtained, empiric antibiotics are prescribed. This has become the standard approach for these patients for the following reasons: most infectious episodes are caused by bacteria; no rapid and accurate technique currently exists to definitively exclude an infection; early initiation of appropriate antibiotic therapy results in a reduced incidence of shock, and a delay in the onset of antibiotic therapy, while awaiting cultural data, can result in the death of the bacteremic patient. The clinician should administer two antibiotics that are bactericidal, synergistic, and capable of inhibiting the growth of the more common gram-positive cocci and gram-negative aerobic bacilli that invade the tissues of the febrile, leukopenic leukemic patient. The antibiotics should be exclusively prescribed by the intravenous route, and the aminoglycoside dosage necessitates regulation by sequential monitoring of serum concentrations. A combination of antibiotics is administered not only to improve the antibacterial spectrum, but also to achieve synergistic activity, particularly for the profoundly and persistently neutropenic patient, and to decrease the emergence of drug-resistant pathogens. An additional reason for prescribing combinations is that each agent exerts antibacterial activity at a different time, thereby assuring more 'around the clock' protection for the compromised leukopenic host. A two-drug regimen leaves some gaps in the antimicrobial spectrum of activity, but no convincing evidence exists that the addition of a third drug improves the therapeutic response.[8] Some investigators have employed single-agent treatment (such as mezlocillin, moxalactam, or ceftazidime), but limited spectrum of activity of these agents and the concern for rapid emergence of resistant strains has diminished enthusiasm for these single agents. At present, however, the fixed dose combination drug, imipenem-cilastatin, is being studied as empiric monotherapy of the febrile leukopenic leukemia patient.

Most physicians initiate antibiotic treatment with an aminoglycoside antibiotic (gentamicin, tobramycin, or amikacin) and an extended-spectrum penicillin with activity for *Pseudomonas aeruginosa* (carbenicillin, ticarcillin). Other physicians prescribe alternative penicillins (mezlocillin, azlocillin, piperacillin, ticarcillin-clavulanic acid), substitute a cephalosporin (cefamandole, moxalactam, ceftazidime) for the penicillin, or, alternatively, elect to administer two beta-lactam antibiotics (carbenicillin with cephalothin, carbenicillin with cefamandole, ticarcillin with moxalactam, moxalactam with piperacillin). The two beta-lactam antimicrobial program diminishes the potential for nephrotoxicity or ototoxicity attributable to the aminoglycoside, but this combination enhances the potential for drug-induced bleeding. Additional concerns of the two beta-lactam antibiotic program are the occasional development of antagonism, the occasional rapid development of bacterial resistance, presumably mediated by inducible chromosome-encoded beta-lactamases, and the potential prolongation of the duration of granulocytopenia.[9]

The selection of initial therapy is a difficult problem for the patient with a history of an immediate or an accelerated hypersensitivity event attributed to prior administration of a beta-lactam (penicillin, cephalosporin, carbapenem) antibiotic. There should be great reluctance to prescribe azlocillin, ticarcillin, mezlocillin, piperacillin or ticarcillin-clavulanic acid to these patients. One approach is to consider oral desensitization with increasing doses of the penicillin drug. Another consideration is to substitute the new monobactam antibiotic, aztreonam, for the penicillin or the cephalosporin drug because initial limited studies suggest minimal, if any, cross-reactivity between aztreonam and other beta-lactam antibiotics.

It is important to appreciate that no specific antibiotic combination has emerged as the preferred initial treatment. In addition, for the patient with an indwelling intravenous line (Hickman catheter), there should be no hesitation to add vancomycin to the empiric antibiotic combination to assure adequate coverage for potential bacteremia caused by *Staphylococcus aureus* or *Staphylococcus epidermidis*.

A recent concern has been the recognition that a number of strains of *E. coli* recovered from these patients are highly resistant to ticarcillin.[10] This organism is one of the most common causes of bacteremia in the febrile leukopenic leukemia patient. Some of these *E. coli* isolates are also resistant to piperacillin. This observation suggests that the agent ticarcillin-clavulanic acid would be preferable to ticarcillin as one component to the empiric two-drug therapy because the *E. coli* are susceptible to ticarcillin-clavulanic acid.

The general approach is to treat patients for 4 days after all signs and symptoms have resolved, which usually amounts to a total antibiotic course of at least 7 to 10 days. Discontinuation of antibiotics after only 3 days has been associated with bacteremia and death. If fever resolves following the initiation of empiric antibiotic therapy and if no infection is detected, antibiotics are continued with the assumption that they are controlling an occult infection, preventing an overwhelming infection, and safeguarding the life of the patient. Some experts recommend that, if the patient has resolution of fever and if no source of an infection is recognized, empiric antibiotics should be continued for 14 days or until the polymorphonuclear leukocytes exceed 500 per microliter.

If the patient remains febrile for more than a week after starting therapy with empiric antibiotics, most, but not all, infectious disease specialists recommend that the antibiotics be continued, particularly if the patient appears ill.[11] In addition, they commence empiric antifungal therapy with amphotericin B. This decision is made with an appreciation of the fact that the continuous fever could be caused by the leukemia, an unrecognized noninfectious inflammatory process, an occult viral infection, or even the antibiotics prescribed. There are numerous reasons for initiating empiric antifungal therapy for persistently febrile neutropenic leukemia patients. Persistent fever can be the only sign of a systemic fungal infection, and fungi are second only to bacteria as a cause of infection-related death in leukemic patients. Early diagnosis of fungal infection in these patients is rarely accomplished before extensive tissue invasion occurs. The signs and symptoms of systemic fungal infections are nonspecific and resemble those of bacterial infections. Blood cultures rarely grow *Aspergillus* species or *Rhizopus* species, and rapid, specific, and sensitive serologic tests are not readily available to detect either these fungi or *Candida* species. In addition, early administration of amphotericin B therapy can be associated with successful treatment and the patient's survival.

There are some concerns about the use of amphotericin B, however. This agent can cause nephrotoxicity. Limited data indicate that sodium loading can improve the renal function of patients receiving amphotericin B.[12] Some researchers have suggested that amphotericin B can initiate an adult respiratory distress syndrome when administered simultaneously with, or just following, granulocyte transfusions in neutropenic patients.[13]

Occult sites of infection should be considered and diligently searched for in the persistently febrile patient who is receiving antibiotics and antifungal agents. Infections such as hepatic candidiasis, splenic abscess, and miliary tuberculosis rarely occur. Their detection, however, is rewarding because these potentially life-threatening disorders can be eradicated with appropriate treatment.

The syndrome of focal hepatic candidiasis, consisting of nausea, abdominal distention, abdominal pain, and diarrhea, often occurs when the patient is in remission.[14] Laboratory abnormalities include respiratory alkalosis and deranged liver chemistries. Striking elevation of the serum alkaline phosphatase, out of proportion to abnormalities of other hepatic enzymes, often occur. Hepatic defects are sometimes identified on computed tomography scans, and liver biopsy establishes the diagnosis. Usually the fungi are seen on histologic preparations and are not grown, but on occasion, the reverse occurs. Prolonged treatment, more than 2 g, with parenteral amphotericin B is the preferred therapy. Some specialists would also prescribe 5-flucytosine by mouth.

Fungal splenic abscesses, usually caused by *Candida* species and, less commonly, by *Aspergillus* species, can cause persistent fever in the leukemic patient receiving broad spectrum antibiotic therapy.[15] Some of these patients experience localized left upper quadrant pain. Technetium (^{99m}Tc)-sulfurcolloid, ^{67}gallium citrate scan, and computed tomography provide invaluable diagnostic information. Definitive therapy often consists of splenectomy.

Treatment with amphotericin B complements splenectomy because patients can harbor additional disease, particularly in the liver.

In the appropriate epidemiologic setting (history of prior tuberculosis, family history of tuberculosis, risk factor(s) for the development of tuberculosis), consideration should be given to the possibility of miliary tuberculosis. This disease is usually unsuspected in the febrile leukopenic patient because the chest X-ray is often free of the anticipated miliary pattern. If the patient does not have uncorrectable bleeding test abnormalities, the diagnostic procedure of choice is the percutaneous liver biopsy. Alternatively, trephine bone marrow biopsy should be performed. Recommended initial therapy of suspected or documented miliary tuberculosis consists of isoniazid, rifampin, and streptomycin until susceptibility patterns are available. No study has documented the superiority of a triple-drug regimen compared to a double-drug program, but most experts prefer this approach when miliary tuberculosis occurs in leukemia.

References

1. Love LJ, Schimpff SC, Schiffer CA, Wiernik PH. Improved prognosis for granulocytopenic patients with gram-negative bacteremia. Am J Med 1980; 68:643.
2. Pizzo PA, Robichaud KJ, Wesley R, Commers JR. Fever in the pediatric and young adult patient with cancer. Medicine 1982; 61:153.
3. Kramer BS, Pizzo PA, Robichaud KJ, Witebsky F, Wesley R. Role of serial microbiologic surveillance and clinical evaluation in the management of cancer patients with fever and granulocytopenia. Am J Med 1982; 72:561.
4. Walsh TJ, Belitsos NJ, Hamilton SR. Bacterial esophagitis in immunocompromised patients. Arch Intern Med 1986; 146:1345.
5. Moir CR, Scudaniore CH, Benny WB. Typhlitis: selective surgical management. Am J Surg 1986; 151:563–566.
6. Overholser CD, Peterson DE, Williams LT, Schimpff SC. Peridontal infection in patients with acute nonlymphocytic leukemia. Arch Intern Med 1982; 142:551.
7. Wolfson JS, Sober AJ, Rubin H. Dermatologic manifestations of infections in immunocompromised patients. Medicine 1985; 64:115.
8. Lawson RD, Gentry LO, Bodey GP, Keating MJ, Smith TL. Randomized study of tobramycin plus ticarcillin, tobramycin plus cephalothin and ticarcillin, or tobramycin plus mezlocillin in the treatment of infection in neutropenic patients with malignancies. Am J Med Sci 1984; 287:16.
9. Neftel KA, Hauser SP, Muller MR. Inhibition of granuloporesis in vivo and in vitro by beta-lactam antibiotics. J Infect Dis 1985; 152:90.
10. Klastersky J, Glauser MP, Schimpff SC, Zinner SH, Gaya H, EORTC antimicrobial therapy project group. Prospective randomized comparison of three antibiotic regimens for empirical therapy of suspected bacteremic infection in febrile granulocytopenic patients. Antimicrob Agents Chemother 1986; 29:263.

17 | INFECTIONS CAUSED BY NEW PATHOGENS— *CORYNEBACTERIUM* GROUP JK, *CRYPTOSPORIDIUM*, *CAPNOCYTOPHAGA*, AND *AEROMONAS*

NELSON M. GANTZ, M.D., F.A.C.P.

How frequently a microbiology laboratory reports "no pathogens identified" or "culture negative" depends on its ability to recognize "new pathogens". Some of these new pathogens are previously recognized microorganisms that recently have emerged as having importance as a result of improved methods for laboratory detection as well as because of increasing clinical reports showing their importance in human disease.

Four unrelated organisms, *Cryptosporidium*,[1-4] *Aeromonas*,[5,6] *Capnocytophaga*,[7,8] and *Corynebacterium* group JK,[9,10] have assumed increasing importance as causes of opportunistic infections. In addition, *Aeromonas* and *Cryptosporidium* frequently produce disease in normal hosts. Although these organisms are not truly new, an increasing number of reports have emphasized their recognition as frequent etiologic agents of human infection.

Diarrhea remains a major problem in both developed and developing countries. Etiologic agents still remain to be identified. In a recent study of adults with diarrhea in Chicago, only half of the patients had a causative agent isolated on smear or culture.[11] One pathogen in which there has been a sudden increase in interest is *Cryptosporidium*.

CRYPTOSPORIDIUM

Cryptosporidium was recognized as a cause of diarrhea in animals, especially calves, for over half a century. While disease attributable to this organism was occasionally documented by veterinarians caring for infected animals, it was not until the acquired immunodeficiency syndrome (AIDS) epidemic in the 1980s that *Cryptosporidium* was recognized as a frequent cause of diarrhea in that setting.[4] The organism also can produce infection in immunocompetent individuals, e.g., children who attend day-care centers,[12] and should be added to the list of pathogens that are responsible for traveler's diarrhea. Waterborne outbreaks of cryptosporidiosis, as noted with giardiasis, have been described. Finally, this parasite may cause nosocomial diarrhea in health care workers caring for patients with cryptosporidiosis.[13]

Cryptosporidium is a protozoan parasite with a defined life cycle. The oocysts excreted in the feces are infective immediately after shedding and are resistant to many disinfectants. No intermediate host is necessary to complete the life cycle. The disease is transmitted by the fecal-oral route, and common source outbreaks have been attributed to infected water. Normal children infected with *Cryptosporidium* can excrete the organism for approximately 11 days. In comparison, prolonged excretion occurs in patients with AIDS, with a median duration of 5 months and a range of 1 to 22 months. The clinical manifestation of cryptosporidiosis is dependent on the status of the host. Patients with AIDS often have life-threatening diarrhea, which is both severe and protracted. In the immunocompetent host, the illness is less severe and usually lasts up to 14 days. Occasionally, symptoms last for months and a malabsorption syndrome can occur. Abdominal pain that mimics acute appendicitis can be present. Bloody diarrhea is unusual. The pathogenesis of the diarrhea has not been defined, but the process appears to be a secretory one involving the small intestine. Patients with AIDS can lose as much as 17 L of fluid per day. Disruption of the integrity of the epithelium of the small intestine does not occur and blood cultures are not positive. Asymptomatic cryptosporidiosis has been described, but its frequency is unknown.

Cryptosporidial oocysts also have been found in the lungs of patients with AIDS, presumably from the aspiration of gastroesophageal parasites. Although some of these patients have interstitial pneumonia, it is unclear if the cryptosporidial parasites are responsible for pulmonary disease.

The precise incubation period is not known, but for travelers it appears to range from 3 to 12 days with a mean of 6 days.

The diagnosis is made by identification of the oocysts in biopsied intestinal specimens and, far more often, by the presence of the organism in feces. The parasite can be identified in a wet mount of stool stained with iodine or, by using the Kinyoun acid-fast stain of a fecal smear, as a red-stained round organism. The oocysts are small, 4 to 5 microns in diameter. If these tests are negative a concentration technique using sugar flotation can be helpful. Serologic tests and tissue culture techniques appear promising, but are not yet generally available.

Many different antiparasitic agents, antimicrobial agents, and immunostimulants have been used unsuccessfully to treat this infection in patients with AIDS. Except for an occasional success with spiramycin, a macrolide antibiotic given in a dose of 1 g orally four times per day, few drugs are available to treat this devastating illness. In the immunocompetent host, the infection is self-limited and therapy consists of fluid and electrolyte replacement. Care should be taken in handling stools of patients with cryptosporidiosis since person-to-person transmission occurs. Contaminated instruments should be autoclaved to destroy the oocysts. The oocysts are resistant to most disinfectants including glutaraldehyde. Future studies are anxiously awaited to better control this important emerging pathogen.

AEROMONAS

Another organism that appears to be an emerging cause of diarrhea is *Aeromonas* species. *Aeromonas* species are aerobic, gram-negative, motile, oxidase-positive bacilli that cause infection in both immunocompromised and normal individuals. Several species have been recognized, but most infections are due to *Aeromonas hydrophilia*. Another closely related organism, *Plesiomonas shigelloides*, have been implicated in acute gastroenteritis, bacteremia, and meningitis. *Aeromonas* organisms can be recovered easily from both salt and fresh water, soil, and a number of animals such as fish, turtles, reptiles, and frogs. The organism does not comprise part of the normal human fecal flora. Both community-acquired and nosocomial infections with this organism have been reported.[14] In the hospital setting, the organism has been found to survive for 2 weeks on moist but not dry surfaces including sinks, soap, and hospital water sources. Most of the community-acquired infections occur in the summer and fall seasons. Hospital-acquired infections occur mainly in patients who are immunocompromised.

Aeromonas hydrophilia can cause a wide spectrum of clinical infections. Infected wounds resulting from traumatic water or soil injuries should raise the possibility of an *Aeromonas* species infection. Bacteremia with skin lesions, ecthyma gangrenosum, can occur with *Aeromonas* species and are most commonly reported with *Pseudomonas aeruginosa* sepsis. Endocarditis and pneumonia associated with drowning also have been reported. The organism rarely has been isolated from intra-abdominal abscesses, decubiti, surgical wounds, and the cerebrospinal fluid after neurosurgery. Of this clinical syndrome, skin and soft tissue infection (cellulitis) directly associated with traumatic water or soil injuries has been reported most often. The organism has been isolated significantly more often from patients with travelers' diarrhea compared with controls. In one study, prophylactic doxycycline prevented *Aeromonas hydrophilia* diarrheal disease in travelers to Thailand, compared with a control group of travelers who received placebo (8% versus 42%).[15] Oral administration of the organism has failed to produce diarrhea in monkeys, and further studies are needed to define the role of this organism as a gastrointestinal pathogen in humans.

A number of antibiotics demonstrate activity against *Aeromonas* including chloramphenicol, some third generation cephalosporins such as moxalactam, the aminoglycosides, tetracycline, and trimethoprim-sulfamethoxazole. The penicillins such as ampicillin, piperacillin, or nafcillin have little activity against the organism. The therapy of choice as yet has not been defined, and either a third generation cephalosporin in combination with an aminoglycoside or trimethoprim-sulfamethoxazole could be used. The gastrointestinal illness is usually self-limited in a normal host and responds to fluid replacement.

CAPNOCYTOPHAGA

Recently, a gram-negative rod, Capnocytophaga, has gained attention as a cause of bacteremia in patients with granulocytopenia and oral mucosal defects.[7,8] This organism previously was known as *Bacteroides ochraceus*, or Centers for Disease Controls biogroup DF-1. *Capnocytophaga* species are fusiform gram-negative rods that grow either aerobically in the presence of 5 to 10 percent, CO_2 (capnophilic) or under strict anaerobic conditions. The organisms grow relatively slowly and cultures may require 3 to 5 days to become positive. The organism comprises part of the normal oral flora and is a cause of periodontal disease. *Capnocytophaga* can readily be isolated from supragingival plaque. The majority of reported infections with this organism have been life-threatening bacteremias in immunocompromised hosts. Most of the patients have had associated gingivitis, mucositis, or oral ulcers. Infection may occur more often in children than adults.[8] The organism also rarely can cause empyema, osteomyelitis, and bacteremia in a normal host. The organism is susceptible to a number of antibiotics including penicillin, ampicillin, carbenicillin, erythromycin, clindamycin, chloramphenicol, cefoxitin, tetracyline, and metronidazole. Strains are resistant to vancomycin, the aminoglycosides, and the semisynthetic penicillins such as nafcillin. A bactericidal drug such as penicillin should be selected in the compromised host. The organism produces a dialyzable toxin that inhibits granulocyte motility in vitro, but whether this is relevant in vivo to disease pathogenesis is unclear.[16]

CORYNEBACTERIUM GROUP JK

Corynebacterium group JK is another organism that has been increasingly recognized as a cause of bacteremia in the immunocompromised host and, less often, in patients with prosthetic devices. *Corynebacterium* group JK are aerobic, nonspore-forming, gram-positive bacilli. The organism on Gram stain may appear as coccobacilli or may resemble streptococci. Repeated isolations of a "diphtheroid" by the laboratory in an immunocompromised patient should raise the possibility of *Corynebacterium* group JK. These organisms should not be dismissed as contaminants. Most of the infections caused by this species of *Corynebacterium* occur as nosocomial infections. In one bone marrow transplant center, this organism was responsible for 11 percent of the bacteremias.[17] The organism infrequently (12%) colonizes the skin of normal persons; however, about one-third of cultures from skin areas of immunosuppressed hosts yielded this organism.[10] Skin sites from which the organism can be recovered most frequently are the inguinal, rectal, toe web, and axillary areas.[10] Skin carriage of this organism may persist for weeks to months, and interestingly, adult males may harbor this organism more often than adult females.[10,17] No clear explanation exists for the latter finding. In addition to male sex, prior use of broad-spectrum antibiotics as well as prolonged duration of hospitalization favor colonization of patients with group JK bacteria.[17] Most of the infections caused by this organism are bacteremias that originate at an intravenous site in patients with granulocytopenia. Prosthetic valve endocarditis also has been attributed to the JK group. Other reported infections include wound infections, skin cellulitis at an intravenous site, and meningitis. A characteristic feature of group JK bacteria is their high degree of antibiotic resistance to penicillins, cephalosporins, and aminoglycosides. All strains tested to date have been susceptible to vancomycin. Some isolates are susceptible to erythromycin, but vancomycin is the drug of choice.

References

1. Tzipori S. Cryptosporidiosis in animals and humans. Microbiol Rev 1983; 47:84–96.
2. Navin TR, Juranek DD. Cryptosporidiosis: Clinical, epidemiologic, and parasitologic review. Rev Infect Dis 1984; 6:313–327.
3. Wolfson JS, Richter JM, Waldron MA, et al. Cryptosporidiosis in immunocompetent patients. N Engl J Med 1985; 312:1278–1282.
4. Payne P, Lancaster LA, Heinzman M, McCutchan JA. Identification of *Cryptosporidium* in patients with the acquired immunodeficiency syndrome. N Engl J Med 1983; 309:613–614.
5. Davis WA, Kane JG, Garagusi VF. Human *Aeromonas* infections. A review of the literature and a case report of endocarditis. Medicine 1978; 57:267.
6. Freij BJ. *Aermonas*: biology of the organism and disease in children. Pediatr Infect Dis J 1984; 3:164.
7. Parenti DM, Syndman DR. *Capnocytophaga* species. Infections in nonimmunocompromised and immunocompromised hosts. J Infect Dis 1985; 151:140.
8. Warren JS, Allen SD. Clinical, pathogenetic, and laboratory features of *Capnocytophaga* infections. Am J Clin Pathol 1986; 86:513–518.
9. Young VM, Meyers WF, Moody MR, Schimpff SC. The emergence of coryneform bacteria as a cause of nosocomial infections in compromised hosts. Am J Med 1981.

GASTROINTESTINAL DISEASE

18 | DYSPHAGIA

KARIM A. FAWAZ, M.D.

Dysphagia is defined as difficulty in swallowing. In most instances the term dysphagia should be used whenever the patient describes a sensation of "sticking" of an ingested bolus of food or liquid. However, the term dysphagia is also used when the patient describes an inability to initiate swallowing or an inability to transfer food from the mouth to the esophagus. Dysphagia is different from odynophagia, which implies the presence of pain on swallowing, although the two conditions may coexist in certain disorders.

An accurate clinical history is extremely useful in categorizing the cause of dysphagia and in planning for diagnostic steps and therapy. There are two major categories of disorders that cause dysphagia, mechanical and neuromuscular. In general, difficulty in swallowing only solids suggests a mechanical disorder, while difficulty in swallowing both solids and liquids suggests a neuromuscular disorder. Rapidly progressive dysphagia is consistent with an expanding lesion causing progressive mechanical narrowing of the lumen, while episodic dysphagia associated with specific solid foods suggests a fixed, nonprogressive narrowing.

Remember that there is no good correlation between the location that the patient identifies as, "The food sticks here," and the actual site of pathology. A lesion in the esophagus may cause a sensation of sticking that corresponds to the site of pathology or to anywhere proximally along the esophagus, but never distal to the lesion.

There are many causes of dysphagia (Table 18-1). In this discussion, the conditions that are commonly seen in consultation will be discussed in more detail than the rarer causes of dysphagia. In my experience, benign peptic stricture of the esophagus, lower esophageal ring, and carcinoma account for approximately 90 percent of all cases of dysphagia.

TABLE 18-1   Causes of Dysphagia

Mechanical

Intrinsic
Benign peptic stricture
Carcinoma
Lower esophageal ring (Schatzki's ring)
Candidal esophagitis
Esophageal web
Stricture secondary to endoscopic sclerotherapy
Benign tumor
Caustic injury
Zenker's diverticulum

Extrinsic
Malignant tumors (direct extension or metastasis)
Retrosternal thyroid
Vascular compression

Neuromuscular

Smooth muscle disorders
Achalasia
Diffuse esophageal spasm
Scleroderma
Chagas' disease
Hypothyroidism

Striated muscle disorders
Cricopharyngeal achalasia
Polymyositis
Myasthenia gravis
Myotonia dystrophia
Thyrotoxicosis

Neural disorders
Brain stem lesion or stroke
Demyelinating disease
Degenerative disease

MECHANICAL CAUSES OF DYSPHAGIA

Benign Peptic Stricture

Peptic stricture of the esophagus usually is the result of chronic reflux of gastric acid into the esophagus. The acid reflux causes the sensation of heartburn and the pathologic entity of esophagitis. If untreated, the esophagitis becomes chronic and scarring sets in, thereby leading to the formation of a stricture. When a stricture forms, the patient may lose the symptom of heartburn and acquire a new symptom, namely dysphagia. The dysphagia is usually to solid food only unless the lumen becomes so narrow that even liquids have trouble passing.

The diagnosis is usually made by performing a barium swallow that shows a tapered narrowing of the lumen with smooth edges in the distal third of the esophagus. If the stricture is of longstanding duration, dilatation of the esophagus proximal to the stricture may be seen. Endoscopy and esophageal biopsies should be performed if the history or barium swallow provide the slightest suspicion of malignancy. The best treatment is prevention of acid reflux (by vigorous treatment of esophagitis) before a stricture develops.

Once a stricture develops, several different therapeutic options are available, depending on the diameter of the stricture: 1. anti-reflux measures such as antacids, H_2-blockers, elevation of the head of the bed, avoidance of alcohol and cigarettes, a low fat diet, and avoidance of an increase in intra-abdominal pressure; 2. anti-reflux measures plus dilation of the esophagus with bouginage; 3. surgical treatment; and 4. preoperative dilation followed by surgery.

A note of caution is in order concerning patients with longstanding reflux. They are prone to the development of the so-called Barrett's esophagus, which is considered a premalignant condition.[1] The disease involves a metaplastic change in the chronically inflamed squamous epithelium of the esophagus, which leads to replacement of this epithelium by columnar cells. Most commonly, the stricture in Barrett's esophagus occurs in the middle third of the esophagus in contrast to the usual benign peptic stricture, which occurs in the lower third of the esophagus. The presence of a stricture in the upper or middle third of the esophagus is a definite indication for endoscopy, cytology, and biopsy to rule out a malignancy. Unfortunately, neither medical nor surgical treatment of reflux has been shown to cause regression of Barrett's epithelium.

Carcinoma

A history of rapidly progressive dysphagia points to the presence of carcinoma of the esophagus until proven otherwise. Associated symptoms include weight loss and anorexia. By far the most common histologic type of esophageal cancer is squamous cell carcinoma.

Squamous cell carcinoma of the esophagus occurs with almost equal frequency in the upper, middle, and lower thirds of the esophagus. The diagnosis is made by a barium swallow that reveals an intraluminal, irregular, ulcerated mass. Sometimes the radiographic picture is one of smooth narrowing, which is difficult to distinguish radiologically from a benign stricture. It is in such instances that the location of the stricture assumes great importance. Benign strictures occur in the lower third of the esophagus, while malignant strictures can occur anywhere along the esophagus. A stricture in the upper or middle third of the esophagus thus should be considered malignant until proven otherwise. Endoscopy, biopsy, and cytology are a must in this latter group.

A smaller group of patients (less than 10 percent) have adenocarcinoma of the esophagus. Adenocarcinoma is confined to the distal third of the esophagus except if it arises in Barrett's epithelium. It is often difficult to differentiate between a primary esophageal adenocarcinoma and one arising from the fundus of the stomach and secondarily invading the lower esophagus. In both instances, dysphagia is the major symptom.

Unfortunately for patients with esophageal cancer, when they start complaining of dysphagia the lesion is already large and has spread at least locally, thereby making prognosis dismal no matter what type of therapy is employed. In general, tumors in the lower third of the esophagus are best treated by surgical resection with or without preoperative irradiation, while tumors of the upper and middle third are treated by irradiation unless surgical resection is thought to be technically possible. The prognosis is poor for all patients, with less than a 5 percent 5-year survival rate.[2]

Lower Esophageal Ring

The classic symptom of a lower esophageal ring is episodic dysphagia to solid food. The presence of daily dysphagia or progressive dysphagia over days is not suggestive of the presence of a lower esophageal ring. A typical history is one of dysphagia to meat, relieved by vomiting, followed by an asymptomatic period of weeks or months. A protracted history of symptoms of reflux esophagitis is uncommon and should alert the physician to the presence of a peptic stricture, rather than a lower esophageal ring. The diagnosis of a lower esophageal ring is cinched by a barium swallow that reveals a concentric mucosal ring, 2 to 4 mm in thickness, projecting into the lumen of the distal esophagus.

The prevalence of the lower esophageal ring is reported to be between 6 and 14 percent as seen on routine barium swallow; however, only 0.5 percent of patients with a ring suffer from dysphagia.[3] Most patients with rings measuring 13 mm or less in diameter are symptomatic. Rings 13 to 17 mm in diameter may produce dysphagia, but patients with rings greater than 17 mm in diameter are usually asymptomatic. The treatment of a lower esophageal ring is usually rewarding to the physician and the patient. Esophageal dilation with bougies is successful in most cases and affords relief for a prolonged period. Treatment may have to be repeated in months or years and the result is equally good. Only on rare occasions is surgery required.

Candidal Esophagitis

Most patients with acute esophagitis caused by *Candida albicans* complain of dysphagia. This clinical picture is in contrast to patients with herpetic esophagitis who complain of odynophagia. The diagnosis should be suspected in diabetic patients, immunocompromised hosts, and patients receiving steroids. The presence of oral thrush makes the diagnosis of a Candida infection much more likely.

Chronic candidal esophagitis may occur in patients with chronic mucocutaneous candidiasis, a disease characterized by chronic involvement of the skin, nails, and oral cavity. In this condition, the major symptom of esophageal involvement is also dysphagia, while odynophagia is uncommon. The diagnosis may be suspected following a barium swallow that reveals esophagitis, ulceration, or intramural pseudodiverticulosis or stricture. The diagnosis is confirmed by endoscopy and demonstration of the organism by cytology or culture of the brushing or biopsy performed at endoscopy. The most common mode of therapy is oral Ketoconazole (200 to 400 mg daily for 2 weeks), which provides excellent results.[4] In mild cases, oral Nystatin (400,000 to 600,000 units four times a day) may be used, and in severe cases that do not respond to Ketoconazole, low-dose intravenous amphotericin B may have to be prescribed.

Esophageal Web

Esophageal web may be single or multiple and may occur anywhere along the esophagus. The most common type is a single web in the postcricoid region of the upper third of the esophagus, which, when associated with dysphagia, is referred to as the Plummer-Vinson syndrome. Esophageal web has a higher incidence in females and an association with iron deficiency anemia, autoimmune disease, and postcricoid carcinoma.[5] The most common presenting symptom is dysphagia to solids, which may be accompanied by regurgitation and aspiration. Diagnosis is made by barium swallow or by cineradiography. Treatment is by dilation with mercury bougies.

Stricture Secondary to Endoscopic Sclerotherapy

Endoscopic sclerotherapy of esophageal varices is becoming the treatment of choice for bleeding esophageal varices. However, complications of this procedure include esophageal ulcers and stricture formation. Patients who develop strictures complain of dysphagia to solids.

The treatment is esophageal dilation with mercury bougies, the results of which are usually excellent. Theorectically, one would expect bleeding to be a frequent complication of esophageal dilation in such patients; fortunately this has not been the case.

NEUROMUSCULAR CAUSES OF DYSPHAGIA

Achalasia

Achalasia is a motor disorder of the esophagus that results from a marked decrease in Auerbach's ganglion cells. Dysphagia to both solids and liquids is the most common presenting symptom in achalasia. Onset is usually between the ages of 20 and 40 years, although it has been reported in infancy and in the elderly. Regurgitation of food or liquid, particularly in the recumbent position, is the next commonest symptom in achalasia. This may lead to repeated spells of coughing and, when severe and recurrent, may lead to pneumonia. The combination of progressive dysphagia to solids and liquids coupled with regurgitation of material ingested hours or days earlier should alert the physician to a motor abnormality such as achalasia.

The radiologic picture of late achalasia is quite specific, although not absolutely diagnostic. A barium swallow usually reveals a dilated, aperistaltic esophagus that terminates with a very narrow segment referred to as a "beak." The diagnosis is confirmed by esophageal manometry that typically shows hypertensive lower esophageal sphincter, absence of contractions in the esophagus, and incomplete relaxation of the lower esophageal sphincter on swallowing.

Occasionally a carcinoma of the cardia of the stomach with submucosal invasion of the distal esophagus may mimic achalasia radiographically and manometrically. Although endoscopy is not necessary to establish a diagnosis of achalasia, it is advisable in order to differentiate true achalasia from a high gastric ulcer.

Until recently, treatment of achalasia was either by pneumatic dilation (rupture of the lower esophageal sphincter with aid of fluoroscopy or with direct endoscopic vision) or by Heller's myotomy. Both modes of therapy provide relief of symptoms in a majority of patients.[6] Recently, pharmacologic treatment of achalasia with nitrates and calcium-channel blockers has shown promising results.[7] A reasonable approach to treatment is to start with pneumatic dilation, to add pharmacologic therapy if the response is not satisfactory, and to reserve surgery for patients who fail multiple attempts with conservative measures.

Diffuse Esophageal Spasm

Diffuse esophageal spasm is a motor abnormality that usually presents after age 40, but it does occur at an earlier age. The clinical presentation includes chest pain and dysphagia. The dysphagia does not necessarily accompany the chest pain, and the chest pain is not necessarily related to the act of swallowing. The dysphagia is to solids and liquids and is intermittent rather than progressive. Symptoms of dysphagia and/or chest pain may be triggered by very hot or very cold liquids.

A barium swallow may be normal at a time when the patient is asymptomatic, or it may show tertiary contractions, which, when extreme, give the appearance of a "corkscrew" esophagus. Esophageal manometry in a typical patient shows simultaneous high amplitude, prolonged waves called tertiary contractions. A group of patients with similar symptoms has been reported in whom barium swallow appearance is normal, and in whom primary peristaltic waves recorded on esophageal manometry also appear normal. However, the contractions are of extremely high amplitude and are prolonged. This group of patients is considered a variant of diffuse esophageal spasm.

The results of therapy in this disorder are less than desirable. Some patients may respond to pharmacologic agents such as nitrates and calcium-channel blockers. Others may respond to dilations, and those with severe symptoms may have to undergo a long esophageal myotomy.[6]

Several investigators of esophageal motor dysfunction believe that achalasia and diffuse esophageal spasm are at opposite ends of the spectrum of one disease entity.

Scleroderma

The clinical presentation of the motor defect in the esophagus of a patient with scleroderma is one of dysphagia and heartburn. The presence of Raynaud's phenomenon with these symptoms makes the diagnosis of scleroderma almost a certainty. Unlike achalasia, a barium swallow is not diagnostic. It may show a dilated esophagus, a decrease in or absence of contractions in the lower two-thirds of the esophagus, and gastroesophageal reflux. The diagnosis is confirmed by esophageal manometry that reveals a weak lower esophageal sphincter and absent peristalsis in the lower two-thirds of the esophagus.[8]

The two etiologies underlying dysphagia in scleroderma are motor disorder and esophageal stricture secondary to chronic gastroesophageal reflux. There is no specific treatment for scleroderma. Treatment is directed toward preventing esophagitis and stricture formation by antireflux measures including antacids, H_2-blockers, and metoclopramide. In severe cases, antireflux surgery may be indicated.

Other Neuromuscular Disorders

Dysphagia may be associated with diseases of striated muscle such as polymyositis, myasthenia gravis, and myotonia dystrophia. Dysphagia is evoked by both solids and liquids. Neurologic disorders such as a brain stem lesion of stroke, multiple sclerosis, and Parkinson's disease may cause dysphagia. The dysphagia results from an inability to initiate a swallow to transfer food from the mouth to the esophagus. Invariably, the dysphagia is accompanied by choking and aspiration because of trickling to the larynx, especially when liquids are swallowed. Cineradiography, rather than an ordinary barium swallow, is the examination of choice in the preceding conditions. Treatment is directed to the primary disease.

References

1. Cho KJ, Hunter TB, Whitehouse WM. The columnar epithelial-lined lower esophagus and its association with adenocarcinoma of the esophagus. Radiology 1975; 115:563–568.
2. Earlam R, Cunha-Melo JR. Esophageal squamous cell carinoma: I. A critical review of surgery. Br J Surg 1980; 67:381–390.
3. Goyal RK, Glancy MB, Spiro HM. Lower esophageal ring. N Engl J Med 1970; 282:1298–1305.
4. Fazio RA, Wickremesinghe PC, Arsura EL. Ketoconazole treatment of candida esophagitis. Am J Gastroenterol 1983; 78:261–264.
5. Chisholm M. The association between webs, iron, and post-cricoid carcinoma. Postgrad Med 1974; 50:215–219.
6. Vantrappen G, Hellemans J. Treatment of achalasia and related motor disorders. Gastroenterology 1980; 79:144–154.
7. Gelfoud M, Rozen P, Gilat T. Isosorbide dinitrate and nifedipine treatment of achalasia: a clinical, manometric and radionuclide evaluation. Gastroenterology 1982; 83:963–969.
8. Clements PJ, Kadell B, Ippolite A, Ross M. Esophageal motility in progressive systemic sclerosis. Dig Dis Sci 1979; 24:639–644.

19 | CHRONIC ABDOMINAL PAIN

SANJEEV ARORA, M.D.
KARIM A. FAWAZ, M.D.

Abdominal pain is an unpleasant subjective sensation produced by noxious stimuli from most intra-abdominal and some extra-abdominal organs. Noxious stimuli such as burning, cutting, or crushing produce severe pain when applied to the skin. The visceral organs, however, are insensitive to these stimuli. Visceral pain is produced by stimuli such as distension, ischemia, inflammation, or neoplastic infiltration. The rate of distension is important because slow distension as seen in malignant biliary obstruction is painless, whereas rapid distension as seen in gallstone or renal colic is often extremely painful. Ischemia to intra-abdominal organs produces pain by slowing the rate of blood flow and therefore allowing the accumulation of tissue metabolites around the sensory nerves. Inflammation causes increased local production of hormones such as prostaglandin, bradykinin, and serotonin, which in turn can cause pain by stimulating the peripheral nerve endings. Neoplastic infiltration of peripheral sensory nerves as seen in carcinoma of the pancreas can produce severe and unrelenting abdominal pain.

For purposes of this discussion, we will define chronic abdominal pain as discomfort that has lasted longer than 2 weeks or that has been intermittently recurring for a period greater than 2 weeks. We will therefore exclude causes of acute abdominal pain such as acute appendicitis, acute pancreatitis, or perforated viscus.

A detailed history and a careful physical examination are essential when consultation is done on a patient for chronic abdominal pain. Emphasis on the history can avoid many unnecessary and expensive diagnostic tests and can aid in early diagnosis by focusing the diagnostic work-up.

HISTORY

Site and Nature of Pain. Most upper abdominal organs such as stomach, duodenum, gallbladder, common bile duct, and pancreas are innervated by nerves from dermatome T6 to T10.[1] These organs are innervated bilaterally and therefore cause pain at or near the midline anteriorly. Pain from a gastric ulcer is located in the midline or slightly to the left in the epigastric region, whereas pain from an ulcer in the duodenal bulb may be slightly to the right of midline. Pain originating from the jejunum and the ileum, as seen in Crohn's disease, is often located in the midline near the umbilical region. Colonic pain is usually poorly localized and present in the lower mid-abdomen. Gallbladder or common bile duct pain is present in the mid-epigastric region or in the right upper quadrant and may radiate to the back. Visceral pain from these organs is often associated with other autonomic symptoms such as nausea or sweating. Pancreatic pain is usually a dull ache and can radiate to the back. Table 19-1 summarizes various causes of chronic abdominal pain.

Duration. Pain that lasts for several years without weight loss or other complications suggests irritable bowel syndrome. Persistent and worsening mid-abdominal pain that is present for several weeks or months with associated weight loss suggests cancer of the pancreas.

TABLE 19-1 Chronic Abdominal Pain

Clinical Diagnosis	Site of Pain	Description
Peptic ulcer	Epigastric region: right of midline = duodenal ulcer; left of midline = gastric ulcer	Gnawing pain, burning pain, hunger pain, nocturnal pain, relief with food and antacids
Biliary colic	Epigastric region, right upper quadrant radiating to back, interscapular region	Recurrent pain, rapid onset, severe intensity, duration of several hours, associated nausea and vomiting
Pancreatic carcinoma	Epigastric region, right or left of midline, band-like pain around abdomen	Anorexia and weight loss, constant pain, increasing severity, radiation to back
Chronic pancreatitis	Epigastric region, left of midline	Persistent or episodic pain, radiates to back, history of alcoholism
Crohn's disease	Umbilical region, right lower quadrant	Colicky pain, postprandial vomiting, weight loss
Chronic intestinal ischemia	Umbilical area	Postprandial pain 20 to 30 minutes after meals, lasts 60 to 90 minutes, weight loss
Irritable bowel syndrome[3]	Umbilical region, left lower quadrant, or diffuse pain	Diarrhea or constipation, longstanding symptoms, no nocturnal pain, no weight loss, negative diagnostic tests

Relationship to Meals—Aggravating and Relieving Factors. Relief of pain with ingestion of food suggests peptic ulcer disease. It is difficult to differentiate gastric ulcer from duodenal ulcer based on historical data alone. Colicky abdominal pain brought on by meals may indicate gallbladder disease, obstructing inflammatory bowel disease (e.g., Crohn's disease), or pyloric channel ulcer producing gastric outlet obstruction. In an elderly individual with diffuse vascular disease, mid-abdominal pain beginning 20 to 30 minutes after meals in association with weight loss may be caused by chronic intestinal ischemia. Relief of pain with use of antacids is seen in peptic ulcer disease. Pancreatic pain is often aggravated by lying supine and is partially relieved by bending forward. Crampy lower abdominal pain with tenesmus that is relieved by a bowel movement indicates a colonic source of pain.

Radiation. Radiation of abdominal pain to the back is seen with pancreatic disease, gallbladder disease, and disease of the common bile duct.

Associated Symptoms. A history of weight loss associated with abdominal pain should alert the physician to serious disease. In the elderly, malignancy such as pancreatic, gastric, or colonic carcinoma has to be considered. In the young, inflammatory bowel disease may be the etiologic cause.

The presence of hematochezia associated with abdominal pain can indicate colonic carcinoma or diverticulosis in the elderly. In the young, inflammatory bowel disease such as Crohn's disease may be responsible.

Alternating diarrhea and constipation in a young patient with abdominal pain suggests irritable bowel syndrome. In the middle-aged or elderly, however, the diagnosis of irritable bowel syndrome should not be entertained as a primary diagnosis unless investigations of the intestine have excluded neoplasms.

Vomiting associated with abdominal pain may indicate subacute intestinal obstruction, e.g., Crohn's disease, or gastric outlet obstruction, e.g., pyloric channel ulcer. Colicky pain caused by acute distension of the gallbladder, the common bile duct, or the renal pelvis and ureter can also produce vomiting attributable to autonomic stimuli

The presence of abdominal pain with menstrual bleeding may represent menstrual cramps or intra-abdominal bleeding caused by endometriosis.

Family and Personal History. The patient should be queried about a family history of peptic ulcer disease, gallstones, inflammatory bowel disease, and malignancy. A strong history of smoking in a patient with abdominal pain predisposes the patient to peptic ulcer disease and carcinoma of the pancreas. A history of alcoholism may indicate chronic pancreatitis as a cause for chronic abdominal pain.

PHYSICAL EXAMINATION

A physical examination may yield useful clues to the diagnosis of chronic abdominal pain. The presence of icterus and a palpable gallbladder (Courvoisier's sign) may indicate carcinoma in the head of the pancreas. The presence of arthritis and erythema nodosum is suggestive of inflammatory bowel disease. Diminished peripheral pulses and abdominal bruits are often detected in patients who are later diagnosed to have chronic intestinal ischemia. A palpable abdominal mass obviously aids in the diagnosis. The presence of occult blood in the stool should lead to a search for inflammatory or malignant lesions of the gastrointestinal tract.

DIAGNOSTIC TESTS AND PROCEDURES

When the history and physical examination suggests peptic ulcer disease as the most likely etiologic factor for abdominal pain, it is reasonable to attempt a therapeutic trial with H_2-blockers, e.g., cimetidine or ranitidine, before any further investigations are done. If the initial manifestations are atypical or of new onset in an elderly individual, an upper gastrointestinal (GI) endoscopy is the procedure of choice. Although this approach is more expensive than a roentgenogram of the stomach and duodenum, it is much more sensitive and specific than upper GI x-rays for the diagnosis of ulcer disease.[2] In addition, endoscopy allows a biopsy to be done in patients with gastric ulcers.

When biliary tract disease is being investigated, an ultrasound of the abdomen is the procedure of choice to diagnose gallstones because of its high sensitivity and lack of any radiation hazard. Ultrasound has mostly replaced the oral cholecystograms as the first procedure for diagnosis of gallstones. The test is also sensitive to detect obstruction of the biliary tree. Hepatobiliary scans, or liver and spleen scan, are of little use in the investigation of chronic abdominal pain. If stones in the common bile duct are suspected, the procedure of choice is an endoscopic retrograde cholangiogram because neither the ultrasound, the computed tomography (CT) scan, nor the intravenous cholangiogram are sensitive tests to diagnose common bile duct stones.

For neoplastic disease of the pancreas and retroperitoneum, CT scan of the abdomen, though expensive, is the most sensitive preferred primary diagnostic test. Ultrasound of the abdomen is also a good test; however, it is often unable to visualize the entire pancreas and may be limited because of technical problems. The use of ultrasound as a first test often necessitates a CT scan as a follow-up test, and therefore voids its cost advantage and lack of radiation.

TABLE 19-2 Diagnostic Procedures for Chronic Abdominal Pain

Clinical Suspicion	Condition	Diagnostic Test or Procedure
Stomach and duodenum	Peptic ulcer	Therapeutic trial or upper GI endoscopy
	Obstruction, e.g., pyloric obstruction	Upper GI x-ray with barium
Small intestine	Crohn's disease Obstruction Crohn's Tumors Adhesions	Upper GI x-ray and small bowel follow-through
Biliary tract	Gallbladder stone disease	Ultrasound of right upper quadrant
	Common duct stone	ERCP
Pancreas and retro-peritoneum[4]	Chronic pancreatitis	Flat plate abdomen-calcification and/or ERCP
	Carcinoma of pancreas	CT scan of abdomen and/or ERCP
Colonic disease	Diverticulosis Neoplasms	Barium enema Colonoscopy or flexible sigmoidoscopy and barium enema
	Inflammatory bowel disease	Colonoscopy

An endoscopic retrograde cholangio-pancreatography (ERCP) or a needle biopsy of the pancreas may be necessary to confirm diagnostic impressions on a CT scan. Table 19–2 summarizes diagnostic procedures for chronic abdominal pain.

References

1. Way LW. Abdominal pain. In: Sleisenger MH, Fordtran JS, eds. Gastrointestinal disease: pathophysiology, diagnosis, management. 3rd ed. Philadelphia: WB Saunders, 1983:207.
2. Wilson DI. Evaluation of patients with upper abdominal pain. Pract Gastroenterol 1984; Vol. VIII, 5:6–17.
3. Swarberick ET, et al. Site of pain from the irritable bowel. Lancet 1980; 2:443–446.
4. Currie DJ. Abdominal pain. New York: Hemisphere, 1979.

20 | UPPER GASTROINTESTINAL BLEEDING

KARIM A. FAWAZ, M.D.

Upper gastrointestinal bleeding (UGI bleeding) is a common, serious medical emergency. In spite of remarkable improvements in diagnostic techniques and accuracy in the determination of the bleeding site, UGI bleeding continues to carry a mortality rate of up to 10 to 20 percent.[1] The mortality rate increases with age and with the presence of other serious diseases. The diagnosis and management of such patients requires close cooperation among the internist, the surgeon, and the radiologist.

GENERAL REMARKS

The approach to a patient who presents with UGI bleeding depends on the general condition of the patient. The sequence of steps in the diagnosis and management of a patient with massive bleeding and shock is different than the sequence followed in a patient with melena for a few days without orthostatic hypotension. Although the diagnostic steps may be the same, the former scenario requires an immediate and vigorous approach with an emphasis on resuscitative measures that include (1) intravenous access adequate for rapid infusion of saline and blood products, (2) withdrawal of blood for typing, cross matching, and measurement of hemoglobin, hematocrit, platelets, prothrombin time, partial thromboplastin time, urea nitrogen, and creatinine. The primary goal of the physician in the treatment of such patients is the restoration of blood volume, regardless of the diagnosis. Initially either normal saline or Ringer's lactate may be used until blood is available. The use of albumin and plasma expanders is not necessary unless bleeding is continuous and massive and packed cells are not available. While replenishing the blood volume is the most important goal, care should be taken not to "over expand" the blood volume in elderly patients and in those at risk of congestive heart failure. In such patients, it is advisable to monitor central venous pressure (CVP) and to gauge fluid replacement accordingly.

The cardiovascular response to volume loss correlates with the rapidity and severity of blood loss, but is modified by age, medications, previous cardiovascular disease, and other associated diseases. A prompt examination of the pulse and blood pressure allows the physician to roughly estimate the magnitude of blood loss. In general, in an otherwise healthy person the following guidelines apply[2]: (1) a systolic blood pressure below 100 mm Hg or a pulse above 100 beats per minute indicates a 20 percent volume loss, (2) an increase in the pulse of 20 beats per minute or a decrease in the blood pressure of more than 10 mm Hg in response to a postural change indicates a 20 percent volume loss.

These measurements should be repeated frequently while saline is being administered. Caution, however, should be exercised in performing postural signs in the elderly because such maneuvers may precipitate a cerebrovascular ischemic attack.

After a quick examination is performed to estimate blood loss, and after vigorous saline and blood administration have restored the blood pressure and pulse to normal, a nasogastric (NG) tube should be introduced and the stomach contents aspirated. Aspiration of the stomach contents serves several purposes: (1) it identifies the site of bleeding, (2) it provides a more accurate index about the rate of blood loss, (3) it establishes whether bleeding continues or has stopped, and (4) it prevents aspiration, a known complication of UGI bleeding, especially in the elderly.

There are some controversies regarding the use of nasogastric tubes in UGI bleeding. Should a nasogastric tube be introduced in a patient who is suspected of having bleeding esophageal varices? Does gastric lavage help stop bleeding? If gastric lavage is to be done, what type of fluid should be used and at what temperature? Most gastroenterologists believe that the presence of esophageal varices is not a contraindication to a nasogastric tube since there is no evidence that the tube initiates or prolongs bleeding. Gastric lavage is performed as a force of habit, rather than on the basis of objective data. It is empirically believed that lavage with cold fluids helps to stop the bleeding, but no such data exist. Further, there is no evidence that saline is superior to tap water, nor is there evidence that cold fluid is superior to room temperature fluid. My personal bias is to perform gastric lavage with tap water initially in order to know whether bleeding persists, and prior to diagnostic endoscopy in order to have a clearer view.

Measurement of hemoglobin and hematocrit on admission and in 6 to 12 hours is essential to follow the progress of a bleeding patient. Initial values are often misleadingly high, however, because compensatory physiologic mechanisms to reestablish intravascular volume, such as the release of aldosterone and antidiuretic hormone, lag behind. The initial level of hemoglobin and hematocrit do not fall because the blood lost has the same concentration of red blood cells as the blood remaining. The fall in these measurements with time is often the consequence of hemodilution secondary to saline or to ingested fluid.

The measurement of platelets, prothrombin time, and partial thrombo-plastin time is important in order to rule out a bleeding diathesis. The bleeding disorder could be primary or could be secondary to medications, liver disease, consumption coagulopathy, or autoimmune disease.

HISTORY AND PHYSICAL EXAMINATION

After resuscitative measures are instituted and the patient is relatively stable, a detailed history should be taken and a physical examination performed. A history of drug intake, such as salicylates, nonsteroidal anti-inflammatory agents, anticoagulants, and antineoplastic drugs, should be taken. A history of previously known diseases such as alcoholism, chronic liver disease, blood dyscrasias, neoplasm, and arthritis may help in narrowing the differential diagnosis. The following findings are of high diagnostic value:

1. Hematemesis indicates bleeding above the ligament of Treitz; however, patients with bleeding duodenal ulcers may present with melena only.
2. Hematemesis shortly after forceful vomiting should raise the possibility of a Mallory-Weiss tear.
3. A history of epigastric distress and pain for several days prior to bleeding suggests peptic ulcer disease or gastritis.
4. Trauma, burns, or surgery hours to days prior to bleeding suggest stress ulcerations as the cause of bleeding.
5. Previous surgical procedures, such as partial gastrectomy, raise the possibility of an anastomotic ulcer.
6. Dysphagia suggests esophageal lesions such as esophagitis, esophageal ulcer, or carcinoma.
7. The presence of signs of portal hypertension, such as splenomegaly, ascites, abdominal collateral circulation, and spider nevi, suggests the possibility of bleeding esophageal varices.
8. Examination of the skin, mucous membranes, and finger tips is important for the diagnosis of hereditary hemorrhagic telangiectasia, Peutz-Jeghers syndrome, and blue rubber bleb nevus. All of the preceding may present with bleeding.

THE ROLE OF ENDOSCOPY IN UGI BLEEDING

UGI endoscopy has been proven to be the quickest and most accurate means of finding the source of UGI bleeding. In controlled trials the diagnostic yield of UGI endoscopy is 75 to 90 percent, while the yield for barium x-rays is

20 to 50 percent.[3,4] Since earlier and more accurate diagnosis is provided by endoscopy, one might expect a reduction in the mortality rate of UGI bleeding. Unfortunately, controlled studies have failed to show a difference in mortality rate between patients undergoing routine early endoscopy and those who do not.[5] Thus, while giant strides have been made by endoscopy towards accurate diagnosis, treatment of UGI bleeding remains inadequate and lags behind. Newer medications, such as H_2-blockers, are not effective in the treatment of mucosal UGI bleeding. Other medications, such as prostaglandins, are being investigated. Heater and bipolar probes and laser treatment via endoscopy are promising, but the final verdict on such invasive endoscopic procedures is not yet in.

The fact that endoscopy does not reduce mortality does not mean that the procedure should be abandoned. For instance, endoscopic sclerosis of varices is effective in treating bleeding esophageal varices. Endoscopy remains the first and, usually, the only diagnostic procedure that is performed. When should endoscopy be performed? Recent studies have shown that there is no significant difference between the yield of emergency endoscopy and that done within 24 to 48 hours of admission. However, when endoscopy is performed beyond 48 hours, the diagnostic yield declines significantly. Endoscopy should be performed on a more emergent basis when bleeding is suspected to be from esophageal varices because treatment hinges on the correct diagnosis.

Although there is agreement on the diagnostic value of endoscopy, there are situations when it is relatively contraindicated. An endoscopy performed on a patient with massive, active hematemesis may cause aspiration without identifying the source of bleeding (because of inadequate visualization). Endoscopy also is not indicated in an elderly patient with severe hypoxic pulmonary disease who has recently been diagnosed to have a duodenal ulcer. The risk of performing endoscopy in such situations often outweighs the benefit.

RADIOLOGY

Three diagnostic radiologic techniques are useful in patients with gastrointestinal bleeding: radionuclide imaging, barium x-rays, and angiography. I follow the scheme illustrated in Figure 20–1 for the evaluation of patients with UGI bleeding.

Radionuclide Imaging

This technique is the least invasive and the most useful in lower gastrointestinal bleeding. Its yield in UGI bleeding is low, and therefore, radionuclide imaging is rarely used in UGI bleeding.

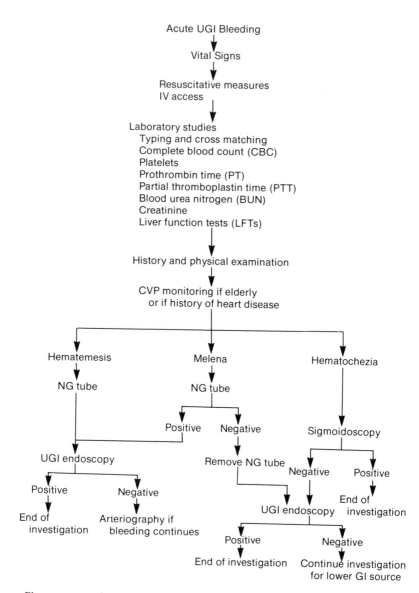

Figure 20-1 Schema for the investigation of a patient with upper gastrointestinal bleeding.

Barium X-rays

Barium studies are inferior to endoscopy in UGI bleeding. In addition, the use of barium has some disadvantages. First, endoscopy or angiography performed soon after a negative barium study is difficult because barium coats the mucosa and adequate visualization is precluded. Second, a barium study may show only one of two coexisting lesions, and that lesion may not be the bleeding site. In general, a barium study is indicated only when endoscopy is contraindicated and active bleeding has ceased.

Angiography

The development of better endoscopic techniques and equipment has led to a marked decline in the use of angiography in UGI bleeding. Studies have demonstrated that peripheral infusion of vasopressin (antidiuretic hormone [ADH]) is as effective as selective arterial infusion of ADH, and have thus further reduced the need for angiography. In general, I reserve angiography for situations where endoscopy is contraindicated or has failed to reveal the source of bleeding, yet active bleeding continues.

INCIDENCE OF THE VARIOUS CAUSES OF UGI BLEEDING

The incidence of the various causes of UGI bleeding varies from one hospital to another and depends on the type of patients the hospital caters to and attracts. Table 20–1 provides a list of the possible sources of UGI bleeding.

In a review and analysis of 2,014 patients with UGI bleeding, Domschke reported the following incidence of endoscopically diagnosed sources of bleeding:[6] gastric and stomal ulcers, 25.1 percent; duodenal ulcer, 24 percent; esophageal and gastric varices, 18.1 percent; Mallory-Weiss tear, 10 percent; esophagitis, 9.5 percent; gastric erosions, 9.1 percent; gastric neoplasm, 3.8 percent; Osler-Weber-Rendu disease and telangiectasia, 0.4 percent. These figures seem representative, but in my experience in an inner city, tertiary care hospital, the incidence of bleeding from gastritis and gastric erosions is higher and that from Mallory-Weiss tear is lower.

In the following discussion, I will concentrate on the diagnosis and management of the most common sources of bleeding.

TABLE 20-1   Sources of UGI Bleeding

Mucosal disease
  Duodenal ulcer and duodenitis
  Gastric ulcer and gastritis
  Stomal or anastomotic ulcer
  Superficial stress ulcers or erosions

Vascular
  Varices: esophageal, gastric, and upper intestinal
  Vascular malformations
  Telangiectasia
  Mesenteric ischemia
  Vasculitis
  Postbypass aortoduodenal fistula

Mechanical or traumatic
  Mallory-Weiss tear
  Strangulated hiatus hernia
  Hemobilia
  External trauma

Neoplasia
  Benign
    Polyps
    Leiomyoma
  Malignant
    Carcinoma
    Melanoma
    Lymphoma
    Leiomyosarcoma

Miscellaneous
  Blood dyscrasia
  Iatrogenic anticoagulation
  Uremia
  Radiation enteritis
  Intestinal lymphangiectasia
  Parasitic infection, e.g., strongyloidiasis

Ulcer Disease

The presentation and management of ulcer disease at any site in the upper gastrointestinal tract are similar. Typical epigastric pain of ulcer disease may preceed bleeding for days or weeks. When bleeding occurs, however, the pain usually disappears because blood is a good buffering agent. Bleeding gastric ulcers more commonly result in hematemesis and melena, while melena alone more commonly results from duodenal ulcers. A negative (for blood) nasogastric tube aspirate eliminates the presence of a bleeding gastric ulcer, but not of a duodenal ulcer. In some instances, a competent pylorus prevents regurgitation of blood into the stomach; the nasogastric tube aspirate thus remains negative for blood. These patients obviously present with melena or hematochezia only.

The diagnosis of ulcer is best achieved by endoscopy. In addition to its accuracy, endoscopy provides valuable information regarding the likelihood of recurrent bleeding. The finding of what endoscopists refer to as a "visible vessel" is associated with a high incidence of recurrence of bleeding during the same hospitalization. Storey reported a 56 percent incidence of rebleeding in patients with a visible vessel compared to 8 percent in patients without a visible vessel.[7]

Regardless of the site, the treatment of bleeding ulcers is the same. We clinically refer to acid-neutralizing agents (antacids), acid-reducing agents (H_2-blockers), and ulcer-coating agents (sucralfate) as treatment. However, there is considerable doubt if they play any role in stopping bleeding or in preventing its recurrence. Fortunately, the majority of bleeding ulcers cease bleeding spontaneously. Anticholinergics are contraindicated.

Since pharmacologic treatment is ineffective, investigators have moved on to more invasive techniques to stop bleeding in an attempt to avoid surgery. These investigative techniques all use some form of electrocoagulation via endoscopy, such as heater and bipolary probes and laser treatment. Although preliminary results seem promising, these methods cannot currently be recommended because of the lack of convincing data and the paucity of technical expertise.

Surgical intervention is the last resort in the treatment of bleeding ulcers. However, the surgical service should be consulted on admission. Close cooperation between the medical and surgical teams is imperative, especially if a visible vessel is seen on endoscopy. No general rule exists as to when to intervene surgically. Although one hopes to avoid surgery, the decision should not be delayed until the patient is moribund. In general, in an otherwise healthy individual, I suggest surgery in the patient whose blood requirement has exceeded 10 units in 24 hours and in the patient who rebleeds during the same hospitalization and whose initial endoscopy showed a visible vessel.

Gastritis and Gastric Erosions

While epigastric pain may be a prominant symptom in ulcer disease prior to bleeding, pain is much less common in patients who have gastritis or gastric erosions. The offending agents or situations that are usually associated with this condition are alcohol, salicylates, nonsteroidal anti-inflammatory agents, stress, neurologic and/or neurosurgical insults, and possibly steroids. A careful history and immediate discontinuation of any potentially offending agent are mandatory. The diagnosis is made by endoscopy; barium x-rays usually miss these superficial lesions.

The treatment of gastritis and gastric erosions, as for ulcer disease, is unproven. Electrocoagulation holds less promise because the lesions are multiple and diffuse. Intravenous vasopressin has been used, but with mixed results. Care should be taken with vasopressin use in the elderly because of possible complications, such as coronory and cerebral vasoconstriction. Surgery should be avoided, if possible, especially when the erosions are in the fundus or are diffuse because the operative procedure increases in magnitude and in risk.

Mallory-Weiss Tear

The most common setting for a Mallory-Weiss tear is in the alcoholic who develops hematemesis after vomiting forcefully. However, neither alcoholism nor initial nonbloody vomitus is a requirement for its presence. In one study of 40 patients with this lesion, 17 (42 percent) had an associated hiatus hernia.[8]

Endoscopy is the diagnostic method of choice. The tears are usually seen in the gastric side of the gastroesophageal junction, especially if there is an associated hiatus hernia. The tear also may extend to the distal esophagus. Medical treatment for this lesion is limited. Fortunately, most patients stop bleeding spontaneously. Intravenous vasopressin has been shown to be effective in case reports and is worth trying before surgery in the minority of patients whose bleeding does not cease spontaneously. Medical treatment is successful in more than 80 percent of cases. Surgical treatment consists of oversewing the laceration.

Bleeding Varices

Bleeding from varices is one of the most serious complications of portal hypertension. Esophageal varices are the most common site of bleeding; however, gastric varices and varices along the rest of the intestinal tract may bleed. Most patients suffer from cirrhosis, but extrahepatic causes, such as portal and splenic vein thrombosis and Budd-Chiari syndrome, are also possible. A history of chronic alcoholism and other chronic liver diseases, as well as signs of portal hypertension (e.g., splenomegaly, ascites, abdominal collateral veins, and spider nevi) should alert the physician to varices as the possible source of bleeding. However, it should not be assumed that every bleeding, cirrhotic patient is actually bleeding from varices. Endoscopy has demonstrated that, even when esophageal or gastric varices are present, 50 percent of cirrhotic patients bleed from other causes, such as gastritis, duodenitis, a Mallory-Weiss tear, peptic ulcer, or esophagitis. Because of this observation (and the resulting difference in management) urgent endoscopy is indicated in patients with cirrhosis and UGI bleeding.

The initial treatment of bleeding varices is not different from any other type of UGI bleeding. However, because of the high incidence of coagulopathy associated with severe liver disease, the need for fresh frozen plasma and platelets is much more common.

Several specific means of treatment for bleeding varices are available, such as intravenous or selective arterial vasopressin infusion, balloon tamponade, percutaneous transhepatic embolization, endoscopic sclerotherapy, and emergency portal decompression surgery. None of these therapies except surgery provides a predictable and consistent lasting effect, not even for the length of the same hospitalization. However, emergency surgery carries a mortality rate of 80 percent. Endoscopic sclerotherapy probably helps in the prevention of rebleeding on a long-term basis, but only after several sessions. Its role in stopping acute bleeding is questionable at present.

I generally adhere to the following plan when treating variceal bleeding.

1. If bleeding is stopped or decreased by the first attempt of endoscopic sclerotherapy, another treatment is undertaken 5 to 7 days later and then every 2 to 4 weeks until obliteration of the varices is accomplished.
2. If massive bleeding continues, a continuous infusion of 0.2 to 0.4 units of vasopressin per minute is started. If bleeding does not cease after vasopressin, a Sengstaken-Blakemore tube is introduced and balloon tamponade is attempted. If all the preceding efforts fail and if bleeding remains massive, thus precluding any endoscopic sclerotherapy, then emergency surgery is the last resort. If any of these medical therapeutic modalities stops bleeding or decreases it enough to allow adequate endoscopic visualization, then endoscopic sclerotherapy should be attempted.

References

1. Schiller KFR, Colton PB. Acute upper gastrointestinal haemorrhage. Clin Gastroenterol 1978, 7:595–604.
2. Law HD, Watts DH. Gastrointestinal disease. Philadelphia: WB Saunders, 1978:219.
3. Hoare AM. Comparative study between endoscopy and radiology in acute upper gastrointestinal haemorrhage. Br Med J 1975; 1:27–30.
4. McGinn FP, Guyer PB, Wilken BJ, Steer HW. A prospective comparative trial between early endoscopy and radiology in acute upper gastrointestinal haemorrhage. Gut 1975; 16:707–713.

5. Peterson WL, Barnett CC, Smith HJ, Allen MH, Corbett DB. Routine early endoscopy in upper-gastrointestinal-tract bleeding: a randomized controlled trial. N Engl J Med 1981; 304:925–929.
6. Domschke W, Lederer P, Lux G. The value of endoscopy in upper gastrointestinal bleeding: review and analysis of 2,014 cases. Endoscopy 1983; 15:126–131.
7. Storey DW, Bown SG, Swain CP, Salmon PR, Kirsham JS, Northfield TC. Endoscopic predication of recurrent bleeding in peptic ulcers. N Engl J Med 1981; 305(16):915–916.
8. Michel L, Serrano A, Malt RA. Mallory-Weiss syndrome: evaluation of diagnostic and therapeutic patterns over two decades. Ann Surg 1980; 192(6):716–721.

21 | RECURRENT LOWER GASTROINTESTINAL BLEEDING

KARIM A. FAWAZ, M.D.

Lower gastrointestinal bleeding, a serious and life-threatening condition, can have a wide variety of causes (Table 21–1). Many of these causes (e.g., inflammation, infection, and neoplasm) are relatively easy to diagnose by sigmoidoscopy, colonoscopy, barium x-rays, stool cultures, and stool microscopy. These conditions will not be discussed. Rather, I will focus in this chapter on the difficult problem of *recurrent* lower gastrointestinal bleeding. A definitive diagnosis usually cannot be made either on initial presentation or during subsequent episodes of bleeding. In spite of marked improvement in our diagnostic tools, most gastroenterologists are haunted by a small cadre of patients with recurrent episodes of lower gastrointestinal bleeding of unknown cause. The fact that most of these patients are elderly and do not tolerate major bleeds well makes the problem more serious and frustrating.

RESUSCITATIVE MEASURES

The initial resuscitative measures for patients with lower gastrointestinal bleeding are the same as for patients with upper gastrointestinal (UGI) bleeding (see *Upper Gastrointestinal Bleeding*).

DIAGNOSIS

The history is extremely helpful in the diagnosis of lower GI bleeding. For instance, a history of tenesmus, abdominal cramping, and diarrhea suggests an inflammatory or infectious etiology. A history of radiation therapy for cancer suggests radiation enteritis. However, in patients with recurrent lower GI bleeding, likely causes are diverticulosis, vascular lesions, and Meckel's diverticulum and history is not helpful. No historical features distinguish these lesions.

I generally follow the schematic plan in Figure 21–1 when investigating a patient with lower gastrointestinal bleeding. I will discuss only diverticulosis (including Meckel's) and vascular lesions (angiodysplasia).

TABLE 21-1 Causes of Lower
Gastrointestinal Bleeding

Diverticulosis

Vascular
    Vascular malformation
    Angiodysplasia
    Vascular ischemia
    Hemorrhoids and fissures
    Ileal and colonic varices
    Vasculitis

Inflammatory bowel disease
    Ulcerative colitis
    Crohn's disease

Infection
    Bacterial
    Parasitic
    Viral
    Toxic

Neoplasm
    Benign
        Polyps
        Leiomyoma
    Malignant
        Carcinoma
        Lymphoma
        Melanoma
        Leiomyosarcoma

Radiation enteritis

Miscellaneous
    Blood dyscrasias
    Meckel's diverticulum
    Solitary rectal ulcer

Diverticulosis

Colonic diverticula are especially common in the older age group. Autopsy studies have shown an incidence of up to 50 percent in patients over the age of 60 years.[1] Diverticula are uncommon under the age of 30 years. Left-sided diverticula are more common than right-sided by a ratio of 10:1. It is important to stress two points in relation to diverticular bleeding. (1) Diverticulitis may be associated with guaiac-positive stools, but rarely presents with massive lower gastrointestinal bleeding. (2) Bleeding from right-sided diverticula is more common than from left-sided diverticula. This observation is in contrast to diverticulitis, which almost always is left-sided.

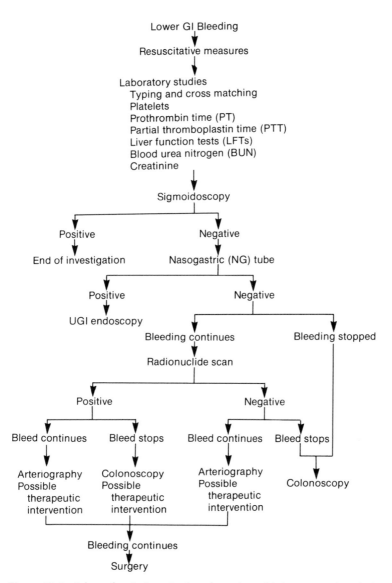

Figure 21-1 Schema for the investigation of a patient with lower gastrointestinal bleeding.

There is some difference of opinion on the diagnostic method of choice in the evaluation of diverticular bleeding, but all investigators agree that it is *not* a barium enema. A barium enema shows diverticula very nicely, but does not identify the bleeding diverticulum. In addition, barium tends to be retained in diverticula, thereby making subsequent tests such as colonoscopy and arteriography difficult to interpret. A barium enema should be performed later in the hospital course to search for colonic lesions other than the identified site of bleeding.

In acute diverticular bleeding colonoscopy also is of little value. During active bleeding, colonoscopy should not be performed because of inadequate visualization of the colon. Colonoscopy may be performed when bleeding stops, but blood, like barium, tends to be retained in diverticula, and identification of the specific bleeding diverticulum is difficult. Radionuclide scanning may help to diagnose the location of the bleeding site, but not the cause of the bleeding.

If conventional barium x-rays, radionuclide scanning, and direct visualization by colonoscopy all are of little use, what diagnostic tool should we use? I strongly believe that selective angiography is the diagnostic test of choice. In addition to its diagnostic superiority, angiography has a potential therapeutic role. Selective arterial infusion of vasopressin has been shown (by angiography) to stop diverticular bleeding.[2]

If bleeding does not respond to vasopressin and remains massive, i.e., greater than 10 units per 24 hours, surgery is indicated. Some investigators believe that selective surgery is indicated after the first massive diverticular bleed, even if the bleeding stops, because of the high incidence (25 to 50 percent) of rebleeding. I do not agree with this opinion.

If arteriography is so accurate, why do many patients with diverticular bleeds remain undiagnosed? The main reason is that, in order to make the diagnosis angiographically, the patient has to be actively bleeding at a rate that exceeds 0.4 ml per minute. Many patients stop bleeding spontaneously before arteriography is carried out, and others bleed in an erratic fashion, thereby eluding diagnosis. Angiography must be done urgently in the patient admitted to hospital with a third or more episode of recurrent lower GI bleeding.

Angiodysplasia

Angiodysplasia, an acquired localized vascular lesion, occurs mainly in the right side of the colon and the distal ileum and can be single or multiple. Histologically, the lesion consists of ectatic submucosal capillaries or veins. There is a strong correlation between angiodysplasia and aging and a weaker association between angiodysplasia and aortic stenosis.

The diagnosis of angiodysplasia can be made by angiography and colonoscopy. In the undiagnosed patient with recurrent lower GI bleeding, angiography is preferable for the reasons discussed in the section on diverticulosis. Again, barium enema is not helpful except to eliminate other lesions. Radionuclide scanning may localize the site of bleeding and aid the angiographer to selectively catheterize the artery suspected of feeding the angiodysplasia.

The treatment of angiodysplasia is endoscopic or surgical. If the bleeding stops and if the angiodysplasia can be identified via colonoscopy, then cauterization with a heater probe, biopolar probe, or laser should be attempted. If bleeding does not stop, then surgical intervention is indicated.

Angiodysplasia is a difficult entity to treat because it may be multiple with a different site of bleeding on different occasions and because it has a tendency to recur, even after surgical resection.

References

1. Hughes LE. Post mortem survey of diverticular disease of the colon. Gut 1969; 10:336–344.
2. Baum S, Rosch J, Dotter CT. Selective mesenteric arterial infusions in the management of massive diverticular hemorrhage. N Engl J Med 1973; 288:1269–1271.

22 | ACUTE DIARRHEA

KARIM A. FAWAZ, M.D.

Diarrhea may be defined in qualitative terms, in which case the consistency and frequency of stools are taken into consideration, or in quantitative terms, where stool volume or weight is measured. The qualitative definition may be misleading because it depends on subjective interpretation by the patient. The quantitative definition considers an individual stool volume of more than 200 ml as diarrhea. To ascertain the presence of true diarrhea is more of a problem in patients who complain of chronic, rather than acute, diarrhea. For the purposes of this discussion, acute diarrhea will be defined as a sudden change in stool consistency that results in liquid stool with a significant increase in stool volume.

THE ROLE OF HISTORY

A detailed history and a complete physical examination are crucial in the differential diagnosis of the various causes of acute diarrhea listed in Table 22-1.

TABLE 22-1   Causes of Acute Diarrhea

Infectious Causes	Noninfectious Causes
Bacterial causes	Inflammatory bowel disease
E. coli	Ulcerative colitis
Shigella	Crohn's disease
Salmonella	
Staphylococcus	Ischemic colitis
Campylobactor	
Yersinia	Lactase deficiency
Clostridium difficile	
	Drugs
Viral causes	Laxatives
Norwalk virus	Antacids
Rotavirus	Antibiotics
	Antimetabolites
Parasitic causes	
Giardia	Acute radiation injury
Ameba	
Cryptosporidium	Mechanical causes
	Fecal impaction
	Partial small bowel
	obstruction

Key questions asked should pertain to the following:

Recent Travel. A history of recent travel to a foreign country suggests an infectious cause for the diarrhea. *E. coli* is the most common offender in traveler's diarrhea, but other bacterial agents, giardiasis, and amebiasis also should be considered.

Recent Restaurant Meal or Intake of Creamy Pastry. This history usually suggests staphylococcus or salmonella gastroenteritis, the illness being caused by a toxin released from that bacteria. The likelihood of this diagnosis is even higher if other members of the family or friends become afflicted at the same time.

Medications. Many drugs can cause diarrhea and the following are some common examples: laxatives, magnesium-containing antacids, digoxin, quinidine, chemotherapeutic agents, and antibiotics, especially penicillin derivatives. The effect of the drug is usually immediate. On the other hand, antibiotic-associated colitis (pseudomembranous colitis) may occur while the patient is receiving an antibiotic such as ampicillin or clindamycin, but it also may present several days to weeks after cessation of therapy.

Radiation Treatment. Acute diarrhea may occur secondary to mucosal sloughing from acute radiation injury. Acute radiation diarrhea follows closely after treatment, unlike the diarrhea secondary to mesenteric vascular injury that may occur months later.

Heart Disease. Patients with congestive heart failure, especially those on diuretic therapy, are prone to develop acute ischemic colitis with bloody diarrhea secondary to a "low-flow" state.

Tenesmus. The presence of this symptom usually indicates rectal involvement. It is a common symptom in inflammatory bowel disease and in infections involving the distal colon.

Bloody Diarrhea. The presence of bloody diarrhea indicates mucosal inflammation and should direct the physician's attention towards inflammatory bowel disease and organisms that cause inflammation or ulceration, such as *Shigella, Campylobactor, Salmonella,* ameba, and *C. difficile*.

Change in Eating Habits. This is a question that is rarely asked by a physician when seeing a patient with acute diarrhea. It is an important question to ask, however, because the answer may prevent a long and expensive diagnostic investigation. Postoperative patients are often put on a liquid diet rich in dairy products. Because some of these patients have a lactase deficiency that they are not aware of, diarrhea develops. I also have seen many patients who have been advised by old timers or by friends that milk is good for their ulcer pain. Large amounts of milk are consumed, thus unmasking lactase deficiency and causing diarrhea.

Rectal Intercourse. Diarrhea occurring after rectal intercourse should direct the physician's attention to infections such as gonorrhea, shigellosis, amebiasis, giardiasis, and *Chlamydia* and *Campylobactor* infections.

Extraintestinal Manifestations of Inflammatory Bowel Diseases. Diarrhea associated with joint pain, iridoscleritis, or skin eruptions such as erythema nodosum and pyoderma gangrenosum suggests the presence of inflammatory bowel disease.

Questions in these ten simple areas help the physician to decide which diagnostic tests, if any, should be ordered and in what sequence. In many instances, however, the patient recovers by the time the diagnosis is made. Detailed investigation need not be done in patients with mild diarrhea until the diarrhea lasts for longer than 2 to 3 weeks.

DIAGNOSTIC TESTS

To reach the correct diagnosis in a patient with an acute diarrheal illness usually requires results from four tests: stool microscopy, stool culture, endoscopic visualization with or without biopsy, and x-ray studies. Not all patients need to undergo all these tests. Furthermore, if barium studies are planned they should be performed last because barium interferes with the detection of ova and parasites for 2 to 3 weeks. In addition, patients with suspected acute severe colitis have a relative contraindication to a barium enema because of the danger of precipitation of toxic megacolon.

In the following discussion I will focus on the clinical presentation, diagnosis, and management of the more common causes of acute diarrhea in adults.

BACTERIAL INFECTION

Bacterial infections, the most common causes of acute diarrhea, are usually caused by contaminated food or water. Acute diarrhea that develops in association with travel to developing countries is referred to as "traveler's diarrhea" and is caused by bacterial infection in the majority of cases.

Escherichia Coli Diarrhea. Most strains of *E. coli* are harmless. However, some strains are pathogenic, such as enteropathic *E. coli*, which are common causes of diarrhea in neonates and infants, and enterotoxigenic *E. coli*, which are responsible for diarrhea in 45 to 85 percent of cases of traveler's diarrhea.[1,2] The diarrhea, usually nonbloody, is associated with abdominal cramps. Systemic manifestations of fever and chills are not common. The incubation period is 2 to 3 days. The diagnosis of *E. coli* diarrhea is not easy to make since it is a normal finding in stool cultures. A presumptive diagnosis may be made if the stool culture grows pure *E. coli*; otherwise special culture techniques are needed to differentiate pathogenic from nonpathogenic strains.

Specific treatment is not necessary in most instances because this illness is usually self-limiting, lasting only a few days. Adequate hydration should be maintained, and nonspecific antidiarrheal agents, such as loperamide or bismuth subsalicylate, may be used if the diarrhea is bothersome. When symptoms are severe and disabling, antibiotic therapy with trimethoprim-sulfamethoxazole (two double-strength tablets) for 3 to 5 days is effective.

Recently, epidemic outbreaks as well as sporadic cases of hemorrhagic colitis associated with *E. coli* strain O157:H7 have been reported.[3] This illness is much more severe than the usual *E. coli* diarrhea and is associated with systemic manifestations and mucosal damage causing bloody diarrhea.

Shigellosis. Shigellosis, referred to as bacillary dysentery, is the cause of diarrhea in 15 to 22 percent of traveler's diarrhea. The incubation period may be as short as 24 hours. The clinical presentation includes abdominal cramping, fever, and diarrhea that often becomes bloody. Fecal leukocytes are present. The findings on sigmoidoscopy depend on the severity of the disease and are indistinguishable from those of idiopathic ulcerative colitis. The diagnosis is made by stool culture.

There is controversy on whether antibiotic treatment is indicated in mild cases of shigellosis. Most investigators agree that severe cases should be treated. The antibiotics of choice are ampicillin (2 g daily for 5 to 7 days) and trimethoprim-sulfamethoxazole (two double-strength tablets for 5 to 7 days). Nonspecific antidiarrheal drugs such as loperamide and diphenoxylate, which act by delaying intestinal motility, should be used with caution because they may prolong the illness by increasing the time of contact between the bacteria and the colon and may precipitate a toxic megacolon in severe cases.

Salmonellosis. *Salmonella* may cause gastroenteritis, typhoid fever, and bacteremia. Our discussion will be limited to salmonella gastroenteritis, which has an incubation period of 12 to 36 hours. *Salmonella* is cultured in 4 to 5 percent of cases of traveler's diarrhea and is a common cause of epidemic forms of gastroenteritis. It is usually a self-limiting illness characterized by abdominal cramps and diarrhea that may become bloody. Systemic manifestations of fever, chills, and headache may be present. Leukocytosis is common, but blood cultures are negative. Sigmoidoscopy may show colitis that cannot be distinguished from idiopathic ulcerative colitis. Diagnosis is established by stool culture. Specific treatment with antibiotics is not indicated; symptomatic treatment and adequate hydration are sufficient.

Campylobacter Enteritis. Campylobacter enteritis recently has emerged as a common cause of acute diarrhea. Most clinical laboratories now look (and should) for *Campylobacter* in addition to *Salmonella* and *Shigella* in routine stool cultures. The clinical picture is that of diarrhea, abdominal pain, and fever; bloody diarrhea occurs in 46 percent of the cases.[4] The stools are positive for fecal leukocytes, and sigmoidoscopy again reveals a colitis indistinguishable from ulcerative colitis. The illness may last longer than salmonella and shigella infection, but is similar in that it is self-limiting in most instances. The diagnosis is made by a positive stool culture. Again, antibiotic treatment is not necessary in most cases, but when the illness is severe or lasts for greater than 7 days, erythromycin (250 mg three times daily for 7 days) should be administered.

Clostridium Difficile Colitis. Many antibiotics cause *C. difficile* colitis, but the most frequent offenders are ampicillin, clindamycin, and cephalosporins. The clinical presentation is the same as with the other bacterial diarrheas. The illness may commence during the course of antibiotic treatment and up to 3 months after cessation of therapy. Sigmoidoscopy may be normal or may resemble ulcerative colitis. The most characteristic finding is the presence of membranous plaques and hence the term pseudomembranous colitis. The diagnosis is made by a positive *C. difficile* stool toxin assay or a positive stool culture. Specific treatment is indicated in this illness; the agents of choice are metronidazole (500 mg three times daily for 7 days) and vancomycin (125 mg four times daily for 7 days).

PARASITIC INFECTION

Giardiasis. *Giardia*, a common cause of diarrhea, is responsible for 3 percent of traveler's diarrhea.[1,2] The most common symptom is diarrhea that is never bloody. Abdominal pain and malabsorption are more common in children. There is an association with dysgammaglobulinemia, especially in IgA deficiency. The diagnosis is made by stool microscopy, duodenal aspiration, or duodenal biopsy. A negative stool examination does not rule out giardiasis because up to 50 percent of cases with a positive duodenal aspirate have a negative stool microscopy.[5] Sigmoidoscopy is negative. Specific treatment is indicated and consists of metronidazole (250 mg three times daily for 7 days) or quinacrine (100 mg three times daily for 7 days).

Amebiasis. Amebiasis may be acute or chronic. Its clinical manifestations vary from an asymptomatic carrier state to severe colitis. The acute form of colitis is similar to ulcerative colitis and bacterial diarrheas discussed earlier. Sigmoidoscopy is helpful when typical discrete ulcers with undermined edges are present, but this picture is not universally present. Trophozoites may be obtained by scraping the base of the ulcers suspected. A serum test for amebic titer by indirect hemagglutination is an adjunct to diagnosis. Specific treatment is indicated and consists of metronidazole (750 mg three times daily for 7–20 days). Diiodohydroxyquin (650 mg three times daily for 20 days) is the treatment for asymptomatic carriers in combination with metronidazole in severe cases.

INFLAMMATORY BOWEL DISEASE

Patients with ulcerative colitis and Crohn's disease may present acutely or have a more insidious presentation. When the initial presentation is acute, it must be differentiated from infectious colitis. The clinical and sigmoidoscopic picture may be the same, but the presence of extraintestinal manifestations, such as arthralgia, arthritis, erythema nodosum, pyoderma gangrenosum, and associated liver disease, suggests inflammatory bowel disease.

In ulcerative colitis only the colon is involved and the rectum is always involved. The disease is diffuse and continuous without "skip" segments. In contrast, Crohn's disease may involve the small or large intestines. The rectum may be spared and "skip" areas of normal mucosa may be present. The diagnosis is established by a process of elimination of specific causes of colitis. Colonic biopsies may be helpful, but are not specific. Involvement of the small intestine favors the diagnosis of Crohn's disease. Treatment depends on the type, severity, and location of the disease. The drugs used are steroids, sulfasalazine, azathioprine, purinethol, and metronidazole.

References

1. DuPont HL, Reves RR, Galindo E, et al. Treatment of travelers' diarrhea with trimethoprim/sulfamethoxazole and with trimethoprim alone. N Engl J Med 1982; 307(14):841–844.
2. Johnson PC, DuPont HL, Ericsson CD. Travelers' diarrhea — common misconceptions. Pract Gastroenterol 1985; 9(3):14–18, 38–40.
3. Remis RS, MacDonald KL, Lee WR, et al. Sporadic cases of hemorrhagic colitis associated with *Escherichia coli* 0157:H7. Ann Intern Med 1984; 101:624–626.
4. Blaser MJ, Wells JG, Feldman RH, et al. Campylobacter enteritis in the United States. Ann Intern Med 1983; 98:360–365.
5. Ament ME, Rulin CE. Relation of giardiasis to abnormal intestinal structure and function in gastrointestinal immunodeficiency syndromes. Gastroenterology 1972; 62:216–226.

23 | CHRONIC DIARRHEA

KARIM A. FAWAZ, M.D.

Chronic diarrhea is defined as recurrent diarrhea or diarrhea that lasts for more than 3 to 4 weeks. Under normal circumstances, 1 to 2 liters of fluid are ingested orally and 7 liters are secreted into the intestinal lumen by the stomach, liver, pancreas, and small intestines in a 24-hour period. Intestinal absorption is so efficient that 99 percent of the fluid ingested and secreted is reabsorbed. In a normal individual, stool weight is less than 200 g per 24 hours, water accounting for about 75 percent of stool weight.

Diarrhea may be caused by any condition that disturbs the delicate balance between secretion and absorption and results in a decrease in net water absorption. In a patient with diarrhea, water rises to 90 percent of stool weight. Since water is the major factor in determining stool weight, diarrhea is defined quantitatively as the excretion of more than 200 g or 200 ml of stools per 24 hours. Exceptions to this quantitative definition are patients with distal colitis or proctitis and patients with the irritable bowel syndrome who may have an increased stool frequency, but a normal stool weight.

Pathophysiologically, diarrhea may be caused by any one of the following mechanisms: increased intraluminal osmotic load (osmotic diarrhea); decreased absorption (malabsorption); exudation of protein, blood, and fluid into the lumen (exudative diarrhea); excessive intestinal secretion of water and electrolytes (secretory diarrhea); and abnormal intestinal motility (motility-related diarrhea).

Table 23–1 lists the specific causes of chronic diarrhea in relation to the preceding pathophysiologic mechanisms. First, I will review my approach to the initial and subsequent evaluation of a patient with chronic diarrhea and then discuss the more common causes of chronic diarrhea.

INITIAL WORK-UP OF CHRONIC DIARRHEA

History. In the evaluation of a patient with diarrhea, the history should direct the physician to the most appropriate tests and the sequence in which they are performed. After establishing that the diarrhea is truly chronic, the following historical features are helpful clues.

1. Stool character and number: A large volume of stools suggests a secretory diarrhea or malabsorption. Greasy malodorous stools are often seen in patients with malabsorption. The presence of blood suggests a neoplastic

TABLE 23-1   Causes of Chronic Diarrhea

Osmotic Diarrhea
  Disaccharidase deficiency (e.g., lactase deficiency)
  Laxatives

Malabsorption
  Small bowel disease

Celiac sprue	Radiation enteritis
Whipple's disease	Intestinal lymphangiectasia
Tropical sprue	Intestinal lymphoma
Giardiasis	Eosinophilic gastroenteritis
Extensive Crohn's	Bacterial overgrowth
disease and/or	Chronic intestinal ischemia
intestinal resection	Infections associated with
Collagenous sprue	immunodeficiency
Amyloidosis	syndromes, including
	AIDS

Maldigestion
  Chronic pancreatitis
  Pancreatic cancer
  Bacterial overgrowth
  Bile acid deficiency
  Cystic fibrosis

Exudative Diarrhea
  Ulcerative colitis
  Crohn's disease
  Colon cancer
  Amebiasis
  Tuberculosis

Secretory Diarrhea
  Cholera
  Pancreatic cholera (VIP-secreting pancreatic tumor)
  Zollinger-Ellison syndrome
  Carcinoid
  Medullary carcinoma
  Drugs (laxatives, theophylline)
  Bile acids
  Villous adenoma
  Partial small bowel obstruction
  Mucosal injury (celiac sprue, inflammatory bowel disease,
    ischemia)

Motility-Related Diarrhea
  Hyperthyroidism
  Carcinoid syndrome
  Scleroderma
  Diabetes
  Irritable bowel syndrome

or inflammatory process. The presence of mucus and pus indicates inflammation. Diarrhea alternating with constipation, or the passage of several small bowel movements within a short period of time in the morning and none afterwards, is most consistent with irritable bowel syndrome.

2. Stool timing: Nocturnal diarrhea almost always indicates the presence of an organic cause of the diarrhea, rather than a functional cause.

3. Associated intestinal symptoms: The presence of tenesmus points to the presence of an inflammatory or neoplastic condition in the rectum. The presence of abdominal cramps that are relieved by a bowel movement is not specific and may occur in functional or organic diarrhea. Flushing or a reddish discoloration of the skin in a patient with chronic diarrhea suggests carcinoid syndrome.

4. Associated extraintestinal manifestations: Diarrhea associated with arthralgia, arthritis, erythema nodosum, pyoderma gangrenosum, and iridoscleritis suggests the presence of inflammatory bowel disease.

5. Weight loss: The presence of weight loss in association with chronic diarrhea points to the presence of malabsorption, neoplasia, or inflammatory bowel disease, rather than irritable bowel or lactose intolerance.

6. Dietary habits: The association of diarrhea after eating dairy products should raise the suspicion of lactose intolerance.

7. Previous abdominal surgery: Gastric surgery with vagotomy may cause postvagotomy diarrhea. Gastrointestinal surgery may result in diarrhea because of a number of problems including bacterial overgrowth, short bowel syndrome, or bile salt malabsorption. Cholecystectomy may lead to postcholecystectomy diarrhea probably induced by bile acids.[1]

8. Other associated diseases: In diabetics, diarrhea, particularly nocturnal, is not uncommon when other manifestations of neuropathy are present. In patients with scleroderma, abnormal small bowel motility may lead to stasis and bacterial overgrowth resulting in diarrhea.

9. Radiation therapy: Pelvic and abdominal radiation damage can cause chronic diarrhea that can occur months to years after radiation treatment.

10. Drugs: Antibiotics and many other drugs may cause acute diarrhea. In addition, regular ingestion of drugs, such as laxatives, lactulose, bronchodilators, magnesium-containing antacids, colchicine, and guanidine, may cause chronic diarrhea.

11. Sexual habits: Male homosexuals are at significantly higher risk of developing chronic amebiasis, giardiasis, and opportunistic infections associated with AIDS.

12. Travel history: Most infectious diarrhea states associated with travel are acute; however, diseases such as amebiasis and giardiasis often lead to chronic diarrhea.

13. Fever: The presence of fever should raise the strong possibility of inflammatory bowel disease or lymphoma since it is uncommon in all other causes of chronic diarrhea.

Physical Examination.   The physical examination is usually less helpful than the history in the work-up of chronic diarrhea, but occasionally it clinches the diagnosis. The presence of a right lower quadrant mass and perianal fistulous disease is almost diagnostic of Crohn's disease. Examination of the skin for pyoderma gangrenosum and erythema nodosum is helpful in the diagnosis of inflammatory bowel disease. Hyperpigmentation of the skin suggests Whipple's disease or Addison's disease.

Stool Examination.   Every patient with chronic diarrhea should have an initial stool examination that includes testing for the presence of blood and white blood cells (WBCs), a Sudan stain for fat, and microscopy for ova and parasites. In contrast to acute diarrhea, the yield from sending stools for culture in patients with chronic diarrhea is extremely low, since most of the organisms that are grown on stool culture cause self-limited, brief illnesses. The exception to this statement is the immunocompromised patient, including the patient with AIDS.

The presence of blood in the stool suggests an inflammatory or neoplastic condition, while the presence of WBCs suggests an inflammatory condition. A Sudan III stain for fat is a good screening test for fat malabsorption. Stool microscopy for ova and parasites should be done two or three times, especially if the index of suspicion for a parasitic infection is high. Remember that stool microscopy for ova and parasites should be performed on fresh specimens *before* any barium x-ray studies are performed because barium may interfere with the yield and lead to false negative results for at least 2 to 3 weeks after the barium x-ray test.

Blood Tests.   WBC and differential studies need to be done to look for an increase in neutrophils or in eosinophils. Obviously, if bloody diarrhea is present, the hematocrit and hemoglobin need to be checked frequently.

Sigmoidoscopy.   A sigmoidoscopy should be part of the initial evaluation of every patient with chronic diarrhea unless the diagnosis of a parasitic infection is made by stool microscopy. Sigmoidoscopy should be performed without cleansing preparation so that the mucosa and any exudate that may be present on it are not distorted.

SUBSEQUENT WORK-UP OF CHRONIC DIARRHEA

The decision to continue the investigation and the sequence of tests that are ordered depend on the results of the initial investigation and the clinical suspicion of the physician. In a young patient whose initial work-up is completely negative and in whom the clinical suspicion for irritable bowel syndrome is high, a therapeutic trial of dietary manipulation and symptomatic treatment is in order before embarking on a "mega-work-up". Similarly if the clinical suspicion of lactose intolerance is high, a 2-week trial of a lactose-free diet is the next logical step to take. On the other hand, chronic diarrhea that occurs in a 60-year-old person without a previous history of diarrhea deserves full investigation in spite of a negative initial work-up.

The following is a list of tests that may be indicated in the subsequent work-up of chronic diarrhea. One or more of these tests may be indicated, depending on the clinical suspicion formulated from the initial work-up:

1. Routine blood work: BUN, creatinine, electrolytes, albumin
2. Special blood work: gastrin, cortisol, vasoactive intestinal peptide (VIP), thyroid function tests, immunoglobulins
3. X-rays: upper gastrointestinal (UGI) series, barium enema, computed tomography (CT) scan of the abdomen, endoscopic retrograde cholangiopancreatography (ERCP)
4. D-Xylose: 2-hour serum sample and 5-hour urine collection
5. Small bowel aspirate: *Giardia*
6. Small bowel biopsy
7. Urine: 5-hydroxyindoleacetic acid (5-HIAA), Vanillylmandelic acid (VMA)

The sequence of tests depends on the initial formulation. In the following section, I review the major causes of chronic diarrhea, my diagnostic approach, and my plan of management.

LACTOSE INTOLERANCE

Lactose intolerance secondary to mucosal lactase deficiency is an acquired condition that manifests itself in early adulthood. It is a common cause of diarrhea worldwide. In the United States 70 to 75 percent of blacks and 5 to 20 percent of whites suffer from this ailment.[2] Its prevalence in Asia and the Middle East is as high as 90 percent. Typically, the patient with lactose intolerance complains of diarrhea associated with bloating, gaseous distention, and crampy abdominal pain. The diagnosis of lactase deficiency should be suspected in any patient who complains of the preceding symptoms after the ingestion of milk or dairy products, but not all patients recognize this association. Remember that patients may be able to tolerate varying amounts of lactose without any symptoms; the mucosal deficiency of lactase is a graded one and not an all-or-nothing phenomenon.

There are several different tests to confirm the diagnosis. The most accurate, but most invasive, and therefore least-used test is a small bowel biopsy with quantitative measurement of mucosal lactase activity. Other less invasive tests include a lactose tolerance test and labeled breath tests that utilize carbon dioxide and hydrogen. I favor utilizing a therapeutic trial of a lactose-free diet for 1 to 2 weeks rather than any of these tests. I resort to the breath test only when the therapeutic trial is inconclusive.

The treatment of lactose intolerance is obviously a lactose-free diet. That does not mean, however, that a patient is condemned to a dairy-free diet forever. There are commercial milk products that are pretreated with lactase and enzyme preparations and that can be added to milk products. It is also important to know that the ingestion of yogurt by such patients does *not* cause symptoms because, in the process of producing yogurt, bacterial lactase digests the lactose present in the milk.

CELIAC SPRUE

Celiac sprue is also known as gluten sensitive enteropathy. It is the gluten, and particularly the gliadin moiety in gluten, that is toxic to the intestinal mucosa of patients who suffer from this condition. The result is flattening of the intestinal villa, thereby leading to malabsorption. The most common symptoms in celiac sprue are diarrhea, abdominal distention, and weight loss. Abdominal pain is unusual. The causes of diarrhea in these patients are multiple and include malabsorption of carbohydrate, protein, fat, water, and electrolytes; fat reaching the colon and being broken to hydroxy fatty acids by bacteria. Hydroxy fatty acids in turn cause water to be passively secreted into the intestinal lumen; and active secretion of water and electrolytes in the small intestine.

The diagnosis of celiac sprue is based on the following findings: increased 72-hour stool fat (greater than 7 g per 24 hours); abnormal serum and urine D-Xylose test (2-hour serum sample greater than 25 percent and urine greater than 5 g per 5 hours collection); abnormal laboratory findings such as iron and folate deficiencies, prolonged prothrombin time, and low calcium and B_{12}; abnormal small bowel pattern with dilated proximal loops; and flat mucosa with absence of villi on small bowel biopsy, which is the test I rely on most heavily.

The treatment of celiac sprue is a gluten-free diet. It is essential for every patient suspected of having this condition to have a small bowel biopsy to confirm the diagnosis. The patient should also meet with a dietitian to get proper instructions on a gluten-free diet. The treatment is simple in concept, but following a strict gluten-free diet is not easy because gluten is present in so many additives and preservatives in addition to natural food. The clinical response to treatment is relatively quick, but the histologic improvement lags months behind.

CHRONIC PANCREATITIS

Pancreatic exocrine insufficiency, a frequent complication of chronic pancreatitis, causes malabsorption and hence diarrhea. The scenario is usually one of chronic abdominal pain with acute exacerbations for years before the development of diarrhea. Typically, more than 90 percent of the pancreas is destroyed before diarrhea sets in. The pathophysiologic mechanism is maldigestion of protein, carbohydrates, and fat secondary to insufficient enzyme production by the diseased pancreas.

The diagnosis should be suspected when a patient presents with diarrhea after a long history of abdominal pain. Findings such as calcification of the pancreas on kidney, ureter, and bladder (KUB) studies and elevated 72-hour stool fat confirm the diagnosis. In some patients, calcification of the pancreas may not occur and ERCP is required to establish a diagnosis. Recently, the Bentiromide test[3] has gained acceptance as a more specific and less cumbersome test than the 72-hour stool fat test. Bentiromide is a synthetic peptide that is cleaved by chymotrypsin in the small intestine. This results in the release of para-aminobenzoic acid (PABA), which in turn is absorbed and excreted in the urine. The test consists of giving 500 mg of bentiromide after an overnight fast and collecting urine for 6 hours. In normal people, greater than 50 percent of PABA is recovered in the urine. This test has a 5 percent false positive and a 20 percent false negative result.

INFLAMMATORY BOWEL DISEASE

Chronic diarrhea is the most prominent symptom in ulcerative colitis and Crohn's disease. The pathophysiologic mechanisms are multiple and include exudation of protein, blood, and mucus from inflammatory sites, malabsorption, and net fluid secretion. The diarrhea is frequently bloody and may contain pus. Nocturnal diarrhea is not unusual. Abdominal cramping is often an accompanying symptom.

The diagnosis is made by sigmoidoscopy, colonoscopy, and barium x-rays singly or in combination. Caution is necessary during the investigation of patients with inflammatory bowel disease, especially acute ulcerative colitis. A limited sigmoidoscopy without bowel preparation is sometimes the only indicated procedure in patients with severe bloody diarrhea and accompanying systemic manifestations and physical findings such as fever, tachycardia, hypotension, and a distended and tender abdomen. A barium enema or complete colonoscopy are contraindicated because of possible precipitation of a toxic megacolon, which is a life-threatening condition.

The treatment options include sulfasalazine, steroids, azathioprine, and 6-mercaptopurine, depending on the type of disease and its severity.

COLON CANCER

Symptoms in colonic cancer are not uniform; they vary according to the site of the lesion. A change in bowel habits manifested by constipation or alternating constipation and diarrhea are much more common in left-sided colonic lesions than in right-sided ones. Diarrhea occurs more frequently in distal colonic lesions. If gross blood or guaiac-positive stools accompany these symptoms, it becomes mandatory to rule out colonic cancer. The diagnosis of colonic cancer can be made by a sigmoidoscopy and a barium enema or colonoscopy.

IRRITABLE BOWEL SYNDROME

Abdominal pain and constipation are more common than diarrhea in this common syndrome. However, diarrhea alternating with constipation or steady diarrhea occurs in a significant number of patients. The diarrhea is more frequent in the morning, especially after breakfast, and in the early evening. The bowel movements are usually multiple, small in volume, and "mucusy." Nocturnal diarrhea that wakes the patient up from sleep is extremely rare, and dehydration and weight loss do not occur. The condition usually occurs in early adulthood. The onset of similar symptoms for the first time in middle-aged and older persons is rare and should alert the physician to search for a more serious organic condition.

The pathophysiologic mechanism is presumed to be a motility disturbance. However, studies have not been conclusive. The personal experience of many gastroenterologists, as well as epidemiologic studies, suggest that stress and emotional tensions play a role in precipitating this condition.[4]

There is no diagnostic test that clinches the diagnosis, so the diagnosis is made by a consistent clinical picture and by exclusion of other conditions, such as villous adenoma and inflammatory bowel disease. The history of emotional stress in patients with an episodic bowel pattern is also helpful. The management of patients suffering from the irritable bowel syndrome is often difficult. It is of paramount importance to stress to the patient the benignity of this condition. Alterations in diet, anticholinergics, and antidiarrheal agents may be used, but controlled studies have failed to show a beneficial long-term effect for any particular regimen.

CHRONIC DIARRHEA OF UNKNOWN CAUSE

A cause of chronic diarrhea is usually found in most patients. However, every gastroenterologist is referred an occasional patient who remains undiagnosed in spite of an extensive work-up, including routine blood tests, stool examinations, malabsorption work-up, endoscopic procedures, x-ray studies dietary manipulation, and therapeutic trials.

The list of etiologic causes in these unusual patients is long, but among the conditions that must be considered are laxative abuse, bile acid diarrhea, neuroendocrine tumors such as VIP-secreting pancreatic tumors, idiopathic secretory diarrhea, microscopic colitis, intestinal lymphoma, and irritable bowel syndrome. In a prospective study of 87 such patients[5], the most common diagnoses in order of frequency were laxative abuse (20), irritable bowel (14), idiopathic secretory diarrhea (13), and bile acid diarrhea (9).

Certain additional tests are needed in this group of patients. I usually perform them in the following sequence.

1. Alkalinization of the stools (to test for laxatives containing phenolphthalein)
2. Serum hormone levels (VIP, calcitonin, gastrin)
3. 48-hour fasting (to determine that the diarrhea is secretory and not related to absorption)
4. Stool electrolyte levels and osmolarity
5. Colonoscopy and multiple biopsies (to diagnose microscopic colitis)
6. Levels of fecal excretions of ^{14}C-cholylglycine (to diagnose bile acid diarrhea), or a therapeutic trial of cholestyramine, which binds bile acids.

In summary, the work-up of a patient with chronic diarrhea requires a sound understanding of the pathophysiologic mechanisms underlying the different causes of diarrhea, an accurate history, and common sense in choosing the right test in the right order. Haphazard testing or a course of "order everything on the check list" is frustrating, time consuming, expensive, and unrewarding.

References

1. Hutcheon DF, Bayless TM, Gadacz TR. Post-cholecystectomy diarrhea. JAMA 1979; 241:823–824.

2. Bayless TM, Rothfeld B, Massa C, et al. Lactose and milk intolerance: clinical implications. N Engl J Med 1975; 292:1156–1203.
3. Toskas PP. Bentiromide as a test of exocrine pancreatic function in adult patients with pancreatic insufficiency. Gastroenterology 1983; 85:565–569.
4. Medeloff AI, Monk M, Siegel CI, et al. Illness experience and life stresses in patients with irritable colon and with ulcerative colitis. N Engl J Med 1970; 282:14–17.
5. Krijs GJ, Fordtran JS. Chronic diarrhea of unknown origin. In: Sleizenger MH, Fordtran JS, eds. Gastrointestinal disease. Philadelphia: WB Saunders, 1983:269.

24 | ELEVATED TRANSAMINASES

KARIM A. FAWAZ, M.D.

Measurement of the serum levels of hepatic enzymes, aminotransferases (transaminases), provides sensitive assessments of liver cell injury. Elevation of alanine aminotransferase (ALT), formerly referred to as serum glutamic-pyruvic transaminase (SGPT), is more specific for liver cell injury. Elevation of aspartate aminotransferase (AST), formerly referred to as serum glutamic-oxaloacetic (SGOT), also may be seen in myocardial and skeletal muscle injury. I am frequently asked to interpret the significance of elevated aminotransferases in a variety of clinical settings. The ease or the difficulty of correctly interpreting the data depends on a number of factors, including the availability of previous measurements, the results of other liver function tests, the results of serologic tests for hepatitis A and B, and the general medical condition of the patient.

Aminotransferases normally are present in the serum in concentrations of less than 30 to 40 units per liter. Although the rise in serum aminotransferases does not correlate well with the severity of liver disease, the level of aminotransferase elevation does frequently correlate with the type of liver cell injury. In general, elevations of up to eight to ten times the upper limit of normal are seen in any type of acute or chronic liver disease. Values in the low thousands or above are seen exclusively in disorders associated with acute extensive hepatocellular necrosis, such as viral and drug hepatitis and acute cardiocirculatory collapse.

The variety of liver diseases that result in elevated serum aminotransferases is extensive. In order to focus the differential diagnosis, I divide the aminotransferase elevations into two sections, i.e., below or above 500 units per liter. This is an arbitrary, but convenient, way of highlighting the types of liver disease that a physician should first consider. However, considerable overlap does exist between the two groups.

AMINOTRANSFERASES ABOVE 500 UNITS

Aminotransferase elevations above 500 units are seen almost exclusively in conditions that are associated with acute hepatocellular necrosis. Acute viral hepatitis, the most common cause of acute hepatocellular necrosis, accounts for the vast majority (>95 percent) of cases. Other likely causes include drug hepatitis and acute cardiocirculatory failure.

Acute Viral Hepatitis

Three main types of viral hepatitis—A, B and non-A, non-B—account for more than 95 percent of all episodes of acute viral hepatitis. Acute hepatitis attributable to the Epstein-Barr virus and to cytomegalovirus account for the remaining episodes. The prodromal symptoms of all types of hepatitis are similar and consist of anorexia, nausea, malaise, and fatigue. A serum sickness-like syndrome may be seen with hepatitis B. The physical examination usually reveals tender hepatomegaly. Splenomegaly and typical lymphocytes are more common in Epstein-Barr virus and cytomegalovirus infections. The amino-transferases are usually above 500 units, except in the extremely early stages of the illness, but can rise to as high as several thousand units. The AST to ALT ratio is of no value in the differentiation of one type of hepatitis from the other. Aminotransferases tend to be lowest when the disease is caused by cytomega-lovirus, Epstein-Barr virus, and hepatitis non-A, non-B; higher when caused by hepatitis A; and highest when caused by hepatitis B. Serum bilirubin elevation depends on the severity of the disease. Alkaline phosphatase is usually only mildly elevated, but in a third of patients with Epstein-Barr virus infection, it is disproportionately elevated (with respect to the rise in bilirubin).

The diagnosis of a particular type of viral hepatitis is established by serologic tests. Type A hepatitis is diagnosed by the presence of a positive IgM antibody to hepatitis A (anti-HAV, IgM). The presence of a positive IgG antibody to hepatitis A (anti-HAV, IgG) indicates either past exposure to, or present infection with hepatitis A.

The diagnosis of hepatitis B is made by the presence of a positive hepatitis B surface antigen (HBsAg). The physician, however, should remember that an acute hepatitis of a different type may be superimposed on a carrier state of hepatitis B in patients with a high risk of developing multiple episodes of viral hepatitis, such as male homosexuals, intravenous drug addicts, hemophiliacs, and dialysis patients.

Epstein-Barr virus and cytomegalovirus hepatitis are best diagnosed by the presence of a rising titer of the corresponding antibody.

Non-A, non-B hepatitis is a diagnosis that currently is made only by exclusion because of the lack of an available marker. A presumptive diagnosis of non-A, non-B hepatitis is made on the basis of elevated serum aminotrans-ferases, negative markers for hepatitis A, B, Epstein-Barr virus, and cytomega-lovirus, and the absence of other causes of aminotransferase elevations (e.g., drugs or acute cardiocirculatory collapse). The presumptive diagnosis is strengthened further if there is a history of intravenous drug use or of recent transfusion. Non-A, non-B hepatitis accounts for more than 90 percent of post-transfusion hepatitis in the United States.

Drug Hepatitis

Drugs may cause three types of reaction in the liver: (1) an hepatocellular necrosis; (2) a cholestasis; and (3) a mixed hepatocellular and cholestatic picture.

Aminotransferase levels above 500 units, in the range of acute viral hepatitis, are commonly seen with drugs that cause hepatocellular necrosis; in this setting the alkaline phosphatase level is normal or only slightly elevated. The degree of hyperbilirubinemia depends on the severity of the hepatitis. Aminotransferase values that are one to ten times normal are seen with drugs that cause a predominantly cholestatic picture; there is a concomitant moderate to marked elevation of the alkaline phosphatase and the bilirubin. Drugs that cause a mixed picture are associated with a wide range of aminotransferase values.

Drugs that cause hepatocellular necrosis produce their damage by two mechanisms.

1. Direct hepatotoxicity. This is a dose-dependent type of hepatotoxicity that affects all subjects who are exposed to the offending agent. Examples of such agents are acetaminophen, carbon tetrachloride, and poisonous mushrooms.
2. Hypersensitivity or metabolic idiosyncrasy. The liver injury caused by drugs that belong to this group by definition is not dose-dependent. Liver injury produced by a hypersensitivity to a drug usually manifests itself clinically within 1 to 4 weeks and is frequently accompanied by fever, rash, and eosinophilia. When rechallenged with the drug, subjects exhibit immediate aminotransferase elevations. Common examples of such drugs are sulfonamides and para-aminosalicylic acid.

    On the other hand, some drugs cause injury by the slow accumulation of toxic metabolites. The duration of exposure may be weeks or months and the response to a rechallenge may be delayed. Isoniazid is a prime example of a drug that causes drug hepatitis by this mechanism. Both mechanisms of idiosyncrasy are suspected with some drugs, such as halothane and phenytoin.

The list of drugs that can cause hepatitis is virtually endless. In the following discussion I will review the more commonly used agents that may cause hepatitis with aminotransferase elevations above 500 units.

Acetaminophen

This is a safe analgesic when taken in the usual therapeutic doses. However, ingestion of an overdose is a common method of attempted suicide.

Hepatic necrosis and marked aminotransferase elevations may be seen in subjects who ingest more than 6 g. Doses that exceed 15 g are reported in 80 percent of fatal cases. Signs of hepatic necrosis appear when the plasma acetaminophen level exceeds 300 mg per milliliter at 4 hours after ingestion.[1] A correct, early diagnosis is crucial because therapy with acetylcysteine (Mucomyst) within 12 hours of ingestion of an acetaminophen overdose can be lifesaving.

Halothane

This is a widely used and relatively safe anesthetic, but on rare occasions it can cause fatal hepatitis. Obese, elderly females seem to be more susceptible. Halothane and related compounds should always be considered in the differential diagnosis of postoperative aminotransferase elevations. The average time between exposure to halothane and the onset of aminotransferase elevations is 1 week for a first exposure and as short as 3 days for repeat exposures. Fever, anorexia, vomiting, and eosinophilia are the most common associated findings. There is no treatment.

Isoniazid (INH)

INH itself is not hepatotoxic, but its metabolite hydrazine has been implicated in the production of liver necrosis. Hydrazine produces subclinical hepatic injury in 12 to 20 percent of recipients. However, the aminotransferases are usually less than six times normal and eventually return to normal in the majority of subjects in spite of continuation of the drug.[2] Hepatitis from this agent is more common in patients of increasing age and in Orientals. The time of the onset of liver disease is within 2 months of the start of drug therapy in 50 percent of cases, but may be as late as 12 months after drug commencement. I recommend that patients receiving isoniazid have liver function tests at monthly intervals.

Acute Cardiocirculatory Failure

Aminotransferase elevations in the acute viral hepatitis range (and even higher) may be seen in patients who suffer from acute heart failure or from circulatory collapse. The distinguishing feature of this entity is the fact that the aminotransferases quickly return to normal if the patient's circulation is restored to normal. It is not unusual to have values as high as 10,000 units fall to 100 to 200 units in 3 to 4 days. Such rapid recovery is not encountered in any other type of liver disease.

AMINOTRANSFERASES BELOW 500 UNITS

Alcoholic Liver Disease

The majority of patients with alcoholic liver disease have a typical pattern of serum aminotransferase elevation. In 95 percent of cases, the AST is higher than the ALT, and both usually are below 300 units. Even in patients with severe acute alcoholic hepatitis, which carries a mortality rate of 20 percent, the aminotransferases are rarely above 300 units. The lower serum ALT level reflects the decreased synthesis of ALT in the liver secondary to a deficiency of pyridoxal phosphate in alcoholic liver disease.[3] Pyridoxal phosphate is required for ALT synthesis in the liver more than for AST synthesis.

The AST to ALT ratio is usually of little value in distinguishing the different types of liver disease, except in alcoholic liver disease. If the ALT is below 300 units, then an AST to ALT ratio of more than two is suggestive of alcoholic liver disease, and a ratio of more than three is highly suggestive of alcoholic liver disease.[4]

Long-term heavy alcohol intake causes fatty infiltration of the liver in all subjects, but only 10 to 15 percent of those subjects develop alcoholic hepatitis and/or cirrhosis. Fat accumulation in the liver may cause an enlarged liver, but does not usually lead to abnormalities in liver function tests except for occasional mild aminotransferase elevations. Symptomatic alcoholic hepatitis is usually associated with bilirubin elevation in addition to aminotransferase elevations. Such patients usually complain of fatigue, anorexia, nausea, and fever, and have tender hepatomegaly and leukocytosis. The prothrombin time may be elevated and the serum albumin may be low. Alcoholic hepatitis is a potentially reversible condition if cirrhosis has not yet developed. Alcoholic cirrhosis is manifested by hepatomegaly, splenomegaly, palmar erythema, and spider nevi. Liver function tests are the same as in alcoholic hepatitis, but a lower serum albumin level is more common with cirrhosis.

The diagnosis of alcoholic liver disease may be suspected by the history and the typical AST to ALT ratio, but it is established by liver biopsy. The decision to do a liver biopsy should be made on an individual basis after weighing the risks and benefits of the procedure. For example, the risk of bleeding following a liver biopsy outweighs the benefit in a patient with a history of chronic heavy alcohol intake and the presence of massive ascites, a low platelet count, and a prothrombin time 3 seconds or more above control.

Chronic Hepatitis

Chronic hepatitis is defined as a chronic inflammatory disease of the liver that persists for at least 6 months. It is almost always associated with mild to moderate aminotransferase elevations. The most common etiology of chronic hepatitis is viral; however, other causes include drugs, autoimmune disease, and by exclusion, idiopathic hepatitis.

One has to rely on the history and the results of serologic tests in order to determine the etiology of elevated aminotransferases in chronic hepatitis. An accurate history is of paramount importance. Key information includes the duration of symptoms, medications, sexual habits, transfusions, and intravenous drug use. The most important serology test is hepatitis B. The presence of a positive HBsAg usually clinches the diagnosis of chronic hepatitis B, except in rare circumstances when the patient is a chronic carrier of hepatitis B and has a superimposed non-A, non-B or drug hepatitis. The presence of a positive antinuclear antibody is consistent with autoimmune chronic hepatitis, but its absence does not rule out this condition.

Chronic Viral Hepatitis

Type A hepatitis does not cause chronic hepatitis because it is never associated with the presence of a chronic carrier state. In contrast, both types B and non-A, non-B hepatitis are common causes of chronic hepatitis and account for more than 95 percent of all cases of chronic hepatitis. Between 5 to 10 percent of patients with acute hepatitis B remain as chronic carriers. The chronic carrier state occurs predominantly in males and is more common in male homosexuals. The incidence of chronic hepatitis after an acute episode of non-A, non-B hepatitis is 30 to 40 percent.

The presence of considerable overlap makes it impossible to differentiate between chronic persistent hepatitis (benign form) and chronic active hepatitis (may progress to cirrhosis) on the basis of the degree of aminotransferase elevations.

In general, however, aminotransferases are usually below 250 units in chronic persistent hepatitis. When these levels are above 250 units, chronic active hepatitis is more likely. Occasionally, aminotransferases above 500 units are encountered during exacerbation of chronic active hepatitis B. Patients with chronic persistent hepatitis do not show any abnormalities in other liver function tests. In contrast, patients with chronic active hepatitis may have low albumin levels and/or elevated bilirubin, globulin, and alkaline phosphatase levels and an elevated prothrombin time. The physical examination usually reveals an enlarged liver in both conditions. When splenomegaly is present, chronic active hepatitis is much more likely. Remember, however, that patients with either condition may have only elevated aminotransferase levels, and the diagnosis of either cannot be established, short of performing a liver biopsy.

Autoimmune Chronic Hepatitis

This type of chronic hepatitis most commonly affects young women and was formerly referred to as "lupoid hepatitis" because of the frequent presence of a positive lupus erythematosus (LE) cell in the serum. The distinguishing feature of this type of chronic hepatitis is its frequent association with extrahepatic manifestations, such as arthralgia, arthritis, skin rash, fever, and amenorrhea. An elevated sedimentation rate, an increase in gamma globulin, and a positive antinuclear antibody are frequent associated laboratory findings. Serum aminotransferases are usually below 500 units, but they may become higher during an acute exacerbation. Other liver function tests initially may be normal, but with progression of the disease the albumin level decreases and the bilirubin level rises. The correct diagnosis is important because this entity is the only known form of chronic hepatitis that responds to treatment.[5] Treatment consists of corticosteroids and azathioprine.

Chronic Drug Hepatitis

In general, most drugs cause an acute hepatitis; however, several drugs have been shown to cause chronic hepatitis. The common offenders are alpha methyldopa, oxyphenisatin, isoniazid, and nitrofurantoin.

Cirrhosis

The degree of aminotransferase elevation in cirrhosis depends on the etiology and the activity of the disease. Patients with cirrhosis secondary to alcohol, schistosomiasis, hemochromatosis, and alpha-one anti-trypsin deficiency tend to have a mild elevation of aminotransferases. Patients with cirrhosis secondary to chronic active hepatitis, Wilson's disease, sclerosing cholangitis, and primary biliary cirrhosis tend to have higher elevations.

As any of these diseases reach an end-stage inactive form, the aminotransferases decrease and may even become within the normal range. Therefore, a decline in aminotransferases should not always be interpreted as a good prognostic sign. The serum bilirubin and the liver function tests that reflect the synthetic ability of the liver, such as albumin and prothrombin time, are the more important and useful tests to follow in the patient with progressive cirrhosis. The diagnosis of cirrhosis is established by the performance of a liver biopsy, but it should be emphasized that the etiology of the cirrhosis cannot always be determined by the biopsy.

Bile Duct Obstruction

Bile duct obstruction secondary to gallstones, tumor, pancreatitis, and postoperative strictures may be accompanied by mild aminotransferase elevations. Occasionally, high values reaching 1,000 units may be seen in the first 24 to 48 hours after an acute bile duct obstruction secondary to gallstones. However, these values usually drop to below 300 units soon thereafter. As the aminotransferases drop, the alkaline phosphatase and the bilirubin rise if the obstructing stone does not pass spontaneously. A right upper quadrant ultrasound is the first screening test if common bile duct obstruction is suspected.

Congestive Heart Failure

Patients with congestive heart failure may have mild aminotransferase elevations accompanied by an elevated alkaline phosphatase two to three times normal and, in some instances, a mild bibirubin elevation. The presence of congested neck veins, tender hepatomegaly, and a positive hepatojugular relux on physical examination should alert the physician to this condition as the cause of aminotransferase elevations. Liver biopsy shows passive congestion around the central veins, but biopsy is only rarely indicated.

Fatty Infiltration of the Liver

Fat accumulation in the liver (with hepatomegaly) secondary to alcohol, diabetes, obesity, hyperlipemia, and postintestinal bypass surgery may cause a rise in aminotransferases up to six to eight times normal. The diagnosis requires a liver biopsy. In patients with hyperlipemia, control of the serum lipids by diet and/or by medications is advised before a liver biopsy is performed. A return of the serum aminotransferases to the normal range with normalization of the serum lipids is the rule rather than the exception, and biopsy can be obviated.

Other Conditions

Other conditions that cause mild serum aminotransferase elevations are intravenous hyperalimentation, granulomatous hepatitis, primary or metastatic liver cancer, sarcoidosis, amyloidosis, hepatic vein thrombosis, pericholangitis associated with inflammatory bowel disease, primary sclerosing cholangitis, myocardial infarction, hemolysis, and myositis. In the latter three conditions the AST is significantly higher than the ALT and should be differentiated from alcoholic liver disease (in which the AST is also higher than the ALT).

References

1. Hamlyn AN. The spectrum of paracetamol (acetaminophen) overdose: clinical and epidemiological studies. Postgrad Med J 1978; 54:400–404.
2. Mitchell JR, Zimmerman HJ, Ishak KG, et al. Isoniazid liver injury: clinical spectrum, pathology, and probable pathogenesis. Ann Intern Med 1976; 84:181–192.
3. Diehl AM, Potter J, Boitnott J, et al. Relationship between pyridoxal 5'-phosphate deficiency and aminotransferase levels in alcoholic hepatitis. Gastroenterology 1984; 86:632–636.
4. Matloff DS, Selinger MJ, Kaplan MM. Hepatic transaminase activity in alcoholic liver disease. Gastroenterology 1980; 78:1389–1392.
5. Czaja AJ, Beaver SJ, Shiels MT. Sustained remission after corticosteroid therapy of severe hepatitis B surface antigen-negative chronic active hepatitis. Gastroenterology 1978; 92:215–219.

25 | CLINICAL APPROACH TO JAUNDICE

KARIM A. FAWAZ, M.D.

Bilirubin, a breakdown product of heme, is produced in the reticuloendothelial system. The sequence of the reaction is as follows:

$$\text{Heme} \xrightarrow[\text{oxygenase}]{\text{heme}} \text{biliverdin} \xrightarrow[\text{reductase}]{\text{biliverdin}} \text{bilirubin}$$

Fat-soluble, but water-insoluble, bilirubin has to be bound by albumin in order to be transported in blood to the liver where it is conjugated to glucuronic acid. The conjugated bilirubin, now water-soluble, is transported into the bile canaliculi via an energy-requiring process than seems to be the rate-limiting step in bilirubin metabolism.

The traditional Van den Bergh assay for measuring bilirubin, still used in most laboratories, measures both the total bilirubin and the direct fraction; the indirect fraction is the difference between the total and direct levels. The direct and indirect fractions are approximate determinations of the conjugated and unconjugated bilirubin respectively. Newer and more accurate methods of bilirubin measurement are replacing the Van den Bergh method in some laboratories. One such method that is increasingly gaining acceptance is based on photographic film technology. Three fractions of bilirubin are reported by this method: unconjugated bilirubin, conjugated bilirubin, and delta bilirubin; the delta bilirubin is conjugated bilirubin bound to albumin.[1]

The fractionation of bilirubin differentiates between jaundice caused by hemolysis or by Gilbert's disease (indirect hyperbilirubinemia) and jaundice caused by hepatobiliary disease (direct hyperbilirubinemia). The challenge to the physician lies primarily in the differential diagnosis of direct hyperbilirubinemia. The central clinical question is: "Is the elevated direct bilirubin secondary to liver disease or to bile duct obstruction, i.e., is the jaundice medical or is it surgical?"

The evaluation of the patient who presents with jaundice must be rigorous, thorough, and systematic. The initial impression is based on the history and physical examination. Liver function tests help to confirm or refute the initial clinical impression and to point to the next step. If common bile duct obstruction is suspected, noninvasive radiologic studies are required to confirm the suspicion. Invasive radiologic or endoscopic diagnostic procedures may be indicated, depending on the results of the work-up to that point.

If hepatocellular disease is suspected, serologic tests should be ordered and, depending on the clinical picture, a liver biopsy may be required to make a definitive diagnosis.

CLINICAL CLUES

History

In taking a history, several features such as age, exposure, and type of presentation help formulate the initial impression. Viral hepatitis is more common in the younger age group, while malignant obstruction is more common over the age of 60. Alcoholic liver disease is not common before the age of 30, but may occur at any time later. Choledocholithiasis is more common over the age of 40. A history of exposure to friends or to family members with known viral hepatitis, a history of needle sticks, a history of exposure to dialysis patients, a history of intravenous drug use, and a history of blood transfusion should direct attention towards the strong possibility of viral hepatitis. A history of heavy alcohol intake suggests alcoholic liver disease, while a history of a recent or a chronic drug intake makes drug-induced hepatitis a likely contender.

The type of onset of jaundice and the associated symptoms also are helpful in formulating the initial clinical impression. The sudden onset of jaundice, preceded or accompanied by constitutional symptoms of fatigue, loss of appetite, nausea, and vomiting is typical for hepatitis. On the other hand, the gradual onset of jaundice without constitutional symptoms is typical of malignant obstruction and is sometimes recognized by relatives or friends, rather than the patient. The presence of fever, chills, and colicky abdominal pain associated with jaundice is suggestive of choledocholithiasis. High grade fever and abdominal pain are not common in parenchymal liver disease, with the exception of alcoholic hepatitis and infectious mononucleosis. Itching, more common in obstructive jaundice, can be the earliest symptom in primary biliary cirrhosis and is common in other conditions causing intrahepatic cholestasis.

A history of dark urine indicates the presence of direct bilirubin in the urine. Patients with hemolysis and Gilbert's disease do not excrete dark urine because the elevated bilirubin is indirect and hence bound to albumin, which does not traverse the glomerular barrier. Postoperative jaundice, especially after long abdominal or cardiac surgery with large transfusion requirements, should alert the physician to the possibility of benign postoperative jaundice. Prolonged hypotension during surgery or associated with cardiac shock makes the diagnosis of ischemic liver damage the most likely cause of jaundice.

Physical Examination

The size of the liver is not an important differentiating sign between parenchymal and obstructive liver disease because hepatomegaly occurs in both conditions. A firm and nodular liver is seen in cirrhosis and in primary or metastatic cancer of the liver. While an enlarged spleen suggests the presence of portal hypertension (and hence the presence of chronic liver disease), splenomegaly also is present in infectious mononucleosis and in up to 20 percent of patients with acute hepatitis. The presence of ascites and stigmata of chronic liver disease, such as abdominal collaterals, spider nevi, and palmar erythema, are diagnostic of cirrhosis. A gallbladder not tender to palpation suggests malignant obstruction of the common bile duct below the take-off of the cystic duct. When the gallbladder is palpable and tender, empyema of the gallbladder, secondary to cystic duct obstruction by a stone, should be suspected.

Hemogram

A sudden drop in hematocrit without evidence of bleeding suggests a hemolytic process as the cause of jaundice; the majority of the bilirubin should be indirect. Leukocytosis with a left shift, commonly seen in choledocholithiasis and alcoholic hepatitis, is uncommon in viral hepatitis and malignant obstruction. The presence of pancytopenia should alert the clinician to the possibility of chronic liver disease, portal hypertension, and hypersplenism. Atypical lymphocytosis is seen in viral infections, particularly infectious mononucleosis. Finally, eosinophilia should raise the possibility of drug-induced hepatitis.

Liver Function Tests

Although an individual liver function test abnormality may be characteristic of a certain type of hepatobiliary disease, it is essential that it be interpreted in the context of other liver function test abnormalities (Table 25–1), the time period from the onset of the illness, and the whole clinical setting. A perfect example is acute common bile duct obstruction secondary to a stone. In the first 24 to 48 hours the aminotransferases may be markedly elevated and in the range of hepatitis, while the bilirubin and alkaline phosphatase may be minimally elevated. With time, however, the aminotransferases drop quickly, while the bilirubin and alkaline phosphatase continue to rise.

Bilirubin.   Elevation of the serum bilirubin level may occur in response to the following pathophysiologic mechanisms:

1. Overproduction of bilirubin, e.g., hemolysis
2. Impaired uptake or conjugation of bilirubin, e.g., Gilbert's syndrome

TABLE 25-1 Liver Function Test Abnormalities in Various Conditions

Condition	Bilirubin	Alkaline Phosphatase	Aminotransferases
Hemolysis	2 to 6 × N*	N	N
Defects in Bilirubin Metabolism			
Gilbert's syndrome	2 to 6 × N[1]	N	N
Dubin-Johnson syndrome	2 to 6 × N	N	N
Rotor's syndrome	2 to 6 × N	N	N
Hepatocellular Disease			
Viral Hepatitis	N to 40 × N	N to 3 × N†	10 to 100 × N (ALT>AST)
Drug-induced hepatitis	N to 40 × N	N to 3 × N	5 to 100 × N (ALT>AST)
Alcoholic hepatitis	N to 40 × N	N to 3 × N	2 to 8 × N (AST>ALT)
Chronic active hepatitis	N to 15 × N	N to 3 × N	2 to 10 × N
Cirrhosis	N to 20 × N	N to 3 × N	N to 3 × N
Cholestatic Liver Disease			
Drug-induced hepatitis	N to 40 × N	2 to 10 × N	N to 8 × N
1° biliary cirrhosis	N to 40 × N	3 to 20 × N	N to 5 × N
Sclerosing cholangitis	N to 40 × N	3 to 10 × N	N to 10 × N
Extrahepatic Obstruction			
Common bile duct stone	N to 15 × N	2 to 15 × N	N to 8 × N‡
Malignant obstruction	N to 40 × N	3 to 10 × N	N to 5 × N
Infiltrative Disease			
Tumor	N to 5 × N	2 to 15 × N	N to 8 × N (AST>ALT)
Sarcoidosis	N to 5 × N	2 to 8 × N	N to 5 × N

* Indirect bilirubin
† Higher in Epstein-Barr virus infection
‡ Initially increased
N: normal; ×: times

3. Impaired hepatic excretion of bilirubin, e.g., Dubin-Johnson syndrome, obstruction, or cholestasis
4. Regurgitation of unconjugated and conjugated bilirubin from damaged liver cells, e.g., hepatitis

In general, the presence of an elevated bilirubin level without any other abnormality in liver function tests indicates the presence of hemolysis or a genetic abnormality in bilirubin metabolism. The exception to this rule is the occasional patient with inactive stable cirrhosis. Fractionation of the bilirubin narrows the differential diagnosis; indirect hyperbilirubinemia *only* suggests hemolysis or Gilbert's syndrome, whereas direct hyperbilirubinemia *only* suggests Dubin-Johnson syndrome or Rotor's syndrome. When hyperbilirubinemia is associated with other liver function test abnormalities, the degree of elevation is not helpful in the differential diagnosis.

Alkaline Phosphatase. Extrahepatic obstruction and intrahepatic cholestasis stimulate the de novo production of the hepatic enzyme alkaline phosphatase. Thus, the serum alkaline phosphatase is moderately to markedly elevated (three to ten times normal) in such instances. On the other hand, acute or chronic hepatocellular disease is associated with only minor elevation of alkaline phosphatase, usually less than three times normal.

Aminotransferases. The aminotransferases, alanine aminotransferase (ALT) (formerly serum glutamic-pyruvic transaminase [SGPT]) and aspartate aminotransferase (AST) (formerly serum glutamic-oxaloacetic transaminase [SGOT]) are usually much higher in acute hepatocellular diseases than with extrahepatic obstruction and intrahepatic cholestasis. The values are highest in acute viral hepatitis and drug-induced hepatitis; usually the ALT is higher or equal to the AST (ten to 100 times normal). There are some exceptions to this rule; the two most frequent exceptions are alcoholic liver disease and acute gallstone obstruction of the biliary tract. Although acute alcoholic hepatitis is a hepatocellular disease, the aminotransferases are rarely above 300 units (less than eight times normal) and, characteristically, the AST is higher than the ALT. On the other hand, acute gallstone obstruction of the common bile duct may be associated with marked elevation of the aminotransferases, particularly in the first 48 hours (up to 25 times normal). However, they drop quickly to less than eight times normal. Hepatic enzymes, other than aminotransferases, often are measured in a battery of liver function tests. One example is the lactic dehydrogenase, the highest levels of which are seen in hepatocellular carcinoma and liver metastases.

Prothrombin Time. Prothrombin, produced by the liver, requires vitamin K for its production. The prothrombin time could be elevated in hepatocellular and obstructive liver disease because of different mechanisms. An elevated prothrombin time that does not correct with the intramuscular injection of vitamin K indicates severe liver disease because it reflects the inability of the diseased liver to produce prothrombin. On the other hand, if the prothrombin time returns to normal following the administration of vitamin K, the presence of vitamin K malabsorption is indicated. Vitamin K, being fat-soluble, may be malabsorbed in obstructive jaundice because of inadequate micelle formation owing to the lack of bile salts in the small intestine.

Serum Proteins. Generally, serum protein determinations are not helpful in the differential diagnosis of acute jaundice. They may, however, be helpful in cirrhosis. In severe cirrhosis the serum albumin is usually low, whereas hypergammaglobulinemia is more characteristic of Laennec's cirrhosis and of autoimmune chronic active hepatitis.

Serologic Studies. When acute or chronic hepatitis is suspected as the cause of jaundice, serologic tests such as antibody to hepatitis A virus (anti-

HAV), hepatitis B surface antigen (HBsAG), and delta hepatitis antibody (anti-HDV) are indicated. If primary biliary cirrhosis is suspected, antimitochondrial antibody (AMA) should be done. Other tests such as antismooth muscle antibody and antinuclear antibody are not specific and are not helpful.

Radiologic Noninvasive Studies

The history, physical examination, and laboratory tests provide the data for the initial impression. If common bile duct obstruction is suspected, one of two noninvasive radiologic studies is indicated—ultrasonography (ECHO) or computerized tomography (CT) scanning. Both techniques give the needed information regarding the size of the bile duct. Ultrasonography is more readily available, quicker, and cheaper. Its disadvantage is that overlying gas often hinders adequate visualization of the pancreas and retroperitoneal structures. The CT scan provides more information about the pancreas, retroperitoneum, and liver; its disadvantage lies in its high cost and lack of availability. I believe that the best screening test to rule out extrahepatic obstruction is ultrasonography.[2] The common bile duct is considered dilated if it measures more than 8 mm in diameter. False negative results can occur with both techniques if the obstruction is intermittent or of short duration.

Invasive Endoscopic or Radiologic Studies

The decision to perform an invasive procedure to visualize the biliary system usually is made after finding a dilated bile duct by ultrasonography or by CT scan. These procedures, however, may be indicated when the noninvasive radiologic tests are equivocal or when the clinical suspicion of biliary tract obstruction is high. The two invasive techniques that visualize the biliary tree are endoscopic retrograde cholangiopancreatography (ERCP) and percutaneous transhepatic cholangiography (PTC). These techniques have diagnostic as well as therapeutic capabilities.[3,4,5] Endoscopic sphincterotomy of the ampulla of Vater, stone extraction, and biliary stent placement may be accomplished via an ERCP, while external and internal drainage may be accomplished via a PTC. Several factors deserve consideration before one of these procedures is carried out:

1. Suspected cause of the obstruction
2. General condition of the patient
3. Availability of the test
4. Skill of the operator in diagnostic and therapeutic maneuvers
5. Long-term plan of treatment

For example, if a common bile duct stone is suspected, the procedure of choice is an ERCP with an endoscopic sphincterotomy, provided the technical expertise is available. If cancer of the pancreas or chronic pancreatitis causing common bile duct obstruction is suspected (and the patient is a good surgical candidate), an ERCP is superior because it may visualize the pancreatic duct, help to confirm the diagnosis, and delineate the extent of the disease prior to surgery. If a proximal common bile duct obstruction is suspected and surgery is *not* being considered, then a PTC is a more desirable test to perform because of its ability to provide biliary tract drainage.

Liver Biopsy

Liver biopsy is not indicated in acute hepatitis, but is desirable if chronic hepatitis or cirrhosis is suspected. Biopsy helps to differentiate the different types of cirrhosis, such as Laennec's cirrhosis, postnecrotic cirrhosis, primary biliary cirrhosis, hemochromatosis, and Wilson's disease.

In conclusion, I believe the approach to the jaundiced patient must be a stepwise one using the information initially obtained by the history, physical findings, and liver function tests. Recent advances in radiologic and endoscopic techniques have markedly improved our diagnostic accuracy and provided nonsurgical therapeutic options not available a decade ago.

References

1. Weiss JS. The clinical importance of a protein-bound fraction of serum bilirubin in patients with hyperbilirubinemia. N Engl J Med 1983; 309:147–150.
2. Matzen P, Malchow-Moller A, Brun B, et al. Ultrasonography, computed tomography, and cholescintigraphy in suspected obstructive jaundice—a prospective comparative study. Gastroenterology 1983; 84:1492–1497.
3. Elias F, Hamlyn AN, Jain S, et al. A randomized trial of percutaneous transhepatic cholangiography with the Chiba needle versus endoscopic retrograde cholangiography for bile duct visualization in jaundice. Gastroenterology 1976; 71:439–443.
4. Zimmin DS, Chang J, Clemett AR. Advances in the management of bile duct obstruction. Med Clin North Am 1979; 63:593–609.
5. Kozarek RA, Sanowski RA. Nonsurgical management of extrahepatic obstructive jaundice. Ann Intern Med 1982; 96:743–745.

26 | HEPATIC ENCEPHALOPATHY

SANJEEV ARORA, M.D.
KARIM A. FAWAZ, M.D.

Hepatic encephalopathy is a neuropsychiatric syndrome that includes all changes in mental status that occur directly because of liver dysfunction. The clinical manifestations are diverse and range from subtle personality changes to deep coma (Table 26–1). In the early stages, the sleep pattern changes markedly, resulting in insomnia at night and somnolence during the day. Loss of affect, depression, euphoria, or mild intellectual impairment occur frequently. These emotional and behavioral abnormalities may be apparent only to the family members or to a physician who has been caring for the patient for a period of time. As the encephalopathy progresses, the patient becomes drowsy, confused, and disoriented. Light coma is the penultimate phase; the patient appears comatose, but is arousable. The final stage is deep coma; the patient is unresponsive even to painful stimuli.

DIAGNOSIS

In order to make the diagnosis of hepatic encephalopathy, it is obligatory to establish the presence of liver disease. Liver disease of any type can cause

TABLE 26–1 Stages of Hepatic Encephalopathy

Stage	Symptoms	Signs
I	Personality changes, loss of affect, euphoria, apathy, inappropriate behavior, altered sleep pattern, insomnia with daytime somnolence	Constructional apraxia, difficulty in writing
II	Mental confusion, disorientation to time and place	Asterixis, fetor hepaticus
III	Severe mental confusion, light coma, may appear comatose, but is arousable by stimuli	Asterixis, fetor hepaticus, rigidity, hyperreflexia, extensor-planters, grasping reflexes
IV	Deep coma, unresponsive to stimuli	Fetor hepaticus, unarousable, diminished muscle tone, decreased reflexes

encephalopathy, from acute hepatic failure, as seen in fulminant viral hepatitis, drug toxicity (e.g., acetaminophen), Reye's syndrome, and fatty liver of pregnancy, to chronic liver disease such as alcoholic liver disease or post-hepatitic cirrhosis.

When a patient with suspected hepatic encephalopathy is seen, a detailed history should be obtained from the family of the patient. Special emphasis should be placed on a history of previously diagnosed liver disease, a history of alcohol abuse, or a history of hepatitis. In addition, a family history of liver disease should be taken to search for familial diseases such as Wilson's disease and hemochromatosis. A prior history of blood transfusions or intravenous drug abuse may suggest chronic non-A, non-B hepatitis as an etiology for liver disease. Use of hepatotoxic drugs such as methyldopa, nitrofurantoin, or isoniazid may be the cause of chronic liver disease, whereas a large dose of acetaminophen or a history of recent halothane anesthesia may be responsible for fulminant hepatocellular necrosis. The presence of hepatic failure in a female during the third trimester of pregnancy suggests fatty liver of pregnancy or hepatic toxemia as possible etiologies. A complete history should be taken to try to exclude other causes of metabolic encephalopathy such as uremia, carbon dioxide narcosis, or drug overdose as part of a suicide attempt.

During the physical examination of a patient with suspected hepatic encephalopathy, the physician should look for the characteristic stigmata of liver disease. The presence of icterus, spider nevi, gynecomastia, testicular atrophy, and ascites usually indicates advanced liver disease. Distended veins on the anterior abdominal wall with flow of blood away from the umbilicus caput medusae indicate the presence of portal hypertension, thus providing confirmatory evidence for the presence of serious liver disease.

A neurologic examination during the early stages of encephalopathy usually reveals constructional apraxia (inability to reproduce simple diagrams, such as a five-pointed star) and writing difficulty. During light coma the patient usually has asterixis (flapping tremor of the hand elicited by having the patient extend his wrist with fingers held apart). Other physical findings in the stage of light coma are rigidity of the limbs, hyperreflexia, the presence of grasping and sucking reflexes, and fetor hepaticus. Fetor hepaticus is a sweet musty odor in the breath caused by sulphur-containing mercaptans. In the stage of deep coma, there may be a loss of muscle tone and diminished deep tendon reflexes. It is important to look for the presence of focal neurologic signs or of physical signs of head trauma; it would be a grave error to miss an intracranial hematoma in a comatose alcoholic who also has liver disease.

The laboratory tests that are most valuable in assessing the degree of hepatocellular function are the serum albumin level and the prothrombin time because they reflect hepatocellular synthetic function. The serum bilirubin level, aminotransferase levels (see *Elevated Transaminases* and *Clinical*

Approach to Jaundice), hematocrit level, and platelet count are always helpful. Hepatitis serologic tests and blood toxicology screens may help in certain circumstances. Serum ammonia levels usually are elevated in patients with hepatic encephalopathy, but the level of serum ammonia does not correlate with the degree of encephalopathy. A patient with severe encephalopathy thus may have normal or only mildly elevated levels of serum ammonia. In contrast, some patients with extremely high levels of ammonia have either minimal or no encephalopathy. In an individual patient, the level of serum ammonia, if raised at the baseline, may be useful to follow the progress of encephalopathy. In following a patient with hepatic encephalopathy, we believe that the degree of constructional apraxia and the presence (or absence) of asterixis are better indicators of the level of encephalopathy than sequential serum ammonia levels.

Electroencephalogram (EEG) often shows high-amplitude, low-frequency waves without any focal changes. Triphasic waves in paroxysmal bursts and paroxysms of delta waves (1.5 to 3 Hz) are common. Although these EEG changes are characteristic, they are not diagnostic of hepatic encephalopathy. Patients with other metabolic encephalopathies such as uremia and carbon dioxide narcosis may have similar findings. We do not believe that most patients with hepatic encephalopathy need an EEG. The diagnosis is made clinically by the findings just discussed. In a complicated case, an EEG may be helpful to distinguish hepatic encephalopathy from postepileptic states or from focal intracranial lesions such as cerebrovascular accidents or hematomas.

PATHOPHYSIOLOGY

The liver plays a central role in the metabolism of the body. It is therefore not surprising that hepatic failure is associated with changes in mental status. Though investigated intensively for many years, the pathophysiology of these changes is not well understood. There is a vast amount of experimental data to support various postulated mechanisms.[1]

1. A failure of the liver to detoxify potentially neurotoxic products such as ammonia and short chain fatty acids,
2. Abnormal neurotransmitter balance, which results in increased concentrations of inhibitory neurotransmitters such as gamma-aminobutyric acid (GABA), octopamine, and serotonin,[2]
3. Increased permeability of the blood brain barrier, and
4. Alteration in brain energy metabolism.

These mechanisms are probably not mutually exclusive and may act synergistically to produce the clinical syndrome of hepatic encephalopathy.

MANAGEMENT

Hepatic encephalopathy can be brought on by gradually worsening liver disease or by a sudden deterioration in liver function as occurs in fluminant hepatitis. Another clinical situation in which hepatic encephalopathy is common is a patient with stable chronic liver disease who develops hepatic encephalopathy because of a superimposed precipitating event.[3] The usual precipitating factors are:

1. Gastrointestinal bleeding: Presence of blood in the gastrointestinal (GI) tract can acutely induce hepatic encephalopathy by presenting an unusually large protein load to the gastrointestinal tract. Every 100 ml of blood provides 15 g of protein, which is then broken down to produce ammonia (NH_3) and other toxic nitrogenous products.
2. Azotemia: Because of the presence of ascites and other hemodynamic changes associated with advanced liver disease (which, in turn, cause decreased renal perfusion), this group of patients is more susceptible to the development of azotemia than is the general population. Injudicious use of diuretics, large-volume abdominal paracentesis, use of nonsteroidal anti-inflammatory drugs, or gastrointestinal bleeding can all produce renal insufficiency. During azotemic states there is increased intestinal secretion of urea, which is then broken down by colonic bacteria to produce ammonia. The ammonia, when reabsorbed, may produce encephalopathy.
3. Sedatives: Patients with cirrhosis of the liver are not able to effectively metabolize usual doses of sedatives. Drugs such as diazepam may have an extremely long half-life in this group of patients. In addition, these patients are very sensitive to the central nervous system effect of these drugs.
4. Electrolyte and acid-base disturbances: The most common acid-base disturbance seen in patients with cirrhosis is metabolic alkalosis, attributable either to diuretics or to loss of acid gastric juice. In addition, diuretics produce hypokalemia. Cirrhotics often suffer from respiratory alkalosis as well, perhaps because of the central effect of NH_3 on the respiratory center. Mixed metabolic and respiratory alkalosis also occurs; both alkalemia and hypokalemia tend to worsen hepatic encephalopathy.
5. Infection: The development of infection such as spontaneous bacterial peritonitis can be responsible for rapid development of hepatic encephalo-

pathy. This is usually attributable to an increased catabolic state associated with serious infections.

6. Others: Excessive dietary protein and presence of constipation can also precipitate encephalopathy.

The first goal in the management of a patient with hepatic encephalopathy is to correct or reverse any precipitating factors that are present. If blood is present in the GI tract, it should be evacuated with a nasogastric (NG) tube and/or laxatives. Hypokalemia and alkalosis should be corrected with intravenous potassium chloride administration. Volume depletion should be corrected if present. Saline is appropriate if the patient does not have ascites. If ascites is present, the administration of saline simply makes it worse; colloids (e.g., blood, albumin) should be given as required. A deliberate search should be made to detect infections. Patients with ascites should have a diagnostic paracentesis to rule out the presence of spontaneous bacterial peritonitis.

The next step in management is the prevention of absorption of nitrogenous breakdown products present in the digestive tract; lactulose (1,4 galactosido-fructose) is the most accepted drug to achieve this goal.[4] Lactulose is broken down by colonic bacteria to form lactic acid, formic acid, acetic acid, and carbon dioxide. These acids lower the pH of the colonic contents to about 5.5, which prevents the absorption of ammonia by converting it into the ammonium ion. In addition, the lower pH results in movement of intracellular ammonia into the colonic lumen where it is excreted as the ammonium ion. Lactulose is also a laxative and thus helps evacuate the colon. The aim of therapy is to produce two to three soft stools per day. The usual dose of the drug is 60 to 120 ml per day in divided doses. Lactulose can also be administered in the form of an enema (300 ml of lactulose is mixed with 700 ml of water and administered as a high colonic enema). Avoid severe diarrhea since excessive fluid losses could produce hypernatremia, hypovolemia, and azotemia, all of which can exacerbate encephalopathy.

Neomycin, a nonabsorbable antibiotic, was the drug of choice before the widespread use of lactulose. Neomycin reduces the bacterial counts of urea-splitting organisms in the colon, thereby reducing the load of ammonia and other nitrogenous products that are absorbed into the systemic circulation. Neomycin is a valuable adjunct to lactulose in some patients with refractory encephalopathy who are not totally improved with lactulose alone. Other patients may respond better to neomycin than to lactulose. The usual dose of neomycin given orally is 2 to 4 g per day in divided doses. One to 3 percent of orally-administered neomycin is absorbed. Therefore it has the potential for ototoxicity and nephrotoxicity, especially in patients with renal failure. For this reason lactulose is the preferred first line drug for management of hepatic encephalopathy.

Patients with hepatic encephalopathy should be fed a protein-restricted diet. Patients with stage I or stage II encephalopathy can be given small amounts, such as 30 to 40 g per day. In patients with stage III or IV encephalopathy, dietary protein should be withheld until there is clinical improvement. New and expensive modalities of treatment, such as intravenous infusions of branched chain amino acids, remain unproven.

In summary, the management of patients with hepatic encephalopathy is based on an aggressive search for and reversal of precipitating factors, as well as on the reduction of the absorption of nitrogenous breakdown products. The latter is accomplished by the reduction of protein intake and by the use of lactulose and/or neomycin.

References

1. Fraser CL, Arieff AI. Hepatic encephalopathy. N Eng J Med 1986; 313 (14):865–873.
2. Jones EA, et al. The neurobiology of hepatic encephalopathy. Hepatology 1984; 4:1235–1242.
3. Schenker S, Hoyumpa AM Jr. Pathophysiology of hepatic encephalopathy. Hosp Prac 1984; September:99–121.
4. Conn HO, Lieberthal MM, eds. The hepatic coma syndrome and lactulose. Baltimore: Williams and Wilkins, 1984.

RENAL DISEASE

27 | HYPONATREMIA AND HYPERNATREMIA

ANDREW S. LEVEY, M.D.

Hyponatremia and hypernatremia occur frequently in hospitalized patients and usually indicate disturbances in osmolality and in water metabolism. Although disturbances in the serum sodium concentration may coexist with disorders of sodium metabolism, serum sodium concentration does not indicate total body sodium content or extracellular fluid (ECF) volume. Mild hyponatremia and hypernatremia are rarely associated with serious symptoms or complications and are usually corrected by treatment of the underlying condition. Severe hyponatremia or hypernatremia, however, may be life-threatening and are medical emergencies. Proper diagnosis and treatment require a clear understanding of the factors that regulate osmolality and water metabolism.

OSMOLALITY OF BODY FLUIDS

Water constitutes approximately 60 percent of body weight. Since most cell membranes are permeable to water, body fluid compartments are in osmotic equilibrium. The normal range for serum osmolality is 280 to 295 mOsm per kilogram. In practice, osmolality usually can be estimated from the serum sodium concentration[1].

Within the ECF, sodium (and an approximately equal concentration of anions), glucose, and urea are the most abundant solutes. As shown in the following equations, if blood glucose and blood urea nitrogen (BUN) concentrations are normal, the serum sodium concentration may be used to calculate serum osmolality.

Osmolality (mOsm/kg)

$$= 2[Na^+]\,(mEq/L) + \frac{[glucose]\,(mg/dl)}{18} + \frac{[BUN]\,(mg/dl)}{2.8}$$

$$= 2[Na^+] + \frac{90}{18} + \frac{14}{2.8}$$

$$= 2[Na^+] + 10$$

In normal circumstances, the estimated serum osmolality closely approximates (i.e., within 10 mOsm/kg) the measured serum osmolality. A discrepancy or "osmolar gap" between the estimated and the measured values may occur in two conditions: (1) if water is displaced from the serum by increased concentrations of protein or lipid, or (2) if additional solute is present in the serum. In the first case, the additional colloid introduces an error in the measurement of serum solute concentrations. The value for sodium is artifactually low (psuedohyponatremia), thus leading to underestimation of serum osmolality; however, the measured value for osmolality is normal. Although these patients appear to have hyponatremia, they do not have a disorder of osmolality or of water metabolism and do not require treatment for the low serum sodium concentration. In the second case, the presence of additional solute raises plasma osmolality, draws water into the plasma, and lowers the serum sodium concentration. These patients have true hyponatremia, but are hyperosmolar and may require urgent treatment to reverse the underlying disorder. Hyperosmolar conditions are discussed later in this chapter.

A review of the normal mechanisms for the regulation of osmolality and of water balance is necessary before the causes and treatment of hyponatremia and hypernatremia are discussed. Osmolality is normally maintained within narrow limits by thirst, antidiuretic hormone (ADH), and the renal concentration mechanism.[2] A reduction in total body water from either decreased water intake or increased water losses leads to an increase in osmolality. This increase stimulates thirst and the release of ADH, which in turn leads to increased water intake, decreased renal water excretion, and restoration to normal of total body water and serum osmolality. Conversely, an increase in total body water from either increased intake or impaired excretion results in decreased osmolality, reduced thirst, and release of ADH. The subsequent decreased water intake and increased water excretion reduce body water and raise serum osmolality to normal. Figure 27–1 shows the normal relationships among serum osmolality, plasma ADH, urine concentration, and urine volume.[3,4] In most patients the cause of hyponatremia and hypernatremia can be diagnosed accurately from the measurement of urinary specific gravity and of urine volume. Rarely, the measurement of ADH level is necessary. Measurement of serum ADH is now performed in only a few diagnostic laboratories, but in the future this test is likely to be widely available.

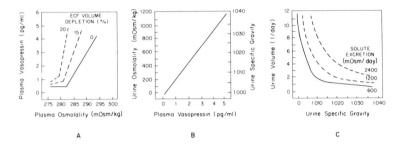

Figure 27-1 Approximate relationships among serum osmolality, plasma antidiuretic hormone level, urine concentration, and urine volume. The bold lines represent normal relationships. The dotted lines in panel *A* indicate altered relationships in ECF volume depletion. The dotted lines in panel *C* indicate relationships during solute administration.

HYPONATREMIA

Hyponatremia, defined as a serum sodium concentration less than 130 mEq per liter, is probably the most common electrolyte abnormality and affects approximately 2.5 percent of hospitalized patients.[5] In most patients, the hyponatremia is mild (serum sodium between 120 and 130 mEq/L) and asymptomatic. However, patients with severe hyponatremia (serum sodium less than 120 mEq/L) frequently have signs and symptoms of hypo-osmolality, including nausea, vomiting, diarrhea, confusion, and seizures, and they may develop permanent neurologic damage.[6] In patients with serious underlying medical illnesses, such as heart failure or cirrhosis, hyponatremia is associated with a more severe pathophysiologic disturbance and a poorer prognosis.[7] Rapid diagnosis is the key to successful treatment, regardless of the cause or the severity of hyponatremia.

Approach to the Patient

A practical approach to the diagnosis of hyponatremia is shown in Figure 27-2. The cause usually can be established in less than an hour by using this approach. Most patients with hyponatremia are hypo-osmolar; measurement of serum osmolality is necessary only if pseudohyponatremia or hyperosmolar conditions are suspected. In patients with hypo-osmolality, water intake has exceeded water excretion, thus resulting in a relative excess of water. Meas-

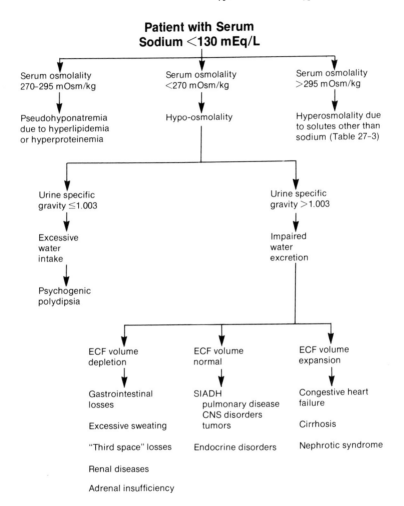

Figure 27-2   Diagnostic approach to the patient with hyponatremia.

urement of urinary specific gravity is then necessary to determine whether the underlying pathophysiologic defect is excessive water ingestion or inadequate water excretion.

Most patients with hyponatremia have impaired water excretion. As discussed, an abnormality in serum sodium concentration is not necessarily indicative of an abnormality in sodium metabolism or in ECF volume. Nonetheless, disorders of sodium metabolism may impair renal water excretion secondarily, thus leading to water retention and hyponatremia. For this reason, an assessment of the state of ECF volume is necessary in order to determine the cause of inadequate water excretion. A recent history of fluid losses, diuretic use, or weight loss and physical findings of diminished skin turgor, postural hypotension, or tachycardia usually indicate ECF volume depletion. In contrast, a recent history of fluid administration, weight gain, jugular venous distension, peripheral edema, pulmonary congestion, hepatic ascites, or pleural effusions indicate ECF volume expansion. Occasionally, measurements of central venous or pulmonary capillary wedge pressures are necessary to assess the state of ECF volume.

Although this approach to the diagnosis of hyponatremia is based principally on evaluation of the urine specific gravity and on physical examination, evaluation of other serum electrolytes and of renal function provides valuable diagnostic information (Table 27–1). In the following paragraphs, the diagno-

TABLE 27-1 Serum Composition in Hypo-osmolar Syndromes

Disorder	Sodium	Potassium	Chloride	Bicarbonate	BUN	Creatinine	Uric Acid
Excessive water drinking	L	N	L	N	N-L	N-L	N-L
ECF volume depletion							
Vomiting	L	L	VL*	H	H	N-H	H
Diarrhea	L	L	L-N†	L	H	N-H	H
Diuretics	L	L	VL*	H	H	N-H	H
K-sparing diuretics	L	H	L	N	H	N-H	H
ECF volume excess	L	N‡	L‡	N‡	H	N-H	H
Normal ECF volume	L	N-L	L	N	L	L	L

N = normal, L = low, VL = very low, H = high

* Value for chloride is reduced proportionately more than sodium because of the metabolic alkalosis.

† Value for chloride is reduced proportionately less than sodium because of the nonanion gap (hyperchloremic) metabolic acidosis.

‡ Value may be altered by diuretic therapy.

sis and the treatment of the specific disorders and the use of hypertonic saline for severe hyponatremia are discussed.

Hyponatremia with Normal or Increased Osmolality

These disorders account for approximately 15 percent of cases of hyponatremia[5] and are recognized easily from the patient's history and clinical presentation. In patients with hyponatremia attributable to hyperlipidemia or to hyperproteinemia, the serum osmolality is normal. Typically, the serum sodium concentration is stable, there are no symptoms of hypo-osmolality, and serum concentrations of potassium, chloride, bicarbonate, BUN, and creatinine are proportionately reduced. In these patients, measurement of serum osmolality is necessary to confirm the diagnosis of pseudohyponatremia.

Patients with hyponatremia attributable to the presence of another solute usually are symptomatic from the underlying disorder and, in addition, may have symptoms of hyperosmolality, including polyuria, thirst, lethargy, coma, or seizures. Moreover, these patients often have accompanying disorders in acid-base and potassium metabolism and in renal function. These conditions are reviewed in the discussion of hyperosmolality. In patients with hyponatremia caused by hyperglycemia, serum sodium is reduced by 2 to 3 mEq per liter for each 100 mg per deciliter elevation above normal of the blood glucose.

Hyponatremia Attributable to Excessive Water Intake

Excessive water intake is a rare disorder seen in patients with underlying psychiatric disorders (psychogenic polydipsia). If renal function is normal, maximal water excretion is 10 to 12 L per day, or 400 to 500 ml per hour. Hyponatremia develops only if the rate of water ingestion exceeds this amount. While it is extremely rare for a patient to drink this volume of water continuously, a transient binge of water drinking (2 or 3 gallons) may temporarily exceed the maximal rate of water excretion and lead to severe hyponatremia. If renal water excretion is impaired, hyponatremia develops with less extreme water intake. Patients with psychogenic polydipsia are easy to recognize by a history of excessive water drinking, polyuria, and very low values for urinary specific gravity. ADH levels, if measured, would be minimal. BUN and serum creatinine concentration are usually below normal. Serum potassium also may be reduced. Acid-base parameters usually are normal (see Table 27–1).

The diagnosis may be obscured if the history is not available either because of encephalopathy owing to severe hypo-osmolality or because of the patient's unwillingness to acknowledge the water drinking behavior. The usual clinical picture may be further complicated by simultaneous ingestion of antipsychotic drugs that alter ADH release, or by superimposed acid-base and electrolyte disorders from self-induced vomiting or from ingestion of cathartics or diuretics. Even in these patients, however, the response to treatment is usually characteristic.

Treatment is restriction of water intake. If renal function is normal, polyuria continues and the serum sodium rises rapidly. For example if urine output is 400 to 500 ml per hour in a 70-kg patient, serum sodium concentration would rise from 110 mEq per liter to 120 mEq per liter in 6 to 8 hours. Treatment with hypertonic saline is necessary only if serum sodium concentration is less than 120 mEq per liter, if the patient has neurologic symptoms, and if the urine output is less than 300 ml per hour.

Hyponatremia Attributable to ECF Volume Depletion

ECF volume depletion is the cause of approximately 20 percent of cases of hyponatremia in hospitalized patients.[5] Two pathophysiologic factors contribute to impaired water excretion: (1) direct stimulation of ADH release, and (2) reduced renal perfusion. The relationships among serum osmolality, ADH level, and ECF volume are shown in Figure 27–1.[2] For any level of serum osmolality, reduction in ECF volume results in a higher ADH level, and consequently a higher urine concentration and a reduced rate of water excretion. Hyponatremia develops if the intake of water exceeds the reduced water excreting capacity even transiently.

Diagnosis is made by findings of a urinary specific gravity greater than 1.003 and of clinical features associated with ECF volume depletion. Typically the BUN is elevated; the serum creatinine concentration may be within the normal range, but is usually higher than the patient's baseline value. Measurement of urinary sodium concentration is helpful in establishing the route of ECF losses. Urinary sodium concentration exceeds 40 mEq per liter if renal sodium wasting is ongoing, as in patients with renal diseases or adrenal insufficiency or in those taking diuretics. Urinary sodium concentration is less than 20 mEq per liter if the losses are "non-renal", as in patients with vomiting, diarrhea, gastrointestinal drainage, third space losses, or heat exposure.

Treatment is replacement of the ECF deficit with isotonic saline and correction of the underlying disorder. When ECF volume is restored, the ADH level declines, renal blood flow improves, and the excess water is excreted. Hypertonic saline should be administered if hyponatremia is severe. Other electrolyte and acid-base disorders frequently result from ECF losses and also must be repaired.

Hyponatremia with ECF Volume Expansion

Signs of ECF volume expansion are found in approximately 20 percent of hospitalized patients with hyponatremia.[5] In congestive heart failure and in liver disease, the two most common causes of hyponatremia, the underlying renal pathophysiology is similar to that found in patients with volume depletion. Altered systemic hemodynamics result in the release of ADH and reduced renal perfusion, thereby leading to impaired water excretion. Typically, hyponatremia develops late in the course of the disease and indicates severe circulatory abnormalities. Development may be earlier, however, as a consequence of diuretic administration.

The diagnosis is usually clear cut. Urinary specific gravity is greater than 1.003, the patient has signs of ECF volume excess, the BUN is elevated, and serum creatinine also may be increased. Urinary sodium concentration is typically less than 20 mEq per liter unless diuretics are being administered. Management of these patients is difficult. In general, it is best to reduce diuretic dosage and to restrict total oral and intravenous fluid intake to 1 L per day. Definitive treatment must be directed at improving the underlying medical condition. For patients with heart failure, measures should be taken to improve cardiac output by augmenting myocardial contractility and by optimizing afterload and preload. For patients with cirrhosis, albumin can be infused to increase the serum protein concentration transiently. If such attempts are unsuccessful, hyponatremia and edema persist. Fluid restriction should be maintained and diuretics continued at the lowest doses that maintain the patient's comfort. If hyponatremia is severe, hypertonic saline with an increased dosage of diuretics may be administered judiciously. Although this regimen provides temporary improvement of hyponatremia, it often worsens edema.

Hyponatremia with Normal ECF Volume

These disorders were first characterized in 1957 by Schwartz and Bartter, who defined them as a syndrome of inappropriate ADH secretion (SIADH). Now they are recognized as the most common cause of hyponatremia among hospitalized patients, accounting for approximately one-third of cases.[5] The pathophysiology of impaired water excretion is fundamentally different in two respects from the disorders discussed previously: (1) ADH level usually is elevated, but there is no physiologic stimulus for ADH release (i.e., patients are neither hyperosmolar nor volume depleted), and (2) renal perfusion is normal or increased; thus, there is no stimulus for sodium retention. The cause of the disorders is excessive release of ADH from the pituitary caused by certain drugs (Table 27–2) or by endocrine, central nervous system, and

TABLE 27-2 Drug-Induced SIADH

Antidiuretic Hormones
  Vasopressin
  Oxytocin

Thiazide diuretics

Antidepressants and Antipsychotic Agents
  Monoamine oxidase inhibitors
  Tricyclic antidepressants
  Tetracyclic antidepressants
  Phenothiazines
  Thioxanthenes
  Butyrophenones

Anticonvulsants
  Carbamazepine

Oral Hypoglycemics
  Chlorpropamide
  Tolbutamide
  Glyburide

Antineoplastic Agents
  Vincristine
  Cyclophosphamide

Analgesics and Anti-Inflammatory Agents
  Narcotic analgesics
  Nonsteroidal anti-inflammatory agents

Others
  Clofibrate

pulmonary disorders, or by ectopic production of ADH by some tumors. The disorders can be mimicked by drugs that increase the sensitivity of the kidney to ADH (clofibrate) or by selective impairment of the urinary dilution mechanism (thiazide diuretics).

The clinical features include urinary specific gravity greater than 1.003 and apparently normal ECF volume. In contrast to patients with hyponatremia and altered ECF volume, serum concentration of BUN, creatinine, and uric acid are low, thereby reflecting increased renal perfusion, increased glomerular filtration, and decreased tubular reabsorption (see Table 27-1). Urinary sodium concentration is usually greater than 40 mEq per liter unless the patient is following a low salt diet. Initial treatment is restriction of total water intake to 1 L per day. With this regimen, the hyponatremia and all other features of the disorder should resolve. Severe hyponatremia should be treated with hypertonic saline and diuretics.

If the underlying disease cannot be improved, long-term therapy to prevent the redevelopment of hyponatremia is necessary. Although long-term water restriction is effective, most patients are not compliant. Recently several alternative measures to increase renal water excretion have been proposed.[7] The most useful method is administration of demeclocycline (Declomycin), a tetracycline that induces a mild urinary concentrating defect. Doses of 900 to 1,200 mg per day are usually well-tolerated and effective. Mild azotemia may occur, but is reversible when the dose is reduced. Demeclocycline should not be used for the treatment of hyponatremia caused by heart failure or cirrhosis because, in these patients, renal failure has been reported as a complication of this therapy.

Emergency Treatment of Severe Hyponatremia

Death or permanent neurologic impairment may result in patients with severe symptomatic hyponatremia.[8] Treatment with hypertonic saline should be considered if serum sodium is less than 120 mEq per liter and if neurologic symptoms are present. The goal of therapy is to raise the serum sodium level judiciously (1 mEq per liter per hour) to a final value of not more than 130 mEq per liter. Some authors have cautioned that this treatment may be associated with a devastating neurologic complication, central pontine myelinolysis. Apparently, however, development of this lesion is associated with the rapid elevation of the serum sodium concentration to normal or elevated levels.[9,10] Hypertonic saline should be administered cautiously because of the potential danger of rapid correction or overcorrection of hyponatremia, and serum sodium should be monitored frequently during therapy. As discussed earlier, treatment with hypertonic saline is usually necessary only in patients with impaired water excretion. Administration of 400 to 800 ml of 3 percent saline (520 mmol per liter) over 4 hours would directly raise the serum sodium level by 5 to 10 mEq per liter. In patients with ECF volume depletion, the restoration of ECF volume would reduce ADH secretion, improve renal perfusion, and increase water excretion, thus further raising the serum sodium concentration. In patients with normal or expanded ECF, administration of hypertonic saline poses a risk of precipitation of pulmonary congestion. In such patients, loop diuretics, for example furosemide 80 mg, should be administered intravenously to reduce ECF volume prior to infusion of hypertonic saline.[11] In addition, the water diuresis that results further increases the serum sodium concentration. Serum potassium concentration usually declines and must be carefully monitored during this therapy. Repeat measurement of serum electrolytes should be obtained within 12 hours as a guide to further therapy.

HYPERNATREMIA

Hypernatremia, defined as a serum sodium concentration greater than 145 mEq per liter, always indicates hyperosmolality. Hyperosmolality is usually the result of reduced total body water, but in some cases it is the result of solute excess. Regardless of the cause, hyperosmolality is a potent stimulus to thirst; thus, persistent hyperosmolality also signals either a disorder of thirst or an inability to obtain water. Hyperosmolality may coexist with either hypernatremia or hyponatremia, depending whether sodium or another solute is present in relative excess in serum. Regardless of the serum sodium concentration, severe hyperosmolality (serum osmolality > 330 mOsm per kilogram) may lead to neurologic alterations including delirium, coma, and permanent brain damage.[6,12] The causes of hyperosmolality are listed in Table 27-3. In this chapter, only disorders associated with hypernatremia will be discussed.

Mild hypernatremia (serum sodium 146 to 155 mEq per liter) attributable to inability to obtain water in postoperative or debilitated patients usually poses no difficulty for recognition or treatment. Severe hypernatremia (serum sodium greater than 155 mEq per liter) is associated with severe hyperosmolality and requires urgent diagnosis and therapy. Regardless of the severity, the cause of hypernatremia can be diagnosed quickly with a few readily available measurements.

Approach to the Patient

The approach to the patient with hypernatremia demonstrated in Figure 27-3 should establish the diagnosis within an hour. Patients with hypernatremia are hyperosmolar. Measurements of urinary volume and specific gravity allow classification of hyperosmolar syndromes according to the pathophysiologic defect: impaired water intake, solute excess, or renal water losses. Renal water conservation is normal in patients with impaired water intake, thereby resulting in a reduced volume of highly concentrated urine. In patients with solute excess, urinary solute excretion is elevated, the urine is isotonic with plasma, and the urine volume is increased. In patients with renal water losses, the urine is dilute or slightly concentrated and the urine volume is not increased. The cause of the renal defect is assessed by observation of the patient after administration of exogenous ADH. Measurement of the plasma level of ADH is helpful as well. The following paragraphs describe the various causes of hypernatremia and the approach to treatment. The concluding section describes the calculation of the water deficit and the method of water administration to correct the hypernatremia.

TABLE 27-3 Serum Composition in Hyperosmolar Syndromes

Disorder	Sodium	Potassium	Chloride	Bicarbonate	Anion Gap	BUN	Creatinine	Glucose	Osmolar Gap
Hyperglycemia	L*	N†	L	N†	N†	H	N-H	H	H
Mannitol	L*	N	L	N	N	H	N-H	N	H
High protein tube feedings	L*	N	L	N	N	VH	N-H	H	H
Ethanol	N	N	N	N	N	N	N	N	H
Methanol	N	N	N	L	H	N	N	N	H
Ethylene glycol	N	N	N	L	H	H‡	H‡	N	H
Severe renal failure	N-L	H	N	L	H	VH	VH	N	H
Sodium bicarbonate administration	H	N	N	H	N	H§	H§	N	N
Water deprivation	H	N	H	N	N	H	N-H	N	N
Neurogenic diabetes insipidus	H	N	H	N	N	H	N-H	N	N
Nephrogenic diabetes insipidus	H	N	H	N	N	H	N-H	N	N

N = normal, L = low, H = high, VH = very high
* Osmotic diuresis, hypernatremia, and severe hyperosmolality may develop.
† If ketoacidosis is present, values will be altered.
‡ Acute renal failure
§ Value is usually elevated because of acute renal failure following resuscitation.

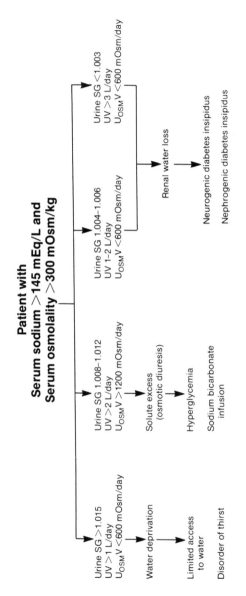

**Patient with
Serum sodium >145 mEq/L and
Serum osmolality >300 mOsm/kg**

Urine SG >1.015
UV >1 L/day
U_{OSM} V <600 mOsm/day

Water deprivation

Limited access
to water

Disorder of thirst

Urine SG 1.008–1.012
UV >2 L/day
U_{OSM} V >1200 mOsm/day

Solute excess
(osmotic diuresis)

Hyperglycemia

Sodium bicarbonate
infusion

Urine SG 1.004–1.006
UV 1–2 L/day
U_{OSM} V <600 mOsm/day

Urine SG <1.003
UV >3 L/day
U_{OSM} V <600 mOsm/day

Renal water loss

Neurogenic diabetes insipidus

Nephrogenic diabetes insipidus

Figure 27–3 Diagnostic approach to the patient with hypernatremia.

Hypernatremia from Inadequate Water Intake

Inadequate water intake is probably the most common cause of hypernatremia. The diagnostic features include the patient's inability to obtain water, maximal urine concentration, and reduced urine volume. Typically, urinary specific gravity is 1.025 to 1.035 and urine volume is 500 ml per day or less. However, in elderly or malnourished patients, maximal urine specific gravity may be reduced to 1.018 to 1.020, thus resulting in a urine volume of 500 to 1,000 ml per day. Treatment is provision of sufficient water to restore and maintain normal osmolality.

Hypernatremia from Solute Excess

Hypernatremia from solute excess results from one of two mechanisms: (1) Administration of hypertonic sodium salts directly raises serum sodium concentration and expands ECF volume. If renal function is impaired, these patients may develop ECF volume excess. (2) Administration or generation of solutes other than sodium raises serum osmolality, and initially lowers the serum sodium concentration (see Table 27–3); however, the ensuing osmotic diuresis impairs the renal concentration and dilution mechanism and leads to water losses and the subsequent development of hypernatremia. Moreover, the sodium and chloride losses that accompany osmotic diuresis may lead to extreme contraction of the ECF volume.[13]

Patients with solute excess are usually easy to recognize. There is a history of recent development of diabetic hyperglycemia or of hypertonic solute administration, such as saline, sodium bicarbonate, dextrose, high protein nasogastric tube feedings, intravenous hyperalimentation fluid, or mannitol. Typically, urinary specific gravity is 1.008 to 1.012, urine volume is greater than 2 L per day, and solute excretion exceeds 800 mOsm daily. Treatment is discontinuation of solute administration and, in the case of diabetic hyperglycemia, provision of insulin. In patients with hypotension owing to ECF volume depletion, isotonic sodium chloride should be administered first. Once vital signs are stable, hypotonic solutions should be administered to lower the serum osmolality. Deficits of other electrolytes also must be replaced, for example, potassium and phosphorus in diabetic hyperglycemia. In patients with ECF volume expansion, ongoing solute diuresis restores ECF volume, but administration of hypotonic solutions is necessary to lower serum osmolality. Hypotonic solutions should be given carefully to avoid development of pulmonary edema. Diuretics may be necessary to increase solute excretion, but may further increase serum osmolality. If renal function is impaired, dialysis may be necessary to lower ECF volume and serum osmolality.

Hypernatremia from Renal Water Loss

These disorders are recognized by the occurrence of hypernatremia without excess solute excretion and by failure to concentrate the urine maximally. Sometimes, diagnosis can be based on usual clinical features and on urinary specific gravity. In many cases, however, accurate diagnosis requires performance of an overnight water deprivation test[4,14] and administration of exogenous ADH (vasopressin).[10]

Neurogenic Diabetes Insipidus

Pituitary secretion of ADH is absent or, if present, reduced. The most common causes of neurogenic diabetes insipidus are head trauma, neurosurgery, brain tumor (especially pituitary adenoma and craniopharyngioma), and idiopathic disease of young adults. Many patients can be diagnosed by their neurologic and endocrinologic features.

If ADH levels are extremely low (less than 1 pg per milliliter), urinary specific gravity is less than 1.003 and urine volume is 3 to 5 L per day or more. Rapid dehydration and extreme hyperosmolality result if access to water is limited. In these circumstances, urinary specific gravity may rise as high as 1.012. In adults this extreme defect is seen only in neurogenic diabetes insipidus. With milder defects in ADH secretion, ADH levels are higher than 1 pg per milliliter, but are still abnormally low for the elevated serum osmolality. Urinary specific gravity may be as high as 1.012 and urine volume as low as 2 to 3 L per day even without development of extreme dehydration and hyperosmolality. Clinically, these patients may be difficult to distinguish from patients with nephrogenic diabetes insipidus. To make the diagnosis, it is usually necessary to perform an overnight water deprivation test and to assess the response to vasopressin.[14] In neurogenic diabetes insipidus, urinary specific gravity rises only slightly after water deprivation, but increases promptly after administration of vasopressin. Treatment is correction of the underlying disorder if possible. Emergency treatment is subcutaneous administration of arginine vasopressin in oil (Pitressin Tannate) every 12 hours to maintain urine volume at approximately 3 L per day. Long-term treatment is intranasal administration of short-acting lypressin (lysine vasopressin) or long-acting desmopressin[15] (DDAVP) to maintain the desired urine volume, usually 2 to 4 L per day. Partial defects in ADH excretion may be treated by chlorpropamide or clofibrate, which increase ADH release and the renal response to ADH, respectively.

Nephrogenic Diabetes Insipidus

ADH levels are normal for the degree of hyperosmolality, but the urinary specific gravity is not increased appropriately. Nephrogenic diabetes insipidus is the result of renal disorders that interfere with the urine concentration mechanism and the response to ADH. In adults, common causes are metabolic disturbances (hypokalemia and hypercalcemia), drugs (lithium, demeclocycline, amphotericin B, loop diuretics), and parenchymal renal diseases causing prominent tubulointerstitial damage (Table 27-4). In addition, any chronic parenchymal renal disease associated with marked reduction in renal function (serum creatinine greater than 4 mg per deciliter) results in impaired urinary concentration and may lead to hypernatremia if water intake is reduced.

In most cases, the renal defect is not severe, and urinary concentration may achieve specific gravity as high as 1.012. Therefore, urine volume is typically 2 to 3 L per day. As discussed earlier, the diagnosis may be difficult to distinguish from mild neurogenic diabetes insipidus. However, in contrast to neurogenic diabetes insipidus, urinary specific gravity remains 1.012 or less after an overnight water deprivation test and administration of vasopressin. Treatment is correction of the underlying cause of renal impairment, if possible. If the defect is severe, thiazide diuretics (hydrochlorothiazide 100 mg per day) can be used to promote mild ECF volume contraction and to increase urine concentration. With this regimen, urinary specific gravity can reach 1.012, and urine volume can be reduced to 2 to 4 L per day.

TABLE 27-4   Nephrogenic Diabetes Insipidus from
Renal Diseases with Prominent Tubulointerstitial
Damage

Acute pyelonephritis
Obstructive nephropathy
Acute tubular necrosis (diuretic phase)
Sickle cell nephropathy
Sjögren's syndrome
Amyloidosis
Myeloma kidney and light chain nephropathy
Lead nephropathy

Repairing the Water Deficit

Hyperosmolality, whether the result of solute excess or of water loss, indicates a water deficit relative to the amount of solute. The magnitude of the water deficit is estimated from the patient's present weight and serum osmolality by application of the following formula:

$$\text{water deficit (L)} = \text{normal total body water} - \text{current total body water}$$

$$= \frac{\text{osmolality (mOsm/kg)}}{290 \text{ (mOsm/kg)}} \times \text{current weight (kg)}$$

$$\times \ 0.6 \ \text{ (L/kg)} - \text{current weight (kg)} \times 0.6 \ \text{(L/kg)}$$

$$= \text{current weight} \times 0.6 \times \left(\frac{\text{osmolality}}{290} - 1 \right)$$

This calculation is based on the assumption that there has been no change in total body solute content. This assumption is generally valid in hyperosmolality attributable to water deprivation or to neurogenic and nephrogenic diabetes insipidus. In cases of solute excess and osmotic diuresis, however, this assumption is not valid. The solute gains or losses may be estimated by comparing the patient's calculated normal weight with the actual weight before the development of hyperosmolality. As discussed earlier, repair of solute excess or deficit should begin prior to correction of the relative water deficit. The preferred solution for correction of the water deficit is 5 percent dextrose in water. If hyperosmolality has developed over several days, water administration should proceed slowly in order to prevent the development of cerebral edema. Not more than half the water deficit should be infused during the first 24 hours. The serum sodium should be measured every 12 hours during therapy.

References

1. Gennari FJ. Serum osmolality: uses and limitations. N Engl J Med 1984; 310:102–105.
2. Bichet DG, Levi M, Schrier RW. Polyuria, dehydration, overhydration. In: Seldin DW, Giebisch G, eds. The kidney: physiology and pathophysiology. New York: Raven Press, 1985:951.
3. Robertson GL, Shelton RL, Athar S. The osmoregulation of vasopressin. Kidney Int 1976; 10:25–37.
4. Levev AS, Harrington JT. Polyuria. In: Taylor RB, ed. Difficult diagnosis. Philadelphia: WB Saunders, 1985:392.
5. Anderson RJ, Hsiao-Min C, Kluge R, Schrier RW. Hyponatremia: a prospective analysis of its epidemiology and the pathogenetic role of vasopressin. Ann Intern Med 1985; 102:164–168.

6. Arieff AI, Guisado R. Effects on the central nervous system of hypernatremic and hyponatremic states. Kidney Int 1976; 10:104–116.

7. Schrier RW. Treatment of hyponatremia. N Engl J Med 1985; 312:1121–1123.

8. Narins RG. Therapy of symptomatic hyponatremia: does haste make waste? N Engl J Med 1986; 314:1573–1575.

9. Ayus JC, Krothapalli R, Arieff AI. Changing concepts in the treatment of severe symptomatic hyponatremia: rapid correction and its possible relation to central pontine myelinolysis. Am J Med 1985; 78:897–902.

10. Ayus JC, Krothapalli RK, Arieff AI. Treatment of symptomatic hyponatremia and its relation to brain damage: a prospective study. N Engl J Med 1987; 317:1190–1195

11. Hartman D, Rossier B, Zohlman R, Schrier RW. Rapid correction of hyponatremia in the syndrome of inappropriate secretion of antidiuretic hormone: an alternative to hypertonic saline. Ann Intern Med 1973; 78:870–875.

12. Snyder NA, Feigal DW, Arieff AI. Hypernatremia in elderly patients: a heterogenous, morbid, and iatrogenic entity. Ann Intern Med 1987; 107:309–319.

13. Gennari FJ, Kassirer JP. Osmotic diuresis. N Engl J Med 1974; 291:714–720.

14. Zerbe RL, Robertson GL. A comparison of plasma vasopressin measurements with a standard indirect test in the differential diagnosis of polyuria. N Engl J Med 1981; 305:1539–1546.

15. Richardson OW, Robinson AG. Desmopressin. Ann Intern Med 1985; 103:228–239.

28 | HYPOKALEMIA AND HYPERKALEMIA

ANDREW S. LEVEY, M.D.

The serum potassium concentration normally is maintained within a narrow physiologic range, from 3.5 to 5.0 mEq per liter. Alterations in serum potassium concentration are frequent, especially in hospitalized patients. Hypokalemia occurs during the course of hospitalization in 30 percent of patients and has been noted in up to 50 percent of acutely ill patients at the time of admission.[1,2] By comparison, hyperkalemia is a less frequent complication, but still occurs in up to 10 percent of hospitalized patients.[3] Consultation usually is requested if the alteration in potassium level is severe or persistent or if the etiology is not easily recognized. The proper diagnosis is important because the abnormal serum potassium concentration is usually a clue to the diagnosis of a serious underlying disorder or a complication of treatment and because the resulting alteration in cellular transmembrane potential may cause life-threatening complications, such as cardiac arrhythmias and muscle paralysis. This chapter will focus on the pathophysiology and the etiology of hypokalemia and hyperkalemia. The treatment of these disorders will be discussed briefly; more detailed considerations of therapy have been reviewed elsewhere.[4,5]

PATHOPHYSIOLOGY OF DISORDERS OF POTASSIUM METABOLISM

Disorders in serum potassium concentration are the result of either altered internal distribution, increased intake, or decreased excretion of potassium.[6,7] A review of several features of normal potassium metabolism is important before the specific disorders are discussed. Total body potassium content is approximately 50 mEq per kilogram body weight, or 3,000 to 3,500 mEq in adults. Potassium is the most prevalent intracellular cation, its concentration being approximately 150 mEq per liter. The majority of potassium is located in skeletal muscle; by contrast, only 2 percent of total body potassium is contained in extracellular fluid. The normal distribution of potassium across the cell membrane is maintained by active transport processes and is influenced by levels of insulin, by adrenergic nervous system activity, by exercise, by alterations in the osmolality and acidity of body fluids, by drugs that affect membrane transport, and by disorders that disrupt cell metabolism or cause cell lysis.

The usual American dietary potassium intake is 50 to 125 mEq per day (equivalent to 2 to 5 g per day). Potassium is present in all animal and vegetable matter, especially meat, certain fruits (bananas, oranges, tomatoes), vegetables, beans, coffee, and cocoa. Gastrointestinal losses of potassium are usually 5 to 15 mEq per day, but increase with diarrhea, chronic renal failure, and hyperaldosteronism. The remainder of ingested potassium is excreted in the urine. Renal excretion of potassium is closely linked to dietary intake and thereby maintains total body content and serum concentration of potassium at normal levels.

Within the kidney, potassium is filtered by the glomerulus, virtually totally reabsorbed in the proximal nephron, and secreted in the distal nephron. The most important sites of potassium secretion are the distal convoluted tubule and the cortical collecting duct. Potassium excretion is regulated by alterations in the rate of potassium secretion. Although the usual potassium excretion is 50 to 125 mEq per day, urinary excretion can vary from 5 to 1,000 mEq potassium per day under circumstances of extreme depletion or loading of potassium. However, these extreme adjustments occur much more slowly than the usual physiologic responses to alterations in intake. The major factors that normally regulate distal nephron potassium secretion include the level of aldosterone, the urine flow rate, and the serum potassium concentration. Potassium secretion is also influenced by alterations in body fluid acidity, by adrenergic nervous system activity, and by drugs and diseases that directly affect renal tubular transport.

After intravenous administration of approximately 50 mEq potassium to normal subjects, 50 percent of the load is excreted in the urine within 4 to 6 hours. Severe hyperkalemia would result if the retained potassium remained confined to the extracellular fluid. In fact, approximately 40 percent of the administered load is taken up into cells; thus the serum potassium concentration rises by only 0.3 to 0.5 mEq per liter. If potassium is administered for several days, increases in cellular uptake and in renal and gastrointestinal excretion of potassium occur, and the rise in serum potassium concentration is less. Therefore, the rise in the serum level after a potassium load depends on the amount, the route and rate of administration, the transcellular distribution, and the renal excretion of potassium.

Conversely, if potassium is withdrawn from the diet, renal excretion of potassium continues and leads to a deficit in total body content and a reduction in the concentration of potassium in cells and in extracellular fluid. Up to 3 weeks are required for maximal renal conservation of potassium. Therefore, the decline in serum potassium concentration depends on the extent of renal losses, the occurrence of gastrointestinal losses, and the factors influencing the transcellular distribution of potassium.

The relationship between the serum level and the total body content of potassium varies widely in disorders of potassium metabolism. If the altered serum concentration is the result of altered transcellular distribution, total body potassium content remains normal. In disorders where the total body content is abnormal, there is a rough correlation between the serum level and the extent of the deficit or surfeit (Table 28-1). The definitions in Table 1 of mild, moderate, and severe alterations in serum potassium concentration are arbitrary; nonetheless, they provide a convenient framework for discussion of the etiology and the treatment of hypokalemia and hyperkalemia. It is important to note that extensive depletion of total body potassium is necessary before moderate or severe hypokalemia results. On the contrary, moderate or severe hyperkalemia may result from much smaller increments in total body potassium content. Data are not available on the potassium surfeit in moderate to severe hyperkalemia, thus the figures given in Table 1 are speculative only. However, common clinical experience has shown that administration of relatively small amounts of potassium (100 mEq) to patients with mild hyperkalemia may precipitate the rapid development of moderate or severe hyperkalemia.

Regardless of the severity of hypokalemia or hyperkalemia, proper recognition and diagnosis are important in order to avoid the development of life-threatening complications. Often more than one disorder of potassium metabolism is present. Determination of the etiology necessitates the identifi-

TABLE 28-1 Correlation Between Serum Potassium Level and Change in Body Potassium Content

Hypokalemia		
Severity	Serum Concentration (mEq/L)	Approximate Deficit (mEq)
Severe	<2.5	500-1,000
Moderate	2.5-2.9	300-800
Mild	3.0-3.4	<300
Hyperkalemia		
Severity	Serum Concentration (mEq/L)	Approximate Surfeit (mEq)
Mild	5.1-5.5	50-75
Moderate	5.9-6.0	>100
Severe	>6.0	>100

cation of all the potential abnormalities in distribution, intake, and excretion of potassium and the assessment of the severity and the temporal development of the hypokalemia or hyperkalemia. The remainder of the chapter will discuss the consequences, the most important causes, and the treatment of hypokalemia and hyperkalemia.

HYPOKALEMIA

Consequences of Hypokalemia

Severe hypokalemia may cause dysfunction in many organs. Polyuria from impaired urinary concentration, marked hyperglycemia from impaired insulin secretion and hepatic gluconeogenesis, and hepatic encephalopathy from increased renal ammonia generation have been reported; however, these disorders are rarely present unless hypokalemia is severe.

The most important effects of hypokalemia are on muscle and nerve tissue. Impaired gastrointestinal motility and skeletal muscle weakness may occasionally result from moderate hypokalemia, and cardiac alterations may occur in the presence of even mild hypokalemia. Electrocardiographic abnormalities are common (Fig. 28–1), and ventricular arrhythmias may occur in patients receiving digoxin. Whether or not mild hypokalemia increases the risk of arrhythmias in patients with acute myocardial infarction or with underlying heart disease is not conclusively determined. Similarly, the frequency of arrhythmias in otherwise healthy subjects with hypokalemia is not known. Currently, it appears that serious arrhythmias attributable to mild hypokalemia are extremely unlikely unless other precipitating factors also are present.[8,9] Mild hypokalemia in hypertensive patients treated with thiazide diuretics has recently been suggested to be associated with a small (3 to 5 mm Hg) elevation in blood pressure.[10] More data are required to evaluate the effect of the serum potassium level on blood pressure in this setting.

Causes of Hypokalemia: Altered Transcellular Distribution

A shift of potassium from extracellular fluid into cells should be considered as a cause of hypokalemia when there is a sudden fall in serum potassium concentration by approximately 0.5 mEq per liter without evidence of a recent loss of potassium. In one recent study, 25 percent of hospitalized patients with sudden hypokalemia had no obvious cause of potassium deficiency, and in many patients, the hypokalemia resolved without specific therapy.[1] A discussion of the most important causes of transcellular shifts of potassium into cells follows.[7]

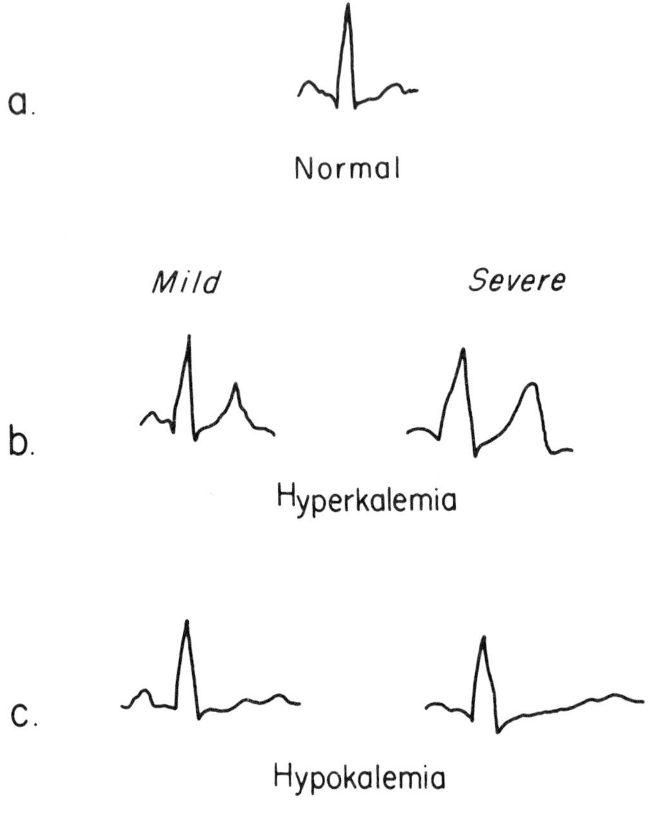

a.

Normal

Mild   *Severe*

b.

Hyperkalemia

c.

Hypokalemia

Figure 28-1 ECG changes in hypokalemia and hyperkalemia. a = normal, b = hyperkalemia. The T wave becomes peaked, followed by loss of P waves and prolongation of the QRS complex, approaching a "sine wave" appearance as serum potassium rises. c = Hypokalemia. The QT interval is slightly prolonged and the ST segment is depressed. The T wave is lower and a U wave is present. Later, the T and U waves fuse, the ST segment becomes more depressed, and the QRS more prolonged as serum potassium decreases. (Reproduced and modified with permission from Beckwith JR. Grant's clinical electrocardiography: the spatial vector approach. New York: McGraw Hill, 1970; 105.)

Beta-Adrenergic Stimulation

Intravenous infusion of epinephrine to raise the serum epinephrine level as high as that found in "acute stress" leads to a transient fall in serum potassium concentration by approximately 0.5 mEq per liter. The magnitude of the decline in serum potassium concentration is similar in subjects who are initially normokalemic or hypokalemic.[11] The hypokalemia is the result of a shift of potassium into muscle and liver cells that is mediated by beta-2 receptor stimulation. Similar declines in serum potassium level have been noted in patients receiving beta-adrenergic agonists for treatment of asthma or for inhibition of labor. Interestingly, recent studies have shown that alpha-adrenergic inhibition also may lower serum potassium owing to a transcellular shift of potassium.[12] Usually no therapy is necessary for the hypokalemia unless the patient also has a potassium deficiency or unless the patient is also at risk for the development of cardiac arrhythmias.

Insulin

Insulin promotes the uptake of glucose and potassium into muscle and liver cells. The administration of glucose and insulin results in a rapid lowering of the serum potassium concentration. Therefore, this combination is utilized in the management of severe hyperkalemia. Hypokalemia that results from a transcellular shift of potassium mediated by glucose and insulin is clinically apparent in two circumstances: (1) In normal (non-diabetic) individuals, administration of glucose in parenteral hyperalimentation solutions raises blood levels of both glucose and insulin and lowers serum potassium concentration. Simultaneous administration of potassium, 80 to 100 mEq per day, is recommended unless renal excretion of potasium is impaired. (2) In diabetics with hyperglycemia, administration of insulin lowers blood glucose and potassium levels. Potassium supplementation is not necessary for patients who are eating normally. However, in patients with diabetic ketoacidosis and non-ketotic hyperosmolar coma, potassium deficiency is common because of renal potassium losses, and moderate to severe hypokalemia may occur during insulin therapy. Administration of 100 to 200 mEq potassium in the first 12 to 24 hours of therapy is indicated in these patients; therapy can begin at the initiation of insulin therapy, unless the serum potassium concentration is initially elevated.

Bicarbonate

Acute elevation of the serum bicarbonate concentration results in a transcellular shift of hydrogen ions from cells into extracellular fluid and of potassium from extracellular fluid into cells. Administration of bicarbonate rapidly lowers serum potassium concentration in patients with severe hyperkalemia. Similarly, in patients with a normal serum potassium concentration, administration of bicarbonate (e.g., for treatment of metabolic acidosis) often leads to hypokalemia. Interestingly, the shift of potassium into cells appears to be influenced more by the increase in serum bicarbonate concentration than by the decrease in hydrogen ion concentration.[13] There is little change in serum bicarbonate concentration in acute respiratory alkalosis, and the serum potassium concentration is characteristically normal.

Hypokalemic Periodic Paralysis

In these rare diseases, episodes of moderate to severe hypokalemia are accompanied by profound muscle weakness.[14] The condition occurs as an inherited dominant trait or as a complication of thyrotoxicosis, particularly in Orientals. Episodes are treated by oral or intravenous administration of potassium, in doses of 40 to 120 mEq, until the muscle weakness and hypokalemia resolve.

Causes of Hypokalemia: Inadequate Intake

Full adaptation of renal conservation of potassium occurs relatively slowly. Therefore, mild potassium deficiency and hypokalemia result from reduced potassium intake. In these cases, urinary potassium excretion is reduced to less than 20 mEq per day. Severe hypokalemia, however, does not occur unless there are additional losses of potassium.

Causes of Hypokalemia: Excessive Excretion

A deficit of potassium may result from increased losses of potassium from either gastrointestinal or renal routes. When hypokalemia is attributable to increased gastrointestinal losses, urinary potassium excretion declines to less than 20 mEq per day. By definition, if urinary potassium excretion exceeds this rate, hypokalemia is the result of renal potassium losses. Therefore, measurement of urinary potassium excretion distinguishes between hypokalemia caused by inadequate intake or by gastrointestinal losses and hypokalemia owing to renal losses of potassium.

Gastrointestinal Losses

The potassium concentration in liquid stool may be as high as 30 to 50 mEq per liter. Large losses of potassium and bicarbonate during severe diarrheal illnesses lead to hypokalemia and metabolic acidosis with a normal anion gap (see *Acid-Base Disorders*). In contrast, the concentration of potassium in gastric, biliary, or pancreatic fluid is only 5 to 10 mEq per liter. The hypokalemia that results from vomiting or from gastric drainage is the result of increased renal potassium excretion that occurs in association with the metabolic alkalosis.

Renal Losses: Diuretics

With the exception of the "potassium-sparing" agents, all diuretics increase the secretion of potassium in the distal nephron as a result of increased delivery of sodium chloride and increased urine flow at this site.[9,15] The magnitude of the diuretic-induced potassium deficit is correlated with the magnitude of the sodium chloride losses. Mild diuretics, such as thiazides and carbonic anhydrase inhibitors, produce mild to moderate hypokalemia, whereas the potent loop diuretics and osmotic agents may result in severe hypokalemia. The magnitude of the potassium deficit is also influenced by the underlying disorder. For example, in nonedematous hypertensive patients, the potassium deficit induced by thiazide diuretics is typically less than 200 mEq, thereby resulting in mild hypokalemia. In only 5 percent of patients does the serum potassium concentration decline to less than 3.0 mEq per liter.[15] However, in patients treated with diuretics for edematous conditions, such as congestive heart failure, cirrhosis, nephrotic syndrome, or venous insufficiency, aldosterone levels are typically high and further increase the secretion of potassium, thereby augmenting the potassium deficiency.

Guidelines for the treatment of diuretic-induced hypokalemia are based on the severity of the potassium deficit. In edematous patients and in patients treated with loop diuretics, prescription of potassium chloride, 80 to 120 mEq per day, or potassium sparing diuretics is usually necessary to prevent potassium deficiency. Patients treated with carbonic anhydrase inhibitors may also develop metabolic acidosis and require alkali therapy in addition to potassium supplements. In nonedematous hypertensive patients treated with thiazide diuretics, the need for potassium supplementation is controversial.[8,9,15,16] The presently available data do not indicate that the risk of serious complications of mild hypokalemia warrants prophylactic supplementation of dietary potassium or prescription of potassium. Instead, prescription of potassium chloride or potassium-sparing diuretics appears necessary only for patients (1) who are taking digoxin, (2) who have symptoms related to the potassium deficit, or (3) whose serum potassium concentration is persistently below 3.0 mEq per liter. Treatment of these patients with potassium chloride, 40 to 60 mEq per day, is required to restore serum potassium to normal and to correct the potassium deficit.[17]

Renal Losses: Chronic Metabolic Acidosis and Metabolic Alkalosis

Urinary potassium excretion is usually increased in chronic metabolic acid-base disorders.[18] In metabolic acidosis, the increased excretion in the urine of anions, such as salicylate, lactate, or ketoacid anions, facilitates secretion of potassium by the distal nephron, thereby causing hypokalemia. Important exceptions include the acute metabolic acidosis associated with administration of mineral acid (ammonium chloride, arginine hydrochloride, or hydrochloric acid) and the metabolic acidosis of acute and chronic renal failure. In these conditions, serum potassium is typically normal or elevated.[13] In metabolic alkalosis, the increased reabsorption of sodium in the disal nephron and the relative depletion of chloride secondarily increase potassium secretion, thereby causing hypokalemia. Treatment of hypokalemia in metabolic acid-base disorders includes correction of the underlying disorder and replacement of the potassium deficit. In metabolic acidosis, potassium should be provided with alkali; in metabolic alkalosis, potassium should be provided with chloride.

Renal Losses: Hyperaldosteronism

The primary action of aldosterone on the distal renal tubule is to increase reabsorption of sodium and to increase secretion of potassium and of hydrogen ions. High levels of aldosterone and other mineralocorticoid hormones lead to potassium depletion, hypokalemia, and metabolic alkalosis. A wide variety of disorders increase secretion of adrenal steroids and lead to hypokalemia (Table 28–2). Primary hyperaldosteronism is the result of an adrenal adenoma (Conn's syndrome), bilateral adrenal hyperplasia, or adrenal carcinoma and is characterized by asymptomatic mild to moderate hypokalemia, hypertension, and mild metabolic alkalosis. Women are more frequently affected; the usual age is 30 to 50 years. The diagnosis is established by findings of elevated serum or urinary aldosterone in association with low plasma renin activity that cannot be raised by maneuvers that normally stimulate renin release, such as upright posture or diuresis. By definition, secondary hyperaldosteronism is the result of increased plasma renin activity. The most common causes are abnormalities in extracellular fluid volume (congestive heart failure, cirrhosis, volume depletion, Bartter's syndrome), renal damage from malignant hypertension, and high renin essential hypertension. High levels of glucocorticoid hormones, as seen in Cushing's syndrome, also stimulate distal tubular secretion of potassium and lead to hypokalemia. Treatment of the underlying condition and replacement of the potassium deficit resolves the hypokalemia. Spironolactone or other potassium-sparing diuretics are effective in preventing ongoing potassium losses in patients with primary hyper-

TABLE 28-2   Disorders of Potassium Metabolism Attributable to Alterations in the Renin-Angiotensin-Aldosterone System

Disorder	Hypokalemia	Hyperkalemia
Abnormal aldosterone secretion	Primary hyperaldosteronism Adrenal adenoma Adrenal hyperplasia Adrenal carcinoma Exogenous adrenal steroids Licorice Iatrogenic	Primary hypoaldosteronism Congenital biosynthetic defect Addison's disease Drugs Heparin Angiotensin converting enzyme inhibition
Abnormal renin secretion	Hyperreninemic Hyperaldosteronism Congestive heart failure Cirrhosis Nephrotic syndrome Volume contraction Bartter's syndrome Malignant hypertension High renin essential hypertension	Hyporeninemic Hypoaldosteronism Diabetes Renal diseases Prostaglandin synthetase inhibition Beta-adrenergic blocking agents
Abnormal ACTH secretion	Cushing's syndrome Pituitary adenoma Ectopic ACTH secretion	

aldosteronism or with Cushing's syndrome. Inhibitors of prostaglandin synthesis are useful to reduce the elevated plasma renin activity in patients with Bartter's syndrome. Long-term therapy with potassium supplements, 80 to 160 mEq per day, is frequently necessary for patients with secondary hyperaldosteronism.

Renal Losses: Renal Tubular Disorders

A number of diseases or drugs may cause hypokalemia by increasing renal tubular secretion of potassium by a variety of mechanisms. These disorders include renal tubular acidosis, resolving acute tubular necrosis, postobstructive diuresis, multiple myeloma, light chain nephropathy, and nephrotoxicity from amphotericin B and platinum. In addition to increased potassium excretion, sodium conservation and hydrogen ion secretion may be impaired. Acute myelogenous leukemia, hypomagnesemia, and administration of carbenicillin may cause hypodkalemia without other tubular disorders.

Treatment

Treatment of hypokalemia is guided by the severity and cause of the hypokalemia and by the patient's other medical conditions. As already discussed treatment is usually not required for mild, transient hypokalemia attributable to transcellular shift of potassium or for mild hypokalemia owing to thiazide diuretic therapy for hypertension. However, treatment should be prescribed if the patient is at risk for cardiac arrhythmias or if the serum potassium is below 3.0 mEq per liter.

The other causes of hypokalemia require treatment to restore the serum potassium concentration to normal and to restore the deficit in total body potassium. Two types of treatment are available: potassium supplements and potassium-sparing diuretics. Serum potassium levels rise slowly during therapy with potassium-sparing diuretics; thus these agents are not indicated for treatment of moderate to severe hypokalemia. Potassium supplements are more reliable. The preparation of potassium depends on the cause of the hypokalemia. Hypokalemia owing to inadequate intake may be treated with foods rich in potassium or with potassium supplements containing either chloride or alkali. Diuretic-induced hypokalemia attributable to renal potassium losses generally should be treated with potassium chloride, while hypokalemia caused by diarrhea and by renal tubular disorders should be treated with alkalinizing potassium salts. Comparative doses and costs for currently available commercial preparations are described elsewhere.[4]

The route and the speed of potassium administration depend on the patient's ability to tolerate oral or enteral medication, the renal function, and the severity of the hypokalemia. The vast majority of patients should be treated by oral administration of liquid solutions of 10 percent or 20 percent potassium chloride, 40 mEq per dose. For prevention of hypokalemia, potassium chloride wax-matrix or microencapsulated tablets and potassium-sparing diuretics are also useful. For severe hypokalemia, potassium chloride may be given intravenously. The concentration of potassium in intravenous fluid should not exceed 40 to 60 mEq per liter. The serum level should be measured again after 80 to 100 mEq are administered. Usually not more than 150 to 200 mEq should be given in one day. Higher rates of administration of potassium are occasionally necessary. Potassium chloride, 10 to 20 mEq, may be diluted in 100 ml of intravenous fluid and administered "piggy back" into another intravenous solution over 1 hour for the prevention of cardiac arrhythmias in hypokalemic patients taking digoxin or during acute myocardial infarction. For life-threatening hypokalemia (serum potassium less than 2.0 mEq per liter, ventricular arrhythmias, paralysis), potassium chloride may be infused at 30 to 40 mEq per hour with continuous monitoring of the electrocardiogram.[19] The serum potassium should be measured after 2 to 3 hours. The need for such rapid intravenous infusions rarely arises.

The principal risk of potassium therapy is hyperkalemia. The prevalence of hyperkalemia is 4 percent in hospitalized patients receiving potassium therapy; life-threatening hyperkalemia develops in 0.4 percent of patients.[20] The risk of life-threatening hyperkalemia is increased to 5 to 9 percent in patients who are over age 50 and have a blood urea nitrogen concentration (BUN) greater than 50 mg per deciliter or who receive both oral and intravenous potassium. The prevalence of hyperkalemia in hospitalized patients receiving potassium-sparing diuretics is 10 percent; the risk of life-threatening hyperkalemia is 3 percent.[21] The risk of life-threatening hyperkalemia is increased to 16 percent in patients receiving both potassium-sparing diuretics and potassium chloride and is further increased to 42 percent if the BUN is greater than 50 mg per deciliter. These considerations argue for judicious use of potassium supplements and of potassium-sparing diuretics for treatment and prevention of hypokalemia.

HYPERKALEMIA

Consequences of Hyperkalemia

Hyperkalemia causes disturbances in cardiac and skeletal muscle. If hyperkalemia is severe, parasthesias and weakness of the arms and legs may be followed by ascending symmetrical flaccid paralysis and may lead to hypoventilation. Interestingly, muscles of the head and neck and sensation are not altered. The most serious consequences of hyperkalemia are cardiac arrhythmias. Changes in the electrocardiogram (ECG) are only roughly correlated with the severity of hyperkalemia. Nonetheless, because of the potential for life-threatening cardiac arrhythmias, the ECG is used as a guide in determining the need for and effectiveness of treatment of hyperkalemia (see Fig. 28–1). In general, changes in the ECG first appear when the serum potassium concentration exceeds 6.0 mEq per liter. Thereafter, the serum potassium level may rise precipitously, and the progression from mild ECG changes to ventricular fibrillation may occur rapidly. Thus, an ECG must be obtained in patients with severe hyperkalemia, and treatment must be initiated at once if changes of hyperkalemia are present.

Causes of Hyperkalemia: Factitious Hyperkalemia

The serum potassium concentration in this condition is elevated in the blood sample tube, but not in the patient. Potassium is released into the serum from white blood cells and from platelets during in vitro blood coagulation or from in vitro lysis of red blood cells. Normally, the serum concentration of potassium exceeds the plasma concentration by 0.2 to 0.3 mEq per liter as a result of in vitro blood coagulation, but severe elevation of the potassium level may occur in patients with extreme thrombocytosis (platelet count greater than 1 million per mm^3) or leukocytosis (white blood cell count greater than 100,000 per mm^3). In hyperkalemia attributable to in vitro blood coagulation, the concentration of potassium is elevated in serum, but not in plasma. In vitro hemolysis is easily detected by an examination of the serum after centrifugation. Of course, it is important to distinguish in vitro hemolysis from in vivo hemolysis, which may cause true hyperkalemia. In factitious hyperkalemia, there are no ECG abnormalities and treatment is not necessary. In fact, the absence of changes in the ECG of patients with severe hyperkalemia should arouse suspicion that the hyperkalemia is factitious.

Causes of Hyperkalemia: Altered Transcellular Distribution

There are many causes of hyperkalemia owing to a shift of potassium from cells to extracellular fluid.[7] Because of the increased renal tubular secretion of potassium that occurs when serum potassium concentration is elevated, the hyperkalemia caused by transcellular shifts of potassium is usually mild. Serum potassium concentration rarely exceeds 6.0 mEq per liter unless there also is a defect in renal potassium excretion. The hyperkalemia may be transient or sustained, depending on the cause. Typically, the hyperkalemia attributable to exercise, to acidemia, and to glucose infusion in diabetics is transient. Drug-induced hyperkalemia is usually transient, but in the case of hyperkalemia caused by beta-adrenergic blockers, the alteration in serum potassium concentration is sustained as long as the medications are continued.

Exercise

Potassium is released during depolarization of muscle cells. Vigorous exercise may result in a transient elevation of the serum potassium concentration by 1 to 2 mEq per liter and ECG abnormalities of hyperkalemia.

Acidosis

The elevation in serum potassium concentration consequent to acidemia is highly variable and is related to the cause and severity of the acidosis.[13] Clinically significant hyperkalemia occurs only in acute metabolic acidosis attributable to the administration of mineral acid and in acute severe respiratory acidosis (pH less than 7.00). By contrast, there is virtually no rise in the serum potassium concentration in acute lactic acidosis and ketoacidosis or in mild acute respiratory acidosis. As discussed earlier, chronic metabolic acidosis results in increased potassium excretion and is associated with hypokalemia.

Glucose

As previously discussed, administration of glucose to nondiabetic subjects increases insulin levels and lowers serum potassium concentration. However, in diabetics, infusion of approximately one to two ampules of 50 percent dextrose (25 to 50 g) raises the serum potassium concentration by 0.2 to 2.0 mEq per liter.[22] The mechanism of hyperkalemia is thought to be a transcellular shift of potassium owing to extracellular fluid hyperosmolarity. Glucose-induced hyperkalemia in diabetics may occur following administration of hypertonic dextrose for treatment of presumed hypoglycemia coma. Severe hyperkalemia may result if renal potassium excretion is impaired owing to renal disease and hypoaldosteronism.

Beta-Adrenergic Inhibition

Long-term treatment with beta-adrenergic receptor blocking agents results in dose-dependent mild hyperkalemia. The average rise in serum potassium concentration is 0.5 mEq per liter, and the serum potassium concentration rarely exceeds 6.0 mEq per liter.[22] Severe hyperkalemia has been reported in patients taking beta-blockers in association with vigorous exercise or with ingestion of an exogenous potassium load and in patients with diabetes, renal disease, and hypoaldosteronism. Because the hypokalemic effect of epinephrine is mediated by beta-2 receptor stimulation, selective beta-1 receptor blockade does not raise serum potassium to the same level as nonselective beta blockade. Selective beta-1 blocking agents might be more appropriate agents for patients at risk for hyperkalemia.

Other Drugs

Succinylcholine, arginine monohydrochloride, and alpha-adrenergic stimulation raise serum potassium concentration and may cause severe hyperkalemia in patients with other risks for hyperkalemia.[22] Massive digitalis overdose (20 to 40 times the therapeutic dose) also causes severe hyperkalemia.

Hyperkalemic Periodic Paralysis

In this form of periodic paralysis, the serum potassium concentration is elevated during the attack of muscle weakness.[14] Either mild or severe hyperkalemia may occur. The condition occurs as an inherited dominant trait with the usual age of onset between 5 and 10 years. Treatment is oral administration of glucose. If hyperkalemia is severe, additional measures to lower serum potassium concentration are necessary.

Causes of Hyperkalemia: Excessive Intake

Increased potassium intake is accompanied by increased renal tubular secretion of potassium. If renal function is normal, sustained hyperkalemia from excessive intake occurs only if the potassium load is extremely large or rapid. The potassium load may be exogenous, as in the case of increased dietary intake or of prescription of potassium-containing medications, or it may be endogenous, as in the case of cell lysis. An increased endogenous load is included as a form of increased intake because the extracellular fluid is presented with an increased load of potassium that cannot shift back into cells and that therefore must be excreted.

Increased Dietary Intake

Although all foods containing animal or vegetable matter contain potassium, an elevated serum potassium concentration is virtually impossible to sustain from increased intake of usual food if renal function is normal. By contrast, in patients with reduced renal capacity for potassium excretion, hyperkalemia is frequent unless potassium intake is restricted. Potassium intake can be assessed from dietary records or from measurement of 24-hour urinary potassium excretion. Urinary potassium excretion closely reflects dietary potassium intake in patients whose serum potassium concentration is stable and who are not oliguric or markedly catabolic. If potassium intake is greater than 75 to 100 mEq per day, dietary potassium should be restricted to 50 to 75 mEq per day (2 to 3 g per day). Nutritional counseling is essential to encourage compliance with diets restricted in potassium. However, further restriction is not warranted if potassium intake is 50 to 75 mEq per day or less, as diets extremely low in potassium are severely restricted in most natural foods and are not practical for more than a few days.

In addition to potassium in usual foods, other dietary sources must be considered. Salt-substitutes contain 15 to 70 mEq potassium per teaspoon and have been implicated as contributing factors to the development of hyperkalemia in patients with inadequate renal excretion.[23] Other unusual sources of potassium include food supplements and herbal remedies.

Potassium-Containing Medications

Potassium chloride is the most important medicinal source of potassium. In a large survey of hospitalized patients, potassium chloride administration was implicated in 96 percent of episodes of hyperkalemia; in contrast, hyperkalemia occurred in only 0.4 percent of patients not receiving potassium.[20] The risk of hyperkalemia from therapeutic use of potassium chloride has been discussed in a previous section of this chapter. Other sources of potassium include alkalinizing potassium salts, potassium penicillin (1.7 mEq potassium per million units), and blood (3 to 4 mEq potassium per unit).

Cell Lysis

Acute tumor lysis, rhabdomyolysis, and hemolysis result in an outpouring of potassium from necrotic cells into extracellular fluid. Occasionally, these disorders are accompanied by acute renal failure, which delays excretion of the potassium load and exacerbates the rise in serum potassium concentration. However, even in the absence of renal failure, severe hyperkalemia has been reported after chemotherapy for remission induction in patients with a large tumor burden.[22] In these disorders hyperkalemia peaks in the first 24 hours, and dialysis may be necessary to lower potassium level. Other complications from the liberation of intracellular contents include hyperphosphatemia, hyperuricemia, and metabolic acidosis. Prior administration of allopurinol and intravenous hydration with saline and sodium bicarbonate reduce the complications from tumor lysis.

Causes of Hyperkalemia: Inadequate Excretion

In most patients with hyperkalemia, renal excretion of potassium is defective due to a variety of causes.

Chronic Renal Failure

In most chronic renal diseases, serum potassium is usually normal or only mildly increased unless renal function is severely impaired (glomerular filtration rate less than 15 ml per minute, corresponding to serum creatinine concentration greater than 5 to 7 mg per deciliter). The principal mechanism of this adaptation of potassium homeostasis is increased distal tubular secretion of potassium.[6] A quantitatively less important mechanism is an increase in colonic secretion of potassium. If renal function is more severely impaired, moderate to severe hyperkalemia is commonly observed. Restriction of dietary potassium intake to 2 to 3 g (50 to 75 mEq) per day is usually successful in preventing hyperkalemia if the patient is compliant. However, noncompliance is frequent and oral administration of the cation exchange resin, sodium polystyrene sulfonate (Kayexalate), 50 to 75 g per day, may be necessary. Each gram of resin binds 0.5 to 1.0 mEq potassium and releases 2 to 3 mEq sodium. The resulting sodium load may precipitate extracellular fluid volume overload in patients with severe renal impairment. If glomerular filtration rate is normal or only moderately reduced, the development of hyperkalemia indicates an impairment of renal tubular secretion of potassium. A discussion of the causes of impaired renal tubular potassium secretion follows.

Acute Renal Failure

The causes of hyperkalemia in acute renal failure are multiple and include severe reduction in glomerular filtration rate, oliguria, accelerated catabolism, acute acidemia, and inadvertent administration of potassium chloride.[6] Hyperkalemia occurs in aproximately 50 percent of patients with acute tubular necrosis and is generally an indication for dialysis. In patients with prerenal azotemia, medical measures that are successful in improving renal function and in raising the urine volume also lower the serum potassium concentration.

Hypoaldosteronism

Hyperkalemia is the most frequent manifestation of hypoaldosteronism. Primary hypoaldosteronism is due to adrenal disorders. Although it is rare, Addison's disease should be considered in all cases of hyperkalemia because life-threatening complications may be prevented by appropriate hormonal replacement. A wide variety of conditions are associated with secondary hypoaldosteronism (see Table 28-2). Numerous examples of drug-induced hyperkalemia owing to interference with the renin-angiotensin-aldosterone system have recently been recognized.[22] Among the most important are inhibition of renin secretion by beta-adrenergic blockers and by nonsteroidal anti-inflammatory drugs, inhibition of converting enzyme by captopril and enalapril, inhibition of aldosterone biosynthesis by heparin, and inhibition of aldosterone action by spironolactone (see following). Nonetheless, not all causes of secondary hypoaldosteronism are due to drug effects. In one series[24], the mean age of patients with hypoaldosteronism was 65 years, although the range was from 32 to 82 years. Mild renal insufficiency was present in 70 percent and diabetes was present in 50 percent. Sustained hyperkalemia was found in 75 percent of patients and metabolic acidosis was present in 50 percent, but salt-wasting was rare. Most patients were asymptomatic, but muscle weakness and arrhythmias were each documented in 25 percent of patients. Investigation into the cause of the hypoaldosteronism revealed that most patients had normal glucocorticoid function, but that 80 percent of patients had abnormally low plasma renin activity. The cause of suppressed renin was not elucidated.

Treatment is recommended if serum potassium exceeds 5.5 mEq per liter because of the risk of cardiac arrhythmias in these patients. A variety of treatments have been proposed. Restriction of dietary potassium to 2 to 3 g (50 to 75 mEq) per day is usually sufficient. Other treatments include administration of a loop diuretic, such as furosemide 40 to 80 mg once or twice daily, to facilitate renal potassium excretion. Supplementary dietary sodium chloride is sometimes necessary to prevent extracellular volume contraction. Correction of metabolic acidosis, if present, may lower serum potassium concentration. Cation exchange resins also are useful. Administration of pharmacologic doses of the exogenous mineralocorticoid fludrocortisone acetate (Florinef), 0.4 to 1.0 mg per day, usually increases potassium excretion, but frequently results in sodium retention manifested by weight gain, hypertension, and edema.

Potassium-Sparing Diuretics

Two fundamentally different classes of drugs inhibit sodium reabsorption in the distal nephron and thereby reduce potassium secretion.[22] Spironolactone competes with aldosterone for binding to a cytoplasmic receptor in renal tubular cells. Amiloride and triamterene bind reversibly to the luminal membrane of the distal tubule, block reabsorption of sodium, and reduce secretion of hydrogen ions and potassium. This effect is independent of aldosterone. As discussed in *Edema*, the diuretic potency of amiloride is greater than that of spironolactone and triamterene. The latter two agents are used principally to prevent hypokalemia in patients treated with other diuretics. The most important side effect of all three drugs, however, is hyperkalemia. As discussed earlier, patients who have renal insufficiency or who are receiving potassium chloride are at particularly high risk of hyperkalemia from potassium-sparing diuretics. Thus, these agents should be avoided in patients with risks for the development of hyperkalemia, such as renal insufficiency, diabetes, and ingestion of drugs that impair transcellular potassium distribution, suppress the renin-angiotensin system, or directly reduce renal potassium secretion.

Renal Tubular Secretory Defects

Hyperkalemia may be the result of renal parenchymal diseases that markedly impair tubular potassium secretion, even though glomerular filtration rate is only mildly decreased.[6] In general, these diseases are associated with prominent tubulointerstitial damage and sometimes also cause a defect in hydrogen ion secretion that results in hyperchloremic metabolic acidosis. Serum aldosterone levels are elevated appropriately for the elevation of serum potassium concentration. The most common examples include sickle cell nephropathy, lupus nephritis, partial obstruction of the urinary tract, acute and chronic kidney transplant rejection, and toxicity from cyclosporine and lithium. Treatment is correction of the underlying disorder if possible. Administration of loop diuretics is usually sufficient to maintain serum potassium levels below 5.5 mEq per liter. Sometimes, cation exchange resins or dietary potassium restriction are necessary.

Treatment

The goal of treatment of hyperkalemia is to prevent the development of cardiac arrhythmias, to restore the serum level of potassium to normal, and to reduce the surfeit, if any, in total body potassium. No treatment is necessary for factitious hyperkalemia or for mild hyperkalemia attributable to transcellular shifts. In patients with normal renal function, it is usually not necessary to discontinue beta-adrenergic blocking agents, angiotensin converting enzyme inhibitors, nonsteroidal anti-inflammatory agents, or heparin because of mild hyperkalemia. However, patients should be warned about the possible dangers of vigorous exercise and advised to avoid excessive dietary potassium intake, salt substitutes, potassium supplements, and potassium-sparing diuretics. Serum potassium should be monitored regularly. In patients with chronic renal failure, restriction of dietary potassium usually is not necessary unless serum potassium is greater than 5.5 mEq per liter. However, patients must be warned to avoid excessive intake of potassium rich foods, of potassium supplements, of salt substitutes, and of drugs that reduce excretion or impair transcellular distribution of potassium. Serum potassium must be monitored frequently.

For moderate hyperkalemia (serum potassium 5.5 to 6.0 mEq per liter), potassium intake should be reduced and drugs that impair transcellular distribution or excretion of potassium should be discontinued. If the serum potassium concentration is rising or if the patient's medical condition is unstable, treatment should be instituted immediately in order to avoid precipitous further rise in potassium level. For severe hyperkalemia (serum potassium concentration greater than 6.0 mEq per liter or ECG changes of hyper-kalemia), immediate treatment is also necessary.

Treatment may be divided into three general categories: (1) reversal of the effect of hyperkalemia on cell membranes (calcium); (2) a shift of potassium from extracellular fluid into cells (glucose, insulin, bicarbonate); and (3) removal of potassium from the body (loop diuretics, cation exchange resins, dialysis). The treatment selected depends on the severity of the hyperkalemia, the ECG, and the patient's condition. If the serum potassium concentration is 6.0 to 6.4 mEq per liter and if the ECG is normal, treatment is directed at removing potassium from the body. Intravenous administration of furosemide 40 to 80 mg, ethacrynic acid 50 to 100 mg, or bumetanide 1 to 2 mg generally results in excretion of 75 to 100 mEq potassium in 2 L of urine in 1 to 2 hours. In oliguric patients, loop diuretics are usually not effective; kayexalate, 25 to 50 g, should be administered orally with 35 to 70 percent sorbitol, 100 to 200 ml. In postoperative patients who are unable to take oral medications, cation exchange resins can be administered as a retention enema with or without sorbitol. If serum potassium concentration is 6.5 mEq per liter or greater and if the ECG shows only peaking of the T wave, glucose 25 g, regular insulin 5-10 units, and sodium bicarbonate 50 mEq should be administered intravenously. Loop diuretics or cation exchange resins should be administered at the same time. However, if the ECG shows widening of the QRS complex, 10 percent calcium gluconate, 10 ml should be given intravenously together with glucose, insulin, bicarbonate, and either diuretics or cation exchange resins. Additional calcium can be given at 10 to 15 minute intervals. The ECG should be moni-tored continuously until the QRS complex returns to normal. If the cause of hyperkalemia can be corrected, usually one or two doses of diuretics or resin are sufficient to lower serum potassium to 5.5 mEq or less. However, dialysis is necessary if the response to diuretics or resin is inadequate, if the cause of the hyperkalemia cannot be corrected, or if the serum potassium is expected to increase again. During dialysis, the ECG and the serum potassium concen-tration should be monitored every 2 to 4 hours. Additional details of the treatment of hyperkalemia are discussed elsewhere.[5]

References

1. Morgan DB, Young RM. Acute transient hypokalemia: New interpretation of a common event. Lancet 1982; 2:751–752.
2. Lawson DH, Henry DA, Lowe JM, Gray JMB, Morgan G. Severe hypokalemia in hospitalized patients. Arch Intern Med 1979; 139:978–980.
3. Shemer J, Ezra D, Modan M, Cabili S. Incidence of hyperkalemia among hospitalized patients. Isr J Med Sci 1983; 19:659.

4. Levey AS, Harrington JT. Hypokalemia. In: Glassock RJ, ed. Current therapy in nephrology and hypertension 1984-1985. Philadelphia: BC Decker, 1984:21.
5. Katz LD, DeFronzo RA. Hyperkalemia. In: Glassock RJ, ed. Current therapy in nephrology and hypertension 1984-1985. Philadelphia: BC Decker, 1984:13.
6. Cohen JJ, Gennari FJ, Harrington JT. Disorders of potassium balance. In: Brenner BM, Rector FC Jr, eds. The Kidney. Philadelphia: WB Saunders, 1981:908.
7. Alexander EA, Perrone RD. Regulation of extrarenal potassium metabolism. In: Maxwell M, Kleeman CR, Narins RG, eds. Clinical disorders of fluid and electrolyte metabolism. New York: McGraw-Hill, 1987:105–117.
8. Harrington JT, Isner JM, Kassirer JP. Our national obsession with potassium. Am J Med 1982; 73:155–158.
9. Tannen RL. Diuretic-induced hypokalemia. Kidney Int 1985; 28:988–1000.
10. Kaplan NM, Carnegie A, Raskin P, Heller JA, Simmons M. Potassium supplementation in hypertensive patients with diuretic-induced hypokalemia. N Engl J Med 1985; 312:746–749.
11. Struthers AD, Whitesmith R, Reid JL. Prior thiazide diuretic treatment increases adrenaline-induced hypokalemia. Lancet 1983; 1:1358–1360.
12. Williams ME, Gervine EV, Rosa RM, Landsberg L, Young JB, Silva P, Epstein FH. Catecholamine modulation of rapid potassium shifts during exercise. N Engl J Med 1985; 312:826–827.
13. Adrogre HJ, Madias NE. Changes in potassium concentration during acute acid-base disturbances. Am J Med 1981; 71:456–467.
14. Layzer RB. Periodic paralysis. Ann Neurol 1982; 11:547–552.
15. Kassirer JP, Harrington JT. Diuretics and potassium metabolism: A reassessment of the need, effectiveness and safety of potassium therapy. Kidney Int 1977; 11:505–515.
16. Kaplan NM. Our appropriate concern about potassium. Am J Med 1984; 77:1–4.
17. Schwartz AB, Swartz CD. Dosage of potassium chloride elixir to correct thiazide-induced hypokalemia. JAMA 1974; 230:702–704.
18. Gennari FJ, Cohen JJ. Role of the kidney in potassium homeostasis: Lessons from acid-base disorders. Kidney Int 1975; 8:1–5.
19. Pullen H, Doig A, Lambie AT. Intensive intravenous potassium replacement therapy. Lancet 1967; 2:809–811.
20. Lawson DH. Adverse reactions to potassium chloride. Q J Med 1974; 43:433–400.
21. Greenblatt J, Koch-Weser J. Adverse reactions to spironolactone. JAMA 1973; 225:40–43.
22. Ponce SP, Jennings AE, Madias NE, Harrington JT. Drug-induced hyperkalemia. Medicine 1985; 64:357–370.
23. Ricardella D, Dwyer JD. Salt substitutes and medicinal potassium sources: Risks and benefits. J Am Diet Assoc 1985; 85:471–474.
24. DeFronzo RA. Hyperkalemia and hyporeninemic hypoaldosteronism. Kidney Int 1980; 17:118–134.

29 | ACID-BASE DISORDERS

ANDREW S. LEVEY, M.D.

Acid-base disorders signify alterations in the metabolic, renal, and pulmonary processes responsible for the maintenance of normal body acidity.[1] The importance of early recognition and treatment is two-fold: First, the presence of an acid-base disorder is a valuable clue to the diagnosis of a serious underlying disturbance. Second, the alteration of body acidity may itself give rise to serious disorders requiring urgent treatment. This chapter will review the principles of diagnosis and of treatment of the four cardinal acid-base disorders: metabolic acidosis, metabolic alkalosis, respiratory alkalosis, and respiratory acidosis. Mixed acid-base disorders will also be reviewed briefly.

ACID-BASE PHYSIOLOGY

The Henderson equation shown here relates the equilibrium concentrations of hydrogen ions (H^+), bicarbonate ($HCO3^-$), and partial pressure of carbon dioxide ($PaCO_2$):

$$[H^+] \, (nEq/L) = 24 \times PaCO_2 \, (mm \; Hg)/[HCO3^-] \, (mEq/L)$$

Given the normal values for $PaCO_2$ (40 mm Hg) and bicarbonate (24 mEq/L), the normal hydrogen ion concentration is 40 nEq per liter, corresponding to a pH of 7.40. From inspection of the Henderson equation it is clear that alterations in either $PaCO_2$ or bicarbonate result in alterations in hydrogen ion concentration and, therefore, in pH. Primary alterations in $PaCO_2$ are defined as respiratory acid-base disorders. Primary alterations in bicarbonate are defined as metabolic acid-base disorders.

Normal metabolic processes generate approximately 15,000 mmol of CO_2 each day that are excreted by the lungs. Normal $PaCO_2$ is maintained by alterations in the rate of alveolar ventilation that match alterations in the rate of CO_2 production. Deviations from normal indicate impaired alveolar ventilation attributable to disorders in the central or peripheral nervous system or to disordered respiratory mechanics. In addition to CO_2, nonvolatile acids such as phosphoric acid, sulfuric acid, and ammonium (approximately 1 mEq per kilogram body weight per day) are liberated into the body fluids, are titrated by bicarbonate and other body buffers, and finally are excreted by the kidneys. Normal serum bicarbonate concentration is maintained by renal filtration and reabsorption of bicarbonate and by excretion of acid in the urine, thereby regenerating bicarbonate lost during titration of nonvolatile acids. Deviations in bicarbonate concentration indicate disorders in the rate of addition of acid to the body fluids or in the renal tubular processes of bicarbonate reabsorption and acidification of the urine.

In addition to primary alterations in $PaCO_2$ or bicarbonate, in each acid-base disorder there are secondary physiologic adjustments that diminish the deviation in hydrogen ion concentration that results from the primary disorder. In metabolic acid-base disorders, the alteration in body acidity initiates secondary changes that alter the rate of ventilation and therefore the $PaCO_2$. In metabolic acidosis, the primary decline in serum bicarbonate is followed immediately by a secondary decline in $PaCO_2$. As a result, the rise in hydrogen concentration is blunted, but not nullified. Conversely, in metabolic alkalosis the primary elevation in serum bicarbonate is followed immediately by a secondary elevation in $PaCO_2$, thus reducing, but not preventing, the fall in hydrogen ion concentration. In respiratory alkalosis the primary decline in $PaCO_2$ is accompanied by a secondary decline in serum bicarbonate concentration. As the serum bicarbonate declines, the reduced hydrogen ion concentration returns toward normal but remains low. In respiratory acidosis the primary increase in $PaCO_2$ leads to a secondary increase in serum bicarbonate concentration, thus reducing the attendant elevation in hydrogen ion concentration. It is important to note that the secondary changes in the $PaCO_2$ and the bicarbonate concentrations reduce the severity of the primary alteration in hydrogen ion concentration, but do not restore it to normal. Thus the net change in hydrogen ion concentration (and pH) always reflects the primary acid-base disturbance.

In summary, each of the cardinal acid-base disorders is defined by a primary and a secondary alteration in the $PaCO_2$ and the bicarbonate concentrations and by the resultant effects on hydrogen concentration and pH. The direction and magnitude of these primary and secondary alterations are given in Table 29-1 and Figure 29-1.

APPROACH TO ACID-BASE DATA

The first step in the diagnosis of acid-base disorders is to identify the disorder by use of the definitions in Table 29-1. An arterial blood sample is necessary for measurement of pH and $PaCO_2$. From the data obtained, the value for plasma bicarbonate concentration is calculated and reported by most laboratories. The measured value for venous serum total CO_2 concentration is

TABLE 29-1 Definition of Acid-Base Disorders

Disorder	Primary Alteration	Secondary Alteration	Overall Effect on Body Acidity
Metabolic acidosis	$\downarrow HCO_3^-$	$\downarrow PaCO_2$	$\uparrow H^+$ ($\downarrow pH$)
Metabolic alkalosis	$\uparrow HCO_3^-$	$\uparrow PaCO_2$	$\downarrow H^+$ ($\uparrow pH$)
Respiratory alkalosis	$\downarrow PaCO_2$	$\downarrow HCO_3^-$	$\downarrow H^+$ ($\uparrow pH$)
Respiratory acidosis	$\uparrow PaCO_2$	$\uparrow HCO_3^-$	$\uparrow H^+$ ($\downarrow pH$)

usually within 3 to 4 mEq per liter of this calculated value for bicarbonate concentration. If not, a measurement error is likely and another sample of arterial and venous blood should be obtained.

The next step is to determine if the acid-base data indicate a simple (single) or mixed (two or more) acid-base disorder. Figure 29-1 indicates the 95 percent confidence bands for the simple acid-base disorders. Values for $PaCO_2$ and bicarbonate concentration within these bands are consistent with the diagnosis of a simple acid-base disorder. Values that lie between the bands are the result of two or more primary acid-base disorders. However, acid-base values that lie within a band do not necessarily indicate a simple acid-base disorder because, sometimes in mixed disorders, the values may lie within a band for a simple acid-base disorder.

The final step is to make a differential diagnosis for each disorder. The most important causes of each disorder are given in the subsequent sections of this chapter. History, physical examination, and review of fluid intake and output are usually sufficient to narrow the list of diagnostic possibilities to two or three alternatives. Additional laboratory data usually are necessary for definitive diagnosis. Partial pressure of oxygen (PaO_2) is measured as part of the blood gas analysis and is necessary for accurate diagnosis of respiratory acid-base disorders. Serum electrolytes (sodium, potassium, and chloride), renal function tests (BUN and serum creatinine), and urine pH should also be obtained in all patients. It is sometimes necessary to measure serum levels of lactate, ketones, or salicylate, urine chloride concentration, or drug metabolites in blood and urine. Based on these results, appropriate treatment may be initiated. However, further evalutation is usually required to confirm the diagnosis of isolated renal tubular defects and adrenal diseases.

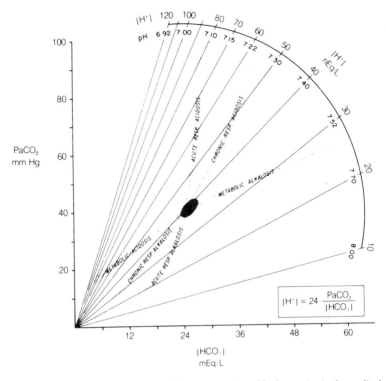

Figure 29-1 Range for serum bicarbonate, $PaCO_2$, and hydrogen ion in the cardinal acid-base disorders. (Reprinted with permission from Cohen JJ, Kassirer JP. Acid base. Boston: Little, Brown, 1982.)

METABOLIC ACIDOSIS

The normal metabolic processes liberate hydrogen ions into body fluids and therefore tend to lower serum bicarbonate concentration. Maintenance of the normal bicarbonate concentration requires urinary excretion of the daily endogenous acid load. The normal response to a primary decrease in serum bicarbonate concentration is to lower the urine pH to minimal values (4.5 to 5.0) and to increase renal acid excretion. Metabolic acidosis, defined as a primary decrease in serum bicarbonate concentration, is the result of increased production or addition of nonvolatile acids to the body fluids, reduced renal acid excretion, or loss of bicarbonate.[1] These disorders reduce serum bicarbonate concentration, acidify the body fluids, and lead to a secondary increase in ventilation.

In distinguishing among the various causes of metabolic acidosis, it is first necessary to calculate the anion gap (AG), defined as:

$$AG = [Na^+] - ([Cl^-] + [HCO_3^-])$$

$[Na^+]$ and $[Cl^-]$ are the serum concentrations of sodium and chloride respectively. The normal value for the anion gap is 8 to 14 mEq per liter and is the result of negatively charged serum proteins, principally albumin. Tables 29–2 and 29–3 list causes of metabolic acidosis with an elevated and a normal anion gap, respectively.[1,2]

An elevated anion gap in metabolic acidosis indicates addition, overproduction, or retention of acid in association with anions other than chloride. In most cases, the disorders can be recognized by their accompanying clinical and laboratory features. Confirmation by measurement of the anion in serum is usually necessary only for drug intoxications and for atypical cases of alcoholic ketoacidosis and lactic acidosis.

A normal anion gap in metabolic acidosis indicates addition of acid in association with chloride, loss of bicarbonate, either in urine or intestinal fluids, or failure of renal acid excretion. The urine pH is a valuable clue to the differential diagnosis of a normal anion gap metabolic acidosis. If the cause of metabolic acidosis is the addition of hydrochloric acid or the loss of bicarbonate in intestinal fluids (diarrhea, small bowel, biliary, or pancreatic drainage), renal acid excretion is increased and the urine pH is acid (4.5 to 5.0). If, on the other hand, the cause of metabolic acidosis is the urinary loss of bicarbonate or the failure of renal tubular hydrogen ion secretion, the urine pH may be any value within the normal range (4.5 to 7.5) and reflects the specific tubular defect.[1,3]

For accurate measurement of urine pH, the urine should be tested immediately after collection and should be free of infection with ureaseproducing bacteria. The evaporation of carbon dioxide or the addition of ammonia alkalinize the urine and obscure the renal contribution to urine pH. In most circumstances the urine dipstick provides the necessary information. However, if the value for pH is borderline (5.5), the urine should be collected under oil and tested with a pH electrode.

As indicated in Table 29–3, the serum potassium concentration is also a helpful clue in the differential diagnosis of a normal anion gap metabolic

TABLE 29-2 Causes of Metabolic Acidosis with an Elevated Anion Gap (AG > 14 mEq/L)

Disorder	Causes of Elevated AG	Clinical Characteristics	Confirmatory Tests
Ketoacidosis			
Diabetes	Acetoacetate, beta-hydroxybutyrate	Serum glucose ↑, urine and serum ketones strongly positive	Serum beta-hydroxybutyrate
Alcoholism	Beta-hydroxybutyrate	History of alcoholism, urine and serum ketones weakly positive	Serum beta-hydroxybutyrate
Starvation	Acetoacetate, beta-hydroxybutyrate	Very mild acidosis, urine and serum ketones weakly positive	
Lactic acidosis	Lactate	Hypoxia, shock, tumor	Serum lactate
Renal failure	Sulfate, phosphate, other endogenous anions	Azotemia	Serum creatinine >4 mg/dl
Drug Intoxications			
Aspirin	Salicylate, unknown endogenous anions	Primary respiratory alkalosis, tinnitus	Serum salicylate level
Ethylene glycol	Glycolate	Coma, seizures, renal failure, urinary calcium oxalate crystals, osmolar gap ↑	Serum ethylene glycol level
Methanol	Formate	Dimming of vision, abdominal pain, osmolar gap ↑	Serum methanol level
Paraldehyde	Unknown	Distinctive breath odor	Serum paraldehyde level

TABLE 29-3 Causes of Metabolic Acidosis with a Normal Anion Gap (AG <12 mEq/L)

Disorder	Urine pH	Serum Potassium	Clinical Characteristics	Confirmatory Tests
Acid ingestion	≤5	↑	History of treatment with hydrochloric acid, ammonium chloride, amino acids	
Diarrhea or intestinal fluid losses	≤5	↓		
Urinary-intestinal Anastomosis	>5	↓	History of treatment for urinary obstruction or reflux	
Mild renal disease	≤5	N or ↑	Serum creatinine 2–4 mg/dl	
Renal tubular acidosis (RTA)				
Type I (distal)	>5	↓	Serum creatinine normal, renal stones, bone disease	Acid loading test
Type II (proximal)	≤5	↓	Serum creatinine normal	Alkali loading test
Adrenal Disease				
Hyporeninemic Hypoaldosteronism (Type IV RTA)	≤5	↑	Mild renal disease, diabetes	Aldosterone ↓, renin ↓
Adrenal insufficiency	<5	↑		Cortisol ↓
Carbonic anhydrase inhibition	>5	↓	History of treatment with acetazolamide	

acidosis. Serum potassium concentration is usually increased in adrenal insufficiency and following the administration of hydrochloric acid. Serum potassium is usually decreased in intestinal bicarbonate losses and renal tubular defects.[1,4]

Treatment of Metabolic Acidosis

In some circumstances, the acidosis itself has serious consequences and requires urgent therapeutic intervention in addition to specific treatment for the disorders that lead to metabolic acidosis. The most important consequences include secondary hyperventilation, disturbances in myocardial function, and alterations in the serum potassium concentration. Most patients experience labored respirations if the systemic pH declines to less than 7.20 (serum bicarbonate concentration less than 12 to 14 mEq/L). In addition, depression in myocardial contractility and reduction in the threshold for ventricular fibrillation may occur if the pH is below 7.20. Based on these considerations, intravenous administration of sodium bicarbonate is recommended to raise the pH to this level. The following guidelines should be followed during therapy with sodium bicarbonate:

1. The dose of sodium bicarbonate should be estimated from the bicarbonate deficit and the rate of ongoing losses. The bicarbonate deficit is calculated as follows:

$$\begin{array}{ccc} \text{bicarbonate} & & \text{space of} \\ \text{deficit} & = & \text{distribution} \times (\text{target value} - \text{current value}) \\ (\text{mEq}) & & (\text{L}) & (\text{mEq/L}) \end{array}$$

Ongoing losses of bicarbonate are calculated as follows:

$$\text{bicarbonate loss (mEq/day)} = \text{fluid loss (L/day)} \times \text{fluid } [HCO_3^-] \text{ (mEq/L)}$$

These calculations provide a rough estimate only. Usually half of this dose should be administered initially and repeat measurements should be obtained in 4 to 8 hours.

2. The space of distribution for administered bicarbonate is usually approximately 50 percent of body weight (0.5 L per kilogram). However, in extreme acidosis (pH less than 7.10), the space of distribution usually exceeds this value and may be as high as 80 to 100 percent of body weight.[5]

3. If the reduction in $PaCO_2$ is appropriate for the reduction in serum bicarbonate concentration, the target value for bicarbonate concentration should be 12 to 14 mEq per liter. In patients with mixed acid-base disorders, the target value should be estimated from the Henderson equation and Figure 29-1 and should be based on the assumption that the $PaCO_2$ will not change initially.

4. Serum potassium generally declines during bicarbonate therapy. Potassium supplementation should begin immediately in hypokalemic patients and

in normokalemic patients without renal failure. Potassium therapy should be withheld initially in patients with hyperkalemia or in normokalemic patients with renal failure. In all circumstances, serum potassium should be monitored at 8 to 24-hour intervals during therapy. Further discussion of potassium therapy is included in *Hypokalemia and Hyperkalemia*.

5. "Overshoot alkalosis" frequently occurs during therapy as a result of three factors: (1) persistent hyperventilation owing to persistent cerebral spinal fluid acidosis that results from slow equilibration of administered bicarbonate between plasma and cerebral spinal fluid. (2) metabolism of organic anions (ketoacids, lactate) to bicarbonate after correction of the underlying condition, and (3) continuing renal acid excretion and regeneration of bicarbonate.

6. In lactic acidosis, bicarbonate administration may actually increase lactate production and blood lactate levels may rise; however, this increase has not been shown to have deleterious clinical consequences.[6,7]

For these reasons it is important to limit bicarbonate therapy to cases of severe acidemia and not to exceed the target value of 12 to 14 mEq per liter for the serum bicarbonate concentration.

METABOLIC ALKALOSIS

Metabolic alkalosis is defined as a primary elevation in the serum bicarbonate concentration. Although many disorders may lead to an increase in the serum bicarbonate concentration, the alkalosis persists only if the increased bicarbonate concentration is sustained. In discussing metabolic alkalosis, the processes that initiate a rise in serum bicarbonate concentration must be distinguished from those that sustain it. This is especially important since, in metabolic alkalosis, unlike other acid-base disorders, the disorder may persist even after resolution of the initiating factors.

Metabolic alkalosis may be initiated by addition of bicarbonate, loss of hydrogen ions, or loss of chloride with subsequent contraction of the extracellular fluid volume.[1] The most common causes of metabolic alkalosis include antacid ingestion, vomiting, nasogastric suction, and diuretic administration. These disorders raise the serum bicarbonate, alkalinize body fluids, and lead to a secondary decrease in ventilation. Two normal processes operate to reduce the elevated bicarbonate level. First, the ongoing generation of endogenous acids titrates bicarbonate. Second, the normal response to a primary increase in the serum bicarbonate concentration is a decrease in renal acid excretion. Therefore, factors that may sustain the metabolic alkalosis include persistent bicarbonate administration or acceleration of renal acid excretion caused by increased secretion of mineralcorticoid hormones or by contraction of the extracellular fluid volume in combination with a low salt diet.

The patient's history usually discloses the factors that initiated the metabolic alkalosis. In distinguishing among the factors that sustain the alkalosis, measurement of urine pH and of chloride concentration provide valuable clues to the diagnosis and a rationale for treatment. Table 29–4 lists the causes of metabolic alkalosis separated on the basis of these measurements.

A urine pH greater than 6.0 discloses the presence of bicarbonate in the urine and suggests that alkali administration is ongoing. Because of the high

TABLE 29–4   Causes of Metabolic Alkalosis

Disorder	Clinical Characteristics	Confirmatory Tests
Alkali Administration (Urine pH >6)		
Milk-alkali syndrome	Serum calcium ↑, serum creatinine ↑	
Administration of large amounts of sodium bicarbonate	Hypertension	
Combined therapy with nonabsorbable antacids and cation exchange resins	Renal insufficiency	
Chloride-Responsive (Urine Cl <10 mEq/L)		
Gastric fluid loss	Serum potassium ↓	
Diuretic therapy	Serum potassium ↓	
Following relief of hypercapnea	Serum potassium ↓	
Colonic villous adenoma	Serum potassium ↓	
Chloride-Resistant (Urine Cl >20 mEq/L)		
Primary hyperaldosteronism	Hypertension, serum potassium ↓	Aldosterone ↑, renin ↓
Cushing's syndrome	Hypertension, hirsutism, serum potassium ↓	Cortisol ↑
Bartter's syndrome	Serum potassium ↓	Aldosterone ↑, renin ↑
Idiopathic	Serum potassium ↓	

rate of bicarbonate excretion that may be achieved by the normal kidney, metabolic alkalosis rarely results from alkali administration unless the glomerular filtration rate is impaired. It is important to note that other factors may raise the urine pH in patients with metabolic alkalosis. As discussed earlier, evaporation of carbon dioxide or infection with urease-producing bacteria also alkalinize the urine. In addition, transient elevation of the urine pH may occur during vomiting and during alkali administration, even if the administered alkali is not responsible for sustaining the alkalosis. Thus, the finding of an alkaline urine must be interpreted in light of the patient's clinical history.

A urine pH less than 6.0 indicates that ongoing renal acid excretion is the cause of sustained metabolic alkalosis. Measurement of the urine chloride concentration distinguishes two subgroups of disorders that differ in their pathogenesis and treatment. A urine chloride concentration less than 10 mEq per liter indicates that the patient is ingesting a low salt diet and that contraction of the extracellular fluid volume with relative chloride deficiency is the cause of persistent renal acid excretion. These disorders are termed "chloride-responsive" because of the prompt excretion of bicarbonate in the urine and resolution of the alkalosis when chloride is provided in the diet or in intravenous fluids. In patients with metabolic alkalosis attributable to ongoing diuretic therapy, the urine chloride concentration is transiently elevated during the diuresis. However, the alkalosis is sustained even after the diuretic is discontinued unless chloride is provided. Severe metabolic alkalosis (serum bicarbonate concentration greater than 35 mEq/L) with low urine chloride is usually the result of drainage of gastric fluid or of diuretic therapy for edematous conditions. In contrast, metabolic alkalosis from diuretic administration in nonedematous subjects is usually relatively mild.

A value for urine chloride greater that 20 mEq per liter indicates that the patient has adequate dietary chloride intake and that another factor, such as mineralocorticoid excess, is the cause of sustained renal acid excretion. These disorders are termed "chloride-resistant" because treatment with chloride fails to improve the metabolic alkalosis and, in fact, many worsen the acid-base disorder. In most cases, the metabolic alkalosis is mild; hypokalemia is usually the more marked electrolyte abnormality.

Treatment of Metabolic Alkalosis

In addition to specific treatment for the underlying cause of metabolic alkalosis, therapy to lower the serum bicarbonate may be indicated if the value exceeds 35 mEq per liter. The rise in systemic pH in metabolic alkalosis is not extreme because of secondary hyperventilation. Indeed, the pH does not exceed 7.55 unless the serum bicarbonate concentration is greater than 50 mEq per liter. (see Fig. 29–1). Nonetheless, reduction of the serum bicarbonate concentration to less than 35 mEq per liter is important because of the following considerations:

1. Secondary hypoventilation reduces alveolar oxygen tension. For patients with cardiopulmonary diseases, the resultant decline in PaO_2 may result in clinically significant hypoxia.

2. Transient hyperventilation of even a modest degree strikingly raises systemic pH to severely alkaline values. For example, if serum bicarbonate concentration is 35 mEq per liter, a reduction in $PaCO_2$ from the expected value of 47 mm Hg to 35 mm Hg results in a rise in pH from 7.50 to 7.62. In fact, it follows from the Henderson equation that whenever the values for bicarbonate concentration and $PaCO_2$ are equal, hydrogen concentration is 24 mEq per liter, and corresponds to a pH of 7.62. Extreme alkalemia may be associated with depression of consciousness, delerium, seizures, and tetany. The likelihood of hyperventilation is greatest in patients with cardiopulmonary or liver diseases, with sepsis, and, in the postoperative periods, circumstances in which metabolic alkalosis frequently occurs.

3. Increased urinary potassium excretion and potassium depletion are the consequence of virtually every cause of metabolic alkalosis. In general, the degree of potassium depletion parallels the severity of the alkalosis although the acid-base disturbance is not the cause, per se, of the altered potassium metabolism. In patients with serum bicarbonate 35 to 40 mEq per liter, the serum potassium is often 2.5 to 3.5 mEq per liter, and the potassium deficit is 200 to 500 mEq. Furthermore, renal potassium conservation and repair of the potassium deficit cannot proceed until the underlying acid-base disorder is corrected. During treatment of metabolic alkalosis, it is important to assess the extent of the potassium deficit, to provide adequate potassium therapy, and to monitor carefully the serum potassium concentration.

The treatment for metabolic alkalosis attributable to alkali administration is discontinuation of alkali therapy. If renal function is not severely impaired, the continuing alkaline diuresis rapidly lowers serum bicarbonate concentration. If hypercalemia is also present, as in the milk-alkali syndrome, treatment with sodium chloride and loop diuretics often improves renal function and aids in resolution of the alkalosis. This treatment increases urinary potassium excretion. Treatment with hydrochloric acid or its precursors is necessary (vide infra) if renal function is severely reduced.

Chloride-responsive metabolic alkalosis requires provision of chloride to correct the acid-base disorder and to prevent further renal potassium wasting. The choice of the cation to accompany chloride depends on the severity of the cation deficits, the patient's tolerance to administered cations, and the severity of the alkalosis. As discussed, potassium chloride administration is usually necessary because of the accompanying potassium deficit. In patients with extracellular fluid depletion, sodium and potassium chloride should be prescribed either in the diet or intravenously. In edematous patients, it is necessary to continue sodium restriction and to administer potassium chloride alone. With correction of chloride depletion, renal acid excretion is reduced and bicarbonate is excreted in the urine. However, if serum bicarbonate is markedly elevated, or if renal function is impaired, several days may be required for serum bicarbonate to decline to an acceptable level. In these cases, more rapid lowering of serum bicarbonate may be achieved with infusion of hydro-chloric acid.

In chloride-resistant alkalosis, by definition, treatment with chloride fails to improve both the alkalosis and the potassium deficit. Definitive treatment requires resolution of the underlying condition. Disorders of excess adrenal steroid secretion may be ameliorated by spironolactone, and Bartter's syndrome may improve following treatment with indomethacin. Treatment with large amounts of potassium chloride is sometimes helpful in idiopathic chloride-resistant metabolic alkalosis. The alkalosis is rarely severe, and treatment with hydrochloric acid is rarely necessary.

Extreme metabolic alkalosis (serum bicarbonate concentration greater than 45 mEq per liter), regardless of the cause, should be treated by infusion of hydrochloric acid or one of its precursors. The dose of acid administered should be calculated to reduce the serum bicarbonate to approximately 35 to 40 mEq per liter over an 8 to 24 hour interval. The space of distribution of administered acid may be assumed to be approximately 50 percent of body weight. Various acid solutions are available for intravenous infusion. Ammonium chloride (20 mg/ml) contains 350 mEq per liter hydrogen ions and can be given at rates up to 500 ml per hour. However, ammonium chloride is contraindicated in patients with liver disease. Arginine monohydrochloride (10 percent) contains approximately 500 mEq per liter hydrogen ions and can be given at rates of 300 ml per hour if necessary. Serum potassium levels rise, however, and this therapy is contraindicated in patients with severe renal insufficiency. Dilute hydrochloric acid (0.1 to 0.15 N) contains 100 to 150 mEq per liter hydrogen ions and may be give safely to patients with renal and liver diseases; however, because of its corrosive nature it must be administered into a central vein. Hydrochloric acid is the preferable method of treatment if a central venous catheter is in place. As already discussed, serum potassium should be carefully monitored during therapy and acid-base status should be reassessed in 4 to 8 hours.

RESPIRATORY ALKALOSIS

Respiratory alkalosis, defined as a primary decrease in $PaCO_2$, is synonymous with alveolar hyperventilation and is the most common acid-base disorder. In many cases, the abnormal pattern of respiration is easily detected by clinical observation. Often, however, these signs are overlooked, and hyperventilation is recognized only after an arterial blood gas measurement is performed. Regardless of the cause, a primary decline in $PaCO_2$ alkalinizes body fluids and reduces renal acid excretion, thus leading to a secondary decline in serum bicarbonate concentration. Unlike the rapid respiratory response to metabolic acid-base disorders, the new steady state levels for serum bicarbonate concentration and pH are only achieved 2 to 3 days after the primary change in $PaCO_2$.[1] Thus, the duration of hyperventilation in patients with respiratory alkalosis may be estimated from the values for serum bicarbonate and pH, as shown in Figure 29–1.

Under normal circumstances the rate of alveolar ventilation is regulated by the brain stem respiratory center in response to changes in acidity and in oxygen tension in body fluids. Both hypoxemia and acidosis increase alveolar ventilation. However, these normal regulatory processes may be overridden by drugs that affect the respiratory center and disorders of the central nervous system or of the pulmonary system, thereby leading to hyperventilation despite normal or increased PaO_2 and systemic pH. As shown in Table 29–5, respiratory alkalosis may be caused by a wide variety of disorders.

The approach to the diagnosis is first to determine if hypoxia is the cause of hyperventilation. Alveolar ventilation is stimulated by a decline in PaO_2 to 60 mm Hg or lower. The underlying causes of hypoxemia include ventilation-perfusion mismatching attributable to pulmonary diseases or to right to left cardiac shunts. Tissue hypoxia owing to hypotension (especially when associated with sepsis) or to severe anemia (hemoglobin less than 30 percent of normal) may also result in hyperventilation, even if PaO_2 is normal. Of course, respiratory alkalosis is normally seen in people living at high altitude and is a result of the reduced atmospheric oxygen tension.

In patients without hypoxia, hyperventilation is attributable either to stimulation of respiration by drugs or toxins, to central nervous system or pulmonary disorders, or to mechanical overventilation. It is important to note that respiratory alkalosis is a characteristic feature of normal pregnancy; $PaCO_2$ falls to as low as 28 to 30 mm Hg in the third trimester. The hyperventilation of pregnancy has been ascribed to increased levels of progesterone.

TABLE 29-5   Causes of Respiratory Alkalosis

Hypoxia
   High altitude
   Ventilation-perfusion mismatching
   Right to left cardiac shunt
   Hypotension
   Severe anemia

Central nervous system mediated
   Pregnancy
   Anxiety
   Drugs and toxins (salicylates)
   Neurologic diseases
   Hepatic failure
   Sepsis
   Recovery from metabolic acidosis

Pulmonary diseases
   Pulmonary edema
   Interstitial lung disease
   Pulmonary embolism
   Pneumonia

Mechanical overventilation

Modified from Cohen JJ, Kassirer JP. Acid base. Boston: Little, Brown, 1982.

Treatment of Respiratory Alkalosis

Respiratory alkalosis occurs in a wide variety of clinical settings, ranging from normal adaptations and mild self-limiting anxiety to severe life-threatening disorders. In most cases the respiratory alkalosis itself is a harmless feature of the underlying condition. Reduce $PaCO_2$ causes cerebral vasoconstriction; consequently, mechanical hyperventilation is employed therapeutically in patients with acute neurologic disease to reduce cerebral edema. However, it is unknown whether the decline in cerebral blood flow is responsible for the central nervous system side effects of hyperventilation. Acute severe respiratory alkalosis is associated with parasthesias in the extremities, circumoral numbness, tightness in the chest, and in some cases, seizures. Atrial and ventricular tacharrhythmias may occur in patients with underlying ischemic heart disease. In contrast, there are few clinical manifestations attributable to chronic respiratory alkalosis.

Treatment should be directed at the underlying cause of the disorder. In patients with hypoxemia, elevation of the PaO_2 to 60 mm Hg should be sufficient to suppress the hypoxic respiratory drive and to raise the $PaCO_2$. In patients with anxiety hyperventilation, $PaCO_2$ can be raised transiently by instructing the patient to breathe in and out of a paper bag, thus raising the $PaCO_2$ in the inspired air. In patients with mechanical overventilation, ventilator settings for rate, tidal volume, or dead space may be adjusted to reduce the rate of alveolar ventilation. This subject is discussed in more detail in *Care of the Intubated and Mechanically Ventilated Patient*. If the underlying disorder cannot be reversed (for example, hepatic failure or central nervous system disease), there is little that can be done to suppress ventilation. Usually the alkalemia is not severe unless there is accompanying metabolic alkalosis. In cases of severe alkalemia attributable to mixed acid-base disorders, treatment of the alkalemia itself is best accomplished by treatment of the metabolic alkalosis.

RESPIRATORY ACIDOSIS

Respiratory acidosis, defined as a primary increase in $PaCO_2$, is synonymous with alveolar hypoventilation. The adequacy of alveolar ventilation cannot be assessed on clinical grounds alone; the measurement of $PaCO_2$ in an arterial blood sample is essential for an accurate diagnosis of respiratory acidosis. Regardless of the cause, a rise in $PaCO_2$ acidifies body fluids, secondarily increases renal acid excretion, and elevates serum bicarbonate concentration. The new steady state levels for serum bicarbonate concentration and for pH are achieved 2 to 3 days after a primary change in $PaCO_2$.[1] Thus, acute and chronic respiratory acidosis may be distinguished by the values for serum bicarbonate and for pH, as shown in Figure 29–1. This distinction is especially important in the diagnosis and treatment.

The causes of hypoventilation include a variety of central and peripheral nervous system, thoracic, and pulmonary diseases that suppress the ventilatory response to CO_2, that impair respiratory mechanics, or that obstruct the airway (Table 29–6). Acute respiratory acidosis may result from any of these disorders and constitutes a medical emergency. Chronic respiratory acidosis usually is seen only in patients with chronic obstructive or restrictive lung diseases, kyphoscoliosis, or neuromuscular diseases, and often persists despite maximal therapy.

The approach to the diagnosis is first to examine the patient's respirations. Infrequent shallow respirations in respiratory acidosis indicate depression of the brain stem respiratory center or neuromuscular disorders. It is especially important to discontinue or reverse drugs causing sedation or neuromuscular blockade. Tachypnea and signs of respiratory distress indicate thoracic disorders and obstructive or restrictive pulmonary diseases. The history, a physical examination (including neurologic examination), and a blood gas analysis (including measurement of PaO_2) are usually sufficient to distinguish among the various causes of respiratory acidosis. In some cases,

TABLE 29-6   Causes of Respiratory Acidosis

Acute	Chronic
Airway obstruction Aspiration Laryngospasm Bronchospasm Obstructive sleep apnea Drowning	Chronic obstructive pulmonary disease
Respiratory center depression General anesthesia Sedative-hypnotic drug overdose Central sleep apnea	Obesity hypoventilation syndrome
Circulatory catastrophe Cardiac arrest Severe pulmonary edema	
Neuromuscular defects Cervical spine transection Guillain-Barré syndrome Myasthenia gravis crisis Drugs or toxin (succinylcholine, aminoglycosides)	Poliomyelitis Multiple sclerosis Muscular dystrophy Amyotrophic lateral sclerosis Polymyositis Myxedema
Restrictive defects Pneumothorax Flail chest	Kyphoscoliosis Spinal arthritis Pleural effusion Severe interstitial fibrosis Decreased diaphragmatic movement (ascites, obesity)
Mechanical underventilation	

Modified from Cohen JJ, Kassirer JP. Acid base. Boston: Little, Brown, 1982.

measurement of respiratory mechanics is also necessary. In contrast to metabolic acidosis, measurements of serum electrolytes, renal function, urinary pH, and urinary electrolytes usually are not helpful in distinguishing among the causes of respiratory acidosis.

Treatment of Respiratory Acidosis

The most serious consequences of alveolar hypoventilation are hypoxia and the central nervous system effects of hypercapnea. During acute hypoventilation, severe hypercapnea rarely develops because patients succumb to hypoxia before $PaCO_2$ can rise to extreme levels. If ventilation ceases abruptly, death from hypoxia occurs in less than 5 minutes. Thus, in the absence of supplemental oxygen, $PaCO_2$ values greater than 80 mm Hg rarely occur. If, however, PaO_2 is maintained by supplemental oxygen, $PaCO_2$ may rise to levels in excess of 100 mm Hg. The effects of hypercapnea include cerebral and peripheral vasodilatation and stimulation of the sympathetic nervous system. Clinical manifestations include anxiety, breathlessness, headache, disorientation, and confusion. With extreme hypercapnea ($PaCO_2$ 70 to 100 mm Hg), depression of consciousness, asterixis, and coma may occur. Rarely, there are also signs of increased intracranial pressure, including papilledema and focal neurologic findings. The effects of $PaCO_2$ on neurologic function are highly variable and probably are influenced by the prevailing PaO_2, the pH, the baseline level of $PaCO_2$, and the rate of rise in $PaCO_2$. Acute respiratory acidosis is accompanied by flushing, tachycardia, and diaphoresis; however, these manifestations are not present in chronic respiratory acidosis. Although supraventricular and ventricular tachycardias are frequent in patients with chronic respiratory acidosis attributable to chronic lung disease, it is likely that these arrhythmias are caused by concommitant effects of hypoxia, bronchodilators, and digitalis, rather than by the elevated level of $PaCO_2$ itself.

Acute respiratory acidosis is a medical emergency. Supplemental oxygen and restoration of ventilation must be achieved at once. The most common causes include airway obstruction from aspiration or asthma, depression of the respiratory center from drugs or toxins, severe pulmonary edema, cardiac arrest, cervical spinal cord transection, pneumothorax, and flail chest. Mechanical ventilation must be initiated if the underlying disorder cannot be reversed within minutes.

The most common cause of chronic respiratory acidosis is chronic obstructive pulmonary disease. The degree of airway obstruction correlates poorly with the level of hypercapnea. Chronic CO_2 retention reduces the sensitivity of the respiratory center to CO_2. While provision of supplemental oxygen frequently is necessary for treatment of hypoxemia, elevation of the PaO_2 to values greater than 60 mm Hg may suppress hypoxic respiratory drive and may further suppress ventilation. Therefore, oxygen should be administered initially in a low dose (24 to 28 percent) to patients with chronic respiratory acidosis. Arterial blood gases should be sampled after 20 minutes to guide further oxygen therapy. Treatment of the underlying disorder may improve the CO_2 retention.

MIXED ACID-BASE DISORDERS

A mixed acid-base disorder is defined as the coexistence of two or more primary (simple) acid-base disorders. As discussed earlier, a large number of medical conditions affect the $PaCO_2$ and bicarbonate concentrations. Not surprisingly, the coexistence of several such conditions frequently gives rise to a mixed acid-base disorder. Some examples of common mixed acid-base disorders include: (1) severe pulmonary edema (lactic acidosis and hypoventilation), (2) sepsis (lactic acidosis and hyperventilation), (3) severe renal failure with vomiting (uremic acidosis and metabolic alkalosis), (4) salicylate intoxication (metabolic acidosis and hyperventilation), and (6) improvement after an exacerbation of chronic obstructive pulmonary disease (respiratory acidosis and metabolic alkalosis). Although the diagnosis of mixed acid-base disorders should be suspected in patients with multiple causes of acid-base disturbances, accurate diagnosis requires evaluation of arterial blood gas data and knowledge of the confidence bands in Figure 1. If the acid-base data do not lie within the confidence interval for a simple acid-base disorder, a mixed disorder is necessarily present. However, the converse is not true: a mixed disorder may be present even if the data are consistent with a simple disorder. For example, combined metabolic acidosis and alkalosis may appear as a simple metabolic acidosis or alkalosis, and combined acute respiratory acidosis and metabolic alkalosis may appear as a simple chronic respiratory alkalosis. In these cases the correct diagnosis is surmised from the clinical history, the temporal evolution of the acid-base abnormalities, consideration of the anion gap, and serum potassium concentrations.

In general, the treatment of mixed acid-base disorders should proceed in the same fashion as the treatment of the individual acid-base disorders that are present. It is important to remember that the coexisting primary disorders may have off-setting or aggravating effects on overall hydrogen ion concentration. Therefore, special care is required to select target values for bicarbonate that maintain pH in the desirable range during the administration of acid or alkali.

References

1. Cohen JJ, Kassirer JP. Acid base. Boston: Little, Brown, 1982.
2. Gabow PA. Nephrology forum. Disorders associated with an altered anion gap. Kidney Int 1985; 27:472–483.

3. Sebastian A, Morris RC Jr. Renal tubular acidosis. In: Earley LE, Gottschalk CW, eds. Strauss and Welt's diseases of the kidney. 3rd ed. Boston: Little, Brown, 1979:1029.
4. Fulop M. Serum potassium in lactic acidosis and ketoacidosis. N Engl J Med 1979; 300:1087–1089.
5. Garrella S, Dana CL, Chazan JA. Severity of metabolic acidosis as a determinant of bicarbonate requirements. N Engl J Med 1973; 289:121–126.
6. Graf H, Leach W, Arieff AI. Evidence for a detrimental effect of bicarbonate therapy in hypoxic lactic acidosis. Science 1983; 227:754–793.
7. Madias N. Nephrology forum. Lactic acidosis. Kidney Int 1986; 29:752–774.

30 | DIAGNOSIS OF RENAL INSUFFICIENCY

ANDREW S. LEVEY, M.D.

Renal insufficiency, defined as a decline in glomerular filtration rate (GFR), may be acute or chronic, depending on its duration. This chapter will focus principally on the diagnosis of acute renal insufficiency; the management of acute and chronic renal insufficiency is discussed in the following chapter. Acute renal insufficiency is a frequent and serious problem among hospitalized patients. Consultation usually is requested because of the finding of a sudden increase in the serum creatinine concentration during routine monitoring of an acutely ill patient. Despite the inexact relationship between serum creatinine concentration and GFR (Fig. 30–1A), a rise in serum creatinine concentration is the most reliable and readily available clinical indicator of an acute decline in renal function.[1,2]

HOSPITAL-ACQUIRED RENAL INSUFFICIENCY

In a recent prospective survey of approximately 2,000 patients admitted to the medical and surgical services of a large teaching hospital,[3] acute renal insufficiency was diagnosed in 5 percent of patients; 80 percent of episodes of renal insufficiency were acquired during the course of hospitalization. The prevalence of hospital-acquired acute renal insufficiency was higher in patients with preexisting renal insufficiency: it was 2.9 percent for patients with an initially normal serum creatinine concentration and 14 percent for patients with an initially elevated serum creatinine concentration. The major causes were reduced renal perfusion caused by circulatory disturbances (42 percent), drug toxicity, particularly from aminoglycoside antibiotics and radiographic contrast (20 percent), or a combination of disorders occurring within 72 hours after surgery (18 percent) (Table 30–1). Fortunately most episodes of renal insufficiency were mild; the rise in serum creatinine was greater than 3.0 mg per deciliter in only 19 percent of patients, and dialysis was necessary in only 8 percent. Mortality was approximately 30 percent and was related to the severity of acute renal insufficiency (see Table 30–1). In patients with a rise in serum creatinine concentration less than 3.0 mg per deciliter, mortality was 15 percent; in patients with a rise greater than 3.0 mg per deciliter, mortality was 65 percent. Despite the high mortality rate, only 10 percent of deaths were attributable to renal insufficiency per se.

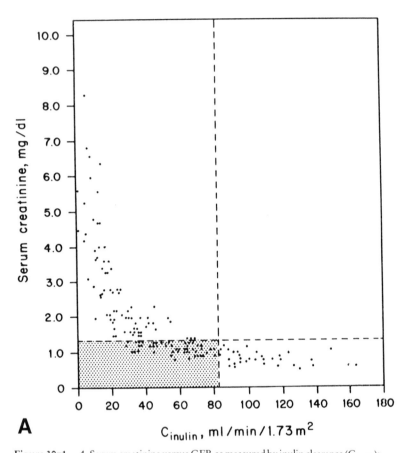

A C_{inulin}, ml/min/1.73 m^2

Figure 30-1 *A*, Serum creatinine versus GFR as measured by inulin clearance (C_{inulin}); and *B*, creatinine clearance ($C_{creatinine}$) versus GFR as measured by inulin clearance (C_{inulin}). The points are data from 171 patients with glomerular disease. In *A*, the broken horizontal line represents the upper limit of normal for serum creatinine. In *B*, the broken horizontal line represents the lower limit for normal creatinine clearance. In *A* and *B*, the broken vertical line represents the lower limit for normal inulin clearance. The shaded area indicates the range in which GFR is reduced, but serum creatinine or creatinine clearance remains normal. (Reproduced with permission from Semesh O, Goldbetz H, Kriss JP, Myers BD. Limitation of creatinine as a filtration marker in glomerulopathic patients. Kidney Int 1985; 28:830–838.)

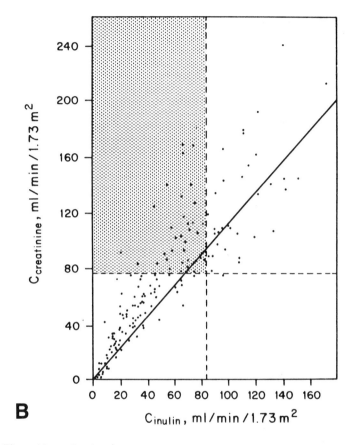

B

Figure 30-1 *Continued*

TABLE 30-1 Causes and Mortality of Hospital-Acquired Renal Insufficiency

	Number of Episodes	Percent of Total	Number of Deaths	Mortality (%)
Decreased renal perfusion		42		
ECF volume contraction	22		2	9
Severe heart failure	18		9	50
Sepsis with hypotension	10		4	40
Hypotension of unknown cause	4		4	100
Therapeutic agents		20		
Aminoglycosides	9		1	11
Contrast media	16		1	6
Platinum	1		0	0
Major surgery		18	3	13
Heart surgery	15			
Aorta surgery	3			
Other surgery	5			
Urinary obstruction	3	2	0	0
Hepatorenal syndrome	5	4	4	80
Multifactorial	4	3	0	0
Miscellaneous and unknown	14	11	4	29
	129	100	32	25

Data from Hou SH, Bushinsky DA, Wish JB, Cohen JJ, Harrington JT. Hospital-acquired renal insufficiency: a prospective study. Am J Med 1983; 74:243–248.

DIFFERENTIAL DIAGNOSIS OF ACUTE RENAL INSUFFICIENCY

Serum Creatinine Concentration

Interpretation of changes in the serum creatinine concentration is complicated by a number of factors.[1,2] First, creatinine is excreted both by glomerular filtration and by tubular secretion; therefore the serum creatinine concentration is consistently below the value that would be obtained if creatinine were an ideal filtration marker (see Fig. 30-1A). Second, creatinine generation is reduced in normal persons with reduced meat intake or with low muscle mass, such as vegetarians, thin women, and the elderly (both sexes), and in patients who are chronically ill or debilitated. Thus, values for serum creatinine concentration within the normal range may be associated with reductions in GFR to as low as 20 ml per minute per 1.73 m² (see Fig. 30-1A). As a result, the serum creatinine correlates only roughly with the absolute value of GFR. Nevertheless, the finding of an elevated serum creatinine in the steady state is a near certain indication that GFR is reduced. An important exception to this rule is the serum creatinine elevation that occurs without a reduction in GFR because of interference, by certain drugs or chemicals, with tubular secretion of creatinine or with laboratory measurement of creatinine[1] (Table 30-2).

Creatinine clearance (C_{cr}) is a more accurate estimate of GFR than is serum creatinine (see Fig. 30-1B). Although GFR may be reduced despite a normal value for creatinine clearance, a reduced value for creatinine clearance virtually always indicates a reduced GFR. Unfortunately, measurement of creatinine clearance requires the collection of a timed urine sample, such as a 24-hour sample, which is usually difficult in sick, hospitalized patients. Alternatively, a variety of formulas and nomograms are available to predict creatinine clearance from the patient's steady state serum creatinine concentration (P_{cr}), age, weight and gender. The formula derived by Cockcroft and Gault is particularly simple to use:[4]

$$\text{Men: } C_{cr} \text{ (ml/min)} = \frac{140 - \text{age (years)} \times \text{weight (kg)}}{72 \times P_{cr} \text{ (mg/dl)}}$$

$$\text{Women: } C_{cr} \text{ (ml/min)} = \frac{140 - \text{age (years)} \times \text{weight (kg)}}{85 \times P_{cr} \text{ (mg/dl)}}$$

However, predicting the GFR from formulas and nomograms also requires caution. First, creatinine clearance exceeds GFR at all levels of renal function (see Fig. 30-1B) because creatinine is excreted by both glomerular filtration and tubular secretion. Second, the predicted value for creatinine clearance exceeds the measured value in patients with obesity, edema, or severe renal insufficiency, in whom body weight is not an accurate estimate of creatinine generation. As a result, the predicted value for creatinine clearance may deviate substantially from the GFR.[5]

TABLE 30-2 Causes of Elevated Serum Creatinine Without Reduced GFR

Inhibition of tubular secretion of creatinine
    Trimethoprim
    Cimetidine
Interference with measurement of creatinine in serum
    Ketones (Jaffe reaction method)*
    Cephalosporins (Jaffe reaction method)*
    Flucytosine (iminohydrolysis method)†

---

* Jaffe reaction is utilized by ACA and SMAC autoanalyzers (Technicon Instruments Corp., Tarrytown, NY).
† Iminohydrolysis method is utilized by EKTACHEM auto analyzers (Eastman Kodak Co., Rochester, NY).

It is important to recall that patients with acute renal insufficiency are generally not in a steady state of creatinine balance. Thus, estimation of GFR or prediction of creatinine clearance from the serum level is not appropriate. If serum creatinine is rising, the creatinine clearance predicted from the equation overestimates true creatinine clearance.[6]

Pathophysiologic Classification of Acute Renal Insufficiency

The causes of acute renal insufficiency are traditionally classified according to the mechanism of the decline in GFR. Circulatory disturbances that reduce blood flow to the kidney and, consequently, reduce GFR are termed "prerenal." Reduced renal blood flow can accompany states of extracellular fluid (ECF) volume excess (for example, congestive heart failure) or volume depletion (for example, dehydration consequent to severe diarrhea). By definition, prerenal disorders do not cause renal parenchymal damage, impaired tubular function, or appearance of tubular cells or casts in the urinary sediment. Most importantly, reversal of prerenal conditions restores renal blood flow, GFR, and serum creatinine concentration to their prior levels. Reduced GFR that persists after relief of prerenal conditions indicates, by definition, the presence of a concomitant postrenal or renal condition.

Conditions that obstruct urine flow in the renal pelvis, ureters, or lower urinary tract are termed "postrenal." The resulting increase in pressure within the renal pelvis leads to hydronephrosis and a decline in GFR. Obstruction that persists for more than a few days may lead to impaired tubular function, parenchymal damage, and urinary sediment abnormalities, which may persist even after obstruction is relieved. Although successful treatment of postrenal conditions relieves the obstruction and raises GFR, recovery of glomerular and tubular function may be delayed or incomplete. Persistent impairment of renal function that is the sequelae of obstruction is defined as postobstructive nephropathy and is more severe in the elderly, in patients with obstruction of long duration, and in patients in whom obstruction is complicated by urinary tract infection or stones. Concomitant prerenal or renal conditions may also be responsible for persistent renal insufficiency following relief of obstruction.

The "renal" causes of acute renal insufficiency include primary renal diseases and systemic diseases that affect the kidneys. These conditions damage renal parenchyma, reduce GFR, impair tubular function, and cause urinary sediment abnormalities. The most important renal causes of acute renal insufficiency are ischemic and drug-induced acute tubular necrosis. Other renal parenchymal diseases are included in Table 30-3. Patients with acute renal insufficiency frequently have multiple disorders. Accurate diagnosis requires consideration of all potential causes of reduced GFR, differentiation of acute

TABLE 30-3   Renal Parenchymal Diseases Causing Acute Renal Insufficiency

Glomerular diseases: Crescentic glomerulonephritis (acute and rapidly progressive glomerulonephritis)*

Low serum complement
Systemic lupus erythematosus
Poststreptococcal glomerulonephritis
Subacute bacterial endocarditis
"Shunt" nephritis
Essential mixed cryoglobulinemia
Idiopathic membranoproliferative glomerulonephritis

Normal serum complement
Polyarteritis nodosa
Hypersensitivity vasculitis
Henoch-Schönlein purpura
Wegener's granulomatosis
Visceral abscess
Goodpasture's syndrome
IgA-IgG nephropathy
Idiopathic crescentic glomerulonephritis

Tubulointerstitial diseases

Marked interstitial inflammation
Severe pyelonephritis
Drug-induced allergic interstitial nephritis
Drug-induced toxic interstitial nephritis

Mild interstitial inflammation
Acute tubular necrosis
Papillary necrosis
Myeloma kidney
Hypercalcemic nephropathy
Uric acid nephropathy

Vascular diseases
Hemolytic-uremic syndrome
Malignant nephrosclerosis
Scleroderma
Atheroembolism
Cortical necrosis
Infarction

* Adapted from Madaio MP, Harrington JT. The diagnosis of acute glomerulonephritis. N Engl J Med 1983; 309:1299–1302 and with permission.

and chronic renal insufficiency, and careful interpretation of selected diagnostic tests.

Differentiation of Acute and Chronic Renal Insufficiency

Acute and chronic renal insufficiency are differentiated by the cause and the time course of the disorder and by measurement of kidney size. The causes of acute renal insufficiency have already been discussed. The principal causes of chronic renal insufficiency are listed in Table 30–4. Note that acute tubular necrosis, the most common cause of acute renal insufficiency, is not listed because it rarely causes permanent reduction in renal function.

The time course of acute renal failure is traditionally divided into three phases: a phase of injury, during which the pathophysiologic events that lead to

TABLE 30–4   Renal Parenchymal Diseases Causing Chronic Renal Insufficiency

Glomerular diseases
  Diabetes mellitus
  Systemic vasculitis
    Systemic lupus erythematosus
    Polyarteritis nodosa
    Wegener's granalomatosis
    Sequelae of Henoch-Schönlein purpura
  Amyloidosis and light chain nephropathy
  Drug-induced diseases
    Heroin, gold, penicillamine, captopril
  Idiopathic diseases
    Membranous nephropathy
    Focal glomerulosclerosis
    Membranoproliferative glomerulonephritis
    IgA-IgG nephropathy

Tubulointerstitial diseases
  Drug-induced diseases
    Analgesic nephropathy
    Allergic interstitial nephritis
  Sickle cell nephropathy
  Multiple myeloma and light chain nephropathy
  Hypercalcemia
  Vesicoureteral reflux nephropathy
  Postobstructive nephropathy
  Urinary tract stones
  Urinary tract infections
    Bacterial infections (associated with obstruction, reflux, stones,
      diabetes, sickle cell disease)
    Tuberculosis

Vascular diseases
  Benign or malignant nephrosclerosis
  Atheroembolism
  Renal artery stenosis
  Scleroderma
  Sequelae of hemolytic-uremic syndrome
  Postpartum renal failure

Hereditary diseases
  Hereditary nephritis (Alport's syndrome)
  Polycystic kidney disease
  Medullary cystic disease

the decrease in GFR are initiated; a maintenance phase, during which the reduction in GFR is sustained; and a recovery phase, during which GFR gradually improves. The maintenance phase is characterized by a rapid rise (over a few days) in serum creatinine concentration; if the reduction in GFR is severe, clinical manifestations of uremia may appear. Oliguria and serious derangements in fluid and electrolyte balance occur in more than one-half of patients.

Chronic renal insufficiency, like acute renal insufficiency, is initiated by a phase of injury. If the injury is sustained, a phase of progression ensues, during which further decline in GFR occurs. In some cases, the decline in renal function is maintained by different mechanisms from those that initiated the injury, and progression therefore advances despite resolution of the initial injury. Eventually, severe renal insufficiency develops, indicated by a phase of uremia. The phase of progression is characterized by a slow rise, over a few weeks to many years, in serum creatinine concentration. However, because of remarkable adaptations in nephron function, oliguria and serious disorders of fluid and electrolyte metabolism generally are absent until GFR has fallen below 10 to 15 ml per minute.

Chronic renal disease leads to fibrosis and atrophy of renal parenchyma with concomitant reduction in kidney size. On the other hand, kidney size is usually normal or slightly enlarged in acute renal insufficiency. Assessment of kidney size by ultrasound examination is a valuable diagnostic procedure in the evaluation of patients with renal insufficiency.

Patients with chronic renal insufficiency therefore typically present with an asymptomatic elevation in serum creatinine, mild hyperkalemia, metabolic acidosis, hyperphosphatemia, hypertension, and a nearly normal ECF volume. Review of past records indicates that serum creatinine has been abnormal for several months or years, and if serum creatinine is approximately 4 mg per deciliter or greater, renal ultrasound examination typically reveals small kidneys with reduced cortical thickness. In contrast, patients with acute renal insufficiency typically have a recent increase in serum creatinine concentration in the setting of an acute medical illness, associated with recent diagnostic tests or therapeutic procedures. Moreover, one-half or more of these patients manifest oliguria, ECF volume overload, hyponatremia, severe hyperkalemia, or severe metabolic acidosis. Kidney size and cortical thickness are normal.

DIAGNOSTIC TESTS

Further evaluation of the patient with acute renal insufficiency includes the following diagnostic tests.

Assessment of Renal Perfusion

Diagnosis of Reduced Renal Perfusion. Renal blood flow is reduced by conditions that lower systemic blood pressure or that increase renal vascular resistance. Even if systemic blood pressure remains within the normal range, an increase in renal vascular resistance leads to a reduction in renal perfusion and GFR. Unfortunately, no single item of the patient's history, physical examination, or laboratory data provides a foolproof assessment of renal perfusion. Table 30-5 includes disorders that are often associated with reduced renal perfusion. Assessment of the status of ECF volume is most important. In particular, evidence of ECF volume depletion should be carefully sought; the presence of one or more findings listed in Table 30-6 usually is associated with a reduction in renal blood flow.

Response to a Volume Challenge. The patient's response to a rapid intravenous infusion of isotonic solution (volume challenge) provides important diagnostic information. The purpose of a volume challenge is to increase intravascular volume, central venous pressure, pulmonary capillary wedge pressure, and cardiac output, and thereby to increase renal perfusion. If reduced renal perfusion is the cause of reduced GFR (prerenal disorders), the improvement in renal perfusion raises GFR, increases urine flow, and lowers serum creatinine concentration. If reduced renal perfusion is not the cause of reduced GFR (postrenal or renal disorders), no improvement occurs in GFR, urine flow, or serum creatinine concentration.

I recommend administering a volume challenge to patients with acute renal insufficiency in whom a prerenal disorder is suspected unless there are signs of intravascular volume excess, such as increased central venous pressure, increased pulmonary capillary wedge pressure, or pulmonary edema. I even suggest careful administration of a volume challenge to patients with ECF volume excess in whom intravascular volume depletion is suspected, for example, patients with burns or gastrointestinal ileus. In all cases, it is necessary to monitor the systemic hemodynamic response as well as the renal response to the volume challenge.

TABLE 30-5   Clinical Settings Associated With Reduced Renal Perfusion

Hypotension
Decreased cardiac output
Hemorrhage
Reduced serum albumin concentration
Congestive heart failure
Cirrhosis
Gastrointestinal ileus
Burns
Decreased extracellular fluid volume

**TABLE 30-6   Causes and Findings in Extracellular Fluid (ECF)
Volume Depletion**

Causes of ECF volume depletion
  Increased fluid losses
    Vomiting
    Diarrhea
    Drainage of stomach, intestinal, pancreatic, or biliary fluid
    Profuse sweating
    Diuretic therapy
  Reduced fluid intake
    Fluid restriction
    Dietary salt restriction
Signs of ECF volume depletion
  Postural hypotension
  Fluid intake less than fluid output
  Recent weight loss
  Reduced skin turgor
  Dry oral mucous membranes and axillary skin
  Reduced central venous pressure
  Reduced pulmonary capillary wedge pressure
  Response to volume challenge (see text)

In patients with overt ECF volume depletion, administration of isotonic
saline is not only a diagnostic test of the cause of acute renal insufficiency, it is
also the appropriate therapy. Monitoring of the supine and sitting blood
pressure and pulse is a sufficient measure of the systemic hemodynamic
response.

In patients with apparently normal or increased ECF volume, further
measurements are required when a volume challenge is performed. In addition
to pulse and blood pressure monitoring, a catheter should be inserted to enable
measurement of central venous or pulmonary capillary wedge pressure every 15
minutes during the volume challenge. Patients with apparently normal ECF
volume should receive 500 to 1,000 ml of isotonic saline over .5 to 2 hours.
Patients with ECF volume excess should *not* receive saline because they
already have a surfeit of salt and water; instead they should receive 12.5 to 25 g
of salt-poor albumin. An increase in arterial and venous pressure during the
volume challenge indicates that sufficient fluid has been administered to alter
the systemic hemodynamic profile. An improvement in urine flow and serum
creatinine concentration indicates that the renal insufficiency is caused by
reduced renal perfusion and that definitive measures should be undertaken to
improve renal perfusion. Whether these measures should include further
administration of intravenous fluids depends on the underlying disorder. No
improvement in urine flow or serum creatinine, despite improvement in the
systemic hemodynamic profile, indicates that renal insufficiency is not caused

by intravascular volume depletion and that postrenal or renal disorders should be considered.

Urine Volume and Pattern of Urination

The normal urine volume of 1 to 2 L per day represents the tiny fraction of the glomerular filtrate (150 to 180 L per day) that is not reabsorbed by the renal tubules. Urine volume cannot decline to less than 400 ml per day if GFR is normal, assuming a normal upper limit of urinary concentration of 1,200 to 1,400 mOsm per kilogram (urinary specific gravity approximately 1.030) and assuming a normal solute load of approximately 600 mOsm per day. Consequently, urine volume less than 400 ml per day, defined as oliguria, is a definite indication of reduced GFR. In approximately two-thirds of patients with acute renal insufficiency, however, the urine volume remains within the normal range because of a reduction in both GFR and tubular reabsorption (nonoliguric acute renal insufficiency). Urine volume less than 50 ml per day, defined as anuria, is the result of a severe reduction in GFR and suggests the diagnosis of total obstruction, bilateral renal vascular occlusion, or specific severe renal diseases including acute glomerulonephritis, cortical necrosis, and hemolytic uremic syndrome. Anuria occurs infrequently during the course of acute tubular necrosis; however, because acute tubular necrosis is the most frequent cause of acute renal insufficiency, it remains the most frequent cause of anuria. The decline in GFR, the frequency of complications, and the mortality are greater in patients with oliguria and anuria than in patients with normal urine volume.[7,8]

The pattern of urination also is normal in most patients with acute renal insufficiency. Symptoms during urination may indicate lower urinary tract abnormalities associated with obstruction. Similarly, erratic intervals between urination or widely varying urine volumes may indicate partial obstruction, even in patients who are asymptomatic. Rectal and pelvic examinations should be performed on all patients with acute renal insufficiency to detect mass lesions that could cause obstruction of the lower urinary tract.

Urinalysis

Dipstick and Urine Sediment Examination. Dipstick testing of the urine for protein and hemoglobin is easily and accurately performed by all hospital laboratories. However, there is no substitute for careful examination of the urine sediment by the consulting physician. In both acute and chronic renal disorders, the presence of significant proteinuria (2+ or greater), renal tubular cells, cellular or coarsely granular casts, or fat in the urine is diagnostic of parenchymal renal damage.[9] In acute renal insufficiency, these findings suggest either an acute renal condition or an acute prerenal or postrenal condition superimposed on a chronic renal condition. Moreover, the types of cells and casts suggest the type of pathologic process that involves the renal parenchyma (Fig. 30-2). For example, red blood cells and red blood cell casts are seen in acute glomerulonephritis and rarely in vascular diseases that also involve the glomeruli, such as hemolytic-uremic syndrome and malignant nephrosclerosis. White blood cells and white blood cell casts usually indicate an inflammatory tubulointerstitial disease, such as acute pyelonephritis or allergic interstitial nephritis. Tubular cells, tubular cell casts, and coarsely granular casts are seen in all forms of acute renal damage, but they are the principal findings in acute tubular necrosis and are found in the urine sediment of 70 to 80 percent of patients with this disorder.[10]

Urine sediment examination results permit an orderly, focussed approach to further diagnostic testing. The approach to patients with acute glomerulonephritis relies on identification of whether the patient has a systemic disease and on the measurement of serum complement.[11] Expectations for serum complement for the most important causes of acute glomerulonephritis are

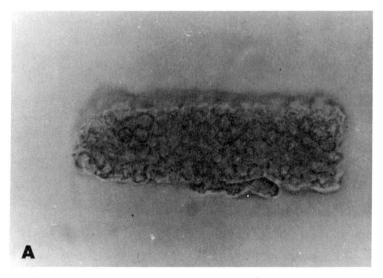

Figure 30-2 Urinary sediment. *A*, Red blood cell cast.

Figure continues on following page

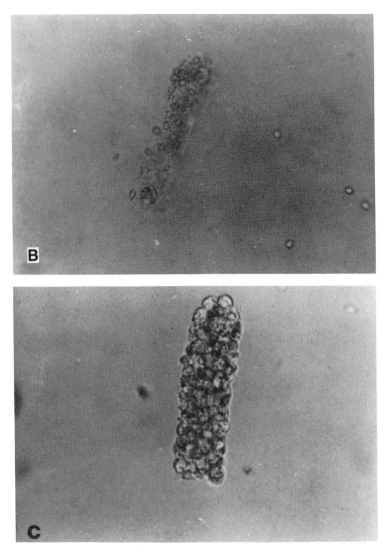

Figure 30-2 (continued) *B*, Red blood cell cast. *C*, White blood cell cast. (*B* and *C* are reproduced with permission from Gennari FJ, Kassirer JP. Laboratory assessment of renal function. In: Early LE, Gottschalk CW, eds. Strauss and Welt's diseases of the kidney. 3rd ed. Boston: Little, Brown, 1979:41.)

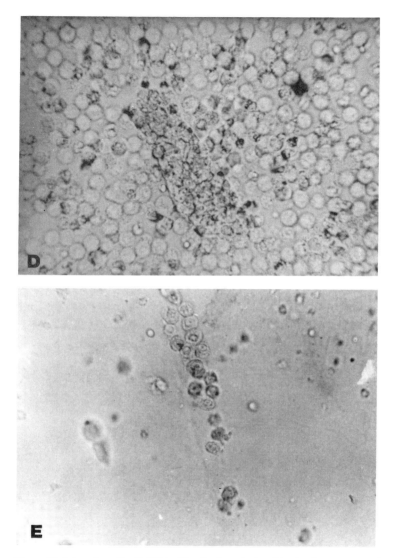

Figure 30-2 (continued) *D*, White blood cells and white blood cell cast. *E*, Renal tubular epithelial cell cast.

Figure continues on following page

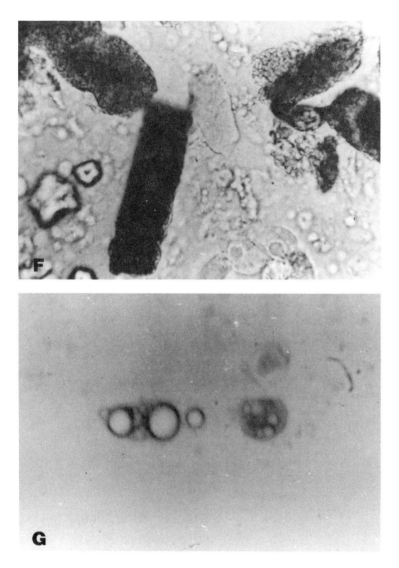

Figure 30-2 (continued) *F*, "Muddy-brown" granular casts. *G*, Oval fat body and free fat.

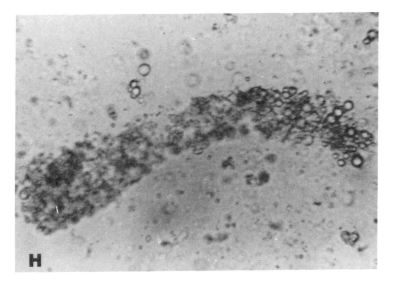

Figure 30-2 (continued) *H*, Fatty cast.

given in Table 30-3. The approach to patients with inflammatory tubulointerstitial diseases includes collection of a urine culture, measurement of eosinophil count, and assessment of possible allergic or toxic reactions to recently administered drugs.[12] Identification of the likely ischemic or toxic insult that caused parenchymal damage is the best approach to patients with acute tubular necrosis. In my experience, the most difficult diagnostic problems arise in two circumstances: 1) The urinary sediment is only mildly abnormal: the patient may have either mild acute tubular necrosis, a noninflammatory tubulointerstitial disorder, or a prerenal condition. 2) The urinary sediment contains red blood cells, renal tubular cells, and granular casts, but no red blood cell casts: the patient may have either acute glomerulonephritis, a vascular disease, an inflammatory tubulointerstitial disease, or a combination of diseases. These circumstances often require a renal biopsy to define the pathology and to guide therapy.

Urinary Specific Gravity. Careful interpretation of the urinary specific gravity in acute renal insufficiency contributes valuable information on the status of tubular function. The specific gravity of glomerular filtrate in normal individuals and in patients with acute renal insufficiency is approximately 1.010 to 1.012. In prerenal conditions, reduced renal perfusion leads not only to reduced GFR, but also to increased reabsorption of sodium and water from tubular fluid. The resulting urine has an increased concentration of nonreabsorbable solutes, such as creatinine and urea, and therefore the urinary specific gravity is greater than that of serum. Patients with acute obstruction or acute glomerulonephritis also may have preserved tubular function and concentrated urine. By contrast, in most other renal conditions, tubular and glomerular function both are impaired; thus the urine is not concentrated (specific gravity 1.010 to 1.012). Similarly, tubular function is impaired soon after the development of renal obstruction; consequently the urine usually is not concentrated in chronic postrenal conditions. The finding of concentrated urine (specific gravity greater than 1.015) in acute renal insufficiency indicates preserved tubular function and usually suggests the diagnosis of a prerenal condition.

The usefulness of the urinary specific gravity may be limited by several factors. Diuretics impair urinary concentration and are frequently administered to patients with acute renal insufficiency. In patients who have been treated with diuretics within the previous 12 to 24 hours, urine specific gravity may remain 1.010 to 1.012, even if acute renal insufficiency is caused by reduced renal perfusion. Conversely, urinary specific gravity is raised by the presence of small solutes in high concentration, such as glucose or mannitol, by large amounts of high molecular weight solutes, such as protein, or by heavy solutes, such as radiographic contrast. If these solutes are present, urinary specific gravity may be elevated even if the concentrating ability of the tubules is impaired.

Ultrasound Examination

A renal ultrasound should be obtained in patients in whom the cause of acute renal insufficiency is not determined by assessment of renal perfusion, urine volume, pattern of urination, and urinalysis. The principal uses of the ultrasound examination are to detect obstruction and to measure kidney size. Hydronephrosis is detected on the ultrasound as the presence of enlarged kidneys with echolucent clusters within the central renal echoes, which corresponds to dilated calyces within the renal pelvis (Fig. 30–3). These findings are found in approximately 95 percent of patients with hydronephrosis.[13] The absence of hydronephrosis on ultrasound examination usually eliminates obstruction as the cause of renal insufficiency. In patients with hydronephrosis, the site and cause of obstruction are sometimes visible on the ultrasound exam. In particular, a postvoiding view of the bladder should be obtained to determine if there is a bladder outlet obstruction.

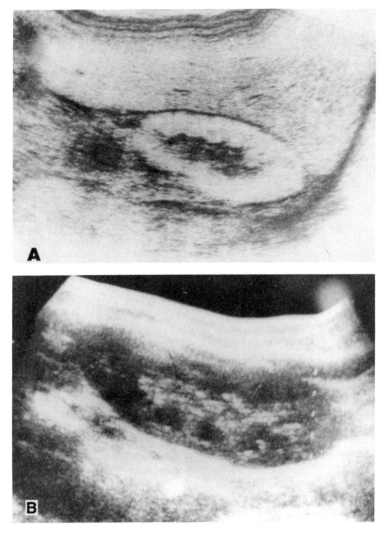

Figure 30-3 Renal ultrasound. *A*, Normal features include peripheral homogeneous thick cortex (white) and central heterogeneous fluid-filled calyces (black). Note that individual calyces cannot be visualized. *B*, In acute hydronephrosis, features include normal cortex (gray) and dilated calyces (gray areas within central white).

As mentioned earlier, kidney size is normal, 11 to 12 cm in length, in most patients with acute renal insufficiency. Small kidneys indicate that renal disease is chronic, while large kidneys are found in only a few specific diseases. Causes of marked kidney enlargement include obstruction and polycystic kidneys. Mild kidney enlargement may be seen in diabetes, acute glomerulonephritis, acute pyelonephritis, and renal infiltration by tumor, especially lymphoma.

Urine Chemistry and Urinary Diagnostic Index

Measurements of urine sodium concentration, fractional excretion of sodium, and the ratio of urine to serum concentration of creatinine are useful to confirm the diagnostic impression based on the investigations already discussed. The fractional excretion of sodium (FE_{Na}) may be calculated from the concentrations of sodium (Na) and creatinine (cr) in samples of serum and urine obtained at approximately the same time. The fractional excretion of sodium is defined as the percent of filtered sodium that is excreted in the urine. Filtered sodium is calculated as the product of the serum sodium concentration and the GFR (as assessed by creatinine clearance).

$$FE_{Na}\,(\%) = \frac{Na\ excreted}{Na\ filtered} \times 100\%$$

$$FE_{Na}\,(\%) = \frac{urine\ Na\ (mEq/L) \times urine\ flow\ (ml/min)}{serum\ Na\ (mEq/L) \times C_{cr}\ (ml/min)} \times 100\%$$

$$FE_{Na}\,(\%) = \frac{urine\ Na\ (mEq/L) \times serum\ cr\ (mg/dl)}{serum\ Na\ (mEq/L) \times urine\ cr\ (mg/dl)} \times 100\%$$

In prerenal conditions, in acute obstruction, and in acute glomerulonephritis, tubular function is intact, the concentration of sodium is low (<20 mEq per liter), the fractional excretion of sodium is low (<1 percent), and the ratio of urine to serum concentration of creatinine is high (>40). By contrast, in most other renal and postrenal conditions tubular function is impaired, urinary concentration of sodium is high (>40 mEq per liter), the fractional excretion of sodium is high (>1 percent), and the ratio of urine to plasma concentration of creatinine is low (<20). Representative values for urine

TABLE 30-7   Urine Chemistries and Urinary Diagnostic Indices in
Acute Renal Insufficiency

	Prerenal Conditions	Oliguric Renal Conditions	Nonoliguric Renal Conditions	Postrenal Conditions
Urine Na (mEq/L)	18 ± *	68 ± 5	50 ± 5	68 ± 10
FE_{Na} (%)	0.4 ± 1	7 ± 1.4	3 ± 0.5	6 ± 2
Urine-serum creatinine ratio	45 ± 6	17 ± 2	17 ± 2	16 ± 4

* Values are expressed as mean ± standard deviation.
Data from Miller TR, Anderson RJ, Linas SL, Henrich WL, Berns AS, Gabow PA, Schrier RW. Urinary diagnostic indices in acute renal failure: a prospective study. Ann Intern Med 1978; 89:47–50.

chemistries and urinary diagnostic indices for several causes of acute renal insufficiency are included in Table 30-7.[14]

References

1. Levey AS, Perrone RD, Madias NE. Serum creatinine and renal function. Annu Rev Med 1988; 39:465–490.
2. Shemesh O, Goldbetz H, Kriss JP, Myers BD. Limitation of creatinine as a filtration marker in glomerulopathic patients. Kidney Int 1985; 28:830–838.
3. Hou SH, Bushinsky DA, Wish JB, Cohen JJ, Harrington JT. Hospital-acquired renal insufficiency: a prospective study. Am J Med 1983; 74:243–248.
4. Cockcroft DW, Gault MH. Prediction of creatinine clearance from serum creatinine. Nephron 1976; 16:31–41.
5. Rolin HA III, Hall PM, Wei R. Inaccuracy of estimated creatinine clearance for prediction of iothalamate glomerular filtration rate. Am J Kidney Dis 1984; 4:48–54.
6. Kassirer JP. Clinical evaluation of kidney function: glomerular function. N Engl J Med 1971; 285:385–389.
7. Anderson RJ, Linas SL, Berns AS, Henrich WL, Miller TR, Gabow PA, Schrier RW. Non-oliguric acute renal failure. N Engl J Med 1977; 296:1134–1138.
8. Myers BD, Moran SM. Hemodynamically mediated acute renal failure. N Engl J Med 1986; 314:97–105.
9. Levinsky NG. The interpretation of proteinuria and the urinary sediment. DM 1969; March:1–40.
10. Levinsky NG, Alexander EA. Acute renal failure. In: Brenner BM, Rector FC Jr, eds. The kidney. Philadelphia: WB Saunders, 1976:806.
11. Madaio MP, Harrington JT. The diagnosis of acute glomerulonephritis. N Engl J Med 1983; 309:1299–1302.
12. Appel GB, Kunis CL. Acute tubulo-interstitial nephritis. In: Cotran RS, Brenner BM, Stein JH, eds. Contemporary issues in nephrology 10: tubulointerstitial nephropathies. New York: Churchill Livingstone, 1983:151.

13. Ellenbogen PH, Schieble RW, Talner LB, Leopold GR. Sensitivity of grey-scale ultrasound in detecting urinary tract obstruction. AJR 1978; 130:731–733.
14. Miller TR, Anderson RJ, Linas SL, Henrich WL, Berns AS, Gabow PA, Schrier RW. Urinary diagnostic indices in acute renal failure: a prospective study. Ann Intern Med 1978; 89:47–50.

31 | MANAGEMENT OF RENAL INSUFFICIENCY

ANDREW S. LEVEY, M.D.

Renal insufficiency, as defined in the previous chapter, is a decrease in glomerular filtration rate (GFR) and may be acute or chronic, depending on its duration. The diagnosis of acute and chronic renal insufficiency is discussed in the previous chapter; in this chapter, the management of acute and chronic renal insufficiency is described. The management of renal failure, defined as a decrease in GFR to a level that is not compatible with life, is not included in this chapter because it requires dialysis and other specialized procedures. Before proceeding, a review of the clinical manifestations of acute and chronic renal insufficiency is necessary.

CLINICAL MANIFESTATIONS

The signs and symptoms of renal insufficiency are determined chiefly by the severity of the decrease in GFR. The normal value for GFR in adults is approximately 125 ml per minute. Patients with GFR above 20 to 25 ml per minute generally have few or no symptoms attributable to renal insufficiency, whereas if GFR is below 5 to 10 ml per minute, the full constellation of uremic symptoms appears. Manifestations that may be seen in both acute and chronic renal insufficiency include pericarditis, gastrointestinal symptoms, and encephalopathy, particularly if the serum urea nitrogen concentration is greater than 100 mg per deciliter. In addition to the severity of renal insufficiency, the duration also influences the clinical manifestations.

Serious derangements in fluid and electrolyte balance are common in acute renal insufficiency. As discussed in the previous chapter, oliguria, extracellular fluid (ECF) volume overload, hyponatremia, severe hyperkalemia, severe metabolic acidosis, or hyperphosphatemia occur in more than one-half of patients. By contrast, in chronic renal insufficiency serious fluid and electrolyte disturbances are uncommon unless GFR is severely reduced. Symptoms that occur more commonly in patients with a long duration of renal insufficiency include weight loss, pruritus, peripheral neuropathy, osteodystrophy, and metastatic calcifications.

Whether renal insufficiency is acute or chronic, severe and persistent manifestations of uremia constitute a medical emergency, and a nephrologist should be consulted at once in order to arrange for dialysis. Thus the first responsibility of the consulting internist in the evaluation of patients with renal insufficiency is to assess their need for dialysis. Indications for initiation of dialysis are given in Table 31-1.

GOALS OF MANAGEMENT

The goals of management of patients with renal insufficiency are to

1. Identify and treat reversible causes of renal insufficiency
2. Prevent complications of renal insufficiency
3. In acute renal insufficiency, provide general supportive care until recovery of renal function
4. In chronic renal insufficiency, delay progression of renal functional decline.

Reversible Causes of Renal Insufficiency

I recommend systematic evaluation of patients with renal insufficiency to detect all treatable causes of renal disease. A list of potentially reversible

TABLE 31-1   Indications for Dialysis in Renal Failure

Indications arising commonly in acute and chronic renal failure
    Pericarditis
    Anorexia
    Nausea
    Vomiting
    Hiccups
    Lethargy
    Seizures

Indications arising most commonly in acute renal failure
    ECF volume overload
    Hyponatremia
    Severe hyperkalemia
    Severe metabolic acidosis
    Hypermagnesemia

Indications arising most commonly in chronic renal failure
    Weight loss
    Pruritus
    Peripheral neuropathy

conditions is given in Table 31-2. Of course, a reversible cause is much more likely to be discovered in patients with acute renal insufficiency. Nonetheless, patients with chronic renal insufficiency frequently suffer acute reductions in GFR: "acute superimposed on chronic" renal insufficiency. Detection and reversal of superimposed causes of renal insufficiency may permit partial recovery of renal function and delay the onset of total renal failure. The differential diagnosis of these conditions is discussed in the previous chapter.

In addition, it is important to avoid further insults to renal function, particularly, as discussed in the previous chapter, because the risk of acute renal insufficiency from diagnostic procedures and therapeutic agents is higher in patients with reduced renal function. If possible, depletion of ECF volume, intravenous radiographic contrast, aminoglycoside antibiotics, nonsteroidal anti-inflammatory agents, and cis-platinum should be avoided in patients with renal insufficiency.

TABLE 31-2 Reversible Causes of Renal Insufficiency

Prerenal conditions
  ECF volume depletion
  Congestive heart failure
  Nonsteroidal anti-inflammatory agents
  Hyperviscosity syndromes

Postrenal conditions
  Bladder outlet obstruction
    Prostatic enlargement
    Pelvic malignancy
  Ureteric obstruction (bilateral)
    Urinary tract stones
    Papillary necrosis
    Retroperitoneal malignancy

Renal conditions
  Glomerular diseases
    Postinfectious glomerulonephritis
    Systemic vasculitis
    Preeclampsia
  Tubulointerstitial diseases
    Urinary tract infection
    Drug toxicity
    Drug allergy
    Hypercalcemia
    Tumor lysis
  Vascular diseases
    Malignant hypertension
    Hemolytic-uremic syndrome
    Renal artery stenosis

Prevention of Complications

Successful prevention of complications of renal insufficiency depends on prescription of appropriate dietary and fluid restrictions, adjustment of drug dosages, and timely initiation of dialysis.

Dietary and Fluid Restrictions

The goal of dietary and fluid management in patients with renal insufficiency is to maintain the volume and composition of body fluids as close to normal as possible. Initial evaluation of the patient requires a measurement of weight, a physical examination to determine the status of ECF volume, an assessment of dietary intake, and the serum and urine measurements that are shown in Table 31-3. The dietary prescription is formulated on the basis of this assessment and the severity and duration of renal insufficiency. The assistance of a skilled nutritionist is essential in the assessment of dietary intake and the design of a dietary regimen that fulfills the prescription. My approach to patients with acute and chronic renal insufficiency is summarized as follows and in Table 31-4. References one to five provide additional details.[1-5] Chronic renal insufficiency is described first because the dietary and fluid prescription is simpler than in acute renal insufficiency.

Chronic Renal Insufficiency. The principal manifestation during the progressive phase of chronic renal insufficiency is retention of nitrogenous wastes, such as creatinine and urea. Hypertension, disorders of calcium metabolism, phosphorus retention, and mild electrolyte and acid-base disorders are common, but serious disturbances of fluid and electrolyte balance are not usual. Serum albumin and transferrin concentrations are normal unless the

TABLE 31-3   Serum and Urine Measurements in Patients With Renal Insufficiency

Serum	
Creatinine	Phosphorus
Urea nitrogen	Magnesium
Sodium	Albumin
Potassium	Transferrin
Chloride	Glucose
Bicarbonate	Triglycerides
Calcium	Cholesterol
Urine	
Creatinine	
Urea nitrogen	
Sodium	
Potassium	
Protein	

nephrotic syndrome, nutritional deficiency, or another chronic illness is present. Abnormalities in carbohydrate and lipid metabolism are frequent and manifest as hypertriglyceridemia. Serum glucose and cholesterol concentrations usually are normal.

If serum urea nitrogen concentration is greater than 70 to 80 mg per deciliter, I recommend restriction of dietary protein intake to 0.6 g per kilogram lean body weight per day, with more than one-half of the dietary allowance composed of high biologic value protein, such as meat, poultry, fish, and eggs. Energy intake should be prescribed to maintain lean body weight, usually approximately 35 kilocalaries (Cal) per kilogram per day. The proportion of calories derived from fat and carbohydrate should be adjusted to maintain lipid levels as close to normal as possible. Fluid restriction is not necessary.

Patients with chronic renal insufficiency do not absorb dietary calcium adequately because of deficient renal production of the active form of vitamin

TABLE 31-4 Dietary and Fluid Prescription in Acute and
Chronic Renal Insufficiency

Nutrient	Chronic Renal Insufficiency	Acute Renal Insufficiency
Fluid	No restriction	Restrict intake based on measured losses to maintain normal ECF volume and serum sodium concentration
Protein	Restrict to 0.6 g/kg/day (50% as high biologic value) to maintain serum urea nitrogen <70 to 80 mg/dl	Same as in chronic renal insufficiency
Energy	35 Cal/kg/day to maintain body weight. Adjust proportion of carbohydrate and fat to maintain serum glucose and lipids	At least 1,500 Cal carbohydrate per day. If possible 40 to 50 Cal/kg/day
Calcium	Calcium carbonate, 1,000 to 1,500 per day	No supplements unless serum calcium <8.0 mg/dl
Phosphorus	Calcium carbonate or aluminum hydroxide to maintain serum phosphorus ≤5.0 mg/dl	Aluminum hydroxide to maintain serum phosphorus ≤6.0 mg/dl
Sodium	No restriction unless hypertension or edema	Restrict intake to measured losses or 2 g per day
Potassium	No restriction unless serum potassium >5.5 mEq/L	Restrict intake to measured losses or 2 g per day
Alkali	Calcium carbonate or sodium bicarbonate to maintain serum bicarbonate ≥18 mEq/L	Sodium bicarbonate to maintain serum bicarbonate ≥18 mEq/L

D (1,25-dihydroxycholecalciferol). As a result, negative calcium balance and diminished bone calcium content are universal findings. If serum creatinine is greater than approximately 4 mg per deciliter, it is advisable to prescribe a calcium supplement, usually calcium carbonate 500 mg two or three times daily, unless serum calcium is elevated or serum phosphorus is extremely high, as subsequently described.

I attempt to maintain serum phosphorus below 5 mg per deciliter by dietary restriction and by prescription of phosphorus-binding antacids. Restriction of dietary protein usually results in concomitant reduction in phosphorus intake and serum phosphorus concentration. However, persistent elevation requires further reduction in dietary intake by restriction of foods rich in phosphorus, such as dairy products and cola-colored soft drinks, and by prescription of phosphorus binders, either calcium carbonate or aluminum hydroxide, at initial doses of 500 to 1,000 mg three times daily with meals. Aluminum is not completely excreted in patients with renal insufficiency. Therefore binders containing calcium, rather than aluminum, are preferable. However, if serum calcium is greater than 11.0 mg per deciliter or if serum phosphorus exceeds 6 to 7 mg per deciliter, aluminum hydroxide is preferred over calcium carbonate because of the risk of serious hypercalcemia and metastatic calcification. Magnesium-containing antacids are contraindicated because of the risks of magnesium accumulation and hypermagnesemia.

If blood pressure is elevated, I suggest restriction of dietary sodium to approximately 3 g (130 mEq) per day. It is important to note that patients with chronic renal insufficiency cannot fully conserve sodium. Thus, sharp reduction in dietary sodium may result in negative sodium balance and ECF volume depletion that could possibly lead to further deterioration in renal function. If blood pressure is normal, sodium restriction need not and should not be advised. Instead, dietary sodium content should be estimated from diet records and urinary sodium excretion, and this amount should be prescribed.

Dietary potassium intake should be assessed by the same methods. If serum potassium is normal, patients should be instructed in the potassium content in their diet, and the amount of potassium that they are currently ingesting should be prescribed. If serum potassium is greater than 5.5 mEq per liter, dietary potassium should be restricted to 2 to 3 g (50 to 75 mEq) per day. If hyperkalemia persists, cation-exchange resins, such as Kayexalate 25 to 75 g per day, or loop diuretics, such as furosemide 40 to 80 mg per day, may be prescribed. Kayexalate contains approximately 4.1 mEq sodium per 1 g and thus may contribute to ECF volume expansion. Conversely, diuretics may result in ECF volume depletion. Of course, careful monitoring for these complications is essential.

Treatment of metabolic acidosis is warranted if serum bicarbonate is below approximately 18 mEq per liter. Alkali, 25 to 50 mEq per day, should be prescribed, either as additional calcium carbonate (10 mEq per 500 mg tablet) or sodium bicarbonate (8 mEq per 650 mg tablet).

Acute Renal Insufficiency. Different dietary and fluid restrictions are necessary in patients with acute renal insufficiency because, as previously discussed, this condition is frequently accompanied by serious fluid and electrolyte disturbances. Preservation of fluid balance is of the utmost importance throughout the maintenance and recovery phases. If ECF volume is increased, oral and intravenous fluids should be restricted or withheld and vigorous therapy with loop diuretics should be employed. Conversely, if ECF volume is depleted, isotonic fluid must be administered. If ECF volume appears normal, but the serum sodium concentration is low, oral fluids should be restricted to 500 ml per day and all intravenous solutions should be isotonic. If the patient is euvolemic with a normal serum sodium concentration, the combined oral and fluid intake should be restricted to the amount that is excreted by renal and extrarenal routes. Usual extrarenal fluid loss is attributable to insensible water loss, generally approximately 500 ml per day. Of course, insensible losses are increased in patients with high fever or burns. Additional extrarenal fluid losses may occur through the gastrointestinal tract, for example, in patients with vomiting, nasogastric drainage, or diarrhea. The fluid allowance must be increased in patients with increased extrarenal losses.

The dietary sodium and potassium prescription should be based on measured sodium and potassium losses in urine and other fluids. Typically, in the absence of oliguria or gastrointestinal fluid losses, sodium and potassium should be restricted to 2 g per day each (85 mEq and 50 mEq, respectively). Potassium-sparing diuretics should be avoided and sources of potassium in addition to the diet must also be restricted (see chapter on *Hypokalemia and Hyperkalemia*). The allowance of sodium and potassium must be increased for patients with gastrointestinal fluid losses.

Guidelines for protein intake are similar to those described for chronic renal insufficiency. During the maintenance phase, the serum urea nitrogen concentration should be maintained below 80 to 100 mg per deciliter. Energy needs are higher than in patients with chronic renal insufficiency and range from 40 to 50 Cal per kilogram per day. However, because of the anorexia that typically accompanies acute renal insufficiency, it is difficult for patients to achieve this intake, and parenteral alimentation may be required. A minimum of 1,500 Cal per day, including at least 20 g of essential amino acids, should be provided because of the beneficial effect of preventing complications.[1-3]

During acute renal insufficiency it is usually not necessary to modify energy intake on the basis of serum lipid levels or to provide supplementary calcium. I recommend treatment of hyperphosphatemia with aluminum hydroxide and of metabolic acidosis with sodium bicarbonate, rather than with calcium carbonate.

During the recovery phase of acute renal insufficiency, an increase in fluid, sodium, and potassium allowances is necessary. Protein restriction may be lifted and aluminum hydroxide may be discontinued as serum concentrations of urea nitrogen and phosphorus decline. It may be necessary to continue alkali therapy or potassium restriction temporarily.

Drug Prescribing in Renal Insufficiency

Metabolism and excretion of many drugs are altered in renal insufficiency. Proper prescription of drugs requires knowledge of the usual routes of elimination, the alterations in patients with reduced renal function, the approximate level of renal function in the patient under consideration, and the method of dose adjustment, if any, that is necessary for that level of renal function. Comprehensive reviews of this subject are available[6-8] and should be consulted prior to prescription of *any* and *all* drugs for patients with renal insufficiency.

Drug elimination by the kidneys occurs by glomerular filtration, tubular secretion, and cellular metabolism. Drugs that are hydrophilic, that are not bound to plasma proteins, and that have molecular weight below approximately 10,000 daltons are available for glomerular filtration. Examples include sulfonamides, penicillins, most cephalosporins, aminoglycosides, aspirin, normeperidine (a metabolite of meperidine), digoxin, allopurinol, methotrexate, and cis-platinum. Tubular secretion of other low molecular weight anions and cations, such as cimetidine, trimethoprim, probenecid, hippuric acid, phenobarbital, diuretics, and radiographic contrast, contributes significantly to their renal excretion. Moreover, renal tubular cells are the site of metabolism of several peptides, including insulin. In renal insufficiency, excretion or degradation of these substances is reduced. Consequently, reduction of dosage is necessary to achieve and maintain therapeutic levels and to avoid toxicity.

Dosage may be reduced either by reducing the amount of drug and maintaining the same interval between doses, by lengthening the interval between doses and maintaining the same amount of drug, or by a combination of methods. In general, all methods are acceptable for most agents. Most references provide the appropriate dose reduction or interval change indicated for the level of renal function that is estimated from creatinine clearance. As discussed in the previous chapter, I recommend, using the serum creatinine and the formula of Cockcroft and Gault for the estimation of creatinine clearance in the steady state. Whenever possible, serum drug levels also should be measured directly. If serum creatinine is not stable, but is rising, renal function should not be estimated from this formula. Instead, creatinine clearance should be assumed to be less than 10 ml per minute, and drug levels should be monitored frequently.

Supportive Measures During Acute Renal Insufficiency

In prerenal and postrenal causes of acute renal insufficiency, the maintenance phase continues until the underlying cause of reduced GFR is corrected. In acute tubular necrosis, the most common renal cause of acute renal insufficiency, no treatment is available for the renal disease per se. The duration of the maintenance phase is from a few days to 6 to 8 weeks. In other parenchymal renal diseases, the duration depends on the efficacy of treatment. The reader is referred to general nephrology textbooks for treatment of specific diseases.

Mortality of acute tubular necrosis remains greater than 50 percent, despite advances in nutritional and dialytic support.[9] The principal causes of death are related to the patient's underlying illness that precipitated the renal injury. Potentially preventable causes of death include infections and upper gastrointestinal hemorrhage. I advise careful monitoring of sites of infection (wounds, urinary and respiratory tract), minimizing invasive procedures, and removing indwelling catheters. Routine treatment with cimetidine, ranitidine (in reduced dosages), or aluminum hydroxide is recommended for prevention of upper gastrointestinal hemorrhage.

The hallmark of the recovery phase is an early increase in urine volume, sometimes leading to polyuria, and a gradual decline in serum creatinine concentration. Serious fluid and electrolyte disturbances also may arise during this phase because of incomplete recovery of glomerular and tubular function. If the patient survives, full recovery of renal function is the rule in acute tubular necrosis, in many acute tubulointerstitial diseases, and in reversible prerenal and postrenal conditions. Unfortunately, effective treatment is not available for many of the glomerular and vascular diseases that cause acute renal insufficiency; hence, renal function may not recover fully, and patients may be left with chronic renal insufficiency.

Delaying Progression of Chronic Renal Insufficiency

Patients are typically asymptomatic during the progression phase of chronic renal insufficiency. Treatment efforts during this phase should focus on delaying the progressive decline in kidney function. Because of the reciprocal relationship between serum creatinine and GFR, it is difficult to estimate the rate of decline in renal function directly from the rate of change in the serum creatinine concentration. Recently, however, several investigators have noted that, once the serum creatinine concentration has risen to greater than 2.5 to 3.0 mg per deciliter, the decline of the reciprocal of serum creatinine concentration over time is nearly constant.[10] Thus, it may be possible to estimate the time interval required for the reciprocal serum creatinine, and hence, the serum creatinine, to reach a defined level. However, this estimation is of limited use in predicting the prognosis of an individual patient because of the wide variability of the serum concentration at the onset of uremia. Moreover, because the serum creatinine concentration is influenced by numerous variables in addition to the GFR, the rate of decline in reciprocal serum creatinine provides only a crude guide to the rate of loss of renal function.[11]

Presently, few therapies are available to halt progression of most chronic renal diseases. However, a variety of clinically applicable treatments recently have been found to retard progression in experimental animals.[12] There are now several clinical trials that are evaluating the efficacy of 1) restriction of dietary protein, phosphorus, and fat; 2) control of blood pressure, blood sugar, and blood lipids; 3) administration of a variety of immunosuppressive, anti-thrombotic, and anti-inflammatory agents; and 4) administration of inhibitors of angiotensin coverting enzyme. Thus far, none of these treatments has been shown convincingly to delay progression of renal disease in humans. Because of current uncertainly and expected developments in this area of research, I recommend consultation with a nephrologist for all patients with even mild chronic renal insufficiency.

References

1. Wesson DE, Mitch WE, Wilmore DW. Nutritional considerations in the treatment of acute renal failure. In: Brenner BM, Lazarus JM, eds. Acute renal failure. Phildelphia: WB Saunders, 1983:618.
2. Toback FG. Amino acid treatment of acute renal failure. In: Brenner BM, Stein JH, eds. Contemporary issues in nephrology 6: Acute renal failure. New York: Churchill Livingstone, 1980:202.
3. Kopple JD. Acute renal failure: conservative, non-dialytic management. In: Glassock RJ, ed. Current therapy in nephrology and hypertension 1984-1985. Toronto: BC Decker, 1984:236.
4. Mitch WE, Walser M. Nutritional therapy of the uremic patient. In: Brenner BM, Rector FC Jr, eds. The kidney. 3rd ed. Philadelphia: WB Saunders, 1986:1759.
5. Kopple JD. Chronic renal failure: nutritional and non-dialytic management. In: Glassock RJ, ed. Current therapy in nephrology and hypertension 1984-1985. Toronto: BC Decker, 1984:252.
6. Bennett WM, Aronoff GR, Morrison G, Golper TA, Pulliam J, Wolfson A, Singer I. Drug prescribing in renal failure: dosing guidelines for adults. Am J Kidney Dis 1983; 3:155-193.
7. Glassock RJ. Use of drugs in renal failure. In: Glassock RJ, ed. Current therapy in nephrology and hypertension 1984-1985. Toronto: BC Decker, 1984:294.
8. Maher JF. Pharmacological aspects of renal failure and dialysis. In: Drukker W, Parsons PM, Maher JF, eds. Replacement of renal function by dialysis. Boston: Martinus Nijhoff, 1983:749.

9. Levinsky NG, Alexander EA. Acute renal failure. In: Brenner BM, Rector FC Jr, eds. The kidney. 1st ed. Philadelphia: WB Saunders, 1981:1181.

10. Mitch WE. Measuring the rate of progression of renal insufficiency. In: Mitch WE, Brenner BM, Stein JH, eds. Contemporary issues in nephrology 14: Progressive nature of renal disease. New York: Churchill Livingstone, 1986:167.

11. Levey AS, Perrone RD, Madias NE. Serum creatinine and renal function. Annu Rev Med 1988; 39:465-490.

12. Brenner BM. Nephrology forum: hemodynamically mediated glomerular injury and the progressive nature of renal disease. Kidney Int 1983; 23:647-655.

32 | EDEMA

VINCENT J. CANZANELLO, M.D.

The extracellular fluid (ECF) volume normally comprises one-third of total body water (or approximately 20 percent of body weight). The extravascular, or interstitial, fluid volume contains 75 percent of the ECF, and the plasma volume contains the remaining 25 percent of the ECF. By definition, edema is a pathologic expansion of the interstitial fluid volume. Edema may occur through alterations in the physical forces (Starling forces) that govern fluid movement across the capillary membrane (i.e., the hydrostatic and oncotic pressures of the plasma and the extravascular space) or through a primary change in capillary wall permeability. Congestive heart failure and hypoalbuminemia are examples of the former, and burns or anaphylactic reactions are examples of the latter.

Edema may be localized or diffuse. Venous or lymphatic obstruction is the most common cause of localized edema, whereas dysfunction of the heart, liver, or kidney commonly results in diffuse edema (additional causes are listed in Table 32–1). Regardless of the cause of edema, the common denominator in the maintenance of the edematous state is enhanced sodium reabsorption by the kidney. The result is a state of persistent, positive sodium balance.

The onset of generalized edema frequently is insidious. The interstitial fluid space can accommodate a volume expansion of up to 3 to 5 L before

TABLE 32–1 Conditions Associated With Generalized Edema

Cardiac Causes
   Congestive heart failure
   Pericardial diseases

Cirrhosis

Renal Causes
   Nephrotic syndrome
   Acute renal failure (e.g., acute glomerulonephritis)
   Chronic renal failure

Pregnancy

Premenstrual Syndrome

Drug Related Causes
   Estrogen-containing preparations
   Antihypertensive agents (e.g., minoxidil)
   Nonsteroidal anti-inflammatory drugs

Idiopathic (Cyclical) Edema

edema is detectable. The patient may report an increase in weight, a decrease in urine output, nocturia, or darker urine. Complaints of "tight" shoes, rings, or belts are common. Supine cough or dyspnea suggests an increase in pulmonary interstitial water secondary to myocardial failure, whereas facial, particularly periorbital, puffiness on awakening in the morning is typical of the nephrotic syndrome.

APPROACH TO THE PATIENT WITH GENERALIZED EDEMA

The physician should first consider the underlying disorder (Is it treatable? Is the current treatment regimen optimal?) and should secondly consider the risk-benefit ratio of aggressive saluretic (diuretic) therapy. The underlying disorder or predisposing factors are usually evident by history, physical examination, and routine laboratory studies. Specific treatment of entities such as heart failure, cirrhosis, renal disease, and idiopathic edema will be discussed later. Here, I will focus on treatment principles common to all edematous disorders.

The presence of edema does not, by itself, necessarily warrant aggressive therapy. The goal of therapy should be to increase the patient's comfort and mobility and to prevent or reduce impairment in vital organ function. Such goals include a reduction of pulmonary symptoms in congestive heart failure, a reduction of respiratory embarrassment or abdominal discomfort from massive ascites, prevention of tissue breakdown from pedal edema, and avoidance of genitourinary dysfunction from extensive scrotal, labial, or penile edema. Occasionally, simple bedrest or intermittent elevation of the lower extremities alone is helpful. In most cases, however, therapy must be directed at the proximate cause of edema, namely the state of ongoing positive sodium balance.

In the edematous patient, dietary sodium intake must be lowered below the average American dietary intake of 80 to 200 mEq per day. This intake can be reduced to 70 to 125 mEq per day simply by not using the salt shaker and even further, to 50 to 70 mEq per day, by not adding salt when cooking. This latter value is a reasonable goal. Fluid restriction to approximately 1 L per day is required only if the patient is hyponatremic. A frequent error during dietary planning is the prescription of a 4 g "sodium" diet instead of a 4 g "salt" (sodium chloride) diet. One g of sodium contains 43 mEq of sodium, whereas 1 g of sodium chloride contains about 17 mEq of sodium. Thus, the former diet contain 172 mEq of sodium, and the latter contains a more desirable level of 68 mEq of sodium. Dietary intake in extreme instances can be lowered to 10 mEq per day, but this usually requires hospitalization and specialized nutritional support.

In most cases, the severity of edema, the intensity of renal sodium retention, and poor adherence to salt restriction mandate the addition of one or more diuretic agents to produce negative sodium balance and, hence, to reduce the ECF volume. Table 32-2 classifies diuretics by site of action within the nephron and provides relevant clinical information regarding their use. In this Table, fractional excretion of sodium (FENa) refers to the typical percentage of the filtered sodium load excreted in the urine during therapy with these agents; the loop agents are the most potent and the proximal agents the least potent.

MANAGEMENT OF SPECIFIC EDEMATOUS DISORDERS

Congestive Heart Failure

The mechanisms of enhanced renal sodium reabsorption in patients with congestive heart failure (CHF) have been the focus of extensive investigations and the topic of a recent detailed review.[1] The most critical factor is renal sensing of a reduced effective arterial plasma volume, with subsequent enhanced proximal and distal tubular sodium reabsorption (the latter attributable in part to stimulation of the renin-angiotensin-aldosterone axis). Stimulation of the renal sympathetic nervous system and attenuated release of natriuretic substances, e.g., atrial natriuretic hormone from chronically distended cardiac atria, also may play significant roles.

The primary therapeutic goal in the management of CHF is to improve myocardial contractility (see the chapter entitled *Congestive Heart Failure*). The management of systemic venous congestion, however, frequently requires the use of diuretics. The usual aims are to ameliorate symptoms of pulmonary congestion and to improve exercise tolerance. Massive peripheral edema, itself, may reduce systemic venous compliance and be responsible for the observation that vasodilator therapy alone, in some patients, fails to lower elevated right and left ventricular filling pressures. Successful diuresis increases the venous compliance (demonstrated as a reduction in the ratio of cardiopulmonary blood volume to total blood volume) and reduces cardiac filling pressures.[2]

A thiazide diuretic is an appropriate initial choice for treatment of patients with relatively mild to moderate heart failure and normal renal function. Patients with more severe disease often require a loop diuretic. Furosemide in daily oral doses of 20 to 40 mg should be used and the dose titrated upward as needed, depending on clinical response. Doses of up to 600 mg per day of furosemide (in divided doses) have been effective and well tolerated. Three loop diuretics are currently available in the United States: furosemide, ethacrynic acid, and bumetanide. All share a similar site and

TABLE 32-2 Characteristics of Commonly Used Diuretics

Site of Action	How Supplied	Adult Dose Range (mg/day)	Fractional Excretion of Sodium (%)	Adverse Effects
Proximal				
Acetazolamide	PO 125, 250 mg IV 500 mg/5 ml	250 to 1000	2 to 3	Hypokalemia, metabolic acidosis
Loop				
Bumetanide	PO 0.5 mg IV 0.5 mg/2 ml	0.5 to 10	15 to 20	Volume depletion, metabolic alkalosis, hypokalemia, hypomagnesemia, and ototoxicity. Diarrhea, GI upset more common with ethacrynic acid
Ethacrynic Acid	PO 25, 50 mg IV 50 mg/50 ml	50 to 100	15 to 20	
Furosemide	PO 20, 40, 80 mg IV 10 mg/ml	20 to 600	15 to 20	
Distal (Potassium-Wasting)				
Chlorothiazide	PO 500 mg IV 500 mg/20 ml	500 to 1,000	5 to 8	Volume depletion, metabolic alkalosis, hypokalemia, hypomagnesemia, hypercalcemia, hyperuricemia, glucose intolerance
Hydrochlorothiazide	PO 25, 50 mg	25 to 100	5 to 8	
Metolazone	PO 2.5, 5, 10 mg	2.5 to 10	5 to 8	
Distal (Potassium-Sparing)				
Amiloride	PO 5 mg	5 to 10	2 to 3	Hyperkalemia and metabolic acidosis. Spironolactone may produce gynecomastia, whereas triamterene has been associated with blood dyscrasias and nephrolithiasis
Spironolactone	PO 25, 50 mg	100 to 400	2 to 3	
Triamterene	PO 50, 100 mg	200 to 300	2 to 3	

mechanism of action and none has been shown to be more effective than the others in any of the edematous disorders when used at roughly equivalent doses (40 mg furosemide; 1 mg bumetanide; 50 mg ethacrynic acid).[3,4]

The pharmacokinetics of the most extensively studied loop diuretic, furosemide, appear to be altered in congestive heart failure. Patients with decompensated heart failure who are receiving a single oral dose of furosemide demonstrate a delayed time to peak plasma concentration and a lower absolute value of this peak compared to the same dose administered in the compensated state.[5] Mucosal edema and reduced intestinal motility and/or perfusion have been postulated to explain these observations. The total amount of drug absorbed, however, is not different, and a difference in the absolute amount of natriuresis has not been demonstrated. These findings support the common clinical impression that an intravenous route of administration is indicated for emergent situations such as acute pulmonary edema. In this case, intravenous furosemide doses of 10 to 20 mg for patients not previously receiving diuretics, 40 mg for patients previously receiving diuretics, and 80 to 120 mg for refractory patients appear reasonable.[6]

Cirrhosis

Hepatic venous outflow obstruction from the cirrhotic process that results in augmented hepatic lymph flow into the extravascular compartment appears to be the primary mechanism of ascites fluid formation. Intense renal sodium avidity is also important.[7] In addition, peripheral edema is common in cirrhotic patients as a result of hypoalbuminemia, intense sodium reabsorption by the kidney, and, possibly, the mechanical effect of tense ascites on the inferior vena cava. The use of diuretics in these patients is problematic. The physician should have clearly defined goals in mind and a knowledge of the potential complications resulting from aggressive diuresis in the cirrhotic patient.

Improved patient comfort is the most frequent indication for the use of diuretics since successful diuresis alone does not appear to reduce portal venous pressure or to affect the underlying disease. The decision regarding diuretic use should be tempered by the observation that approximately 30 percent of patients hospitalized for 1 week and maintained on bedrest and salt restriction alone undergo complete disappearance of ascites and/or edema.[8] In cirrhotic patients not responding to conservative therapy, spironolactone, an aldosterone antagonist, is a highly effective diuretic, which presumably reflects the observation that plasma aldosterone levels are frequently elevated in decompensated cirrhotic patients. Stimulation of the renin-angiotensin-aldosterone axis by a reduced effective arterial plasma volume and reduced hepatic clearance of aldosterone may explain this finding. It is unlikely, however, that aldosterone is the only factor in cirrhosis-associated sodium retention since 1. many cirrhotic patients have normal plasma aldosterone levels, 2. others have undergone a spontaneous diuresis without a significant change in plasma aldosterone levels, and 3. blockage of adrenal production of aldosterone with aminoglutethimide does not consistently produce a diuresis.[9] Spironolactone, 150 to 300 mg per day in divided doses for 7 to 14 days, has produced a safe and effective natriuresis in the majority of patients, results that compared favorably to furosemide, 80 to 160 mg per day.[10] Avoidance of thiazide and loop diuretics may lower the risk of hypokalemia-stimulated renal ammonia production and hepatic encephalopathy.

Rapid mobilization of ascites may produce significant intravascular volume depletion manifested clinically by hypotension and decreased renal function. In general, the rate of loss of ascites should not exceed 300 to 900 ml per day. The additional presence of peripheral edema, however, may allow for a more rapid diuresis, at least initially. In a recent study of a spironolactone plus furosemide-induced diuresis in cirrhotic patients with ascites and edema, plasma volume and renal function remained stable despite daily weight losses of 2 kg. Edema fluid was clearly demonstrated to be preferentially mobilized compared to the ascitic fluid compartment (1,800 ml per day versus 700 ml per day). Once the edema disappeared, however, attempts to produce daily weight losses of greater than 0.7 kg resulted in significant reductions in plasma volume and renal function.[11]

In summary, the approach to the diuretic management of symptomatic edema and/or ascites in the cirrhotic patient should follow a step-wise progression, beginning with bedrest and salt and water restriction. Spironolactone, 25 mg four times daily, is an appropriate first choice drug, and the dose should be doubled every 3 to 4 days to a maximum daily dose of 400 mg. Alternatively, amiloride, 5 mg daily, may be used. Unlike spironolactone, amiloride does not produce or exacerbate gynecomastia. Daily weight loss should be no more than 0.5 kg or 2.0 kg in the nonedematous or edematous ascitic patient, respectively. The addition of furosemide, 40 mg daily then doubled every other day up to 400 mg if needed, has produced a significant natriuresis in the majority of patients. Bumetanide in equivalent doses has also been effective.[12] In most clinical studies, symptomatic improvement ordinarily requires 7 to 14 days of gentle diuresis. Orthostatic measurements of blood pressure and pulse must be followed closely, as well as input and output records, weights, serum electrolytes, and renal function tests.

RENAL DISEASE

Nephrotic Syndrome

The edema observed in nephrotic patients is a result of the hypoalbuminemia from urinary loss of protein, coupled with avid sodium retention by the distal nephron. Measurements of the plasma volume in adult patients with the nephrotic syndrome have produced conflicting results, but in general, the volume appears to be well maintained.[13] A thiazide diuretic rarely produces a significant natriuresis in these patients and should be replaced by, or used in combination with, a loop agent. Sensitivity of the renal tubule to the natriuretic effect of furosemide appears to be normal. Binding by the increased quantity of protein within the tubular lumen, however, may reduce the active "free" form of this drug and result in less natriuresis per dose.[13] In addition, avid sodium reabsorption distal to the loop of Henle also is responsible for a suboptimal clinical response to furosemide doses up to 400 to 600 mg per day and may explain the improved results achieved by the addition of a thiazide or other distal-acting diuretic.[14,15]

Patients with severe hypoalbuminemia (serum albumin less than 1.5 g per deciliter), clinical evidence of a reduced plasma volume, and unresponsiveness to the preceding diuretic combinations have been successfully treated with intravenous infusions of concentrated albumin solution. One such regimen (studied mostly in children with minimal change disease) is the infusion of albumin 1 g per kilogram (as a 25 percent solution) followed in 30 minutes by intravenous furosemide, 1 to 2 mg per kilogram.[16] This regimen can be repeated every 8 hours until a clinical response is obtained. This regimen, occasionally needed in adult patients with the nephrotic syndrome, is both expensive and transient in its effectiveness since most of the infused albumin is rapidly excreted in the urine. The use of diuretic combinations and specific treatment of the underlying glomerulopathy remain the primary forms of therapy. Novel approaches such as the successful use of meclofenamate[17] or of captopril[18] to reduce proteinuria recently have been reported in small numbers of patients.

Azotemia

Hypertension and other manifestations of circulatory congestion are common problems in azotemic patients. A decline in renal blood flow, glomerular filtration rate, and tubular function is responsible for decreased delivery of commonly used diuretics to their usual sites of action within the nephron. The result is a progressive need for higher doses of drug to achieve a satisfactory natriuresis. Recently, the effectiveness of a combination of hydrochlorothiazide (25 to 50 mg per day) and furosemide (40 to 480 mg per day) has been demonstrated in eight azotemic patients (serum creatinines 2.3 to 4.9 mg per deciliter).[19] Significant reductions in weight, plasma volume, and blood pressure were achieved at the expense of a moderate deterioration in renal function. This deterioration stabilized after several days, however, and did not progress over several months of observation. Significant hypokalemia (serum potassium less than 3.0 mEq per liter) was common and required potassium chloride supplementation.

The use of potent diuretic combinations in azotemic patients thus is effective, but not without hazard. In most cases, the long-term benefits of blood pressure control and reduced circulatory congestion outweigh a modest, though sustained, reduction in renal function. Minimal doses of potassium-sparing diuretics may circumvent hypokalemia, but mandate detailed patient education regarding dietary potassium restriction and the need for frequent determinations of serum potassium concentration. Clinical and laboratory evaluation should be performed every several days during the initiation of these regimens.

IDIOPATHIC (CYCLICAL) EDEMA

Idiopathic edema is predominantly a disorder of women. A diurnal cycle (worse in the evening) of weight gain and lower extremity edema occurs in a pattern that may be intermittent and characterized by asymptomatic periods. These patients are often concerned about obesity and many have used diuretics to lose weight or to reduce abdominal "bloating" and/or facial puffiness. A paramedical occupation is not unusual. This disorder is not simply a premenstrual phenomenon and has been described in postmenopausal women. In some cases the edema occurs promptly after the sudden discontinuation of diuretics. It reaches a maximum intensity within 10 days and gradually subsides, although postural edema has been reported to persist for up to 2 years in rare cases.[20]

The etiology of this disorder has not been established, although perturbations have been demonstrated in the renin-angiotensin-aldosterone system, the metabolism of dopamine, and the kinin-kallikrein system.[1, 14] A plausible hypothesis suggests that the disorder results from the persistence of a sodium-retaining effector mechanism stimulated by previous diuretic use. All of these described abnormalities could, however, be the result of a reduced plasma volume that is in turn produced by a primary alteration in capillary permeability. Both of these latter abnormalities have been described.[14, 20]

The management of idiopathic edema is symptomatic. Diuretic use, whether persistent or intermittent, should be discouraged. Frequent elevation of the legs and the use of support stockings have been helpful. The need for dietary salt restriction has not been established, although it is probably useful. The converting enzyme inhibitor, captopril (50 mg twice daily), was effective in four women with this disorder.[21] For severe, refractory cases, the dopamine agonist, bromocriptine, 1.25 mg at bedtime and increased slowly to 2.5 mg three times daily, may be effective, but can require several weeks before a response is noted.[22]

THE PATIENT WITH REFRACTORY EDEMA

The evaluation of the patient with refractory edema should begin with a consideration of several possibilities. 1. Dietary salt may not be adequately restricted (a careful dietary history and a 24-hour urine collection for sodium may be helpful). 2. The patient may not be taking the prescribed diuretics because of side effects or inadequate instruction. 3. The underlying illness may be progressing, thereby rendering previously effective drug doses inadequate. 4. There may be interference of diuretic effectiveness by additional medications, e.g., prescribed or over-the-counter nonsteroidal anti-inflammatory drugs, potent vasodilating agents (minoxidil), and estrogen-containing preparations.

ADVERSE EFFECTS OF DIURETIC THERAPY

The more frequently encountered adverse effects of diuretics are described in Table 32-2. Intravascular volume depletion, metabolic alkalosis, and hypokalemia are the most common side effects of loop and distal potassium-wasting diuretics. Hypomagnesemia may occur with chronic use of either of these diuretics, though it more commonly occurs with the loop agents. Concomitant hypokalemia may increase the risk of arrhythmias in susceptible patients, such as those with acute ischemic heart disease or those taking cardiac glycosides. Hyperuricemia is common, but rarely produces clinical gout. Glucose intolerance may be caused, in part, by hypokalemia-related inhibition of pancreatic release of insulin. Significant hypercalcemia (serum calcium above 10.5 to 11 mg per deciliter) during thiazide use is rare and, if present, suggests underlying primary hyperparathyroidism.

The clinician should recall that all of the diuretics listed in Table 32–2, with the exception of ethacrynic acid and the potassium-sparing agents, are sulfa derivatives and may produce hypersensitivity reactions in susceptible individuals. All of the loop agents may produce clinical ototoxicity that, in the case of ethacrynic acid, can be irreversible. These cases have usually been reported in critically ill patients receiving large intravenous doses of these agents in combination with other potentially ototoxic drugs, such as aminoglycosides. With respect to furosemide, ototoxicity seems to be prevented by an intravenous infusion rate of no greater than 4 mg per minute.

Hyperkalemia is clearly the most frequent and serious adverse effect of the potassium-sparing diuretics. The estimated incidence of clinically significant hyperkalemia is 9 to 16 percent and often occurs during the first 10 days of treatment.[23] Hyporeninemic hypoaldosteronism caused by diabetes or by interstitial renal disease is a common predisposing factor, although advanced renal insufficiency of any cause, nonsteroidal anti-inflammatory drug use, or continued use of potassium chloride supplements also have been incriminated.

References

1. Seifter JL, Skorecki KL, Stivelman JC, Haupert G, Brenner BM. Control of extracellular fluid volume and pathophysiology of edema formation. In: Brenner BM, Rector FC Jr, eds. The kidney. 3rd ed. Philadelphia: WB Saunders, 1986:343.
2. Magrini F, Niarchos AP. Hemodynamic effects of massive peripheral edema. Am Heart J 1983; 105:90–97.
3. Bumetanide (Bumex) — A new "loop" diuretic. Medical Letter 1983; 25:61–63.
4. Whelton A. Long-term bumetanide treatment of renal edema. Comparison with furosemide. J Clin Pharmacol 1981; 21:591–596.
5. Vasko MR, Brown-Cartwright D, Knochel JP, Nixon JV, Brater DC. Furosemide absorption altered in decompensated congestive heart failure. Ann Intern Med 1985; 102:314–318.
6. Hutter AM Jr. Congestive heart failure. In: Rubenstein E, Federman DD, eds. Scientific American Medicine. Vol. 2. New York: Scientific American Inc. 1986:1.
7. Epstein M, Perez GO. Pathophysiology of the edema forming states. In: Maxwell MH, Kleeman CR, Narins RG, eds. Clinical disorders of fluid and electrolyte metabolism. 4th ed. New York: McGraw-Hill, 1987:409.
8. Chonko AM, Grantham JJ. Treatment of edema states. In: Maxwell MH, Kleeman CR, Narins RG, eds. Clinical disorders of fluid and electrolyte metabolism. 4th ed. New York: McGraw-Hill, 1987:429.
9. Warnock DG, Boyer TD. Use of diuretics in the treatment of cirrhotic ascites. Gastroenterology 1983; 84:1051–1055.
10. Perez-Ayuso RM, Arroyo V, Planas R, et al. Randomized comparative study of efficacy of furosemide versus spironolactone in nonazotemic cirrhosis with ascites. Gastroenterology 1983; 84:978–986.
11. Pockros PJ, Reynolds TB. Rapid diuresis in patients with ascites from chronic liver disease: the importance of peripheral edema. Gastroenterology 1986; 90:1827–1833.
12. Nicholson G. Treatment of fluid retention: a comparison of bumetanide and furosemide. Curr Med Res Opin 1977; 4:675–679.

13. Geers AB, Koomans HA, Roos JC, Dorhout Mees EJ. Preservation of blood volume during edema removal in nephrotic subjects. Kidney Int 1985; 28:652–657.
14. Berger BE, Warnock DG. Clinical uses and mechanisms of action of diuretic agents. In: Brenner BM, Rector FC Jr, eds. The kidney. 3rd ed. Philadelphia: WB Saunders, 1986:433.
15. Ghose RR, Gupta SK. Synergistic action of metolazone with "loop" diuretics. Brit Med J 1981; 282:1432–1433.
16. Weiss RA, Schoeneman M, Greifer I. Treatment of severe nephrotic edema with albumin and furosemide. NY State J Med 1984; 84:384–388.
17. Velosa JA, Torres VE. Benefits and risks of nonsteroidal antiinflammatory drugs in steroid-resistant nephrotic syndrome. Am J Kidney Dis 1986; 8:345–350.
18. Taguma Y, Kitamoto Y, Futaki G, et al. Effect of captopril on heavy proteinuria in azotemic diabetics. N Engl J Med 1985; 313:1617–1620.
19. Wollam GL, Tarazi RC, Bravo EL, Dustan HP. Diuretic potency of combined hydprochlorothiazide and furosemide therapy in patients with azotemia. Am J Med 1982; 72:929–938.
20. de Wardener HE. Nephrology forum. Idiopathic edema: role of diuretic abuse. Kidney Int 1981; 19:881–892.
21. Docci D, Turci F, Salvi G. Therapeutic response of idiopathic edema to captopril. Nephron 1983; 34:198–200.
22. Vance ML, Evans WS, Thorner MO. Bromocriptine. Ann Intern Med 1984; 100:78–91.
23. Ponce SP, Jennings AE, Madias NE, Harrington JT. Drug-induced hyperkalemia. Medicine 1985; 64:357–369.

33 | RECURRENT URINARY TRACT STONES

ANDREW S. LEVEY, M.D.

Urinary tract stones affect 0.5 percent of the general population. The most common clinical presentation is the passage of a ureteral stone, manifest by colic, microscopic hematuria, and a calcification on a plain x-ray film of the abdomen. Approximately 15 to 20 percent of patients with a stone require hospitalization and instrumentation of the urinary tract because of prolonged pain, persistent obstruction, or development of infection.[1] Consultation with an internist is usually sought when passage of urinary tract stones recurs or when asymptomatic stones are detected on follow-up roentgenograms. In addition to the acute morbidity of recurrently passing stones, chronic renal damage and renal failure may develop.

Remediable metabolic abnormalities contribute to the formation of stones in up to 80 percent of patients with recurrent urinary tract stones.[1] Thus a metabolic work-up should be undertaken in all patients with recurrent stones to determine the cause of the disorder and to guide therapy for prevention of further stones. The prevalence of these disorders is equally high in patients who have formed only a single stone, and these patients are likely to form recurrent stones in the future.[2] Based on these observations, I also advise evaluation of patients who have had only one stone. For all patients, the work-up begins with the identification of the chemical composition of the stone.

TYPES OF URINARY TRACT STONES

Most urinary tract stones form in the kidney. Stones that form in the bladder and prostate are usually the consequence of either an indwelling catheter or chronic prostatic infection. This chapter will discuss only stones that form in the kidney. Table 33–1 lists the chemical composition of the principal types of renal stones, their prevalence and radiologic appearance, and the urinary pH that favors their formation. These characteristics help to identify the type of stone even before it is passed.

Renal stones are the result of formation and growth of crystals in supersaturated urine. Figure 33–1 shows the characteristic appearance of crystals in the urinary sediment. Two major factors contribute to stone formation: (1) an abnormally high concentration of ions in the urine, and (2) an imbalance of

TABLE 33–1 Types of Renal Stones

Chemical Composition	Prevalance* (% of stones)	Radiologic Appearance	Urinary pH
Calcium	70.6		
Calcium oxalate	25.4	Opaque, round	any
Calcium phosphate	7.4	Opaque, round or branched	≥7.5
Mixed calcium	37.8	Opaque, round	any
Struvite (magnesium-ammonium phosphate and calcium phosphate)	21.5	Opaque, round or branched	≥7.5
Uric acid	5.4	Lucent, round or branched	≤6
Cystine	3.5	Opaque, round or branched	≤7.5

* Data on prevalence from Coe FL, Brenner BM, Stein JM, eds. Contemporary issues in nephrology 5: nephrolithiasis. New York: Churchill Livingstone, 1985:1.

promotors and inhibitors of urinary crystallization. Table 33–2 lists the most important abnormalities of urinary composition that lead to stone formation and the most frequent causes of each abnormality. As shown in Tables 33–1 and 33–2, calcium stones are the most common renal stones and are associated with the greatest number of metabolic abnormalities. In the following sections of this chapter, I will discuss the pathogenesis and the treatment of recurrent urinary stones. The less commonly occurring types of stones, struvite, cystine, and uric acid stones, will be discussed briefly first. Calcium stones will then be discussed in more detail.

STRUVITE STONES

The crystallization of calcium, magnesium, and ammonium with phosphate occurs only in the presence of elevated urine pH (see Table 33–1). Elevated urine pH is the result of an increased concentration of ammonia owing to infection with bacteria that produce urease, an enzyme that hydrolyzes urea to ammonia (a strong base) and carbon dioxide. Bacterial species that produce urease include *Klebsiella*, *Proteus*, *Pseudomonas*, and rarely *E. coli*. Patients with struvite stones invariably have a history of recurrent infections with these bacteria and have alkaline urine, but usually do not have other metabolic abnormalities.

TABLE 33-2 Metabolic Abnormalities Associated with Renal Stones

Abnormality	Definition	Types of Stone	Causes
Low urine volume	<1 L/day	Contributes to formation of all stones in susceptible persons	Hot environment, chronic diarrhea
Alkaline urine pH	>7.5	Struvite, calcium phosphate	Infection, distal renal tubular acidosis
Persistently acid urine pH	≤6.0	Uric acid	Diarrhea, high protein intake, gout, idiopathic
Cystinuria	>400 mg/day	Cystine	Homozygous cystinuria
	60 to 300 mg/day	Cystine	Heterozygous cystinuria
Hyperuricosuria	>800 mg/day (men) >750 mg/day (women)	Uric acid, calcium oxalate	High protein intake, gout, myeloproliferative disorders
Hypercalciuria	>300 mg/day (men) >250 mg/day (women)	Calcium oxalate, calcium phosphate	Hypercalcemia, distal renal tubular acidosis, increased dietary calcium intake, idiopathic
Hyperoxaluria	>50 mg/day	Calcium oxalate	Gastrointestinal disease, pyridoxine deficiency
Hypocitraturia	<320 mg/day	Calcium oxalate	Distal renal tubular acidosis, chronic diarrhea, urinary tract infection, thiazide diuretics, idiopathic

Medical therapy for struvite stones is unsatisfactory. In principle, effective antibiotic therapy should eradicate the source of urease, lower the concentration of ammonium, and reduce the abnormally high urine pH. However, antibiotic therapy is rarely effective because bacteria persist within the substance of stones that remain in the renal pelvis. Persistence of infected stones causes episodes of recurrent pyelonephritis, sepsis, and parenchymal renal damage and often culminates in renal failure. Chronic therapy with antibiotics may be prescribed to reduce the risk of bacteremia, but is not successful in the prevention of growth and recurrence of stones or in the prevention of renal damage.

The primary therapy for struvite stones is the complete surgical removal of all stone fragments. However, struvite stones are incompletely removed or

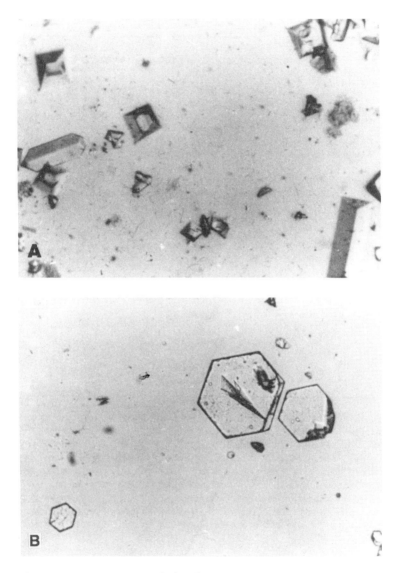

Figure 33-1 *See opposite page for legend.*

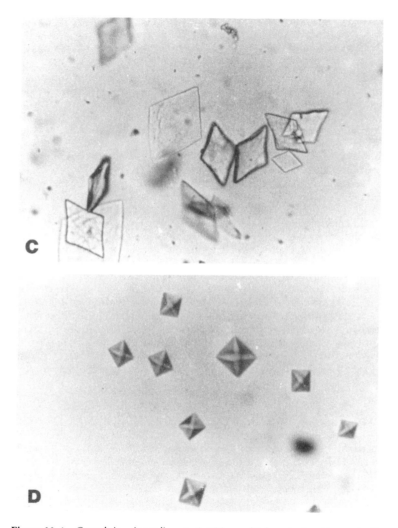

Figure 33-1 Crystals in urine sediment. *A*, "Diamond"-shaped uric acid crystals. *B*, "Envelope"-shaped calcium oxalate crystals. *C*, "Coffin"-shaped struvite crystals. *D*, Hexagonal cystine crystals. (*A* and *D* reprinted from Gennari FJ, Kassirer JP. Laboratory assessment of renal function. In: Earley LE, Gottschalk CW, eds. Strauss and Welt's diseases of the kidney. 3rd ed. Boston: Little Brown, 1979:41.)

recur after 30 percent of renal lithotomies. The efficacy of stone removal is dramatically improved by postoperative antibiotics and by irrigation of the renal pelvis with hemiacidrin (Renacidin, an acid solution of magnesium and organic acids that promotes stone dissolution) through a nephrostomy tube for 2 to 30 days until stone fragments are no longer visible on renal tomograms and until urine is sterile. Using this approach, one investigator has reported that only one of 46 patients with struvite stones developed a recurrence within a mean follow-up interval of 7 years.[3] Early experience with lithotripsy using percutaneous methods or extracorporeal shock waves demonstrates successful fragmentation and passage of struvite stones in 90 percent of patients.[4] Whether these techniques permit complete removal of all stone fragments and freedom from recurrence is not yet known.

Recently, a chemical inhibitor of bacterial urease, acetohydroxamic acid, has been developed. After oral administration, the agent is absorbed and, in patients with normal renal function, is excreted unchanged in the urine. In one small clinical trial, treatment with both acetohydroxamic acid and suppressive antibiotics retarded the growth of stones, prevented the appearance of new stones, and reduced the necessity for surgical intervention when compared to treatment with only suppressive antibiotics.[5] However, stones did not dissolve and half of the patients had side effects that required a reduction in the dosage or the discontinuation of the drug. In view of the need for long-term therapy and the high rate of side effects, acetohydroxamic acid is of limited usefulness. It should be prescribed only for patients in whom surgery or lithotripsy is not advised and in whom continuous antibiotic therapy has failed to prevent stone growth and recurrence. Moreover, this agent should not be used in patients with serum creatinine concentrations greater than 3.0 mg per deciliter because of reduced renal excretion and the possibility of a higher risk of side effects.

CYSTINE STONES

Recurrent formation of cystine stones is the major complication of the metabolic disorder cystinuria. In this autosomal recessive disorder, homozygotes display a marked defect in renal tubular and intestinal transport of the cationic amino acids, cystine, ornithine, lysine, and arginine (COLA). Reduced renal tubular reabsorption of the filtered amino acids results in excessive urinary excretion. Cystine is the least soluble of these amino acids and precipitates if the concentration exceeds 300 mg per liter. As shown in Table 33–2, in homozygotes and in some heterozygotes the urine is saturated with cystine unless the urine volume is high. Recurrent urinary stones is the only clinical complication of cystinuria. Serum levels of the four amino acids are slightly low, but growth and nutrition of affected children appear almost normal. The prevalence of homozygous cystinuria is approximately one in 7,000 infants.

The diagnosis of cystinuria is usually made by the detection of cystine in a urinary stone. As shown in Table 33-1, the prevalence of cystine stones is only 3 to 4 percent. Approximately half of stones formed by patients with cystinuria also contain other salts. Therefore, it is important to examine all urinary stones for the presence of cystine. Furthermore, 5 to 10 percent of stones formed by patients with cystinuria do not contain cystine. The diagnosis also may be made by the measurement of cystine in the urine (the nitroprusside test) or by the detection of cystine crystals in the urine sediment. The nitroprusside test for cystine detects heterozygotes as well as homozygotes and should be performed on all patients with recurrent urinary tract stones. The test is also positive in patients with ketosis. Cystine crystals may be seen in the urine sediment if the concentration of cystine exceeds 250 mg per liter; examination of the first morning urine specimen increases the likelihood of detecting the cystine crystalluria. Crystalluria is sometimes detected in heterozygotes. In patients with a positive nitroprusside test or urine sediment examination, the 24-hour excretion of cystine should be measured. All homozygotes, as well as heterozygotes who have formed stones, should be treated.

The first goal of treatment is to increase the water intake to 5 to 7 liters per day in order to reduce the urinary concentration of cystine to less than 300 mg per liter at all times. Adherence to a strict regimen of high water intake can prevent further stone formation. Alkalinization of the urine with bicarbonate, citrate, or carbonic anhydrase inhibitors markedly increases the solubility of cystine and may be a useful adjunct to therapy for patients who cannot maintain a sufficiently high water intake to prevent recurrent stones. Administration of D-penicillamine (beta, beta-dimethylcysteine) 1 to 2 g daily in three or four divided doses is also effective. This agent undergoes sulfhydryl-disulfide exchange with cystine to form the mixed disulfide of penicillamine and cysteine, which is 50 times more soluble than cystine. During therapy with penicillamine, urinary cystine excretion is reduced and urinary stones dissolve. Because of the high frequency of side effects, penicillamine should be used only in patients who have developed recurrent stones despite attempts at alkalinization of the urine or in patients who have suffered previous complications that have resulted in nephrectomy or renal insufficiency.

URIC ACID STONES

Uric acid is formed by the oxidation of hypoxanthine by the enzyme xanthine oxidase and is the end product of purine catabolism. The usual excretion of uric acid is approximately 600 to 1,000 mg per day, of which one-third is excreted into the gastrointestinal tract and metabolized by bacteria in a process called uricolysis. The remaining two-thirds is excreted in the urine. Under normal conditions, urine is supersaturated with uric acid. The most common causes of uric acid stones are hyperuricosuria and persistently low urine pH.

Hyperuricosuria is found in only one-third of patients with uric acid stones. Uric acid is excreted by the kidney by glomerular filtration, partial reabsorption, and secretion by the tubule. In the steady state, the major determinant of the urinary excretion of uric acid is its rate of production. Hyperuricosuria and the formation of uric acid stones may result from increased dietary purine intake, increased purine turnover as occurs in primary gout, or accelerated cell turnover as occurs in chronic hemolysis or in the tumor lysis syndrome. Interestingly, the prevalence of calcium oxalate stones also is increased in patients with hyperuricosuria and gout. This is discussed in more detail in the section on calcium stones.

Uric acid excretion may be decreased by the restriction of foods rich in purines (especially meat) and by the administration of allopurinol, a competitive inhibitor of xanthine oxidase. The usual dose of allopurinol is 300 mg per day, but up to 900 mg per day may be prescribed for short periods of time, for example, in preparation for chemotherapy of lymphoma or leukemia. During therapy with allopurinol, there is a decline in serum and urine levels of uric acid, and there is a concomitant increase in the levels of xanthine and hypoxanthine. However, urinary stone formation is reduced because the latter compounds are far more soluble than uric acid.

Persistently low urine pH is found in most patients with uric acid stones. Low pH markedly increases the tendency for uric acid to crystalize in urine. Uric acid exists in two forms in the urine: the extremely insoluble undissociated uric acid and the more soluble sodium salt of monohydrogen urate. The pK of the first dissociation of uric acid is approximately 5.5; thus, at lower urine pH values, more uric acid is in the form of the undissociated acid and the risk of crystallization is increased. If urine is persistently acid, crystals grow and stones form. At higher urine pH values, far less undissociated uric acid is present and uric acid crystals dissolve rather than grow.

Chronic diarrhea is one important cause of persistently low urine pH and therefore of uric acid stones. Loss of water and bicarbonate in stool leads to reduced urine volume, increased net acid excretion, and low urine pH. (Calcium stones also occur with increased frequency in patients with chronic diarrhea and gastrointestinal diseases, as is described in more detail later). Another cause of persistently low urinary pH is increased dietary protein intake, which results in increased net acid excretion and decreased urine pH. In other patients, including some patients with primary gout, urine pH is low even though net acid excretion is normal because a lower proportion of acid is excreted as ammonia and a higher proportion is excreted as titratable acidity. The cause of reduced ammoniagenesis in these patients is not understood.

Whatever the cause of persistently low urinary pH, oral administration of alkali, such as sodium bicarbonate 40 mEq per day, results in intermittent excretion of alkaline urine and increased solubility of uric acid. Maintenance of a high urine volume also reduces urine concentration of uric acid. Finally, even if uric acid excretion is not excessive, treatment with allopurinol is effective in lowering uric acid excretion and in preventing recurrent stone formation in patients with persistently low urine pH.

CALCIUM STONES

As shown in Table 33-1, most calcium stones are composed of calcium and oxalate. Normally, urine is saturated with calcium and oxalate, and calcium oxalate crystals may be found during examination of urinary sediment. These findings indicate that the formation of calcium and oxalate stones may be the result of an excessive excretion of calcium or oxalate or the result of an imbalance of promotors and inhibitors of crystallization in urine that usually maintain the urinary tract free of stones. As shown in Table 33-3, one or more

TABLE 33-3   Summary of Metabolic Abnormalities and Treatment in Patients with Calcium Stones

Metabolic Abnormality	Prevalence* (% of patients)	Treatment†
Hypercalciuria		
Primary hyperparathyroidism	5	Surgery
Renal tubular acidosis	1	Alkali
Other causes‡	6	Treat primary disorders
Idiopathic	32	Thiazide diuretics
Hyperoxaluria (enteric)	5	Treat primary disorder Low oxalate diet
Hyperuricosuria	15	Allopurinol
Hypercalciuria and hyperuricosuria	14	Thiazide and allopurinol
Hypocitraturia§	19–63	Citrate

* Data on prevalence from Coe FL, Brenner BM, Stein JM, eds. Contemporary issues in nephrology 5: nephrolithiasis. New York: Churchill Livingstone, 1985:1.

† Increased water intake should be included in therapy for all conditions.

‡ Causes include Paget's disease, sarcoidosis, vitamin D ingestion, and increased calcium intake.

§ Data for hypocitraturia are from Pak CYC.[11] May overlap with other conditions.

treatable disorders are present in 80 percent or more of patients with calcium stones.[6] The following sections of this chapter describe these disorders and their treatment. Table 33–4 describes the suggested metabolic evaluation for patients with calcium stones.

Hypercalciuria

Hypercalciuria is defined as urinary calcium excretion greater than 300 mg per day in men or 250 mg per day in women (see Table 33–3). Other definitions include calcium excretion greater than 4 mg per kilogram of body weight per day or greater than 140 mg per gram of urinary creatinine per day in both sexes. It is important that 24-hour urine samples for the measurement of urinary calcium be collected while the patients are at home and are eating their usual diets.

Increased urinary excretion of calcium may result from increased filtration of calcium by the renal glomerulus, decreased reabsorption of calcium by the renal tubule, or both. Increased glomerular filtration of calcium occurs only if the serum calcium concentration is elevated. Decreased tubular reabsorption of calcium occurs in a variety of conditions, including distal renal tubular acidosis and increased dietary calcium intake. In most patients with hypercalciuria, no cause can be found; this condition is defined as idiopathic hypercalciuria.

Hypercalcemia

Renal stones occur in a number of conditions that cause both hypercalciuria and hypercalcemia. Serum calcium concentration should be measured as

TABLE 33-4   Metabolic Evaluation for Patients
with Calcium Stones

Serum
Calcium
Uric acid
Sodium, chloride, bicarbonate, potassium
Creatinine
Urine (24-hour collection)
Volume
pH
Creatinine
Calcium
Uric acid
Citrate (if no other abnormalities are present)
Oxalate (if gastrointestinal disease is present)

part of the evaluation of patients with a history of even a single calcium stone. The most common cause of hypercalcemia, hypercalciuria, and renal stones is primary hyperparathyroidism. The incidence of stones in this disorder ranges from 40 to 80 percent in various reports and is increased by high dietary calcium intake and high levels of vitamin D. Renal stones may occasionally complicate other disorders in which hypercalciuria and hypercalcemia occur, such as sarcoidosis, vitamin D intoxication, hyperthyroidism, Cushing's syndrome, Paget's disease, and immobilization. In some cases, the hypercalcemia may be minimal or even transient. Correction of the underlying disorder is required to correct the hypercalcemia and hypercalciuria.

Interestingly, not all disorders causing hypercalcemia are associated with hypercalciuria and renal stones. Renal stones are usually not seen in patients with hyperparathyroidism associated with chronic renal failure because the glomerular filtration rate and the urinary calcium excretion are reduced. Renal stones are also uncommon in patients with hypercalcemia attributable to advanced malignancy, perhaps because of the short survival of the patients affected and the reduced glomerular filtration rate seen in association with severe hypercalcemia.[7] Also renal stones do not complicate familial hypocalciuric hypercalcemia. In this disorder, the primary defect appears to be an increased tubular reabsorption of calcium that results in hypercalcemia and hypocalciuria.[8]

Distal Renal Tubular Acidosis

Distal renal tubular acidosis is a rare disorder characterized by a nonanion gap metabolic acidosis, a defect in urinary acidification (inability to lower urinary pH below 6.5), normal glomerular filtration rate, osteopenia, hypercalciuria, and recurrent formation of calcium phosphate renal stones.[9] Measurements of serum electrolytes and urine pH are usually sufficient to detect distal renal tubular acidosis. However, in some patients the metabolic acidosis may be mild and the serum bicarbonate concentration may be in the normal range. Nonetheless, the urine pH is consistently 6.5 or greater. An exogenous acid load can be administered to expose the defect in urinary acidification.

The cause of hypercalciuria in distal renal tubular acidosis is not understood. Some authors hypothesize that metabolic acidosis directly reduces renal tubular reabsorption of calcium and that reduced bone mineral content is secondary to increased renal calcium loss. Other investigators suggest that the hypercalciuria is a secondary effect of the liberation of calcium from bone as a result of buffering of retained acid by alkali in bone mineral. In addition to hypercalciuria, other alterations in urine composition also contribute to stone formation in distal renal tubular acidosis. These include increased urinary pH and decreased urinary citrate excretion, which decreases the solubility of calcium and phosphate in urine. Treatment with alkali (sodium bicarbonate 40 to 60 mEq per day) raises serum bicarbonate, reduces urinary calcium excretion, raises urinary citrate excretion, and reduces the risk of stone recurrence.

Increased Dietary Calcium Intake

The relationship between dietary calcium intake and urinary calcium excretion is shown in Figure 33-2. Within the normal calcium intake range of from 600 to 1,200 mg per day, urinary calcium excretion is approximately 100 to 250 mg per day and is not influenced greatly by alterations in dietary calcium. The relative constancy of urinary calcium excretion throughout the normal range of intake is attributable, in part, to the regulation of intestinal calcium absorption by vitamin D.[10] At low levels of calcium intake, the level of vitamin D and the fraction of ingested calcium that is absorbed are high. At high levels of intake, the level of vitamin D and the fraction of calcium absorbed are reduced. The amount of calcium absorbed is approximately equal to the amount of calcium excreted in the urine; thus calcium balance is

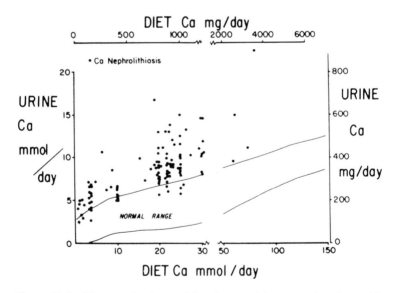

Figure 33-2 Dietary and urinary calcium in normal humans and patients with idiopathic hypercalciuria. (From Lemann J, Adams ND, Gray RW. Urinary calcium excretion in human beings. N Engl J Med 1979; 301:535–541.)

maintained. If excessive calcium is consumed, for example in dairy products, antacids, or vitamin and mineral supplements, the level of vitamin D and the fraction of calcium absorbed decline, yet the absolute amount of calcium that is absorbed by the intestine and excreted in the urine is excessive. The resulting hypercalciuria is associated with an increased risk of stone formation. Patients with hypercalciuria should be referred to a nutritionist for estimation of their dietary calcium intake. If dietary intake is excessive (i.e., greater than 1,000 to 1,200 mg per day), these patients should be advised to restrict dairy products and to discontinue taking antacids and vitamin-mineral supplements that contain calcium. Compliance with the treatment regimen can be assessed by subsequent measurements of urinary calcium excretion.

Idiopathic Hypercalciuria

Idiopathic hypercalciuria affects 5 percent of the general population. The prevalence of renal stones among individuals with this disorder is approximately 4 percent, compared to 0.5 percent in the general population. The disorder may be familial, detectable in childhood, and present as recurrent episodes of gross hematuria without apparent passage of urinary stones. There are no other complications of the disorder. As shown in Figure 33-2, intestinal calcium absorption and urinary calcium excretion are increased at all levels of dietary calcium intake. Thus, patients with idiopathic hypercalciuria appear to have two disorders that result in maintenance of calcium balance: increased excretion and increased absorption of calcium.

Two major hypotheses have been put forward to account for the alterations in calcium metabolism in idiopathic hypercalciuria: (1) In "renal hypercalciuria", it is hypothesized that a primary reduction in tubular reabsorption of calcium leads to hypercalciuria and tends to lower serum calcium concentration, thereby raising parathyroid hormone, vitamin D, and intestinal absorption of calcium. (2) In "absorptive hypercalciuria", it is hypothesized that a primary increase in either vitamin D or intestinal calcium absorption tends to raise serum calcium concentration, thereby lowering parathyroid hormone and renal tubular reabsorption of calcium and increasing urinary calcium excretion. In both disorders the serum calcium concentration is within the normal range. Patients with each primary disorder have been described, but it is not yet clear which disorder is more frequent. Although it is possible to distinguish between renal and absorptive hypercalciuria, in clinical practice it is difficult to make this distinction and is usually not necessary.

Several treatments for idiopathic calciuria have been proposed. Thiazide diuretics are most commonly employed. Urinary calcium excretion is reduced to approximately one-half by doses equivalent to hydrochlorothiazide 25 to 50 mg twice daily, and the rate of formation of new stones is reduced by approximately 90 percent. There are probably two mechanisms of action by which thiazide diuretics reduce calcium excretion. First, thiazides stimulate proximal tubular filtrate reabsorption, including sodium and calcium reabsorption, by inducing mild contraction of the extracellular fluid volume. This effect is blunted if extracellular fluid volume contraction is prevented by excessive dietary sodium intake. Second, thiazides appear to directly stimulate the distal tubular reabsorption of calcium. Short-term effects of thiazides include a transient increase in serum calcium concentration owing to increased serum protein concentration consequent to volume contraction. Serum ionized calcium concentration remains normal. Other side effects of thiazide diuretics include a 1 percent incidence of skin rash, and a 10 percent incidence of nonspecific symptoms that resolve after the dosage is reduced to once daily. Routine potassium supplementation is not necessary.

Factors associated with recurrent stone formation during treatment for idiopathic hypercalciuria include lower urine volume and higher (but normal) urinary calcium excretion. Patients should be encouraged to maintain a high urine volume (2 to 3 L per day) and to restrict dietary sodium intake to 2 to 3 g (approximately 85 to 125 mEq) per day if necessary in order to decrease urinary calcium excretion to less than 2.5 mg per kilogram of body weight per day. Another potential explanation for recurrent stone formation during treatment may be a reduced urinary citrate excretion (see following).

The effects on calcium balance of long-term treatment with thiazide diuretics in idiopathic hypercalciuria remain unknown. In renal hypercalciuria, calcium balance is expected to be maintained with reduced calcium excretion and absorption. In absorptive hypercalciuria, positive calcium balance possibly could develop as a result of reduced excretion in the face of persistently increased absorption of calcium. However, studies of patients treated with thiazides for hypercalciuria (some of whom probably had absorptive hypercalciuria) have not revealed persistent hypercalcemia, soft tissue calcification, osteosclerosis, or other evidence of positive calcium balance. More studies are required to assess the long-term effects on calcium balance.

Some investigators have proposed oral administration of cellulose phosphate as an alternative to thiazide diuretics for treatment of absorptive hypercalciuria. Cellulose phosphate is an ion-exchange resin that complexes intestinal calcium, reduces intestinal calcium absorption, and consequently reduces urinary calcium excretion. When used as a single agent, cellulose sodium phosphate 10 to 15 g per day in divided doses, reduces urinary calcium excretion. However, the frequency of stone formation is not reduced, perhaps owing to decreased absorption and excretion of magnesium and increased absorption and excretion of oxalate, both of which increase the risk of recurrent stone formation. Cellulose sodium phosphate does reduce stone recurrence when combined with a low calcium, low oxalate diet supplemented with magnesium.[11]

Another alternative is therapy with inorganic phosphate salts (orthophosphates), including potassium phosphate (K_2HPO_4) and sodium phosphate (Na_2HPO_4). The mechanism of action of orthophosphates is not clear. There is a slight decline in urinary calcium excretion. This decline may be the consequence of elevated parathyroid hormone and reduced vitamin D that result from the rise of serum inorganic phosphorous concentration. In addition, the urinary excretion of pyrophosphate (an inhibitor of calcium oxalate crystallization) is increased during phosphate administration. Inorganic phosphates, in doses of approximately 2 g elemental phosphorous per day in 3 or 4 divided doses, is effective in reducing recurrent stone formation. However, diarrhea occurs frequently and 10 percent of patients are unable to tolerate the drug, even in reduced dosage. Inorganic phosphates should not be administered to patients with reduced glomerular filtration rate.

In summary, a therapeutic regimen employing thiazide diuretics in conjunction with a high fluid intake and a moderate sodium restriction appears to be the most effective, least complicated, and safest strategy for prevention of recurrent stones attributable to idiopathic hypercalciuria. Protein and sodium restriction *alone* recently has been proposed as an alternative approach.

Hyperoxaluria

Although the vast majority of calcium stones contain oxalate, increased oxalate excretion is rarely found in patients with recurrent calcium stones (see Tables 2 and 3). Oxalate, a low molecular weight organic acid derived principally from the metabolism of ascorbic acid, glycine, and other amino acids, is freely filtered at the renal glomerulus and is also secreted by the tubule. Normally, endogenous oxalate accounts for 85 percent of urinary oxalate; the remaining 15 percent of urinary oxalate is the result of intestinal absorption of dietary oxalate. The most important cause of hyperoxaluria is increased intestinal absorption of oxalate as a result of gastrointestinal diseases; this condition is defined as enteric hyperoxaluria, and is described in more detail below. Other causes of hyperoxaluria are rare and include excessive consumption of dietary oxalate or oxalate precursors (such as ascorbic acid), pyridoxine deficiency, or genetic metabolic disorders (primary hyperoxaluria). Measurement of oxalate in the urine is technically difficult and is necessary only in patients with gastrointestinal disorders or in patients in whom other causes of hyperoxaluria are strongly suspected.

Enteric Hyperoxaluria

Oxalate is absorbed primarily in the small bowel by passive processes. Normally, only 5 percent of dietary oxalate is absorbed because it is complexed with calcium in the bowel lumen. Increased oxalate absorption is associated with hyperoxaluria and recurrent calcium oxalate stones in a variety of gastrointestinal disorders that include regional enteritis, bacterial overgrowth, blind-loop syndrome, nontropical sprue, small bowel resection or bypass, pancreatitis or pancreatectomy, and biliary tract disease. In enteric hyperoxaluria, the colon appears to be the site of increased oxalate absorption. Two hypothesis have been advanced to explain the increased oxalate absorption in gastrointestinal disorders. (1) With steatorrhea, fatty acids form complexes with calcium, thus decreasing the availability of calcium to form complexes with oxalate. The oxalate then becomes available for absorption in the colon. (2) With bile salt malabsorption, colonic mucosa is injured and becomes more permeable to oxalate.

The frequency of stones in these disorders is variable, being approximately 25 percent after intestinal bypass and 5 percent in inflammatory bowel disease. In addition to hyperoxaluria, other factors may contribute importantly to stone formation in gastrointestinal diseases. As a result of chronic diarrhea, mild metabolic acidosis and reduced urine volume, urine pH, and magnesium and citrate excretion are often found. Treatment includes prescription of a high fluid intake and a low oxalate diet, as well as specific measures to control steatorrhea and bile salt diarrhea. Metabolic acidosis, magnesium depletion, and hypocitraturia should be treated if they are present. Allopurinol may also be prescribed to reduce urinary uric acid excretion as described previously.

Hyperuricosuria

Increased urinary excretion of uric acid is found in approximately 30 percent of patients with calcium stones. Hypercalciuria is also present in approximately half of patients with hyperuricosuria (see Table 33–3). One hypothesis for the pathogenesis of calcium stones in patients with hyperuricosuria is heterogenous nucleation of calcium stones by crystals of uric acid or of monosodium urate. Another hypothesis is that crystals of uric acid or of monosodium urate absorb macromolecules that normally inhibit the growth of calcium oxalate crystals.

The most frequent cause of hyperuricosuria in patients with recurrent calcium stones is excessive dietary purine intake. A minority of patients have mild hyperuricemia, and in some patients, the hyperuricosuria is the result of primary gout. Treatment of hyperuricosuria with a low protein diet and allopurinol 100 mg twice daily is effective in reducing uric acid excretion by 30 percent and in reducing the rate of stone formation by 90 percent. In patients with both hypercalciuria and hyperuricosuria, treatment with a combination of thiazides, allopurinol, and a low purine diet is effective in the reduction of recurrent stone formation.

Hypocitraturia

Citric acid, an intermediate in the Krebs tricarboxylic acid cycle, is a low molecular weight organic acid that inhibits the growth of calcium oxalate crystals in urine. Citrate is filtered by the renal glomerulus and reabsorbed by the tubule. Citrate excretion is reduced during metabolic acidosis (including renal tubular acidosis), chronic diarrhea, urinary tract infection, and treatment with thiazide diuretics. Recently recognized is the fact that a large minority of patients with calcium stones have reduced urinary citrate excretion. In some patients, hypocitraturia is the only identifiable metabolic abnormality.

In one report[12], 15 patients with idiopathic hypocitraturia as the sole metabolic abnormality were treated with potassium citrate 60 mEq per day in three divided doses. An additional 10 patients with hypocitraturia and hypercalciuria were also treated with potassium citrate alone. In these 25 patients, urinary citrate excretion rose into the normal range and the frequency of recurrent stone formation decreased by 90 percent. Twelve other patients with hypocitraturia and either hypercalciuria or hyperuricosuria underwent treatment with a combination of potassium citrate and either hydrochlorothiazide or allopurinol. Citrate excretion was increased to normal and stone recurrence was reduced. In another study[13], 13 patients with hypercalciuria and hypocitraturia had recurrent stones despite reduction of urinary calcium excretion during treatment with thiazide diuretics. The addition of potassium citrate raised urinary citrate excretion and reduced the rate of stone formation by 90 percent. Minor side effects of therapy included diarrhea and nausea.

Apparently, some patients with recurrent calcium oxalate stones have idiopathic hypocitraturia, and treatment with potassium citrate is simple, safe, and effective in restoring urinary citrate excretion to normal and in reducing the risk of stone recurrence. Based on these data, measurement of urinary citrate excretion is advisable in patients with calcium oxalate stones who do not have hypercalciuria or hyperuricosuria and in patients who do have these disorders, but who have recurrent stone formation despite thiazide or allopurinol treatment. Patients with hypocitraturia should be treated with potassium citrate 40 to 80 mEq per day in order to raise citrate excretion to normal. The medication is best tolerated when given as a solid preparation during meals.

No Apparent Metabolic Disorder

Approximately 25 percent of patients with recurrent calcium oxalate stones studied by Coe and colleagues had normal serum and urinary measurements of calcium, oxalate, and uric acid.[1] It is hypothesized that these patients have an imbalance between promotors and inhibitors of crystallization that accounts for stone formation. Presumably some, but not all, of the patients had hypocitraturia; however, the data on urinary citrate excretion in these patients have not been reported. Other inhibitors that might be abnormally low include magnesium, pyrophosphate, or glycoproteins (molecular weight 10,000–14,000 daltons). Additional potential causes of stone formation in this group might be an habitually low urine volume or a low pH.

Although the cause of recurrent stones in these patients is unknown, empiric treatment with a combination of thiazides and allopurinol is successful in lowering the excretion of calcium and uric acid by 15 to 30 percent and in reducing the rate of stone formation by 80 percent. Presumably, the risk of recurrent stones is lessened by a reduction of the concentrations of calcium and uric acid. A recent report demonstrates successful therapy with allopurinol alone in a dose of 300 mg per day.[14] Whether thiazide diuretics alone would be equally successful is not known. Because of the morbidity of stones, it seems reasonable to prescribe both agents for patients without an apparent metabolic disorder who form recurrent stones.

References

1. Coe FL, Brenner BM, Stein JM, eds. Contemporary issues in nephrology 5: nephrolithiasis. New York: Churchill Livingstone, 1985:1.
2. Strauss AL, Coe FL, Parks JH. Formation of a single calcium stone of renal origin. Arch Intern Med 1982; 142:504–507.
3. Silverman DE, Stamey TA. Management of infection stones: the Stanford experience. Medicine 1983; 62:44–51.
4. Kahnoski RJ, Lingeman JE, Coury TA, Steele RE, Mosbaugh PG. Combined percutaneous and extracorporeal shock wave lithotripsy for staghorn calculi: an alternative to anatrophic nephrolithotomy. J Urol 1986; 135:679–681.
5. Williams JJ, Rodman JS, Peterson CM. A randomized double-blind study of acetohydroxamic acid in struvite nephrolithiasis. N Engl J Med 1984; 311:760–764.
6. Millman S, Strauss AL, Parks JH, Coe FL. Pathogenesis and clinical course of mixed calcium oxalate and uric acid nephrolithiasis. Kidney Int 1982; 22:366–370.
7. Muggia FM, Heinemann HO. Hypercalcemia associated with neoplastic disease. Arch Intern Med 1970; 73:281–290.
8. Marx SJ. Familial hypocalciuric hypercalcemia. N Engl J Med 1980; 303:810–811.
9. Coe FL, Parks J. Stone disease in hereditary distal renal tubular acidosis. Ann Intern Med 1980; 93:60–61.

10. Lemann J, Adams ND, Gray RW. Urinary calcium excretion in human beings. N Engl J Med 1979; 301:535-541.
11. Pak CYC. A cautious use of sodium cellulose phosphate in the management of calcium nephrolithiasis. Invest Urol 1981; 19:187-190.
12. Pak CYC, Fuller CY. Idiopathic hypocitraturic calcium oxalate nephrolithiasis successfully treated with potassium citrate. Ann Intern Med 1986; 104:33-37.
13. Pak CYC, Peterson R, Sakhaee K, Fuller C, Preminger G, Reisch J. Correction of hypocitraturia and prevention of stone formation by combined thiazide and potassium citrate in the therapy of thiazide-unresponsive hypercalciuric nephrolithiasis. Am J Med 1985; 79:284-288.
14. Ettinger B, Tang A, Citron J, Livermore B, Williams T. Randomized trial of allopurinol in the prevention of calcium oxalate calculi. N Engl J Med 1986; 315:1386-1389.

34 | RECURRENT URINARY TRACT INFECTIONS

VINCENT J. CANZANELLO, M.D.

In the United States, women make approximately 5 million physician visits annually for the management of urinary tract infections (UTI). Recurrent infections, defined as at least two episodes per year, account for the majority of these visits.

Most UTI are caused by a single bacterial species; the presence of two or more organisms usually implies contamination and should prompt a review of specimen collection and handling techniques. In the presence of symptoms, a clean-voided urine specimen containing as few as 10^2 bacterial colonies per milliliter should be considered significant bacteriuria. In the absence of symptoms, colony counts of 10^4 to 10^5 per milliliter are required. Pyuria, defined as at least eight leukocytes per cubic millimeter of uncentrifuged urine or two to five leukocytes per high power field of centrifuged urine, is present in most patients with symptomatic bacteriuria and in a variable number of asymptomatic patients. In evaluating patients with recurrent UTI, *reinfection* (infection either with a different strain of the same bacterial species or with a different species) must be distinguished from *relapse* (infection with the same organism that caused the initial episode). This distinction has important diagnostic and therapeutic implications in the management of patients with recurrent infections (see following). In general, reinfections account for approximately 80 percent of recurrent infections in women and relapses account for the remainder; the converse is true for men.

Three major concerns arise when the clinician is faced with the patient with a recurrent UTI: 1. the discomfort of recurrent, symptomatic episodes and the cost of office visits, diagnostic procedures, medications, and time lost from work; 2. the possibility that recurrent infections may worsen preexisting renal dysfunction; and 3. the possibility that persistent asymptomatic bacteriuria, especially in elderly patients, may be associated with a shortened life span (through, e.g., an increased incidence of bacteremia). These issues will be addressed in the following sections. The appropriate diagnostic and therapeutic approach to recurrent UTI varies among groups of patients. Hence, it is necessary to consider these groups separately.

URINARY TRACT INFECTIONS IN WOMEN

Clinicoepidemiologic Features

Screening studies have shown a prevalence of UTI of 1.2 percent in girls younger than 10 years of age; one-third of these patients were asymptomatic. Following an initial episode of bacteriuria, 80 percent of schoolgirls have one or more recurrences, 80 percent of which are reinfections. Overall, 5 to 6 percent of schoolgirls have at least one UTI between the ages of 5 and 18. The prevalence of bacteriuria in women 15 to 24 years of age is 1 to 3 percent, increasing to about 10 percent by the ages of 60 to 70. For women 24 to 64 years of age, the incidence of dysuria is about 20 percent per year. Fifty percent of these women seek medical attention and, of this 50 percent, two-thirds have significant bacteriuria (defined as bacterial colony counts of 10^5 or more per milliliter); the remaining one-third have the acute urethral syndrome or another cause, such as vaginitis.[1]

What is the clinical impact of recurrent UTI beyond patient discomfort and economic cost? Two careful studies have examined this issue. Freedman and Andriole did not show an increased incidence of renal dysfunction or hypertension in 250 women with bacteriuria (many with persistent or recurrent infection) followed for up to 12 years.[2] Asscher and colleagues followed 107 nonpregnant women with untreated, asymptomatic bacteriuria and 88 matched controls over a period of 5 years.[3] In the absence of preexisting hypertension or obstructive uropathy, progressive renal dysfunction did not occur. It seems likely, therefore, that a UTI that begins in adult life does not, by itself, lead to progressive renal disease or to hypertension. In contrast, in children with vesicoureteral reflux who are less than 5 years of age, UTI is a clear risk factor for the development of renal insufficiency and hypertension, a risk much reduced by maintenance of sterile urine with chronic antibiotic therapy.[1]

Does recurrent or persistent bacteriuria, regardless of symptoms, affect overall patient survival? The population for the study of this question usually has been elderly residents of nursing homes. Data reported for women have been conflicting. One study reported a median survival of 34 months for bacteriuric women between the ages of 70 to 79 years versus 75 months for nonbacteriuric matched residents of the same nursing home.[4] However, a more recent study of a large number of ambulatory and institutionalized elderly patients in Sweden revealed that the 5- and 9-year mortality rates for women were not different in the presence or absence of bacteriuria if corrected for the presence of a chronic indwelling bladder catheter.[5] It thus seems likely that the presence of bacteriuria, at least in elderly women, is simply a marker of the severity of illness and/or of general debilitation and is not an independent contributor to mortality.

Relapse Versus Reinfection

The approach to the nonpregnant woman with recurrent UTI should begin with characterization of the episode as either a relapse or a reinfection. A relapse usually represents an inadequately treated UTI, an unsuspected upper urinary tract infection, or the presence of underlying structural abnormalities such as vesicoureteral reflux, bladder or urethral diverticuli, nephrolithiasis (especially struvite stones), and neuromuscular disorders of the bladder (diabetic autonomic neuropathy, spinal cord injury, multiple sclerosis). Most relapses occur within 4 to 7 days (and almost all within 4 weeks) following either single dose or conventional 10- to 14-day antibiotic therapy of a prior infection. These treatments may have been initiated based on clinical findings that suggested a lower urinary tract infection (simple cystitis). Unfortunately, however, 30 to 50 percent of patients with the acute dysuria-frequency syndrome may have upper tract involvement (determined by antibody-coated bacteria techniques, ureteral catheterization, or bladder washout studies) despite the absence of fever, chills, flank pain, gastrointestinal complaints, and/or macroscopic hematuria.[6] Moreover, chills, fever, and flank pain may be present in patients with only documented lower tract disease or with the acute urethral syndrome.

Reinfections present quite a different clinical picture. In women with recurrent UTI, the overall attack rate for symptomatic bacteriuria is 0.2 infections per month, although up to one-third of infections are followed by an infection-free interval of at least 6 months. Several risk factors predisposing to reinfection have been identified, with varying degrees of certainty. These include genitourinary instrumentation,[7] sexual intercourse,[8] oral contraceptives,[9] diaphragm use,[10] hemorrhoids,[11] and specific bacterial virulence factors.[12]

Diagnostic Evaluation

Evaluation of a woman with recurrent UTI should focus on the frequency, symptoms, and specific treatment of all previous episodes. A history of childhood UTI, concurrent genitourinary tract disease, and one or more of the risk factors that predispose to infection should be sought. The duration of present symptoms and an estimation of the patient's compliance may be important for subsequent management decisions. The time of the present episode in relation to the most recent infection, coupled with the urine culture and sensitivity results, should distinguish relapse from reinfection. Members of the *Enterobacteriaceae* family (especially *E. coli*) account for most UTIs, though several gram-positive cocci, such as the enterococcus and *Staphylococ-*

cus epidermidis, occasionally are isolated. In the acutely symptomatic patient, pyuria and less than 10^2 bacterial colonies per milliliter of urine are sufficient to diagnose the acute urethral syndrome. *Chlamydia trachomatis* infection can be confirmed by culture if this test is readily available and the cost is reasonable.

To distinguish upper from lower urinary tract infection remains a problem. In addition to the clinical findings of chills, fever, and flank pain that suggest upper tract disease, a host of noninvasive studies have been recommended.[1] These studies include measurements of urinary enzymes (lactate dehydrogenase [LDH], beta-glucuronidase, N-acetyl glucosaminidase), plasma C-reactive protein, urinary concentrating ability, and antibody-coated bacterial assays. Many of these tests, however, are nonspecific, difficult to perform, or not widely available. In addition, most have not been compared with the "gold standard" for distinguishing upper from lower tract infection, i.e., ureteral catheterization or bladder washout studies. A relapse occurring shortly after single-dose or conventional therapy may in fact be a more clinically useful indicator of an upper tract infection than any of the urinary enzymes or other factors already referred to.

Intravenous pyelography, cystography, and cystoscopy rarely are indicated in women with recurrent UTI. For instance, in three studies of radiographic evaluation of the genitourinary tract in 443 women with recurrent UTI, only four patients (1.0 percent) had abnormalities (urethral diverticuli in three) that affected subsequent management.[13-15] In view of these data, it is prudent to reserve x-ray studies, cystoscopy, or ultrasound for a small subset of patients: 1. those with acute pyelonephritis who fail to clinically improve after 48 to 72 hours of appropriate antibiotic therapy (to rule out underlying obstructive disease or abscess formation); 2. those who develop a relapse after 6 weeks of antibiotic therapy; and 3. those who develop reinfections while on chronic suppressive antibiotic therapy.

Therapy

Asymptomatic Bacteriuria. The presence of asymptomatic bacteriuria, or its eradication, has not been demonstrated to have positive clinical impact in otherwise healthy patients, with the exception of asymptomatic bacteriuria during pregnancy. In an occasional patient, however, it may predict the subsequent occurrence of symptomatic episodes. In view of this fact, I believe that it is reasonable to utilize single-dose therapy once (see following), but that repeated courses of antibiotic therapy are not indicated.

Acute Dysuria-Frequency Syndrome. I recommend single-dose antibiotic therapy for patients who present without clinical evidence of upper tract infection. Pyuria and bacteriuria should be documented by urinalysis.

The need for urine culture prior to treatment has been debated,[1] although most experts agree on the need for a culture within 4 to 7 days *after* therapy. The absence of pyuria may justify withholding therapy and evaluating the patient for vaginitis. Pyuria without bacteriuria suggests the diagnosis of a chlamydial infection for which a 7-day course of tetracycline or erythromycin is effective. In general, women with dysuria in the absence of pyuria rarely have benefited from antimicrobial therapy.[6]

Currently used single-dose antibiotic regimens are listed in Table 34–1. Success rates of 70 to 95 percent have been obtained with these regimens, a rate equivalent to, but less expensive and better tolerated than, conventional 10- to 14-day therapy. Moreover, at least 50 percent of patients who fail single-dose therapy have also failed conventional treatment. In approximately 200 of the single-dose treatment failures reported, clinical symptoms and signs have been no worse than those initially present, and no subsequent bacteremias, hospitalizations, renal failure, or deaths have occurred.[1]

Single-dose therapy should *not* be used in patients:

1. With clinical evidence suggesting upper tract infection (fever, flank pain or tenderness, gastrointestinal symptoms)
2. With symptoms lasting more than 7 days prior to seeking medical attention
3. Who are potentially unreliable and who may not return for a follow-up urine culture 4 to 7 days following treatment
4. Who are pregnant
5. With underlying renal disease or immunocompromised states

These five groups of patients should be treated with a conventional 10- to 14-day regimen as described in Table 34–2. Patients who relapse following either single-dose or conventional therapy should be treated with 4 to 6 weeks of appropriate antibiotics and reevaluated.

Recurrent Symptomatic Urinary Tract Infections. Women with recurrent episodes of symptomatic urinary tract reinfections should be evalu-

TABLE 34–1 Single-dose Oral Antibiotic Regimens

Drug	How Supplied	Dosage
Trimethoprim-sulfamethoxazole	80 mg trimethoprim/400 mg sulfamethoxazole	4 tablets
	160 mg trimethoprim/800 mg sulfamethoxazole	2 tablets
Trimethoprim	100 mg	2 tablets
Sulfisoxazole	500 mg	4 tablets
Amoxicillin	500 mg	6 capsules

TABLE 34-2 Conventional 10- to 14-Day Oral Antibiotic Regimens

Drug	Dosage
Trimethoprim-sulfamethoxazole	160 mg/800 mg q12h
Trimethoprim	100 mg q12h
Sulfisoxazole	500 mg q6h
Ampicillin	250 to 500 mg q6h
Amoxicillin	250 to 500 mg q8h
Cephalexin	250 to 500 mg q6h
Cefaclor	250 to 500 mg q8h
Nitrofurantoin macrocrystals	50 to 100 mg q6h
Nalidixic Acid	1 g q6h
Carbenicillin*	382 to 764 mg q6h
Norfloxacin	400 mg q12h
Ciprofloxacin	250–500 mg q12h

* Recommended only for treatment of *Pseudomonas* species resistant to other oral agents

ated for the risk factors described previously. If none are present or modifiable, several prophylactic antibiotic regimens are available (Table 34–3).

Chronic urinary acidification with either methenamine mandelate or methenamine hippurate plus ascorbic acid is an effective approach. Its usefulness is limited by the need to take eight (or more) pills daily and to frequently measure urinary pH to ensure a value of 5.5 or lower.

Chronic low-dose antibiotic prophylaxis with either nitrofurantoin, 50 mg daily, or nitrofurantoin macrocrystals, 100 mg daily, also is effective in preventing recurrent infection. Unfortunately, adverse effects, such as acute pulmonary hypersensitivity reactions, chronic interstitial pneumonitis, blood dyscrasias, hepatic toxicity, and neuropathy (the last occurring predominantly in patients with preexisting renal dysfunction), have limited their widespread use. Trimethoprim-sulfamethoxazole (TMP/SMZ), 40 mg trimethoprim/200 mg sulfamethoxazole (1/2 tablet of regular strength Bactrim or Septra) every other day, is probably the most commonly used prophylactic regimen currently employed. In patients allergic to sulfur-containing drugs, trimethoprim 50 or 100 mg every other day is useful.[16]

TABLE 34-3 Prophylactic Antibiotic Regimens

Drug	Dosage
Trimethoprim-sulfamethaxozole	40 mg/200 mg daily or every other day
Trimethoprim	100 mg daily or every other day
Nitrofurantoin macrocrystals	50 mg daily or every other day
Methenamine mandelate*	1 g q6h
Methenamine hippurate*	1 g q12h

* Effectiveness requires acidic urine pH. Concomitant ascorbic acid may be necessary to maintain urine pH below 5.5.

The effectiveness of these treatment regimens has been demonstrated in several studies. In one study, the frequency of recurrent UTI per woman per year treated with placebo, urinary acidification, or TMP/SMZ was 3.4, 1.6, and 0.15, respectively.[17] In a second study comparing TMP/SMZ with nitrofurantoin, the former was slightly more effective at preventing reinfections, but also resulted in a greater emergence of antibiotic resistance in the vaginal and rectal flora.[18] The appropriate duration of prophylactic therapy is unknown. Unfortunately, discontinuation of treatment after 6 to 12 months appears to result in a return to the pretreatment reinfection rate in most patients. In other words, chronic prophylaxis does not appear to have a lasting benefit. Nevertheless, a reasonable approach is to continue prophylaxis for 6 to 12 months, then stop the medication and simply observe the patient. Of interest, a recent study in young women with recurrent symptomatic UTI demonstrated that a patient-administered single-dose antibiotic regimen was equivalent to chronic prophylaxis in terms of clinical effectiveness and economic cost.[19] A subgroup of women with recurrent UTI temporally related to sexual intercourse has been successfully managed with the aforementioned dose of TMP/SMZ taken only following intercourse.

URINARY TRACT INFECTIONS IN MEN

Clinicoepidemiologic Features

Bacteriuria in males is rare before the age of 50 in the absence of prior genitourinary tract instrumentation. By the age of 70, the prevalence of bacteriuria in otherwise healthy men approaches 3 to 4 percent and increases to the 15 to 50 percent range in chronically ill institutionalized patients. Most (80 percent or more) recurrent UTI in adult males are relapses associated with either a prostatic focus of infection or a structural abnormality of the genitourinary tract (e.g., nephrolithiasis, pyelonephritic scarring, or obstructive disease). As in women, men with recurrent bacteriuria without genitourinary tract abnormalities have not developed progressive renal insufficiency during follow-up of up to 10 years.[20] In elderly men, the severity of coexisting disease, and not the presence of bacteriuria, correlates more closely with mortality.[5]

Diagnostic Evaluation

Symptoms of UTI in the male may be difficult to dissociate from those of prostatism. The symptoms include dysuria, frequency, urgency, hesitancy, and nocturia. Although the precise frequency of symptoms associated with UTI is unknown, in one study over 40 percent of patients with recurrent bacteriuria were asymptomatic[21]. Bogginess, tenderness, and/or enlargement of the prostate gland are helpful clinical findings. Pyuria is usually present on urinalysis. The diagnostic evaluation should include urine cultures collected during the initiation and midstream phases of urination, and then during and immediately following prostatic massage. If prostatic secretions are not expressed during massage, ejaculate can provide a suitable alternative for culture. Higher bacterial colony counts in specimens obtained during and after massage than in the voided samples indicate a prostatic site of infection. Additionally, an intravenous pyelogram with postvoid films is recommended for most patients.

Therapy

The choice of antibiotics is dictated by the results of urine culture and sensitivities. Members of the *Enterobacteriaceae* family, particularly *E. coli*, comprise the majority of bacterial pathogens, although enterococci and, rarely, anaerobic bacteria also cause UTI. Patients with acute prostatitis frequently are quite ill and have a high incidence of bacteremia. They should be hospitalized and initially treated with standard intravenous doses of an aminoglycoside and ampicillin until clinical improvement is observed. Subsequently, a 4-week course of TMP/SMZ or trimethoprim alone is recommended for gram-negative infections. Erythromycin or clindamycin is usually effective for gram-positive infections.[22] Similar choices of oral antibiotics are recommended for the treatment of chronic prostatitis. In this circumstance, both single-dose and conventional 14-day regimens are ineffective; 6 to 12 weeks of treatment are required to produce a significant cure rate.[21, 23] Follow-up cultures should be obtained. Relapse is not uncommon despite even these prolonged courses of therapy. Fortunately, most of these relapses are asymptomatic. Sterile urine may be obtained by the use of chronic, low-dose suppressive therapy with nitrofurantoin or, preferably, TMP/SMZ as described previously for women. The absence of symptoms or of significant underlying disease, should temper an overly aggressive approach to antibiotic therapy since the potential clinical benefit of prolonged suppression or prophylactic therapy has not been unequivocally demonstrated in men.

CATHETER-ASSOCIATED URINARY TRACT INFECTIONS

Hospital-acquired urinary tract infections account for 35 percent of all nosocomial infections. Two patients per 100 admissions develop a UTI, thus resulting in an estimated 500,000 infections yearly in the US.[7] The vast majority of these infections are associated with an indwelling urinary catheter.

It is estimated that life-threatening bacteremia develops in 1 percent of these infections (5,000 cases). The occurrence of a UTI in the presence of an indwelling catheter is associated with a substantially increased mortality rate. Platt et al reported a 14 percent excess mortality in such patients compared to uninfected catheterized patients despite similar age, sex, and severity of illness.[24]

Approximately 50 percent of patients with an indwelling catheter develop bacteriuria by the eighth day after insertion. A recent surveillance study in this group demonstrated that the appearance of only a single bacterial colony per milliliter of urine resulted in progression within 24 hours to at least 10^5 colonies per milliliter in 96 percent of cases.[25] Thus, any degree of bacteriuria is of concern. *E. coli* accounts for about 50 percent of these infections with *Proteus*, *Klebsiella*, *Pseudomonas*, *Enterobacter*, and *Serratia* species constituting most of the remaining pathogens. The bulk of these infections are asymptomatic, although *Serratia* and *Klebsiella* are associated with an inordinately high frequency of bacteremia. The risk of infection is about 5 to 10 percent per day and cannot be reduced by either daily meatal care or bladder irrigation with antimicrobial solutions. The incidence of upper tract involvement during these infections is unknown, although assays for antibody-coated bacteria have been positive in up to 30 percent of catheterized bacteriuric patients.[7]

The management of infection in the catheterized patient is clearly difficult. Careful thought must be given before a catheter is inserted, and the catheter should be removed at the earliest possible moment. Asymptomatic bacteriuria should not be treated if the catheter *cannot* be removed since the infection is usually not eradicated or is usually followed by the appearance of another resistant organism. Symptomatic infection should be treated, although the appropriate duration of therapy is unknown; 10 to 14 days with a standard antibiotic regimen appears reasonable. This regimen also is recommended for the treatment of bacteriuria in the presence or absence of symptoms if the catheter can be removed. In general, patients with chronic indwelling catheters rarely become symptomatic unless the catheter becomes obstructed or erosion of the bladder mucosa has occurred.[1] Although intermittent catheterization (estimated risk of infection for a single catheterization is about 0.2 percent) or the use of a suprapubic catheter has been advocated as being associated with fewer infections, there are little data in the form of controlled studies to support these claims. Aseptic insertion, good handwashing, regular emptying of the collection bag (which has been maintained at a level below the patient), and separation of infected patients from uninfected patients are prudent measures that may reduce the incidence of infection.[26] In addition, replacement of a catheter containing visible debris within the collection tubing also is recommended because of the potential for obstruction and/or bacterial colonization.

References

1. Rubin RH, Tolkoff-Rubin NE, Cotran RS. Urinary tract infection, pyelonephritis, and reflux nephropathy. In: Brenner BM, Rector FC Jr, eds. The kidney. 3rd ed. Philadelphia: WB Saunders, 1986:1085.

2. Freedman LR, Andriole VA. The long term follow-up of women with urinary tract infections. Proc 5th Int Congr Neph (Mexico City) 1974; 3:230–235.

3. Asscher AW, Chick S, Radfors N, et al. Natural history of asymptomatic bacteriuria in non-pregnant women. In: Brumfitt W, Asscher AW, eds. Urinary tract infection. London: Oxford University Press, 1973:51.

4. Dontas AS, Kasviki-Charvati P, Papanayiotou PC, Marketos SG. Bacteriuria and survival in old age. N Engl J Med 1984; 304:939–943.

5. Nordenstam GR, Brandberg CA, Oden AS, Svanborg Eden CM, Svanborg A. Bacteriuria and mortality in an elderly population. N Engl J Med 1986; 314:1152–1156.

6. Komaroff AL. Urinalysis and urine culture in women with dysuria. Ann Intern Med 1986; 104:212–218.

7. Turck M, Stamm W. Nosocomial infection of the urinary tract. Am J Med 1981; 70:651–654.

8. Nicolle LE, Harding GKM, Preiksaitis J, et al. The association of urinary tract infection with sexual intercourse. J Infect Dis 1982; 146:579–583.

9. Evans DA, Hennekens CH, Miao L, et al. Oral-contraceptive use and bacteriuria in a community-based study. N Engl J Med 1978; 299:536–537.

10. Fihn SD, Latham RH, Roberts P, Running K, Stamm WE. Association between diaphragm use and urinary tract infection. JAMA 1985; 254:240–245.

11. Shafik A. Role of hemorrhoids in the pathogenesis of recurrent bacteriuria with a new approach for treatment. Eur Urol 1985; 11:392–396.

12. Sobel JD, Kaye D. Host factors in the pathogenesis of urinary tract infections. Am J Med 1984; 76(5A):122–130.

13. Fair WR, McClennan BL, Jost RG. Are excretory urograms necessary in evaluating women with urinary tract infection? J Urol 1979; 121:313–315.

14. Engel G, Schaeffer AJ, Grayback JT, Wendel EF. The role of excretory urography and cystoscopy in the evaluation and management of women with recurrent urinary tract infection. J Urol 1980; 123:190–191.

15. Fowler JE Jr, Pulaski ET. Excretory urography, cystography and cystoscopy in the evaluation of women with urinary tract infection: a prospective study. N Engl J Med 1981; 304:462–465.

16. Stamm WE. Prevention of urinary tract infections. Am J Med 1984; 76(5A):148–154.

17. Harding GKM, Ronald AR. A controlled study of antimicrobial prophylaxis of recurrent urinary infection in women. N Engl J Med 1974; 291:591–601.

18. Stamey TA, Condy M, Mihara G. Prophylactic efficacy of nitrofurantoin macrocrystals and trimethoprim-sulfamethoxazole in urinary infections. N Engl J Med 1977; 296:780–783.

19. Wong ES, McKevitt M, Running K, et al. Management of recurrent urinary tract infections with patient-administered single-dose therapy. Ann Intern Med 1985; 102:302–307.

20. Freeman RB, Smith WM, Richardson JA, et al. Long-term therapy for chronic bacteriuria in men: USPHS cooperative study. Ann Intern Med 1975; 83:133–147.

21. Smith JW, Jones SR, Reed WP, et al. Recurrent urinary tract infections in men: characteristics and response to therapy. Ann Intern Med 1979; 91:544–548.

22. Meares EM Jr. Prostatitis. Kidney Int 1981; 20:289–298.

23. Gleckman R, Crowley M, Natsios GA. Therapy of recurrent invasive urinary-tract infections of men. N Engl J Med 1979; 301:878–880.

24. Platt R, Polk BF, Murdock B, Rosner B. Mortality associated with nosocomial urinary-tract infection. N Engl J Med 1982; 307:637–642.

25. Stark RP, Maki DG. Bacteriuria in the catheterized patient. What quantitative level of bacteriuria is relevant? N Engl J Med 1984; 311:560–564.

26. Kunin CM. Genitourinary infections in the patient at risk: extrinsic risk factors. Am J Med 1984; 76(5A):131–139.

PULMONARY DISEASE

35 | EVALUATION OF PATIENTS WITH HEMOPTYSIS

CHESTER H. MOHR, M.D.
LEONARD SICILIAN, M.D.

Coughing up blood is a common clinical problem and can range in severity from scant blood-streaking in the sputum to life-threatening hemorrhage. Proper therapy requires evaluation of the general health of the patient and the severity of bleeding and identification of the site of hemorrhage and its cause.

DEFINITION

An accurate definition of mild or moderate hemoptysis does not exist. We consider expectoration of more than 200 ml of blood in 24 hours as major hemoptysis. More than 400 ml of blood in 24 hours or 600 ml in 48 hours is defined as massive hemoptysis.[1-3] We will discuss generally the cause and diagnosis of hemoptysis, the initial approach to the patient with hemoptysis, and the evaluation and management of patients with either mild or major hemoptysis.

ETIOLOGY

The most common causes of any hemoptysis in order of frequency are tuberculosis, bronchiectasis, bronchitis and pneumonia, bronchogenic carcinoma, and lung abscess. In large studies done in the United States, the majority of patients with massive hemoptysis had chronic lung disease, primarily tuberculosis and bronchiectasis.[1] Less commonly, hemoptysis may result from pulmonary vasculitis, from foreign body aspiration, and from arteriovenous malformation. Hemoptysis also can occur in cardiovascular disorders, such as congestive heart failure, pulmonary embolism, or mitral stenosis, in which the lung parenchyma or airways are secondarily involved. The severity of hemoptysis in any given disorder varies substantially and, therefore, does not aid in making a diagnosis.

DIAGNOSIS

Determination of the cause and the location of bleeding is essential to proper management. This is facilitated by bronchoscopy, which is mandatory in virtually all cases of hemoptysis. Flexible fiberoptic bronchoscopy (FFOB) can be performed safely in most patients and allows examination of the tracheobronchial tree to the subsegmental level, thereby resulting in precise localization of the bleeding site in the majority of patients.

It is a common misconception that bronchoscopy is useless in the briskly bleeding patient because blood overwhelms the suction capabilities of the instrument and obscures the visual field. However, more than 85 percent of bleeding sites can be identified by bronchoscopy.[1,2,4] In addition, bronchoscopy allows direct collection of bacteriologic, cytologic, and biopsy specimens that can aid greatly in diagnosis. Bronchoscopy also allows the physician to plan therapeutic modalities such as balloon tamponade or to guide the angiographer to the proper lung segment when embolization is planned. FFOB has generally replaced rigid bronchoscopy in the evaluation of hemoptysis. However, the rigid bronchoscope should be considered for use in cases of massive hemorrhage or of hemoptysis attributable to a foreign body because of its superior ability to suction the airway and to remove large objects.

Angiography of the aortic arch and, in some instances, of the pulmonary artery can be used to identify the site of bleeding. Blood loss needs to be in the range of 1 to 2 ml per minute to be visualized. Angiography performed solely to define a bleeding site should be done only in those cases when bronchoscopy cannot accomplish this goal.

INITIAL APPROACH TO THE PATIENT

The occurrence of hemoptysis, even of small amounts of blood, should not be dismissed, but requires prompt, thorough evaluation. The urgency of evaluation is dependent primarily on the rate of bleeding. In several studies the immediate outcome of patients was closely correlated with the rate of hemoptysis. In one series the overall mortality rate was 37 percent in patients expectorating more than 600 ml of blood in 48 hours, and rose to 75 percent in patients losing more than 600 ml of blood in 16 hours.[3] The degree of urgency also is determined in part by the general medical condition of the patient. Since chronic cardiopulmonary disease usually coexists with hemoptysis, the patient needs to be able to tolerate work-up and therapy that often is invasive.

The initial evaluation begins with a thorough, precise history. The duration and estimated volume of the hemorrhage and any prior episodes of bleeding should be determined. The presence of fever, weight loss, cough, or dyspnea should be determined to gain some idea of chronicity and of the extent of any underlying disease. Pertinent environmental exposures, including exposures to tuberculosis and to asbestos, along with a present or past history of cardiovascular disease should be sought diligently.

Physical examination centers around evaluation of the chest and upper airways. Auscultation of the chest may reveal localizing signs such as consolidation or rubs in almost half of the patients. Just as often, however, no localizing signs are present.[1] Abnormal findings must be interpreted with caution because, in a small percentage of cases, inaccurate, equivocal, or bilateral findings may complicate the picture. Bilateral abnormalities on physical examination often arise as a result of aspirated blood from a distant bleeding site that itself remains clinically silent.[1] Examination of the lungs also gives information concerning the presence and severity of underlying pulmonary disease, such as chronic obstructive pulmonary disease (COPD). Cardiac examination may reveal the presence of murmurs or gallops. Clubbing of the digits suggests longstanding pulmonary disease, particularly chronic suppurative disease or thoracic neoplasms. Detailed examination of the nose and oropharynx is essential to exclude a nasopharyngeal source of bleeding where the hemoptysis is caused by aspirated blood being coughed back up.

The presence and degree of respiratory compromise needs immediate assessment because death from hemoptysis usually occurs from asphyxiation rather than from hemodynamic compromise secondary to blood loss. Arterial blood gas (ABG) evaluations reflect the adequacy of gas exchange and the need for supplemental oxygen or mechanical ventilation. Initial laboratory screening must include a hematocrit to help quantitate blood loss. Platelet count and coagulation profile (prothrombin time [PT], partial thromboplastin time [PTT], bleeding time) are necessary to screen for an underlying coagulopathy. The chest roentgenogram localizes the site of bleeding in approximately 60 percent of cases,[1] but can be entirely normal. Furthermore, bleeding may occur at sites anatomically distant from areas of radiologic lung involvement, again as a result of aspiration of blood from a distant site of pathology. Sputum samples must be screened for abnormal cytology and for infectious agents in an attempt to define the cause of the bleeding.

EVALUATION OF MILD HEMOPTYSIS

Blood-streaking of sputum commonly occurs secondary to inflammatory or neoplastic disorders of the lung and to congestive heart failure (CHF) of any cause. Appropriate therapy based on information obtained from the history, the physical examination, and laboratory data should be the initial step in management of this type of hemoptysis (e.g., antibiotics for pneumonia, salt restriction and furosemide for congestive heart failure). Tuberculin skin testing should be performed, and the sputum should be examined for acid-fast bacilli if the skin test is positive or if the chest roentgenogram suggests tuberculosis.

Blood-streaked sputum that is recurrent or persistent commonly presents a dilemma for the clinician, especially if hemoptysis occurs during an upper respiratory infection or bronchitis. The bleeding in these instances could simply be attributable to leakage from engorged vessels in the submucosa of the airways as a result of the hyperemia seen with viral or bacterial infection. Judicial follow-up may be the most appropriate form of management in these cases. On the other hand, the bleeding could be the first sign of a new serious lung disease (e.g., carcinoma) that has been unmasked by an otherwise typical bronchitis. In this case immediate evaluation is indicated. The association of a history of smoking or of constitutional symptoms such as weight loss or fatigue raises the concern of malignancy, and these patients require a more rapid and extensive work-up.

While no simple solution exists to resolve this dilemma, we believe that, if the chest film is abnormal and if the history and clinical findings do not support the diagnosis of an acute treatable infection, then FFOB should be undertaken immediately. FFOB is preferably performed while blood is still present in the sputum since this gives the greatest chance of positively identifying the bleeding site. In any event, biopsies of any suspicious airway lesion or infiltrate noted on the x-ray film should be performed at this time. If no airway lesions are found and if biopsy or cytologic specimens from an infiltrate are not diagnostic for tumor or infection, the patient should be followed closely. Follow-up chest x-ray in 6 to 8 weeks is recommended if FFOB is nondiagnostic and hemoptysis has ceased. A chest film that has returned to normal coupled with an initial FFOB that reveals no evidence of tumor or infection is sufficient to negate further work-up. Finally, if the x-ray film remains abnormal or if any hemoptysis continues, further work-up is necessary and often requires a repeat FFOB, transthoracic needle biopsy, or open lung biopsy, especially if there is a high suspicion of a malignancy.

In patients with mild hemoptysis and a normal chest roentgenogram, we obtain five sputum specimens for cytology and bacteriologic evaluation. If sputum cytology is suspicious for malignancy or if hemoptysis persists for more than 4 weeks, we then perform FFOB. In this setting there is a high likelihood of malignancy, even though there is nothing obvious on the chest film.[5] If the bronchoscopy reveals no evidence of malignancy, the long-term outcome is good and no further work-up is indicated, provided the hemoptysis resolves. We do suggest twice-yearly clinical and radiologic follow-up for a period of 2 years in these patients, even in the absence of symptoms.

We believe that FFOB may be delayed or avoided altogether in nonsmoking patients with streaky hemoptysis who have normal chest roentgenograms. Coagulation profile assessment, thorough otolaryngologic examination, tuberculin testing, and sputum cytology evaluation are mandatory. Close follow-up over a 3- to 6-month period with repeat chest x-ray is an acceptable form of management if the initial evaluation does not find a cause. FFOB should be performed if bleeding recurs at any time or if PPD or chest x-ray indicate a developing pulmonary process.

As defined, hemoptysis of less than 200 ml per 24 hours is minor. As a matter of routine, however, we work up patients with anything more than blood-streaked sputum (e.g., a tablespoonful of blood) as if they had major hemoptysis. It is clear, though, that the short-term prognosis is good since their hemoptysis is not immediately life-threatening.

EVALUATION OF MAJOR HEMOPTYSIS

Major hemoptysis can range in severity from 200 ml of expectorated blood per day to massive hemoptysis with risk of asphyxiation or exsanguination. In general, most patients with bleeding of more than 15 ml in 24 hours should be admitted to the hospital for observation and work-up. If the bleeding is massive or if there is evidence of respiratory or hemodynamic compromise, admission to an intensive care unit is mandatory.

The patient should be placed at bedrest with the site of bleeding (if it is known) in a dependent position to prevent aspiration of blood into the nonbleeding lung. Prior to any radiologic or bronchoscopic documentation, many patients can localize the site of bleeding by pointing to an area on their chest. The physiologic reason for this is not known, but it is always helpful to ask the patient where he or she thinks the blood is coming from. This may aid in proper positioning in bed and may direct the physician to the bleeding site during FFOB.

Additional management includes supplemental oxygen, mild cough suppression, and sedation if necessary. Chest physical therapy and forced expiratory maneuvers should be avoided to prevent exacerbation of bleeding. Empiric treatment should be started while awaiting definitive diagnosis if a specific cause of the hemoptysis (e.g., pneumonia, pulmonary embolus) is suspected, based on the admission history, the physical examination, and the laboratory data.

In general, when indicated, FFOB should be performed as early as possible to facilitate diagnosis as well as to definitively localize the site of bleeding. The latter is important if bleeding does not cease and surgery becomes necessary.

When bleeding is massive, defined as bleeding greater than 50 ml per hour or 400 ml in 24 hours, initial efforts must be directed to ensure that the normal lung and bronchial tree are protected from the bleeding site. As we noted earlier, death with massive hemoptysis most commonly occurs from aspiration of blood into the noninvolved lung with resultant asphyxiation. If positioning of the patient is inadequate to prevent aspiration, the bleeding lung can be isolated by use of a double-lumen endotracheal tube or by insertion of a regular cuffed endotracheal tube into the nonbleeding lung.[6] Either procedure allows independent ventilation of the nonbleeding lung. If bronchoscopy is performed, attempts to tamponade the bleeding can be made by wedging the bronchoscope into the bleeding segment or by placement of a balloon-tipped arterial catheter (Fogarty or a similar type) into the bleeding segmental or subsegmental bronchus under direct visualization. If possible, tamponade should be carried out for 24 to 48 hours.[4] Often, however, the patient's cough displaces the catheter. Reports of successful therapy with Pitressin or with iced saline lavage via the tamponade catheter have been published,[7] but these cannot be recommended as standard procedure.

Patients with massive hemoptysis and adequate pulmonary reserve who do not respond to the aforementioned measures and who have localized disease should be considered for surgical therapy to control bleeding.[8] The decision to perform surgery is not reached easily. The operative mortality is 15 to 30 percent for unstable patients and 12 percent for patients having elective procedures.[2,9,10] The mortality rate, however, is up to 75 percent in patients treated with medical therapy alone.[9] The series reporting these results suffer from bias in patient selection; however, the data generally support surgical intervention in appropriately selected patients with massive hemoptysis.

Determination of who is an appropriate surgical candidate is often problematic. In many instances, little is known about the patient's pulmonary function prior to hemoptysis. Some idea may be obtained by a careful history. Patients with dyspnea at rest or with minimal exertion or those with evidence of cor pulmonale tolerate resection of a bleeding lobe or segment poorly, if at all. Spirometry consisting of forced vital capacity and forced expiratory volume in 1 second (FEV_1) maneuvers gives the best information about surgical risk. Unfortunately, most patients with massive hemoptysis are unable to perform the tests adequately. In cases where the FEV_1 is known prior to the illness, the decision-making process is simpler. In general, patients have sufficient pulmonary reserve to tolerate a lobectomy if their FEV_1 is greater than or equal to 1.6 to 2.0 L. Patients with hypoxemia on room air or with hypercarbia are poor surgical candidates, as are those with hemodynamic compromise secondary to blood loss.

Preoperatively it is mandatory to have accurate localization of the bleeding site and a diagnosis of the cause of bleeding (e.g., carcinoma, foreign body). This usually can be accomplished by bronchoscopy or, in some instances, by angiography. Once identified, definitive surgery consists of removing the involved lobe or segement. Occasionally a pneumonectomy is necessary.

In addition to poor pulmonary reserve, definitive surgical treatment often is precluded by several factors associated with the underlying disease causing the hemoptysis. Patients with far-advanced bilateral or active tuberculosis, bilateral bronchiectasis of any cause (e.g., cystic fibrosis, immunoglobulin deficiency), or end-stage pulmonary fibrosis are not surgical candidates because they usually cannot afford further loss of functioning lung via surgery.[11] In addition, those patients with hemoptysis secondary to unresectable carcinoma are not appropriate for major thoracic surgery. If a specific bleeding site or a localized surgical target cannot be identified, surgery is contraindicated.

Angiography with embolization should be considered for patients who, for whatever reason, are not surgical candidates and who fail to respond to medical therapy. There are several large series of study in which angiographic localization of the bleeding site combined with embolization (with Gelfoam) resulted in control of hemorrhage in more than 80 percent of cases.[12,13] Although bleeding is usually from the bronchial circulation, examination of the pulmonary arterial circulation also is recommended.[13] Embolization is frequently palliative because vascular collaterals often form. Nevertheless, the procedure, if successful, allows for stabilization of the patient and, in certain instances, gives time for any necessary bacteriologic or antineoplastic treatment. A major potential complication of embolization is spinal cord infarction from avulsion or occlusion of the anterior spinal artery, which arises close to the origin of the bronchial artery. This risk appears quite small if strict attention is paid to anatomic detail and if the angiographer is experienced.

Another potential nonsurgical means of controlling bleeding is the use of the neodymium YAG (Nd:YAG) laser to coagulate bleeding sites. This may have as its major use treatment of bleeding associated with bronchial neoplasms in the central airways. There is presently not enough experience with this method of treating hemoptysis, however, to define a specific set of guidelines or indications for use.

References

1. Pursel S, Lindskog G. Hemoptysis. Am Rev Respir Dis 1961; 84:329–336.
2. Crocco J, Rooney J, Fankushen D, DiBenedetto R, Lyons H. Massive hemoptysis. Arch Intern Med 1968; 121:495–498.
3. O'Connor J, Wetstein L. Evaluation and management of hemoptysis. Hospital Physician 1986; Vol. 22:11–16.
4. Saw E, Gottlieb L, Tokoyama T, Lee B. Flexible fiberoptic bronchoscopy and endobronchial tamponade in the management of massive hemoptysis. Chest 1976; 70:589–591.
5. Richardson R, Zavala D, Mukerjee P, Bedell G. The use of fiberoptic bronchoscopy and brush biopsy in the diagnosis of suspected pulmonary malignancy. Am Rev Respir Dis 1974; 109:63–66.
6. Gourin A, Garzon A. Control of hemorrhage in emergency pulmonary resection for massive hemoptysis. Chest 1975; 68:1, 120–121.
7. Magee G, Williams M. Treatment of massive hemoptysis with intravenous pitressin. Lung 1982; 160:165–169.
8. Massive hemoptysis. Br Med J 1978; 1:1570.
9. Gourin A, Garzon A. Operative treatment of massive hemoptysis. Ann Thorac Surg 1974; 18:52–59.
10. McCollum W, Mattox K, Guinn G, Beall A. Immediate operative treatment for massive hemoptysis. Chest 1975; 67:152–155.
11. Muthuswamy P, Akbik F, Franklin C, Spigos D, Barker W. Management of major or massive hemoptysis in active pulmonary tuberculosis by bronchial arterial embolization. Chest 1987; 92:77–82.
12. Remy J, Arnaud A, Fardou R, Volsin C. Treatment of hemoptysis by embolization of the bronchial arteries. Radiology 1977; 122:33–37.
13. Uflacker R, Kaemmerer A, Picon P, Rizzon C, Neves C, et al. Bronchial artery embolization in the management of hemoptysis: technical aspects and long term results. Radiology 1985; 159:637–644.

36 | MANAGEMENT OF ACUTE ASTHMATIC ATTACKS

LEONARD SICILIAN, M.D.

To the generalist, asthma often is perceived as a straightforward disease that is managed simply by a combination of patient education and various bronchodilators. While true for the stable asthmatic, status asthmaticus, defined here as the failure of an acute asthma attack to respond to the patient's usual medications, is a different problem altogether. Acute asthma accounts for over a million days of combined hospitalization and emergency room visits per year in the United States.[1,2] More importantly, unlike chronic bronchitis and emphysema where death usually occurs following a long illness, death in asthma occurs during the acute attack, often before the patient reaches the hospital.[3] Even though the actual number of deaths is small (about 2,000 per year in the United States),[2] the fact that the deaths are, in theory, all preventable and that they occur in patients who otherwise would live many more years makes it obligatory that the physician understand and respect the seriousness of the disease. There is no way to predict either the severity of an asthma attack or which patients are at risk for complications or death.[4,5] Those with prior severe attacks are prone to recurrent episodes, but even patients with apparent mild asthma are not immune to severe attacks. It is therefore incumbent on the physician both to recognize a severe attack and to promptly institute appropriate therapy.

THE LUNG IN STATUS ASTHMATICUS

Pathologically, an acute asthmatic attack is characterized by spasm of the bronchial smooth muscle. If the attack is longstanding, muscular hypertrophy occurs. The precise initiators of the muscle spasm are unknown. Physical agents such as cold air or noxious fumes and gases can directly stimulate smooth muscle contracture. Newer data implicate local mediators of inflammation, especially prostaglandins, as having a central role in the initiation and perpetuation of airway reactivity. If the muscular spasm goes untreated, these local inflammatory mediators produce edema of the mucosa of the airways and increased mucus secretion, thus resulting in plugging of the airways. This biphasic process of muscle spasm followed by hypertrophy, edema, and plugging probably is the reason that early treatment of acute attacks can be accomplished with beta-adrenergic agonists alone, since these drugs are effective in reversing muscular spasm. Beta-agonists, however, are not as effective in opening airways blocked by edema and secretions. This latter situation usually requires the addition of other bronchodilators (xanthines), anti-inflammatory agents (corticosteroids), and physical measures (chest percussion or mucolytic agents) to help reverse obstruction of the airways. The variability in the intensity and type of therapy for acute asthmatic attacks noted in the medical literature is a result of the variability of these many factors in the individual patient at a given moment in time. The longer the duration of the attack prior to treatment, the greater the chance that factors other than simple bronchial smooth muscle spasm are at play and, therefore, the longer and more intense needs be the therapy.[1]

Spasm, edema, and mucus secretions, in turn, lead to increased resistance to airflow, primarily in the large airways. This increased airway resistance results in two pathophysiologic phenomena. First, the work of breathing is increased, resulting in increased oxygen consumption and increased carbon dioxide production. Second, ventilation-perfusion mismatching increases, invariably leading to hypoxemia. As long as the forced expiratory volume in 1 second (FEV_1) remains greater than 25 percent of normal, the increased respiratory rate associated with the acute attack maintains an increased alveolar ventilation. This hyperventilation results in the usual finding of hypocarbia and respiratory alkalosis when arterial blood gases are obtained early in the attack. However, if the FEV_1 falls below this value, alveolar ventilation decreases; the resultant rise in PCO_2 causes respiratory acidosis and heralds ventilatory failure. This, combined with tissue hypoxemia (lactic acidosis), predisposes the patient to cardiac dysrhythmias and sudden death.

ACUTE MANAGEMENT

When a patient in status asthmaticus presents to the emergency room or the physician's office, *immediate* action is mandatory. A quick review of the patient's asthma history should be obtained with emphasis on current medications, compliance, and duration of the present attack. As a rule of thumb, if the patient has been in status for 2 to 3 days and especially if the patient has been unable to eat or sleep, it is unlikely that the attack will be "broken" as an outpatient, and hospital admission is almost certain. The physician also must remember that acute wheezing and dyspnea can be caused by pulmonary edema, upper airways obstruction, and pulmonary embolus, and that consideration must be given to these possibilities before rushing headlong into the treatment of acute asthma.

If at all possible, an arterial blood gas (ABG) sample should be obtained in a severe asthmatic attack. Usually the ABG shows hyperventilation (PCO_2 less than 37 mm Hg), a mild respiratory alkalosis (pH greater than 7.42), and mild to moderate hypoxemia (PO_2 between 60 to 80 mm Hg). Acidosis (pH less than 7.36), carbon dioxide retention (PCO_2 greater than 43 mm Hg), and severe hypoxemia (PO_2 less than 60 mm Hg) should alert the physician that the attack is extremely severe. One of the factors virtually always present in fatal cases is tissue hypoxemia; therefore supplemental oxygen by nasal prongs or face mask should be given immediately. In contrast to patients with chronic carbon dioxide retention whose drive to breathe is based on hypoxemia, in asthma the drive to breathe is based largely on the triggering of irritant receptors in the lung. Therefore, respirations in the asthmatic usually are not suppressed by supplemental oxygen, and oxygen should be administered even before the results of the ABGs are known. Oxygen should be given prior to the use of beta-agonists since these agents cause pulmonary artery dilatation before bronchodilatation, thus resulting in worsening of the ventilation-perfusion mismatch and further hypoxemia. In most cases, 2 to 4 L per minute of oxygen by nasal prongs or a 24 to 35 percent Venturi mask is adequate to prevent severe hypoxemia. The goal of oxygen treatment is a PO_2 in the 70 to 80 mm Hg range, using serial ABG measurements as a guide.

Beta-agonists are the mainstay of status asthmaticus treatment (Table 36-1). Although epinephrine (1/1,000 0.3 to 0.5 ml subcutaneously) given every 20 minutes for three doses is considered the standard first-line therapy, recent studies have shown that all beta-agents, whether inhaled or given subcutaneously, are equally effective.[1] While it is preferable to use the newer, more airway-selective beta$_2$-sympathomimetics, cardiac side effects are common with the frequent dosing used in emergency therapy. Thus, these drugs should be used with caution in patients with preexisting hypertension, heart disease, or dysrhythmias. Although inhaled beta-agents usually are used every 2 to 4 hours, some authors recommend continued usage until the bronchospasm lessens or the pulse rate rises above 140 beats per minute.[1] Patients often state that their "puffer" (metered dose inhaler) is no longer working. This should not dissuade one from using beta-agonists in the acute setting since tachyphylaxis does not occur with the newer drugs.[6] Proper drug delivery depends on proper use of the hand-held nebulizer. The patient should be encouraged to take deep breaths and to hold them as long as possible. It is not necessary to use the nebulizer with each breath, but it should be taken at least once or twice a minute. Therefore, a Y-tube should be employed so that the loss of medication into the atmosphere is minimized.[7] Also a "spacer" of not more than 10 cm in length should be used between the nebulizer and the mouth to facilitate the inhalation of particles of the size that will reach the lower respiratory tract.

Methylxanthines (theophylline or aminophylline) recently have received less attention in the treatment of status asthmaticus,[1] mostly as a result of the

TABLE 36-1 Pharmacotherapy of Status Asthmaticus: Commonly Used Drugs

Drug	Dosage and Route of Administration	Comments
Beta-sympathomimetics*		
Epinephrine	0.3 to 0.5 ml 1/1,000 solution subcutaneously q20 min x 3	Onset of action 1 to 15 min Aerosolized and subcutaneous drug similarly effective
Isoetharine (Bronkosol)	0.25 to 0.5 ml 1% solution† q2 to 4h	Use cautiously in patients with cardiovascular disease
Metaproterenol (Alupent)	0.2 to 0.3 ml 5% solution† q4 to 6h	Side effects similar at high doses despite β 2 selectivity
Albuterol (Ventolin)	0.25 to 0.5 ml 0.5% solution† q6 to 8h	Can increase dosing frequency under close observation to achieve desired bronchodilation
Methylxanthines		
Aminophylline	Loading: 5 to 6 mg/kg IV over 20 min Maintenance: 0.5 to 0.6 mg/kg/hr IV infusion	Maintenance dosage needs to be adjusted based on age, smoking, etc. (see text) Periodic serum levels necessary
Corticosteroids		
Methylprednisolone	40 to 125 mg IV q6h	Dosage not agreed upon
Hydrocortisone	2 to 4 mg/kg IV q6h	Use for ≤ 72 hr, then taper if patient improving
Anticholinergics		
Atropine	0.025 to 0.05 mg/kg† q4 to 6h	Use only when bronchodilation has been documented with spirometry
Ipratropium bromide (Atrovent)	36 μg (2 puffs) metered dose inhaler q4 to 6h	

* Partial list of beta-agonists. Isoproterenol (Isuprel) and terbutaline (Brethine) among others commonly used.

† Via compressed air-driven hand-held nebulizer. Dilute drug with approximately 3 ml of normal saline solution unless premixed unit dosage of drug available.

more aggressive use of beta-agents. However, the bronchodilatory properties of the xanthines are well known. If a significant reduction in symptoms is not forthcoming within 30 minutes of the use of subcutaneous or inhaled beta-agonists, then aminophylline by intravenous infusion should be started. If the patient has not been using an oral theophylline preparation, a loading dose of aminophylline of 5 to 6 mg per kilogram over 20 minutes should be given. If the patient has taken theophylline in the immediate preattack period, then the loading dose may be omitted if less than 18 hours have elapsed since the last dose of a long-acting oral preparation. Eight to 12 hours should pass if a short-acting oral theophylline has been used. With the advent of serum theophylline levels, the guesswork has been taken out of calculating the maintenance dose of aminophylline. Initially, a maintenance dose of 0.5 to 0.6 mg per kilogram per hour should be used in adult nonsmokers. This dose should be halved in patients with known liver disease, alcohol abuse, and congestive heart failure. Children less than 9 years old and current smokers should start at 0.9 mg per kilogram per hour. After the infusion has begun, serum theophylline levels should be obtained at 12 and 24 hours and the dose adjusted to keep the theophylline level in the middle to upper limits of the therapeutic range (10 to 20 μg per milliliter).

The physician should be alert to signs of aminophylline toxicity, nausea and headache being the most common early symptoms. At higher blood levels, seizures, arrhythmias, and cardiopulmonary arrest can occur. These symptoms do not progress in a stepwise fashion, and nausea or headache may not precede an arrhythmia or a seizure. This fact reinforces the need for periodic assays of the serum theophylline level.

Corticosteroids should be given at the outset of the treatment of status asthmaticus. The onset of the anti-inflammatory effect of these drugs may not be for 6 to 12 hours. Recent studies, however, have shown that the number of patients requiring hospital admission was reduced when steroids were given at the time that treatment in the emergency room (ER) was begun.[8] Thus, intravenous corticosteroids (hydrocortisone or methylprednisolone) should be given concomitantly with beta-agonist and aminophylline.[9] The decision to continue corticosteroids is based on the response to all forms of therapy. Even if the patient improves enough to be discharged from the ER, a short, tapering course (7 to 10 days) of corticosteroids usually is well tolerated. The exact dosage of corticosteroids required never has been adequately worked out.[9] I believe that a dose of 125 mg of methylprednisolone (or its equivalent) initially and every 6 hours is more than adequate in most cases of status asthmaticus.

Cromolyn sodium and inhaled corticosteroids have no place in the treatment of status asthmaticus and, in fact, may worsen bronchospasm if used in this setting. Although calcium-channel blockers have bronchodilatory properties, they are not as potent as the beta-agents and xanthines and at present are not recommended for use in status asthmaticus. Anticholinergic drugs (atropine, ipratropium bromide [Atrovent]) can be helpful in certain asthmatics. Their use in the United States has not been extensive thus far, however. I recommend these drugs in status asthmaticus only in patients who are refractory to oxygen, beta-agonists, theophylline, and steroids and who have demonstrated a significant bronchodilatory response by spirometry to these drugs in the past.

WHEN TO ADMIT

While the patient is being treated acutely as already described, a decision whether to admit the patient to the hospital or not needs to be made. Needless to say, this decision has to be individualized, but some guidelines are available. I allow the patient 2 hours (with frequent interim evaluations) to respond to intensive outpatient or emergency room treatment. If the patient has not significantly improved by that time, the patient is admitted. Mild to minimal improvement with therapy presents a dilemma; in these instances, the physician must ask, "Do I expect the patient to be sent home within the next 6 hours?" If the answer to this projection is no, then hospital admission should be arranged.

There are, however, certain instances when immediate admission, usually to an intensive care unit, is warranted. These situations either can be present at the time of initial evaluation or can develop during therapy. The major clinical criteria for immediate admission are (1) a disturbance of consciousness, which usually indicates impending respiratory collapse; (2) evidence of exhaustion, which results from the increased work of breathing; (3) a quiet chest or ineffective cough, indicating such severe airway obstruction that there is insufficient airflow to produce sound and, therefore, insufficient airflow to maintain alveolar ventilation; and (4) cyanosis, indicating severe hypoxemia.

The following laboratory criteria may be used as indication for immediate admission, even though the patient may not appear severely ill. These criteria are (1) infiltrates or atelectasis noted on chest roentgenography; (2) pneumothorax, pneumomediastinum, or subcutaneous emphysema; (3) FEV_1 of 0.5 L or less; and (4) pH less than 7.35, PCO_2 greater than 45 mm Hg, and PO_2 less than 60 mm Hg despite proper therapy.

Fever and a white blood cell count of greater than 15,000 per cubic milliliter unexplained by the use of corticosteroids are other factors that may prompt admission. Infection of any kind increases the demands on the respiratory system and, if present concomitantly with status asthmaticus, can result in exhaustion and respiratory failure.

MISCELLANEOUS FACTORS

There are several diagnostic and therapeutic interventions that are applicable only to certain patients with status asthmaticus. They are, however, important enough that the clinician needs to be aware of them and utilize them when appropriate.

Spirometry, measuring forced vital capacity (FVC), forced expiratory volume in one second (FEV_1), FEV_1/FVC, and peak flow, is a useful tool to determine the severity of the asthma attack (Table 36-2). If the patient is extremely anxious, this may be the most objective way to determine severity. However, patients are usually much more accurate in their own subjective assessment of the severity of their attack.[2] Coupled with this is the fact that

TABLE 36-2   Guide to the Assessment of Severity of an Acute Asthmatic Attack

| Severity | Symptoms | Attack Frequency | Spirometry* | | P_{CO_2} (mm Hg) |
			FEV_1 (L)	Peak Flow (L/min)	
Mild	Minimal, annoying	< 2/month	> 2.0	> 200	—
Moderate	Discomfort, occasionally interferes with normal activity	1 to 2/month	1 to 2	80 to 200	—
Severe	Nocturnal, occasionally in bed	> 3/week	< 1.0	< 80	< 35
Extremely Severe					
A	Refractory, unable to perform normal activity	Daily	~0.75 to 1.0	60 to 80	35 to 45
B	Immediate hospital admission	Continuous	~0.5 or unobtainable	<60 or unobtainable	> 45

* Mild or moderate attacks can severely impair spirometry, but this is transient. Therefore, there is considerable overlap of the parameters mentioned in this table.

accurate spirometry requires patient cooperation, and a patient in status may be too dyspneic to provide that cooperation. An accurate FEV_1 of less than 1 L represents a severe attack, and if values of 0.5 L or less are obtained, this correlates with a profound disturbance of alveolar ventilation.

When carbon dioxide retention occurs, the patient concomitantly develops respiratory acidosis. Lactic acidosis from tissue hypoxemia then can result in a severe combined acidosis in critically ill asthmatics. Treatment of the acidemia requires relief of the bronchospasm and improvement in ventilation and oxygenation. However, when the patient is refractory to treatment, when intubation is imminent, and when acidemia is acute (pH less than 7.15), sodium bicarbonate ($NaHCO_3$) 1 to 2 mEq per kilogram intravenously over 20 minutes may be used as a temporizing measure to prevent more severe acidosis and the fatal arrhythmias that may ensue. It must be remembered that $NaHCO_3$ administered acutely raises P_{CO_2}, thus actually worsening hypercapnia, and its use should be reserved for extreme instances only.

When the patient is obviously fatigued (increased respiratory rate, diaphragmatic paradox, and so on) and alveolar ventilation continues to fall (increased P_{CO_2}), the time has come to intubate and mechanically ventilate the patient. There are no hard and fast criteria as to when this should be done, but it must be emphasized that this decision point can come upon one rapidly since labile bronchospasm can cause a deterioration of an already impaired respiratory system in a matter of a few minutes. The physician must then anticipate the need for mechanical ventilation and intubate the patient before respiratory arrest occurs.

The endotracheal tube is a double-edged sword. Access is provided to the lower respiratory tract to aid alveolar ventilation and secretion removal, but the tube is also an added burden to airway resistance and an irritating foreign body in the trachea that can stimulate further bronchospasm. Therefore, a tube of an internal diameter of at least 8 mm should be used whenever possible to minimize the added airway resistance. In addition, asthmatics do not require a lengthy weaning process from mechanical ventilation prior to extubation. Once the attack is broken and the patient has adequate respiratory mechanics (usually a vital capacity greater than 10 to 15 ml per kilogram and an inspiratory force of less than negative 20 cm H_2O), mechanical ventilation should be stopped and the patient extubated. This eliminates the endotracheal tube itself from being an ongoing cause of bronchospasm.

The use of sedation, paralysis, and general anesthesia occasionally is necessary in the treatment of status asthmaticus. Anxiety and restlessness during an acute asthmatic attack is caused by the sensation of dyspnea and chest constriction. Thus, the treatment is to relieve the bronchospasm. Agitation also can be caused by carbon dioxide retention and impending respiratory failure. The treatment for agitation is not sedatives (especially in the latter instance where it only worsens alveolar ventilation), but treatment of the bronchospasm. If agitation persists after intubation, especially if the patient is "fighting" the ventilator, sedation with a narcotic or a diazepam derivative may be helpful in allowing mechanical ventilation to take place and the respiratory muscles to rest. Occasionally sedatives are insufficient to accomplish this objective, and paralysis with pancuronium bromide (Pavulon)[7] is indicated so that ventilation can be controlled.

Neither of the preceding maneuvers lessen the bronchospasm. Thus, if the patient is sedated, paralyzed, and on maximal bronchodilator therapy and airway resistance is so high that adequate ventilation is still impossible, then a general anesthetic agent, which also aids in bronchial smooth muscle relaxation, should be used.[10] Halothane is currently the drug of choice. Drugs like d-tubocurare and succinylcholine should be avoided in this setting because they can cause histamine release and worsen the bronchospasm.

The clinician always must remember that a paralyzed ventilator-dependent patient is in a dangerous situation since inadvertent disconnection of the ventilator from the endotracheal tube means certain death.

References

1. Summer WR. Status asthmaticus. Chest 1985; 87:875–945.
2. Edelson JD, Rebuck AS. The clinical assessment of severe asthma. Arch Intern Med 1985; 145:321–323.
3. Bernstein IL. Treatment decisions of asthma based on a paradigm of clinical severity. J Allergy Clin Immunol 1985; 76:357–365.
4. Rose CC, Murphy JB, Schwartz JS. Performance of an index predicting the response of patients with acute bronchial asthma to intensive emergency department treatment. N Engl J Med 1984; 310:573–577.
5. Benatar SR. Fatal asthma. N Engl J Med 1986; 314:423–429.
6. McFadden ER Jr. Clinical use of β-adrenergic agonists. J Allergy Clin Immunol 1985; 76:352–356.
7. Cherniack RM. Comprehensive approach to asthma. Chest 1985; 87:945–975.
8. Fanta CH, Rossing TH, McFadden ER. Glucocorticoids in acute asthma. Am J Med 1983; 74:845–851.
9. Siegel SC. Overview of corticosteroid therapy. J Allergy Clin Immunol 1985; 76:312–320.
10. Hopewell PC, Miller RT. Pathophysiology and management of severe asthma. Clin Chest Med 1984; 5:623–634.

37 | RECURRENT PULMONARY INFECTIONS

DOUGLAS T. PHELPS, M.D.
LEONARD SICILIAN, M.D.

The internist frequently is asked to evaluate patients with recurrent pulmonary infections (RPI). Whereas a healthy individual may acquire a lower respiratory tract infection periodically, there are clear instances when the frequency or severity of the pulmonary infection is beyond the norm. Unfortunately, a precise definition of "abnormality" is not possible for this affliction because the spectrum of clinical presentation is so broad. Nevertheless, the first obstacle is to differentiate between recurrent disease that demands investigation and less frequent infection that simply requires acute treatment. The accepted hallmarks of recurrent disease are (1) incomplete clearing followed by recrudescence of clinical illness, (2) infection with the same organism, and (3) infection in the same location. In contrast, patients with less frequent infections have prolonged intervals of good health with clear chest x-rays, different sites of infection, and different organisms.

The entire clinical presentation needs to be taken into account when making a diagnosis of RPI. An arbitrary standard of "infections per year" is useless as a measure of frequency. Comparison of recurrent pneumonia in young adults to recurrent pneumonia in geriatric patients obviously is not helpful, while comparison to peers is more useful. Similarly, pulmonary infection in pediatric nurses exposed to children during respiratory syncytial virus season cannot be directly compared to those without such exposure. Despite these caveats, we believe that any young or middle-aged adult who has more than three or four documented lower respiratory tract infections per year demands at least some investigation. As well as frequency, severity and degree of impairment are important considerations in evaluating RPI. Obviously, a lower respiratory tract infection that lasts 3 or 4 weeks has a different significance than one lasting 3 or 4 days. The unremitting infection should alert the clinician to the possibility of an underlying pathologic process.

NORMAL HOST DEFENSE NETWORK

The host defense network against pulmonary infection is a multitiered system. Mechanical, inflammatory, and immune defenses block access to vital tissues and fluids. Mechanical protection is achieved by filters such as the nose, branching bronchial passages, and bronchial mucus. Multiple mechanical barriers to penetration exist such as the tight bronchial and alveolar epithelial junctions, reflex bronchospasm, and the larynx, which protects the respiratory tract from pharyngeal and upper gastrointestinal secretions. Finally, we have a clearance system comprised of cough, sneeze, and mucociliary escalator action. Together these factors form an impressive mechanical barrier to organisms capable of causing infection.

When barrier action fails, a second line of defense must be mounted. Entrapment and localization is accomplished via reflex vasospasm and dilatation. The resulting inflammatory reaction of swelling and transudation creates an "envelope" containing the spread of infection.

An integrated immune reaction comprises the third line of defense. Cellular immune responses bring polymorphonuclear leukocytes and macrophages to inflamed areas. Local hormonal signals (cytokines) are sent, which recruit T lymphocytes for their modulating and cytotoxic effects. The humoral response then facilitates the localization and destruction of foreign organisms and engorged phagocytes. Immunoglobulin M (IgM) is entrained from the distant blood pool while IgA, IgE, and IgG are synthesized locally. Complement and lymphokines join in as this elegant system overpowers foreign infectious invaders.

When faced with a patient with recurrent respiratory infections, it is necessary to consider a breakdown of these normal host defenses. Most commonly, explanations for RPI can be found in simple mechanical abnormalities (e.g., aspiration following a stroke), concurrent disease processes (e.g., chronic obstructive pulmonary disease [COPD]), or specific exposures. Occasionally there are occult explanations, such as obstructing endobronchial lesions, which can be discovered only with pointed investigation.

GENERAL CONSIDERATIONS

Conditions that interfere with the mechanical protection of the lower respiratory tract readily predispose to RPI. Obstructive diseases such as COPD or endobronchial malignancies result in stasis of bronchial secretions. Exposure to particulate matter may disrupt mucociliary clearance with similar results. Cranial nerve palsies or seizure disorders increase the risk of aspiration, and chronic sinus drainage can flood the normal laryngeal protection.

Disorders of immunity also may present as RPI. Profound immune suppression occurs as a result of steroid use, antineoplastic chemotherapy, and radiation to the chest. Subtle deficiencies can occur with more pervasive entities. Mild to moderate malnutrition can result in T lymphocyte imbalance with a resultant decline in cell-mediated immunity. Alcohol can impair granulocyte adherence at sites of injury. At moderate levels ethanol dulls bactericidal activity of the phagocytes, and at high levels it compromises mucociliary clearance of the respiratory tree. Diabetes, chronic renal failure, or cirrhosis all can lead to RPI through compromise of the immune system.[1]

Inflammatory conditions of the lung lead to RPI by creating a milieu susceptible to secondary infection. Chronic infections with *Mycobacterium* species or Epstein-Barr virus cause a mechanical compromise of clearance, systemic immune depression, and local barriers to immune penetration. Likewise, conditions such as septic or bland pulmonary emboli, sickle cell disease, or collagen vascular disease create conditions favorable to pulmonary infection.

In most of the patients we see for RPI, one or many of these predispositions is obvious and usually elucidated by a careful medical history. Special consideration must be given to the exceptional patient who is young or ostensibly healthy, but suffering from RPI. Likewise, when a patient has a known problem such as asthma, but seems to suffer a disproportionate number of pulmonary infections, one should again consider a more unusual underlying disease. A handful of uncommon entities also present as RPI, including bronchiectasis, immunoglobulin deficiency, immotile cilia syndrome, cystic fibrosis, phagocyte dysfunction, and complement deficiency. The most flagrant examples of these disorders are almost always diagnosed in childhood (e.g., cystic fibrosis), but more subtle presentations often escape diagnosis until adulthood. Therefore, some familiarity with the natural history and means of diagnosis is necessary to facilitate detection of these disorders, and we will now turn to a discussion of these entities.

BRONCHIECTASIS

Bronchiectasis is by far the most prevalent of the aforementioned disorders. This condition is an anatomic anomaly of the bronchial tree characterized by abnormalities in form and function and is the prototype of mechanical dysfunction that results in RPI; it is also the end result of several of the other diseases we will discuss (Table 37-1). The hallmark of bronchiectasis is dilatation of the cartilaginous airways, accompanied by destruction of the cartilaginous support structure, thereby changing a stiff conduit into a floppy tube. Persistent inflammation transforms the columnar mucosa into nonciliated cuboidal or squamous epithelium. This, together with the loss of structural integrity, results in compromise of cough and secretion clearance. In the milder form of cylindrical bronchiectasis the airways involved fail to taper as they branch to the periphery. The more extensive condition of saccular bronchiectasis is seen as dilated airways with multiple outpouchings or pseudo-diverticula.

TABLE 37-1   Causes of Bronchiectasis

Congenital	Acquired
Cystic fibrosis	Prolonged atelectasis
Pulmonary sequestration	Recurrent aspiration
Maunier-Kuhn disease	Foreign body
(tracheobronchomegaly)	Bronchial cancer
Williams-Campbell syndrome	Carcinoid
(bronchial cartilage deficiency)	Right middle lobe syndrome
Kartagener's syndrome	Infections
(bronchiectasis, sinusitis, situs inversus)	Granulomatous
Agammaglobulinemia/	Tuberculosis
hypogammaglobulinemia	Histoplasmosis
Chronic granulomatous disease of	Coccidioidomycosis
childhood	Viral
Yellow nail syndrome	Influenza
(yellow nails, lymphedema,	Varicella
bronchiectasis)	Rubeola
	Adenovirus
	Respiratory syncytial virus
	Bacteria
	Bordetella pertussis
	Acquired hypogammaglobulinemia

The incidence of anatomic bronchiectasis is surprisingly high. One study found that cylindrical bronchiectasis was present in 40 percent of patients with pneumonia. However, this form of bronchiectasis is reversible, and of those patients with pneumonia, only 10 percent had bronchiectasis 3 months after the pneumonitis.[2] Saccular bronchiectasis, on the other hand, is irreversible. The two forms appear to be distinct entities since the cylindrical form rarely progresses to the saccular form.

While anatomic bronchiectasis is relatively common, symptomatic disease is not. Bronchiectasis of the lower and dependent lung zones is usually more symptomatic than the upper lobe variety because gravity drains secretions from the latter location. Upper lobe bronchiectasis, generally caused by granulomatous infections, has hemoptysis as the prominent symptom of this "dry bronchiectasis". The primary symptoms of lower lobe disease are chronic cough and purulent sputum production, both of which may be positional. The quantity and character of the sputum is quite variable. Amounts may vary with time and can range from 20 to 500 ml per day. Typically, the sputum is dark and foul smelling, indicative of stagnation in the airways. Frequently there is hemoptysis of mild to moderate amounts of blood intermixed with purulent sputum. The most frequently cultured bacteria are *Hemophilus influenzae*, *Streptococcus pneumoniae*, and mixed anaerobes.

Localized bronchiectasis may present only as recurrent discrete infections. Pneumonias affecting the same segmental distribution may be separated by months or years without any intervening symptoms belying the chronic nature of the disease.[3] When localized disease is present, it usually affects the left lung (left to right ratio 9:7), presumably because of the smaller caliber of the airways on the left. Frequently, however, more than one lobe is involved and bilateral disease occurs in one-third of all patients.

There are many recognized causes, both congenital and acquired, for bronchiectasis (see Table 37-1). Acquired bronchiectasis results from prolonged or severe inflammatory conditions of the airways. The condition often begins with childhood pneumonias accompanied by atelectasis that leads to entrapment of secretions and suppuration, thus creating the proper environment for destruction of the bronchial walls.

The diagnosis of bronchiectasis is made on clinical grounds with radiographic confirmation. Plain chest roentgenograms are normal 10 percent of the time.[4] When chest films are abnormal, they may reveal clusters of cystic spaces 5 to 10 mm in diameter, ring shadows representing thickened bronchial walls, atelectasis, or the characteristic dilated bronchi with mucus impaction (finger-glove pattern) (Figs. 37-1 and 37-2). Unfortunately, although plain films are often abnormal, their specificity is poor. Confirmation of the diagnosis of bronchiectasis often requires computed tomographic (CT) or bronchographic documentation, especially when surgery is contemplated.[5]

The aim of treating bronchiectasis is to reduce recurrent infection and the resulting fibrosis of lung parenchyma. Usually there is no specific treatment for the underlying cause (except for hypogammaglobulinemia), so the brunt of therapy is aimed at the control of respiratory secretions. Postural drainage and chest physical therapy are the mainstays for keeping the airways clear. Antibiotics should be used when there is change in the amount or character of the sputum. Although there are no definitive studies, we believe that prophylactic antibiotics are efficacious in some patients. Studies in the 1950s showed improvement in cough and reduction in the quantity of sputum produced after treatment with oxytetracycline (500 mg twice a day) or oral penicillin.[6]

Before modern antibiotics, surgical resection of the involved lung was common. Later, enthusiasm waned because of reports that prognosis was unchanged in resected patients.[7] Today some centers perform pulmonary resections for all localized disease (excluding active tuberculosis). In a large series of 2,776 patients with bronchiectasis, le Roux et al report 1,003 (36 percent) surgical resections. In their pediatric group less than 10 years of age, 55 percent were treated with surgery. The procedures done on adults and children were often aggressive, including pneumonectomies, bilateral procedures, and simultaneous congenital heart repairs and pulmonary operations. Results are impressive, with 85 percent achieving satisfactory symptomatic

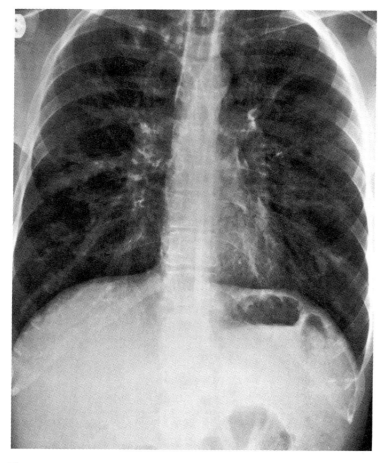

Figure 37-1 A roentgenogram of a 31-year-old male with cystic fibrosis and bronchiectasis. Several streaky densities representing branching bronchi impacted with mucus (arrows) are seen bilaterally.

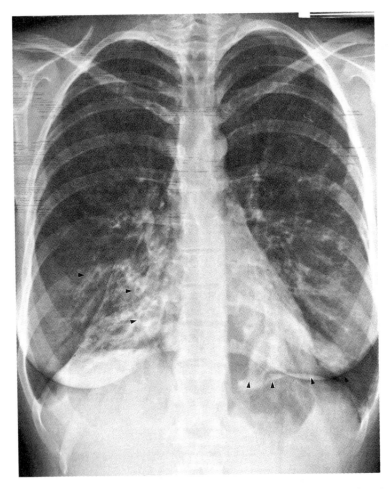

Figure 37–2   A roentgenogram of a 22-year-old woman with bronchiectasis of unknown etiology shows classic changes. In the right lung there is chronic atelectasis of the middle and lower lobes as well as several ring shadows (arrows) representing thickened bronchial walls. In the left chest there is the classic "finger–glove pattern" of mucus-filled ectatic bronchi (arrows).

results with a mortality of 2 percent. The unresected group had a mortality rate of almost 10 percent over 20 years.[4] Despite these impressive results, aggressive use of oral and parenteral antibiotics, especially those with potent gram-negative coverage, is the accepted form of therapy today.

IMMUNOGLOBULIN DEFICIENCY

Deficiencies of humoral immunity, another possible explanation for RPI, most commonly involve selective reduction in IgA levels. The estimated incidence is about 1 in 500 patients with a male to female ratio of 2 to 1. Many of the patients with IgA deficiency are asymptomatic, but as many as 70 percent suffer from RPI,[8] with the sequelae of bronchiectasis and emphysema. In addition, patients often have associated gastrointestinal (GI) problems, such as celiac disease or inflammatory bowel disease, and an increased incidence of autoimmune disorders, such as pernicious anemia, rheumatoid arthritis, lupus, chronic hepatitis, or allergies (asthma, allergic rhinitis, and eczema). Finally, there is also an increased incidence of gastrointestinal and pulmonary tumors with this disorder.[9]

Deficiency of IgG, congenital or acquired, is more unusual than that of IgA and often presents as recurrent infections of the lungs or sinuses. IgG is comprised of four subclasses of immunoglobulin; sometimes a single specific subclass of IgG may be low. Since types 3 and 4 only represent 10 percent of the total IgG level, a specific subclass deficiency may be easily overlooked. For patients with suspicious histories for RPI or bronchiectasis, we recommend quantitation of immunoglobulins, including IgG subclasses. Similarly, a combined IgA-IgG deficiency may be missed on a routine serum protein electrophoresis screen because IgM is often elevated in compensation; hence, the gamma peak appears normal.

Common variable immunodeficiency usually is diagnosed in adulthood. This acquired disorder manifests itself as a depression in one or all of the immunoglobulin classes in the fourth to seventh decades of life. IgG is the most commonly depressed class, but levels may wax and wane during the course of the conditions. Therefore, several determinations may be necessary before this disorder can be excluded. The onset is abrupt and affects males and females equally. The pathophysiology seems to implicate a maturation defect of B lymphocytes.[10] The lack of immunoglobulin results in frequent infections, especially with encapsulated organisms. Areas affected include the lungs, sinuses, middle ear, and GI tract (especially with *Giardia*). The lungs are the only site of infection in up to 50 percent of patients. Bronchiectasis may occur in as many as 30 percent of such patients as a sequelae of recurrent infections. As with IgA deficiency, there is an increased incidence of autoimmune disorders and malignancies in these patients, with tumors of the GI tract, lungs, and lymphatic system representing the leading cause of death.[11]

Early diagnosis of immunoglobulin deficiencies by means of protein electrophoresis and subtype determinations is important because specific therapy is possible. In the case of IgG deficiency, routine infusion of gamma globulin has been shown to reduce the morbidity of recurrent infections.[12] Monthly infusions or intramuscular injections are aimed at keeping IgG levels between 200 and 500 mg per deciliter.

Unfortunately, IgA cannot be replaced. Since secretory IgA is produced locally, systemic infusion is not helpful. Also, there is a high incidence of anaphylactic reaction to immunoglobulin infusion, and therefore, this therapy is relatively contraindicated in the IgA-deficient patient.

IMMOTILE CILIA SYNDROME

The immotile cilia syndrome was first described in 1976 by Afzelius in a group of patients with frequent infections involving the sinuses, middle ear, and respiratory tract.[13] Elegant electron microscopy (EM) showed structural abnormalities of the epithelial cilia and spermatids. Today this syndrome is a recognized cause for RPI, but a rare familial disorder, with an incidence of 1 in 15,000 to 30,000 individuals. Infertility and situs inversus are occasionally seen as part of the affliction. Indeed, Kartagener's syndrome (situs inversus, bronchiectasis, and sinusitis) is the prototype of this anomaly. Normally, ciliated epithelium and sperm have microtubules running through the cilium and flagellum, respectively. These microtubules are arranged with a central pair surrounded by nine additional pairs. These microtubule pairs then have small "dynein" arms that serve to affect movement. When cilia samples from affected patients are examined by cross-sectional EM, there are characteristic abnormalities in either dynein arms or anomalous formations of microtubules.

Immotile cilia syndrome often evades diagnosis until the second or third decades of life. Of course, situs inversus would be an immediate clue to the diagnosis, but more frequently the diagnosis is picked up during evaluations for infertility or recurrent sinopulmonary infections. There are several modalities designed to screen for abnormal mucociliary clearance. Aside from tracking radiolabeled or radiopaque particles and calculating their clearance velocities,[14] the most useful examinations are done directly on a small biopsy of the nasal or bronchial mucosa. Fresh samples can be examined for motility and fixed specimens analyzed by electron microscopy for structural abnormalities. The most sensitive and available test is the contrast examination for motility. A simple screening test may be performed with saccharin by placing a 1-mm particle of saccharin 1 cm back on the inferior turbinate of the nose. The time until the patient can taste the sweetness is then recorded, with times in excess of 30 to 60 minutes being abnormal.[15] The simplest screening procedure for males remains, however, the examination of sperm for motility.

CYSTIC FIBROSIS

Cystic fibrosis (CF), a well-known autosomal recessive disorder, usually is diagnosed in childhood. Severe respiratory infections combined with pancreatic insufficiency and failure to thrive make recognition and diagnosis of this disorder straightforward to the pediatrician. Despite the improved longevity of patients with CF, the average adult clinician has a relatively limited exposure to these patients. Because of the variable penetrance of the gene, there is a broad range of severity in this affliction. Indeed, a patient with a mild condition may escape diagnosis until adulthood. Patients may be virtually asymptomatic until the late teenage years when they develop a chronic productive cough. The milder forms of CF, which present later in life generally lack the GI disturbances that are so characteristic of the infantile presentation.

In the evaluation of a patient with RPI, there may be no specific clues to the diagnosis of CF. Helpful leads to the diagnosis include a family history of CF or sibling morbidity and mortality. However, one may only find a history of siblings with vague chronic respiratory symptoms. Atopy is common in patients with CF, but is nonspecific. Strong consideration of CF should be given in any patient whose respiratory tract is infected or colonized with *Staphylococcus aureus* or *Pseudomonas aeruginosa* (especially if mucoid strains are present). Likewise, if one notes diffuse streaky densities on chest roentgenograms or the classic cystic changes with pulmonary fibrosis, the diagnosis certainly should be pursued.

The most reliable tool for diagnosis of CF is the sweat test. Unfortunately, standard values for older patients are not always reliable. Sweat chloride values generally run higher in patients over 20 years old. Likewise sweat sodium may be elevated in 35 percent of older patients and in parents of children with cystic fibrosis who themselves are not affected. Sweat chloride values above 60 to 80 mEq per liter are consistent with CF, and conventional iontophoresis for sweat electrolytes remains the standard for diagnosis. In adults, high values should always be repeated to establish the diagnosis. Low values in the absence of edema (which may give false negatives) are often sufficient to exclude the diagnosis. The test should only be performed at a laboratory where it is done routinely and on a high volume basis (at least 100 tests per year). Because laboratory error is the most common cause of false positive results, the choice of centers greatly affects diagnostic accuracy. Beyond the technical aspects of the sweat test, it is important to be selective of patients referred for testing.

The specificity and positive predictive value of the test in adults are always dependent on appropriate clinical conditions in addition to the sweat chloride value.[16]

There is no specific therapy for CF; pulmonary toilet and antibiotics are the mainstay of treatment as with other causes of bronchiectasis. Recently, a few patients have undergone heart–lung transplantation to prolong life. In the future this may be a more realistic option in selected CF patients.

PHAGOCYTIC CELL DYSFUNCTION

Disorders of phagocyte function are usually diagnosed in childhood. Occasionally presentation may be delayed until early adult life. Phagocyte dysfunction may come from quantitative or qualitative inadequacies. The problems with reduced numbers of phagocytes are self-evident and manifest routinely in patients with certain hematologic malignancies and in those receiving cancer chemotherapy. Since phagocyte function encompasses chemotaxis, opsonization, ingestion, and intracellular killing, possible qualitative defects are broad and complex. Abnormal chemotaxis is seen in disorders such as the Chédiak-Higashi syndrome or the lazy leukocyte syndrome; it is most unusual for these to present in adulthood.

Intracellular killing of phagocytized organisms is fundamental to phagocyte function. Disorders of impaired intracellular killing include, again, Chédiak-Higashi syndrome, myeloperoxidase deficiency, and chronic granulomatous disease (CGD). Of these, CGD, a hereditary disease transmitted by X-linked or autosomal recessive inheritance, may occasionally present in the second or third decade of life. The most common adult presentation is one of pulmonary fibrosis.[11] History reveals recurrent necrotizing pneumonias, dermatitis, polyarthritis, or glomerulonephritis. Catalase-positive organisms such as staphylococci, *Escherichia coli*, *Aerobacter*, or *Klebsiella* are common pathogens isolated. Physical examination may show lymphadenopathy and hepatosplenomegaly, while blood studies may show leukocytosis and hypergammaglobulinemia. Because there is a problem with hydrogen peroxide production in the phagocytes, this condition is easily screened for with a nitroblue tetrazolium test. Once ingested, this compound is reduced by the polymorphonuclear leukocyte to a blue-black substance that can be seen as intracellular particles. The absence of these particles thus points to the diagnosis of CGD.

COMPLEMENT DEFICIENCY

Complement plays a synergistic role with the phagocyte in the disposal of pathogens. Deficiency of complement factors can arise from depletion and inadequate or dysfunctional production. The spectrum of disease and pathogens encountered with complement deficiency is similar to phagocyte deficiency. Functional abnormalities in, or low levels of, C3, C5, or C3b may result in recurrent pneumonias, ear and sinus infections, sepsis, and meningitis. Pyogenic organisms and fungi predominate the list of pathogens that are frequently isolated. Screening is best achieved with CH50 serum titers and quantitative C3 and C5 levels.[11]

Specific therapy for either complement deficiency or phagocytic cell dysfunction is nonexistent to date.

References

1. Green GM. Integrated defense mechanisms in models of chronic pulmonary disease. Arch Intern Med 1970; 126:500–503.
2. Bachman AL, Hewitt WR, Beckly HC. Bronchiectasis: a bronchographic study of sixty cases of pneumonia. Arch Intern Med 1953; 91:78–96.
3. Crofton J. Diagnosis and treatment of bronchiectasis. I: Diagnosis. Br Med J 1966: 19:721–723.
4. LeRoux BT, Mohlala ML, Odell JA, Whitton ID. Suppurative diseases of the lung and pleural space. Part II: Bronchiectasis. Curr Probl Surg 1986; 23:95–159.
5. Phillips MS, Williams MP, Flower CDR. How useful is computed tomography in the diagnosis and assessment of bronchiectasis? Clin Radiol 1985; 37:321–325.
6. Scalding JG, Crofton JW, Anderson T, et al. Prolonged antibiotic treatment of severe bronchiectasis. Br Med J 1957; 2:255–259.
7. Crofton J. Bronchiectasis. II: Treatment and prevention. Br Med J 1966; 19:783–785.
8. Polmar SH, Woldmann TA, Balestra ST, et al. Immunoglobulin E in immunologic deficiency diseases. I. Relation of IgE and IgA in respiratory tract disease in isolated IgE deficiency, IgA deficiency, and ataxia telangiectasia. J Clin Invest 1972; 51:326–330.
9. Ammann AJ, Hong R. Selective IgA deficiency: presentation of 30 cases and a review of the literature. Medicine 1971; 50:223–233.
10. Hermans PE, Diaz-Buxo JA, Stobo JD. Idiopathic late onset immunoglobulin deficiency in clinical observations in 50 patients. Am J Med 1976; 61:221–237.
11. Dauber JH, Fogarty CM. Immune deficiency states and recurrent respiratory tract infections. In: Fraser RG, Pare JA, eds. Diagnosis of diseases of the chest. 2nd ed. Philadelphia: WB Saunders, 1977:997.
12. Roifman CM, Lederman HM, Lavi S, Stein LD, Levison H, Gelfand EW. Benefit of intravenous IgG replacement in hypogammaglobulinemic patients with chronic sinopulmonary disease. Am J Med 1985; 79:71–74.

13. Afzelius Bjorn A. Human syndrome caused by immotile cilia. Science 1976; 193:317–319.
14. Yergin BM, Saketkhoo K, Michaelson ED, Serafini SM, Kovitz K, Sackner A. A roentgenographic method for measuring nasal mucous velocity. J Appl Physiol: Respir Environ Exerc Physiol 1978; 44:964–968.
15. Stanely P, MacWilliam L, Greenstone M, Mackay I, Cole P. Efficacy of a saccharin test for screening to detect abnormal muco-ciliary clearance. Br J Dis Chest 1984; 78:62–65.
16. Wood RE, Boat TF, Doershuk CF. State of the art—-cystic fibrosis. Am Rev Respir Dis 1976; 113:833–878.

38 | SOLITARY PULMONARY NODULE

LEONARD SICILIAN, M.D.

The solitary pulmonary nodule (SPN) ("coin lesion") is defined roentgenographically as a discrete spherical or oval density located completely within the lung parenchyma and measuring not greater than 4 cm in diameter. The single lesion may have smaller satellite nodules and may also have an irregular border. Original descriptions of SPNs set their size at up to 6 cm in diameter, but more recent data indicate that lesions greater than 4 cm are almost always malignant and therefore do not require the same type of evaluation. Benign in about 60 percent of cases,[1, 2] SPNs most often represent infectious granulomas (many healed), with hamartomas, arteriovenous malformations, cysts, and miscellaneous entities making up the remaining small percentage. Of the 40 percent of SPNs that are malignant, approximately 10 percent represent a metastatic lesion from an extrapulmonary primary cancer.

The goal of evaluation of a patient with a SPN is to determine whether the lesion is malignant or benign (Table 38–1).[3,4] This goal should be accomplished in the least invasive and most cost-effective fashion. The presumption always has been that a malignant lesion discovered when it is small is curable. Indeed, early surgical series reported a cure rate of up to 85 percent. More recent data, however, reveal only a 30 to 50 percent 5-year survival. This difference in outcome may be due to the fact that, theoretically, there are about 30 doublings of a single tumor cell necessary for a nodule to reach a size of 1 cm. Therefore, even small nodules represent established disease, and presumably microscopic metastatic spread accounts for the lower cure rates found in the recent literature.[5] Nevertheless, it is clear that the chance of survival in malignant SPNs is significantly greater than the 15 to 20 percent 5-year survivals for lung cancer in general. This fact, coupled with the usually low mortality and morbidity of resection of a small lung lesion, forces the clinician to begin to think of surgery whenever a SPN is discovered. The following discussion of the clinical, roentgenographic, and biopsy evaluation of the patient with a SPN, should aid the physician in making appropriate decisions regarding the nature of the lesion and its management.

TABLE 38–1 Factors Associated With the Probability of Malignancy of a SPN

Probability	Clinical Characteristics
Low: no further evaluation necessary	Nodules observed to develop in 3 weeks or less
	Central, diffuse, laminar, speckled, popcorn calcification on x-ray
	No change in size compared to chest x-ray 2 years old or more
Intermediate: close observation may be appropriate	Noncalcified nodule in nonsmoker < 35 years old
	Eccentric calcification
	Noncalcified nodule 8 mm diameter or smaller
High: work-up immediately, biopsy or resection usually necessary	Noncalcified nodule in smoker > 35 years of age
	Growth noted compared to chest x-ray >3 weeks and < 2 years old
	Prior pulmonary or extrapulmonary cancer

CLINICAL EVALUATION

The etiology of a SPN rarely is discovered from information obtained by history and physical examination alone. The one exception is an acute or subacute lung injury. (e.g., pneumonia, infarct, hematoma) that heals in the shape of a lung nodule. Here the clinician can follow clinically and roentgenographically the formation of the SPN from its inception and therefore can be certain of its etiology. Short of this unusual situation, less than 25 percent of SPNs are discovered by the symptoms they cause. A thorough history and physical examination can detect systemic disease that may involve the lung (e.g., rheumatoid arthritis with an associate rheumatoid lung nodule). A prior history of extrapulmonary primary cancer is important since a SPN in this setting is likely to be a metastatic lesion in two-thirds of cases.[1] Despite this observation, patients too often have an expensive metastatic work-up done on the assumption that all pulmonary nodules represent metastatic disease. Routine radionucleotide scans, gastrointestinal series, and mammograms result in finding an extrathoracic primary cancer in less than 10 percent of cases in the absence of signs and symptoms discovered by routine laboratory and physical examination (e.g., bone pain, blood in stool, abnormal liver functions, and breast lumps). It is more cost efficient to seek another cancer after resection of the SPN if the histology is diagnostic of a nonlung primary.

Excluding x-ray evaluation, work-up of a SPN is limited. Skin tests or complement fixation studies for granulomatous disease are most helpful only if the results are negative. A positive reaction or result, although clearly indicating exposure, does not ensure that there is a relationship between the SPN and that exposure. Thus, a negative test in the immunocompetent patient effectively eliminates that disease from the differential diagnosis. Sputum must be submitted for cytologic and culture examination in cases where the patient spontaneously produces sputum; these simple inexpensive tests yield a specific diagnosis in up to 25 percent of patients. Because of the low yield, however, it is not worthwhile to induce sputum in patients who do not produce it spontaneously.

Perhaps the most valuable single piece of clinical information is the patient's age. Large series have shown an extremely small percentage (3 percent) of malignancies in individuals less than 35 years of age.[1,2,6] Thus, an asymptomatic SPN in a nonsmoker below age 35 would strongly suggest a benign lesion. Although the SPN should not be forgotten, young patient age at least allows the physician to observe the patient over time to determine if the lesion is static or growing.

ROENTGENOGRAPHIC EVALUATION

The roentgenographic evaluation of a SPN is the cornerstone of patient management. Pulmonary nodules can be detected at a size of 3 to 5 mm on good quality films.[7] Remember that the lesion should be visible on both the anteroposterior and the lateral projections. If not, consideration must be given to an extrathoracic structure (e.g., nipple, skin tag, or nevus). The size of the lesion has some importance. In general, lesions less than 8 mm in diameter are likely to be benign, and those greater than 3 to 4 cm in diameter are virtually always malignant.

The growth of a SPN, as noted in successive chest films, is another important factor. Lesions that have remained static for greater than 2 years are almost always benign and additional work-up can be avoided. Nodules that double in size in less than 3 weeks are also benign and, in most cases, represent acute infectious processes. Between these two extremes lies a vast array of doubling times of tumors and some granulomas. Unfortunately, doubling times of tumors cannot be applied prospectively as a way to follow small suspicious nodules. Thus, earlier chest films are of great importance in determining prior presence and/or growth of a nodule. Old chest roentgenograms *must* be retrieved and reviewed. Reliance on reports alone is poor practice because lesions missed on initial reading can often be found in retrospect.[2]

Calcification is the best roentgenographic evidence of a benign lesion. The pattern of calcification can be central, laminar, diffuse, speckled, or popcorn in appearance. The only pattern of calcification that is questionable for malignancy is eccentric calcification. The concern here is that a malignancy has engulfed a preexisting calcification. Large series, however, have shown that the chance of cancer in an eccentrically calcified lesion is less than 1 percent. In this situation, it is still reasonable to follow closely or to perform a closed biopsy procedure before surgery is considered.

The greatest advance in the evaluation of a SPN has been the application of computerized tomography (CT) of the chest. The chest CT scan, more sensitive in picking up and defining nodules,[8] should be performed in all cases of SPN when the plain films and clinical information do not clearly indicate a benign lesion. The CT scan can more easily detect (1) multiple nodules that are suggestive of metastatic disease; (2) calcification; and (3) mediastinal abnormalities that are suggestive of metastasis and that, therefore, need staging if resection of the SPN is planned. CT scanning does have its drawbacks. Occasionally subpleural nodules smaller than 1 cm in diameter are noted in an otherwise normal scan or in the process of evaluating another SPN. In cases where these lesions have been biopsied, no significant pathology has been found, thus suggesting that a normal lung variant was detected by a sensitive test.

Recently, work has been done using the CT scan density of the SPN to determine whether the lesion is benign.[9] It is thought that microscopic calcification in a benign nodule is detected as an increased density (when compared to water density) by CT scanning in instances where macroscopic calcification cannot be visualized. This work has been hard to reproduce and CT scan "phantoms" have been developed to help clarify this issue.[10] Unfortunately, both these methods are unproven and cannot yet be relied on by the clinician when making decisions. At present, the new modality of magnetic resonance imaging (MRI) has no advantage over a conventional chest CT scan in the evaluation of the SPN.

BIOPSY EVALUATION

Transthoracic skinny needle biopsy and/or bronchoscopic transbronchial biopsy have a variable role in the evaluation of the SPN. They are not always a necessary part of the work-up, although both procedures are safe with minimal morbidity and little or no mortality. One or both usually are considered if the evaluation previously outlined has not revealed a clearly benign lesion.

Transthoracic needle biopsy under CT or fluoroscopic guidance is the method of choice for smaller peripheral lesions and yields positive results in 75 to 90 percent of cancers. Transbronchial biopsy with fluroscopic guidance is less sensitive for small peripheral lesions, but has the same yield for larger or more central lesions. Bronchoscopy has the added advantage of allowing evaluation of the central airways in patients with SPN who have concomitant airway symptoms of cough, hemoptysis, or wheezing and/or stridor. Both procedures allow diagnosis of a specific benign condition less than 40 percent of the time. These procedures, therefore, vary in the extent to which they are performed because a nondiagnostic study is not equivalent to saying the lesion is benign. If clinical and x-ray evaluation of the SPN indicate a moderate or high suspicion of malignancy without evidence of metastatic spread, closed biopsy procedures often are bypassed in favor of an open excisional biopsy and/or resection. Excision should be performed in these cases, whether the closed biopsy is positive or negative for malignancy. However, either of these procedures may be quite helpful in avoiding thoracotomy, and should be done in cases where metastatic disease is suspected or where thoracotomy is contraindicated because of poor pulmonary function. In these instances, a closed biopsy that is diagnostic of metastatic cancer can obviate the need for surgery in the former setting and provide information regarding prognosis in the latter.

OBSERVATION

Often the clinician is faced with the difficult situation where the SPN cannot readily be placed in the high or low probability of cancer category.[4] Similar difficulty arises when the characteristics of the SPN place it in the high probability group, but the patient is a poor risk for either closed biopsy or surgery (e.g., severe cardiac or pulmonary disease or coagulopathy). In these instances, the physician may opt to monitor the patient closely. Follow-up should be at least every 3 months. A plain chest roentgenogram or CT scan at each visit is necessary to evaluate any change in the nodule. Should the patient develop symptoms in the interim, he should be instructed to contact the physician immediately for reevaluation.

Unfortunately, there are few data in the literature on which to base an estimation of the increased risk of a localized resectable cancer becoming metastatic during a period of observation. Therefore, it should be made clear to the patient that some risk of missing a cancer is involved, that the problem must not be ignored, and that close follow-up is mandatory. Even though close observation alone is at times the most appropriate management, it also may be the most anxiety-producing approach for both the patient and physician.

THERAPY

If the SPN cannot be proved to be benign, and if close observation is not chosen because of a high suspicion of malignancy, then the only treatment is thoracotomy with complete excision. As in any lung resection, complete preoperative pulmonary evaluation, including function testing, is necessary to determine if the patient can tolerate the procedure and to assess the probability of postoperative pulmonary impairment.

If CT scans show evidence of mediastinal abnormality in the presence of a SPN, then a staging procedure should be performed to rule out metastatic disease. Staging can be done preoperatively via mediastinoscopy or a small anterior intercostal incision or it can be done intraoperatively by direct visualization and examination of the mediastinum. Flexible bronchoscopy should be performed preoperatively in all patients with airway symptoms to rule out a central tumor, which would necessitate a change in the extent of surgery or would possibly indicate nonresectability.

At thoracotomy, the SPN should not be biopsied, but excised in total. A frozen section should be performed; if a malignancy is found, a curative resection of that lobe or segment (depending on pulmonary function) can then be performed.

Figures 38–1 and 38–2 summarize the management of an individual with a SPN. Figure 38–1 is most applicable to patients with a low probability of malignancy. Figure 38–2 shows a scheme for those cases where surgical excision is the most likely option. At present, there are no data that favor one plan of action over the other.[4] As always, the clinician must individualize each patient and make the best decision based on the specific facts of the case.

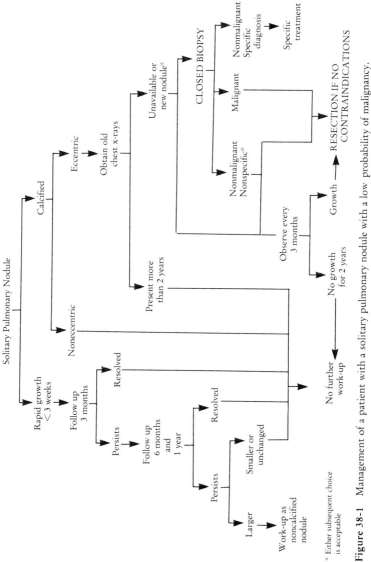

Figure 38-1 Management of a patient with a solitary pulmonary nodule with a low probability of malignancy.

* Either subsequent choice is acceptable

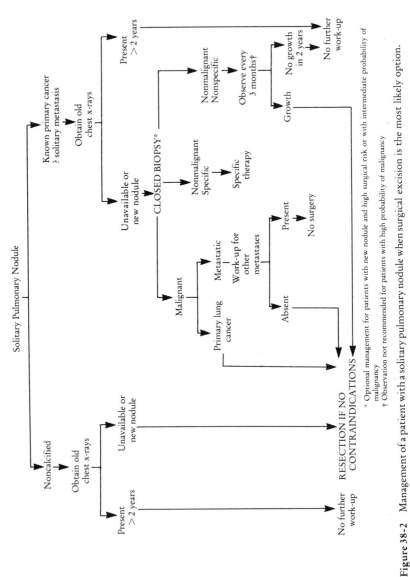

Figure 38-2 Management of a patient with a solitary pulmonary nodule when surgical excision is the most likely option.

* Optional management for patients with new nodule and high surgical risk or with intermediate probability of malignancy

* Observation not recommended for patients with high probability of malignancy

† Observation not recommended for patients with high probability of malignancy

References

1. Lillington GA. The solitary pulmonary nodule 1974. Am Rev Respir Dis 1974; 110:699–707.
2. Lillington GA. Pulmonary nodules: solitary and multiple. Clin Chest Med 1982; 3:361–367.
3. Cummings SR, Lillington GA, Richard RJ. Estimating the probability of malignancy in solitary pulmonary nodule. A Bayesian approach. Am Rev Respir Dis 1986; 134:449–452.
4. Cummings SR, Lillington GA, Richard RJ. Managing solitary pulmonary nodules. The choice of strategy is a "close call". Am Rev Respir Dis 1986; 134:453–460.
5. Weiss W, Boucot KR. The prognosis of lung cancer originating as a round lesion. Data from the Philadelphia Pulmonary Neoplasm Research Project. Am Rev Respir Dis 1977; 116:827–836.
6. Radke JR, Conway WA, Eyler WR, Kvale PA. Diagnostic accuracy in peripheral lung lesions. Chest 1979; 76:176–179.
7. Kundel HL. Predictive value and threshold detectability of lung tumors. Radiology 1981; 139:25–29.
8. Schaner EG, Chang AE, Doppman JL, Conkle DM, Flye MW, Rosenberg SA. Comparison of computed and conventional whole lung tomography in detecting pulmonary nodules: a prospective radiologic-pathologic study. AJR 1978; 131:51–54.
9. Siegelman SS, Zerhouni EA, Leo FP, Khouri NF, Stitik FP. CT of the solitary pulmonary nodule. AJR 1980; 135:1–13.
10. Zerhouni EA, Boukadoum M, Siddiky MA, et al. A standard phantom for quantitative CT analysis of pulmonary nodules. Radiology 1983; 149:767–773.

39 | CARE OF THE INTUBATED AND MECHANICALLY VENTILATED PATIENT

ALEXANDER WHITE, M.B., M.R.C.P.I.
LEONARD SICILIAN, M.D.

Intubation and positive pressure mechanical ventilation are required in critically ill patients when oxygenation and carbon dioxide elimination is severely impaired. Inadequate gas exchange usually results from the rapid onset of respiratory failure in patients with decompensated chronic lung disease (e.g., asthma, emphysema, chronic bronchitis), overwhelming pneumonias, cardiogenic pulmonary edema, and the adult respiratory distress syndrome (ARDS). Ventilatory support also may be necessary in patients with acute chest trauma, drug overdose, and progressive neuromuscular disease when adequate gas exchange can not be maintained spontaneously.

In this chapter we will discuss the routine management of the ventilated patient and review the possible medical complications of ventilatory support. Complications can arise in ventilated patients from the moment of intubation right through to the time of extubation. The airway, the ventilator, or the interaction between patient and machine can generate problems that must be anticipated, prevented, and treated promptly when present.

MONITORING THE PATIENT

Monitoring the respiratory and cardiac status of mechanically ventilated patients is essential to the successful management of patients with respiratory failure.[1] The physician must ensure adequate gas exchange while minimizing the risks of positive pressure. Even though a vast array of sophisticated equipment can be employed to aid in achieving this goal, direct patient observation by the nurse or physician and the interpretation of the arterial blood gas (ABG) levels remain the mainstays. Thus, any new monitoring device must improve our ability to accurately measure pulmonary and cardiac function, thereby leading to improved gas exchange and ventilation of our patients.[2,3]

Table 39-1 lists the four different levels of monitoring. Physical examination (level I) and intermittent monitoring (level II) are most widely used. Although this approach clearly is "low tech" given today's electronics, auscul-

TABLE 39-1 Monitoring of the Intubated and Ventilated Patient

Level of Monitoring	Advantages	Disadvantages
Level I—Physical examination	Always available	Physical changes of end-organ damage occur late in critical illness
Level II—Intermittent Arterial blood gas levels Chest x-ray Spirometry and mechanics (FVC, MIF, $\dot{V}_E$, $\dot{V}_D$, C_{dyn}, C_{st}, R_{aw})*	Widely available May be automated Equipment simple	Changes occur between measurements Some tests require patient cooperation Measurement "crude" compared to controlled laboratory setting
Level III—Continuous Pneumotachography Capnography ($P_{ET}CO_2$)* Oximetry (SaO_2)* Skin/transcutaneous (PO_2, PCO_2, pH) Breath sound analysis Diaphragmatic EMG* Esophageal balloon	Automated Reduces some invasive measurements Detects trends early	Not always available Frequent calibration and equipment check Clinical usefulness still unproven
Level IV—Computer	Rapid processing and display of data Plot trends	Limited availability Costly Clinical usefulness still unproven

*FVC, forced vital capacity; MIF, maximum inspiratory force; $\dot{V}_E$, minute ventilation; $\dot{V}_D$, dead space ventilation; C_{dyn}, dynamic compliance; C_{st}, static compliance; R_{aw}, airways resistance; $P_{ET}CO_2$, partial pressure of end tidal CO_2; SaO_2, arterial oxygen saturation; EMG, electromyography

tation of the chest is still the quickest way to detect a pneumothorax, and respiratory rates greater than 30 to 40 breaths per minute (counted at the bedside) actually correlate very well with more invasive measurements of respiratory muscle fatigue. The drawback to monitoring by physical examination is that signs of end-organ damage occur in the latter stages of injury. For example, hypoxia is far advanced by the time it results in a change in heart rate or rhythm, blood pressure, or level of consciousness.

The ABG measurement is the most useful and widely used form of intermittent monitoring of ventilated patients. This monitoring level also includes serial chest x-rays and serial measures of pulmonary mechanics used to determine the state of the patient's lungs and the ability of the patient to breathe spontaneously. Clearly, the major disadvantage of intermittent monitoring is that changes can occur between measurements, thereby going undetected.

Continuous monitoring (level III), now becoming increasingly available, may be less invasive than intermittent monitoring in some instances. The accuracy of continuous monitoring devices (e.g., oximetry) is dependent on frequent quality checks and calibrations, and their efficacy (defined as improvement in patient outcome) has not been proven. Finally, computer monitoring (level IV) is becoming increasingly popular. At present, the role of computerized equipment is to instantaneously gather, process, and display data derived from all levels of monitoring devices. In the future, direct feedback control may be available. In these instances the computer may directly activate changes (e.g., changes in ventilation rate or inspired oxygen concentration) based on computation from the monitored data (e.g., PCO_2 and PO_2). In patients monitored by these "high tech" approaches, the physician and nurse must resist the tendency to "care for" the equipment rather than the patient. "High tech" monitoring is truly beneficial to the intubated and ventilated patient only when it facilitates optimum decision making and frees the caretakers for more patient contact. Data collection obviously should not be an end-point itself. A more detailed discussion of monitoring patients (and correcting abnormalities discovered) is found in the section on Ventilator Management.

THE AIRWAY: INTUBATION AND ENDOTRACHEAL TUBE MANAGEMENT

Intubation is indicated for (1) relief of upper airway obstruction; (2) protection from aspiration of oropharyngeal contents in patients with impaired sensorium or neuromuscular disease; (3) clearance of pulmonary secretions in individuals who do not have an effective cough; (4) provision of a closed system for mechanical ventilation; and (5) delivery of inspired oxygen (FIO_2) of greater than 60 percent ($FIO_2 > 0.6$). When any of these indications arise, intubation should be carried out rapidly by an individual skilled in this procedure. The majority of complications associated with endotracheal tubes occur at the time of intubation. Thus, if the patient is not cooperative, sedation must be used. Intubation attempts should last no longer than 1 minute since prolonged attempts may result in severe hypoxemia, causing grand mal seizures, and intense vagal stimulation, causing bradycardia and a reduction in cerebral perfusion. If the endotracheal tube is not passed in less than 1 minute, the patient should be ventilated with a bag and mask for 2 to 3 minutes before another attempt is made. Rarely, it is necessary to pass the endotracheal tube into the trachea under direct vision; this is accomplished by placing the endotracheal tube over a flexible fiberoptic bronchoscope, then passing the bronchoscope through the vocal cords into the trachea.[4] Once the bronchoscope is in position, the endotracheal tube can be advanced over the bronchoscope directly into the trachea. The bronchoscope is then removed, and the airway is established.

We recommend avoiding paralysis of the patient (with succinylcholine or pancuronium bromide) to achieve intubation in all but extreme circumstances. Once these medications are given, intubation *must* be accomplished in 1 to 3 minutes since the patient will be left with no respiratory muscle activity and will be subject to hypoxemic injury if he cannot be connected to a mechanical ventilator.

Once the endotracheal tube is placed, the chest should be immediately auscultated. Absent breath sounds bilaterally with abdominal distention suggest esophageal intubation. The tube should be withdrawn and reinserted after a period of ventilation using an Ambu bag. Even if the tube is successfully placed in the trachea, the potential problem of intubation of only the right mainstem bronchus must be considered.

Intubation of the right mainstem bronchus can be suspected from markedly reduced breath sounds on the left compared with the right side. Intubation of the right mainstem bronchus, if left undiagnosed, may cause a number of problems. Hypoxemia may occur due to either inadequate overall ventilation or shunting of blood through the underventilated left lung causing ventilation-perfusion (VQ) mismatch. Other complications include pneumothorax (because all the ventilator volume will be delivered to only one lung), respiratory alkalosis with subsequent predisposition to cardiac arrhythmias, and an inability to suction secretions from the left lung, predisposing the patient to pneumonia.[5] Right mainstem bronchus intubation increases the risk of atelectasis of the left lung. The problem is easily corrected by pulling back the tube a few centimeters and listening to the chest again. A chest x-ray should be taken to confirm correct tube placement; the distal end of the endotracheal tube should be 2 to 3 cm above the carina. The proximal endotracheal tube should be marked at this optimal position at the gum, lip, or anterior nares so that any movement can be easily observed and corrected.

Which type of tube (orotracheal, nasotracheal, or tracheostomy) should be used when a patient requires intubation? As is often the case in medicine, this answer must be individualized. When rapid establishment of an airway is the major goal, orotracheal intubation is the procedure of choice. The exception to this rule is the patient with actual or suspected cervical spine injury; here, manipulation of the neck during tube placement might cause cervical spinal cord damage. In this situation, nasotracheal intubation without neck manipulation or emergency tracheostomy are indicated. Another benefit of an orotracheal tube is that a larger tube can be utilized. The larger tube allows for better suctioning and reduces airways resistance. Both factors are advantageous, especially to patients with preexisting chronic bronchitis or emphysema, the former because secretions are usually a major problem and the latter because the added airway resistance resulting from a small tube may cause respiratory muscle fatigue during weaning. We recommend the placement of at least an 8-mm internal diameter tube in all patients. Tubes less than 7-mm internal diameter markedly increase airways resistance and limit ability to suction secretions from the lower respiratory tract.

Nasotracheal tubes usually have the advantage of making the tube more stable with less chance of accidental extubation or right mainstem bronchus intubation. However, because of the size of the nasal passage, a tube of greater than 7- to 7.5-mm internal diameter rarely can be used. Nasotracheal intubation commonly results in epistaxis, which is usually self-limiting unless the patient has a coagulopathy. Maxillary and sphenoid sinusitis and otitis media are other potential complications seen with nasotracheal intubation. They should be considered in all patients who are intubated and subsequently develop fever or facial and ear pain. Skull x-rays, looking for sphenoid sinusitis, should be done in such patients. Sphenoid sinusitis may be fatal if not promptly diagnosed.[6]

In the successfully intubated patient, a sudden loss of expired volume associated with reduced airway pressure may be due to tube dislodgement or cuff leak. When this occurs with an orotracheal or nasotracheal tube, the tube should be repositioned correctly or, if the cuff is at fault, a new endotracheal tube inserted. In the case of a tracheostomy tube, it may not be possible to replace the tube if the tract is not mature (i.e., less than 72 hours old), and in this case, temporary orotracheal intubation should be performed.

Kinking or blockage of the tube with secretions causes elevation of the peak inspiratory pressure delivered by the ventilator and can usually be corrected by manipulating or repositioning the tube and by suctioning, respectively. Aseptic technique must be followed whenever suction catheters are being utilized to clear secretions from the lower respiratory tract.

Tracheomalacia and tracheal stenosis caused by excessive cuff pressure on the tracheal wall are much less common since the advent of high-volume, low-pressure cuffs. However, it is important to adhere to the correct inflation pressures for endotracheal tubes, i.e., cuff pressure must be below the capillary filling pressure of the trachea, which is less than 25 mm Hg. This goal can be accomplished by attaching an aneroid manometer to the external cuff port and reading the cuff pressure directly to determine if the cuff inflation is in the safe range.

Finally, tracheostomy tubes are usually reserved for elective placement in those patients who require permanent or prolonged intubation. At one time tracheostomy was performed on any patient intubated for more than 72 hours. Now, because of new tube material and cuff construction oro- or nasotracheal tubes may remain in position for 3 to 4 weeks without the need for tracheostomy.[5] Practically, we recommend early tracheostomy to those patients with acute or chronic neuromuscular disease who will have prolonged or lifelong time on ventilatory support. For other patients whose long-term outlook is unclear, we assess them at the end of 2 weeks. If it appears that extubation will not be accomplished in the next 7 to 10 days, we will then schedule the patient for an elective tracheostomy.

Table 39-2 lists the advantages and disadvantages of the three routes of intubation. One can see that, for short periods of intubation, other than tracheostomy, there is little difference among the options. For long-term patients, these differences may become important. Endotracheal and tracheostomy tubes bypass the normal pulmonary defense mechanisms and predispose the ventilated patient to aspiration of material from the nasopharynx. When an intubated patient develops dyspnea, hypoxemia, and radiographic changes in the dependent part of the lung, aspiration pneumonia must be suspected. Care of the oral cavity and oropharynx and good aseptic technique when suctioning help prevent aspiration. Once aspiration occurs, the treatment is mainly supportive, though antibiotics may be required if secondary bacterial infection occurs.[7]

TABLE 39-2 Comparison of the Routes of Intubation

	Endotracheal	Nasotracheal	Tracheostomy
Ease of tube placement	Good with experience	Good with experience	Poor—need controlled surgery
Tube stability	Fair	Good	Good
Access to lower respiratory tract	Good	Good	Good
Resistance to breathing	Varies—depends on tube size	Most—usually smaller tube	Least
Patient acceptance and communication	Poor	Fair	Good

VENTILATOR MANAGEMENT

The ventilator itself is a frequent source of complications. Once successfully intubated and ventilated, sometimes sedated and paralyzed, the patient is dependent on the machine for respiration, literally for life itself. Failure of the machine itself or of the alarms, tubing, valves, and circuitry can seriously impair the patient's respiratory status and may rapidly lead to death. The best way to avoid and treat ventilator problems is to have alert and knowledgeable bedside personnel present at all times. Each patient should be assigned a nurse. In addition, the ventilator (including tubing and equipment) should be checked by a respiratory therapist at least once per nursing shift. The nurse and therapist should check the ventilator more frequently if necessary. A basic hourly checklist for nurses should include FIO_2 tidal volume (V_T), intermittent mandatory ventilation/synchronized intermittent mandatory ventilation (IMV/SIMV) rate, peak inspiratory pressure (PIP), positive end-expiratory pressure (PEEP), and alarms. Ventilator malfunctions include mechanical failure, alarm failure, overheating of inspired air, and ventilator alarm left in the "off" position. Repeated sounding of the alarm unfortunately remains the commonest reason for the alarm being switched off. This must not be allowed! Any alarm warrants immediate evaluation of the patient and the ventilator rather than the alarm being considered a nuisance and simply switched off. Of the items being serially monitored, changes in PIP, V_T, PEEP, and ABG levels are most important.

A sudden rise in airway pressure (PIP) may be due to increased airway resistance or reduced pulmonary compliance. Increased resistance may be a result of malposition or blockage of the tube, as previously discussed, or of bronchospasm. Reduced compliance may result from pneumothorax, pneumomediastinum, or pulmonary edema. Pneumothorax is thought to be due to excessive alveolar pressure resulting in overdistention and rupture of alveoli. Pneumothorax occurs in 3 to 5 percent of patients being given positive pressure ventilation and is more common in those with gram-negative bacterial, *Pneumocystis carinii* pneumonia, and in those requiring PEEP. Physical examination alone is usually insufficient to detect small pneumothoraces; chest x-ray therefore is mandatory, both on a daily basis and when there is a change in the patient's cardiopulmonary status. If a pneumothorax is seen, intercostal chest tube drainage is usually mandatory.

Sudden loss of tidal volume (V_T) can be noted when a discrepancy is detected between the tidal volume setting on the ventilator and the delivered tidal volume. This results in impaired alveolar ventilation and PCO_2 rises. Loss of V_T is usually due to tube malposition or cuff leak, as previously discussed.

Positive end-expiratory pressure (PEEP) increases transpulmonary pressure at end-expiration and thereby increases functional residual capacity

(FRC) of the lung. Reduced FRC is often the most significant factor in pulmonary disease resulting in ventilation-perfusion (VQ) mismatch and systemic hypoxemia. By increasing FRC, PEEP reduces this mismatch and improves oxygenation. By improving FRC, PEEP also improves lung compliance (although excessive PEEP can paradoxically reduce compliance). PEEP improves gas exchange in pulmonary edema and ARDS by increasing alveolar volume, not by moving fluid across the alveolocapillary membrane. At levels of PEEP above 10 cm H_2O, cardiac output can be reduced. Cardiac output falls because of reduced venous return secondary to increased intrapleural pressure and by a direct mechanism of unknown cause. In patients with high PEEP levels, pulmonary capillary wedge pressure readings by Swan-Ganz catheterization become unreliable because the catheter is exposed to high alveolar pressure, resulting in a divergence of wedge and left atrial pressures (i.e., wedge pressure may be read as higher than it actually is). Other effects of PEEP include sodium retention, perhaps from preferential perfusion of juxtamedullary nephrons in the kidney, and changes in atrial natriuretic peptide. Water retention with resultant hyponatremia can occur consequent to increased antidiuretic hormone (ADH) production. Hypotension may occur following institution of positive pressure ventilation, with or without PEEP, and usually responds to volume expansion with normal saline. If this is unsuccessful, other causes of hypotension should be suspected.[8,9]

Most clinical problems occur at levels of PEEP greater than 10 cm H_2O, and all patients being treated at these levels of PEEP should have Swan-Ganz catheters placed to monitor cardiac output and fluid status. PEEP should be used to reduce the inspired oxygen concentration and thus to avoid oxygen toxicity.[9] The lowest level of PEEP that keeps the PO_2 in the 60 to 70 mm Hg range (while the FIO_2 is less than 0.5) and maintains adequate cardiac output should be chosen. This approach helps to prevent the superimposition of lung injury due to oxygen toxicity.

Hyperoxia, a well-known cause of lung damage, acts in two ways: a direct cytotoxic effect mediated by so-called free radicals, and an indirect effect mediated by chemotaxis of polymorphonuclear leukocytes recruited to the site of damage.[10,11] Development of pulmonary oxygen toxicity is directly related to the partial pressure of inspired oxygen and the duration of exposure. Oxygen toxicity must be suspected in any patient receiving an FIO_2 of greater than 0.5 for more than 48 hours. Early symptoms include cough and chest tightness due to tracheobronchitis. As the process progresses, the PaO_2 falls, bilateral parenchymal infiltrates are seen on chest x-ray, and pulmonary mechanics show a progressive restrictive pattern with loss of compliance. It is reassuring that short-term high FIO_2 i.e., for 24 to 48 hours, seems to be associated with little risk of oxygen toxicity.

Respiratory acidosis occurring in a mechanically ventilated patient indicates inadequate ventilation; the patient, endotracheal tube, and ventilator system should be quickly evaluated. Once blockage of the endotracheal tube has been ruled out and excessive secretions, pneumothorax, and new parenchymal lung disease are not found, the ventilator system must be inspected. A leak resulting in loss of inspired V_T should first be sought and corrected. The ventilator setting also should be checked to ensure that the V_T or rate has not been accidently lowered. A common cause of respiratory acidosis in the ventilated patient is poor coordination between patient and machine. Poor coordination results in the machine being unable to deliver the desired V_T. Occasionally sedation or even paralysis of the patient is necessary to restore ventilation control. In all cases of respiratory acidosis resulting from a problem with the mechanical ventilator, the patient should be manually ventilated with an Ambu bag until the problem is resolved.

By definition, respiratory alkalosis is a complication of overventilation. It can cause cardiac arrhythmias, reduced cardiac output, seizures, reduced lung compliance, increased airways resistance, and VQ mismatch, and hence should be rapidly corrected by reducing the V_T or the rate delivered by the ventilator. Agitation caused by the endotracheal tube or the patient's disease can result in increased spontaneous breathing while being mechanically ventilated. In this instance the patient may require sedation or paralysis to control ventilation until the underlying problem can be corrected.

THE VENTILATOR-PATIENT UNIT

In addition to care of the endotracheal tube and care of the ventilator per se, the routine care of the ventilated patient must include the interaction between ventilator and patient. From the physician's point of view, any ventilated patient should be fully examined at least once daily. Patient data must be recorded on a flow sheet hourly (at a minimum), and all recorded information should be assessed at least twice daily by the physician. Limited symptoms may be elicited by asking questions that can be answered by nodding or shaking the head, or a letter board may be used. Full examination must include extremities, especially if an arterial line is inserted, all intravenous sites, pressure areas, calves, and eyes for ulceration. Daily weights are mandatory and are a useful guide to fluid retention because edema may collect in areas not easily seen; input and output charts also should be carefully assessed for evidence of fluid accumulation. All central lines should be changed every 3 days, or sooner if the site appears infected. Swan-Ganz catheters should be removed after 48 hours. Arterial blood gas levels should be checked 30 minutes after the patient has been intubated and a similar time after any readjustments are made in the ventilator. An ABG determination also should be obtained any time a significant clinical deterioration is observed that might be due to a change in pulmonary status.

Chest x-ray must be performed daily and when there is any significant change in the patient's cardiopulmonary status. In particular, the position of the endotracheal tube, Swan-Ganz catheter, and central lines should be noted. The lung pathology should be followed and a pneumothorax and/or pneumo-mediastinum looked for in all ventilated patients, especially those requiring PEEP. Pleural effusion and lobar collapse are sometimes difficult to spot on the supine films that are usually obtained in the intensive care unit. Thus, chest x-rays should be reviewed on a daily basis by the physician with a radiologist. Complete blood count (CBC), electrolyte levels, ABG levels, drug levels, urinalysis, and ECG are usually ordered on a routine basis.

Other measures that should be routinely performed include moving the endotracheal tube from one side of the mouth to the other and retaping it every 12 hours. Endotracheal tube cuff pressure should be checked every 12 hours to ensure it is less than 25 mm Hg. Suctioning is performed as required to maintain patent airways and should be done with strict aseptic technique. Chest physical therapy performed every 4 hours also helps to mobilize secretions. FIO_2, peak inspiratory pressures, tubing, spirometer alarms, humidifier heat and water levels, and temperature of inspired gas should all be checked every hour by nursing staff, and every nursing shift by the respiratory therapists.

The essence of care of the intubated and ventilated patient is regular and routine checking of the patient, the endotracheal tube, and the ventilator. If the physician has the knowledge of all potential problems and the expertise to correct them quickly, the result will be a successful patient outcome.

References

1. Bone RC. Monitoring respiratory function in the patient with adult respiratory distress syndrome. Semin Respir Med 1981; 2:140–150.
2. Fallat RJ. Respiratory monitoring. Clin Chest Med 1982; 3:181–194.
3. Prakash O, Meij S, Zeelenberg C, van der Borden B. Computer based patient monitoring. Crit Care Med 1982; 10:811–822.
4. Messeter KH, Pettersson KL. Endotracheal intubation with the fiberoptic bronchoscope. Anesthesia 1980; 35:294–297.
5. Zwillich CW, Pierson DJ, Creach GE, Sutton FD, Schatz E, Petty TL. Complications of assisted ventilation. A prospective study of 354 consecutive episodes. Am J Med 1974; 57:161–170.
6. Tintinalli JE, Claffey J. Complications of nasotracheal intubation. Ann Emerg Med 1981; 10:142–144.

7. Bartlett J, Gorbach S. The triple threat of aspiration pneumonia. Chest 1975; 68:560–566.
8. Tyler DC. Positive end-expiratory pressure: a review. Crit Care Med 1983; 11(4):300–308.
9. Weisman IM, Rinaldo JE, Rogers RM. Positive end-expiratory pressure in adult respiratory failure. N Engl J Med 1982: 307(22):1381–1384.
10. Jackson RM. Pulmonary oxygen toxicity. Chest 1985; 88(6):900–905.
11. Deneke SM, Fanburg BL. Oxygen toxicity of the lung: an update. Br J Anaesth 1982; 54:737–749.

40 | EVALUATION OF THE PATIENT WITH SUSPECTED OCCUPATIONAL LUNG DISEASE

LEONARD SICILIAN, M.D.

Increased public awareness of the adverse effects of various occupational and environmental agents has resulted in a growing number of patients asking their physicians if a relationship exists between these agents and their illness. To complicate this, often lawyers or insurance companies ask the physician to make the initial assessment. In many instances, the physician is requested not only to diagnose and treat the problem but also to assess the patient's ability to continue work. All of these factors lead to confusion as to the precise role of the practicing physician in the evaluation of occupational lung disease. In actuality, I believe that the physician's role in this case is no different from his or her role in the evaluation of a patient with any disease; thoroughness in the work-up and accuracy in the diagnosis are the primary requirements.

Whether the patient is referred by himself, his physician, his employer, a lawyer, an insurance company, or an administrative agency, some variant of the following critical questions are usually asked.

1. Is there pulmonary disease?
2. Is there impairment and/or disability and to what degree?
3. Is there a cause and effect relationship between the workplace and the disease?

The answers to these questions should be the same regardless of who is asking. This chapter, although it will not discuss specific occupational lung diseases, will give the practicing physician without a background in epidemiology, industrial hygiene, or medicolegal problems a framework in which to approach this facet of pulmonary disease.

IS THERE PULMONARY DISEASE?

The list of occupationally related lung diseases is long, and Table 40–1 represents a summary of the various categories with a few examples of each.[1,2] It is not necessary to know all the possible causes of occupational lung disease to properly evaluate and diagnose a patient. What is crucial is the ability to extract a detailed occupational history. Several problems interfere with obtaining an accurate history. First is variable physician awareness and training. The general internist too often has not been specifically trained to screen for occupational exposures during an evaluation, especially if the patient has another complaint. The fact that exposures can be intermittent or the fact that the disease may have a long latency period following exposure compound this variable. Both facts often cause the patient to dissociate his complaint and his occupation even when directly asked by the physician.

The second major difficulty is that scientific knowledge of a specific agent's pulmonary effects is lacking for many occupational exposures. For example, formaldehyde, clearly an irritant to the respiratory tract, may precipitate an acute attack in patients with asthma. However, the ability of formaldehyde to cause asthma de novo is unknown, even though some animal and epidemiologic studies suggest this.[3]

TABLE 40-1   Classification of Occupational Lung Diseases
(Partial List with Examples)

Inorganic dusts (pneumoconiosis)	
Free silica	Silicosis
Silicates	Asbestosis
Carbon	Coal worker's pneumoconiosis
"Inert" metals	Iron, tin
Biologic dusts (hypersensitivity pneumonitis)	
Animal	Avian protein—pigeon-breeder's disease
Vegetable	Thermophilic actinomyces—farmer's lung, humidifier's lung
Toxic chemicals	
Irritant gases	NO_2—silo-filler's disease
	Phosgene—smoke inhalation
Metals	Beryllium—berylliosis
Dusts, fumes, chemicals causing asthma	
Polyvinyl chlorine (PVC)	Meat-wrapper's asthma
Toluene Diisocyanate (TDI)	
Grains	Baker's asthma
Cotton bract	Byssinosis
Occupational respiratory infections	
Bacterial	Tuberculosis
Fungus	Histoplasmosis—Spelunker's lung
Occupational respiratory carcinogens	
Federally regulated	Asbestos, coke oven emissions
Carcinogenic potential	Uranium, beryllium

A third factor that clouds detection of occupational disease is that, even though the causative agents may be esoteric (avian proteins, cotton bract), the manifestations of pulmonary disease are conventional (bronchitis, fibrosis). Thus, the physician may successfully treat the "asthma" without ever thinking to look for an occupational cause. The converse is also true. The presence of pulmonary disease in the face of exposure to a known pulmonary toxin does not mean that the two are always related. Therefore, the physician must not jump to conclusions and equate exposure with disease. In many instances, smoking-related disease is often the culprit and the exposure is incidental.

Finally, medicolegal issues that often accompany occupationally related diseases are intimidating to the physician and distract efforts aimed at diagnosis and treatment.

As mentioned earlier, a detailed occupational history is the crucial first step in establishing a link between occupation and disease.[4] In almost all cases of occupational lung disease, however, there are no physical or laboratory findings that point specifically to the injurious agent. For example, the wheezing, dyspnea, and airflow obstruction in a patient with occupational exposure to platinum salts are no different from those symptoms seen in a patient with intrinsic asthma. In short, without a proper history, objective data are nonspecific.

A history of exposure can be obtained initially by asking whether the chief complaint is temporally related to the workplace. If the chief complaint is not respiratory in nature or if there are no respiratory questions, the physician should ask during the review of systems whether there has been work in a dusty environment, exposure to fumes, chemicals, or radiation, or work with insulation (asbestos). This questioning often suffices to jog the patient's memory.

A complete occupational history is necessary when there is suspicion that a relationship of respiratory disease to occupation exists;[4] I take such a history in less than 10 minutes. I recommend beginning with the patient's date and place of birth and highest level of education. Home environment, chores after school, and summer jobs held during this time should be explored. Most people begin their careers after school, and thus the patient should be asked about each job from that time to the present. Table 40–2 lists the important questions that must be asked about *each* job. The name, place, and dates of employment should be recorded. Oftentimes temporary jobs are held between major employment, and therefore, if jobs are recorded chronologically, these gaps and the jobs that filled them will be easily picked up. The patient should be asked to describe in his own words the type of work performed. Physicians are usually not familiar with the jargon of industry, and therefore a "layman's" description of the daily work activity is helpful. Job titles or employer's job descriptions are often insufficient to determine potential exposures. Either the common or trade names of the agents to which the patient was exposed should

TABLE 40-2   Essential Questions In a Job History

Name, place and dates of employement.
Describe all positions held and activities performed at each job. Job title alone is insufficient.
Describe agent(s) exposed to—common or trade names.
Describe the job site ventilation and maintenance.
Was any protective equipment worn by the patient or others?
Were others in different areas working with hazardous material?
What is the health of co-workers; do they have similar symptoms?

be obtained. No one expects any physician to know off-hand the properties of all injurious agents, but if the physician has a record of them, they can be researched later to see if their effects are consistent with the present illness.

Next, workplace maintenance, ventilation, and use of protective equipment (masks, respirators, asbestos aprons or gloves) should be recorded. Often the patient may not directly work with an injurious agent, but plant conditions may be such that significant exposure occurred. This certainly was the case with shipyard workers during World War II. Even those who did not work directly with asbestos were exposed by dusty conditions.

Finally, the health of co-workers should be determined. The physician should be tipped off to the possibility of an injurious agent if others in the workplace are reported to have similar medical problems. The practitioner often wonders what to do if he or she believes that the workplace is the source of illness, especially if it has not been reported before. Again, the physician is not expected to organize an investigation.[2] The regional office of the Occupational Safety and Health Administration (OSHA) should be contacted and the problem discussed with an administrator. If indicated, OSHA will initiate an investigation of the workplace and determine what risks, if any, exist. They will advise both employer and employee of any actions that should be taken.

The occupational history is rounded out by obtaining information about exposures that may have taken place during military service or in the course of pursuing hobbies and other recreational activities (e.g., silica exposure from working with ceramics). A description of the present home environment, seeking exposure to chemicals or asbestos insulation among other things, completes this short but comprehensive history.

Because the response of the lung to injury is limited, information obtained from the physical examination is usually not specific enough to make an etiologic diagnosis. Obviously, record all findings, as these abnormalities support the presence of lung disease when backed by the appropriate history. The same can be said for most laboratory data. For example, hypoxemia with secondary polycythemia can be a result of end-stage asbestosis, but without the proper exposure history, hypoxemia can be accounted for by any far-advanced lung disease.

In selected diseases, however, laboratory data can be helpful. In the group of diseases known as hypersensitivity pneumonitis (extrinsic allergic alveolitis), serum precipitating antibodies to organic proteins may be found in the patient's blood. The best-described precipitants are those to thermophilic actinomyces in farmer's lung. In the presence of an exposure history and physical findings of an acute or chronic interstitial lung disease, their presence can confirm the diagnosis.[5,6] However, there are many individuals who work with organic compounds who deelop precipitants but who have no disease. As always, therefore, it is the combination of exposure (history), clinical findings (physical examination), and pertinent laboratory data that makes the diagnosis of hypersensitivity pneumonitis, not laboratory findings alone.

Much work is now being done in the development of immunologic assays for immunoglobulin E-mediated reactions to various agents (e.g., platinum salts, toluene diisocyanate, trimetallic anhydride).[7] Thus far, however, studies indicate that, even when the results are positive, the tests themselves cannot establish the diagnosis. In fact, the "ultimate" pulmonary laboratory test, lung biopsy, is usually not diagnostic unless the presence of an occupational exposure can be established.[1]

I believe that the single most useful objective test for the presence of occupational lung disease is the chest roentgenogram. It is most helpful in the pneumoconioses where the typical patterns (e.g., nodules in silicosis, linear irregular densities in asbestosis) have been well described.[1] Unfortunately, chest x-rays often are of little help in occupational asthma or occupational respiratory infections where the changes are not specific. Whether or not roentgenographic changes are specific, their presence is unrelated to the severity of symptoms, physiologic abnormalities (as measured by pulmonary function testing), or pathologic lesions.

More important than the present chest x-ray is the comparison of the present x-ray with old films. In diseases with long latency periods such as occupational lung disease, the ability to detect the earliest roentgenographic abnormality and follow its progression is crucial to establishing the proper diagnosis. The critical importance of serial x-rays is best exemplified in the case of asbestos-related lung diseases where chronic changes such as pleural plaques or progressive fibrosis (asbestosis) need to be distinguished from new parenchymal cancers or mesotheliomas. Often such a review allows diagnostic and therapeutic decisions to be made. The actual chest films must be obtained and reviewed since small or progressive changes due to chronic disease easily can be overlooked; written reports alone may be misleading.

The final laboratory test that corroborates the presence, but usually not the cause, of occupational lung disease is the pulmonary function test (PFT).

The PFT has major importance in the assessment of the degree of impairment and disability, the second critical question to be answered.

IS THERE IMPAIRMENT AND/OR DISABILITY?

Once pulmonary disease has been detected, the physician then must decide if the patient is "disabled". In truth, the physician cannot answer this question because he can only properly assess the degree of impairment.[8] Impairment has been defined as a medically evaluable condition resulting in a loss of function that may or may not be stable, and that persists after appropriate therapy.[9] The functional loss may have different grades of severity ranging from inability to do any work, to precluding only the most strenuous activities. Impairment at times does not have to result from a loss of function. For example, a health care worker who develops tuberculosis may be unable to work for a certain time because of risk of transmitting the disease, not the inability to perform the job.

In contrast to impairment, disability denotes the total effect of impairment on a patient's life.[9] Disability takes into account age, sex, level of education, social factors, and the economic environment. The latter factors are usually outside of the physician's area of expertise. Thus, a decision regarding disability is usually administratively determined. An obvious example of the difference between disability and impairment is the case of two men with severe emphysema (forced expiratory volume in 1 second less than 1 liter), one who is the owner of a factory, the other with a sixth-grade education who works on the assembly line of that same factory. The former may be able to carry on some, if not all, of his work activities from his desk. The latter will be unable to work because of the energy requirements of the job and low training potential for sedentary work. While both are similarly impaired, their levels of disability are quite different.

These definitions apply only to the United States; different terminology is used in Europe and by the World Health Organizations (WHO).[10]

The degree of impairment is determined by pulmonary function testing. In order to obtain the maximal information, PFTs must be simple for the patient to understand and perform and must be reproducible with little interpreter variability;[11] the tests that fulfill these criteria are listed in Table 40-3. Forced vital capacity (FVC), forced expiratory volume in 1 second (FEV_1), and the ratio of the two (FEV_1/FVC) are the cornerstones of the evaluation. They should be performed before and after bronchodilators if obstructive lung disease is suspected. The single breath diffusing capacity for carbon monoxide (D_{COSB}), next most useful, enables the physician to detect abnormalities of gas exchange that can occur in interstitial lung disease and

TABLE 40-3   Tests for the Assessment of Respiratory Impairment

Recommended
  Forced vital capacity — FVC
  Forced expiratory volume, 1 second — FEV_1
  FEV_1/FVC
  Single breath diffusing capacity for carbon monoxide — D_{COSB}
  Exercise testing

Not recommended
  Maximal voluntary ventilation — MVV
  Arterial blood gas — ABG
  Flow volume loop
  Closing volume — CV

pulmonary vascular disease even when mechanical lung function may be normal. Finally, exercise studies with measurement of maximal oxygen consumption ($\dot{V}O_2$ max) are useful when the simpler studies do not clearly identify severe impairment. The use of exercise testing to identify impairment that is less than severe and to assess remaining work capacity is still controversial.[10] The tests listed in Table 40-3 that are not recommended for use are those that have not been shown or have not yet been proven to give more information than those already mentioned.

It would seem then that impairment should be easy to rate by use of appropriate pulmonary function tests. This is not the case, however. For one reason, there have been several schemes proposed, each of which uses different criteria to determine severe impairment (e.g., Social Security Administration, American Medical Association, Coal Miners Act).[12] The second problem is the assessment of remaining work capacity for those patients whose tests are not normal but also are not consistent with severe impairment.

The American Thoracic Society (ATS) recently has attempted to rectify this situation by suggesting uniform severity criteria and a standard method of evaluation.[9] Table 40-4 lists the criteria by which impairment may be determined for both restrictive and obstructive lung disease. The evaluation should proceed in a stepwise fashion beginning with simple spirometry. If the patient falls below any of the criteria for severe impairment of FVC, FEV_1, or FEV_1/FVC, no further testing is necessary. If test results are better than the criteria for severe impairment, then a D_{COSB} should be obtained, followed by exercise testing if necessary.

TABLE 40-4 Rating of Impairment as Recommended by the American Thoracic Society

	Impairment			
Test	Normal	Mild	Moderate	Severe
FVC	$\geq 80\%$*	60–79%	51%–59%	$\leq 50\%$
FEV_1	$\geq 80\%$	60–79%	41%–59%	$\leq 40\%$
FEV_1/FVC	$\geq 75\%$	60–74%	41%–59%	$\leq 40\%$
D_{COSB}	$\geq 80\%$	60–79%	41%–59%	$\leq 40\%$
$\dot{V}_{O_2}$ max	> 25 ml/kg/min	15–25 ml/kg/min	≤ 15 ml/kg/min	

* Values expressed as % predicted except FEV_1/FVC, which is actual percent.
With permission from American Thoracic Society. Evaluation of impairment and disability. Am Rev Respir Dis 1986; 133:1205–1209.

Exercise testing deserves special mention. Its use in disability and impairment evaluations is not recommended for all individuals since most cases of severe impairment are picked up by the other tests.[9] I believe that exercise testing should be reserved for those individuals who remain symptomatic despite normal or less than severely reduced values of FEV_1, FVC, and D_{COSB}. When exercise is performed, an actual measurement of $\dot{V}_{O_2}$ max is necessary; this value should not be obtained from nomograms even though they exist. An individual can work for extended periods at 40 percent of their $\dot{V}_{O_2}$ max. Tables exist listing the energy requirements ($\dot{V}_{O_2}$ max) of certain jobs. Thus, if 40 percent of the measured $\dot{V}_{O_2}$ max falls below those requirements, the individual is severely impaired.[13] Practically, this turns out to be less than 15 ml per kg per minute $\dot{V}_{O_2}$ max.

As usual there are several exceptions to these guidelines (e.g., asthma, cough syncope, sleep disorders), and these are discussed in the ATS Statement.[9] The practicing physician must use objective data when asked to evaluate impairment. The physician also should state which impairment scheme is being used (e.g., ATS, Social Security, etc). Finally, if there are any extenuating circumstances, these should be reported. These might include the presence of coexisting disease (which might diminish ability to work [e.g., cardiovascular disease]), whether or not the patient has been given proper therapy, or whether the patient has refused to cooperate with the evaluation.

From this discussion one can see that the role of the physician in assessing impairment is not much different from his role in evaluating any disease; that is, the physician must take the objective information, in this case PFTs, and formulate an impression based on this and other information obtained on history and examination. Truly complex "disability" cases will no doubt require the expertise of a pulmonary or occupational disease specialist. However, by using the preceding scheme, the primary physician will be able to initiate the proper work-up and inform the patient regarding the degree of impairment.

IS THE PULMONARY DISEASE CAUSALLY RELATED TO THE WORKPLACE?

The Worker's Compensation System was developed in this country as a no-fault system to reimburse workers for wages lost during a job-related injury. This system works well for acute, short-term injury (usually —traumatic).[14] However, occupational lung disease may occur after several years of exposure and usually results in long-term disability. Worker's Compensation reimburses poorly for this type of injury.[15] When faced with this inequity, individuals have sought other means of financial reimbursement. Many of these actions take the form of personal injury and product liability claims filed not against the employer but against the manufacturer of the agent alleged to cause the lung injury (e.g., Johns Manville Co. for asbestos products). This has had important consequences for physicians for two reasons. First, it often means that lawyers, insurance companies, and administrative agencies either initiate or are heavily involved in the evaluation process. Second, as opposed to Worker's Compensation where the cause of the injury is unimportant in personal injury claims, the causal relationship of the offending agent to the lung disease is crucial in determining responsibility.

Answering this third critical question is foreign to most practicing physicians. The physician's definition of cause and effect (causation) is different than that of lawyers.[16] First of all, physicians look at a cause as being an initiating event, whereas lawyers also look at aggravating events as causes. In addition, physicians are used to examining several potential causes for a given symptom complex and physical findings. Lawyers, on the other hand, are not interested in a differential diagnosis, but in the "one" or proximate cause of the injury. Perhaps the biggest difference in how the two professions assess causation is the determination of probabilities. As physicians we are trained to apply the rules of scientific probability to determine if a causal relationship exists (e.g., $p < 0.05$; that is, a less than 5% probability of two events being related by chance alone). Lawyers and the clients (patients) they represent cannot wait to develop formal scientific proof of causation. Therefore, lawyers and the courts accept a causal relationship as being one in which there is a greater than 50 percent chance of an association (i.e., "more likely than not.") This degree of probability is clearly much more lenient than that accepted by physicians. Physicians, however, think that their opinion for the court must reflect a strict scientific determination of cause. In reality, all that is required is an opinion that states that the association of occupational exposure and lung disease is probable in the legal sense (not possible, which is considered < 50% chance). The physician can do this by combining established scientific fact with objective medical evidence. In essence, this is not unlike a physician making a diagnosis of any disease where the etiology or the pathogenesis is unknown. For example, sarcoidosis can be diagnosed and treated even though its cause is unknown. The largest stumbling block in making the diagnosis of occupational lung disease is the fact that scientific information on many agents is lacking or is derived from animal or epidemiologic data, data difficult to apply to an individual case.

I recommend that clinicians ask themselves four questions when trying to assess causation in alleged occupational lung disease. The initial two questions are epidemiologic. First, is there or has there been exposure to an agent scientifically known or suspected to cause lung disease? Second, is or was there an appropriate temporal relationship between exposure and the lung disease? An example of this latter situation is a patient presenting with dyspnea and an interstitial x-ray pattern 2 years following asbestos exposure. Clearly, asbestos exposure can result in these findings, but it is well known that the latency period for this disease is usually 15 to 20 years. Thus, even though exposure was present, the physician would be suspicious that another disease is present since the temporal relationship is not appropriate.

The last two questions are clinical in nature. The physician first must be able to detect a physical, laboratory, or roentgenographic abnormality. This is a legal prerequisite since without an "effect" there can be no "cause." Once an abnormality is found, the physician must assess whether (1) it is consistent with what has been scientifically reported for that exposure or (2) whether the abnormality can be accounted for by another disease. Again using asbestos exposure as an example, let us consider a patient who is a smoker with dyspnea, a chest x-ray showing hyperinflation, and PFTs with moderate airways obstruction. These findings are not consistent with asbestos-related lung disease, which results in dyspnea, an interstitial x-ray pattern, and restrictive PFTs.

Table 40-5 gives examples of four causation groups (none; possible; probable; definite) that can be obtained by using this schema. The none or possible causation groups would not establish a firm cause and effect relationship, while the probable and definite groups would. One can see from Table 40-5 that it is usually another lung disease not caused by the occupational exposure that prevents the physician from establishing a causal relationship. Thus the physician must not immediately equate exposure with disease.

Practicing physicians are not usually trained to screen for occupational lung disease and often are uncomfortable dealing with the medicolegal aspects of this problem. Yet they represent the initial contact that many patients have

TABLE 40-5 Determination of the Medicolegal Probability of a Causal
Relationship—Examples

	Case 1	Case 2	Case 3	Case 4
Data				
History	Asbestos exposure 1976–1979	Asbestos exposure 1951–1976	Asbestos exposure 1951–1978	Asbestos exposure 1942–1975
Symptoms	Dyspnea, cough	Dyspnea, cough	Dyspnea, cough, chest pain	Dyspnea, cough
Physical examination	Normal	Expiratory prolongation	Crackles	Crackles, clubbing
Chest x-ray	Normal	Hyperinflation	Linear opacities	Linear opacities
PFTs	Normal	Moderate obstruction	Mild restriction	Moderate restriction
Lung biopsy	—	—	—	Fibrosis with asbestos fibers
Four questions				
Exposure	Yes	Yes	Yes	Yes
Temporal relationship	No	Yes	Yes	Yes
Findings due to agent	No	No	Yes	Yes
Findings due to other disease	No	Yes	No	No
Causation	None	Possible	Probable	Definite
Explanation	No lung disease present	Exposure present but findings are result of emphysema	Appropriate history and objective findings: asbestosis	As in Case 3, lung biopsy gives scientific proof of asbestosis

with the entire system. By obtaining a complete occupational history, applying
objective criteria to determine impairment, and giving as accurate an opinion
of causation as possible, the physician will not only diagnose and treat his
patient accurately, but will be able to give reasonable advice as to whether
disability and other medicolegal remedies should be pursued.

References

1. FitzGerald MX, Carrington CB, Gaensler EA. Environmental lung disease. Med Clin North Am 1973; 57:593–622.
2. Brooks SM. An approach to patients suspected of having an occupational pulmonary disease. Clin Chest Med 1981; 2:171–178.
3. Frigas E, Filley WV, Reed CE. Bronchial challenge with formaldehyde gas: lack of bronchoconstriction in 13 patients suspected of having formaldehyde-induced asthma. Mayo Clin Proc 1984; 59:295–299.
4. Goldman RH, Peters JM. The occupational and environmental health history. JAMA 1981; 246:2831–2836.
5. Shatz M, Patterson R, Fink J. Immunopathogenesis of hypersensitivity pneumonitis. J Allergy Clin Immunol 1977; 60:27–37.
6. Fink JN. Hypersensitivity pneumonitis. J Allergy Clin Immunol 1984; 74:1–9.
7. Salvaggio JE. Occupational asthma: overview and mechanisms. J Allergy Clin Immunol 1979; 64:646–649.
8. Richman SI. Meanings of impairment and disability. The conflicting social objectives underlying the confusion. Chest (Suppl) 1980; 78:367–371.
9. American Thoracic Society. Evaluation of impairment and disability. Am Rev Respir Dis 1986; 13:1205–1209.
10. Becklake MR, Rodarte JR, Kalica AR. Scientific issues in the assessment of respiratory impairment. Am Rev Respir Dis 1988; 137:1505–1510.
11. Morgan WKC, Seaton D. Pulmonary physiology—its application to the determination of respiratory impairment and disability in industrial lung disease. In: Morgan WRC, Seaton A. Occupational lung diseases. 2nd ed. Philadelphia: WB Saunders, 1984:18.
12. Epler GR, Saber FA, Gaensler EA. Determination of severe impairment (disability) in interstitial lung disease. Am Rev Respir Dis 1980; 121:647–659.
13. Miller WF, Scacci R. Pulmonary function assessment for determination of pulmonary impairment and disability evaluation. Clin Chest Med 1981; 2:327–341.
14. Balk JL. Problems in providing medical care and economic redress to injured workers: the physician's responsibility: ethical and legal consideration. Ann NY Acad Sci 1979; 330:513–520.
15. An Interim Report to Congress on Occupational Diseases. Submitted to Congress June 1980. U.S. Department of Labor. Assistant Secretary for Policy Education and Research. U.S. Government Printing Office 1980, 0-311-416/4007.
16. Danner D, Sagall EL. Medicolegal causation: a source of professional misunderstanding. Am J Law Med 1977; 3:303–308.

41 | ACUTE INHALATION INJURY

LEONARD SICILIAN, M.D.

The thought of acute lung injury resulting from inhalation of noxious chemicals usually conjures up the image of derailed tank cars billowing thick smoke hundreds of feet into the air and police evacuating the local townspeople. Although this scenario does occur, and at times can account for thousands of deaths (the 1984 Union Carbide plant explosion in Bhopal, India), the injuries that concern most practicing physicians arise from smaller fires and daily chemical use in local businesses and in the home.

As discussed in Chapter 40, environmental or occupational lung injury often is difficult to detect for a variety of reasons. Acute inhalation injury is no exception. Difficulties arise because exposures occur at unpredictable or infrequent intervals, the exact agent is unknown at the time of presentation, the range of clinical manifestations may be wide, and the chronic effects of long-term low levels of exposure to agents usually associated with acute lung injury are unknown or poorly understood.[1,2] As always, a good occupational and/or environmental history is the key to detecting the etiology of lung injury when a chemical spill or smoke inhalation is not obvious.

This chapter focuses on the different types of inhaled agents associated with acute lung injury, the settings in which they occur, their typical manifestations, and the principles of therapy.

GENERAL PRINCIPLES

Considering the wide variety of inhaled agents that are injurious to the lung, there are several principles that physicians must remember and apply.

Although there is a tendency to attribute all inhalation injury to "noxious" or "irritant" gases, very often this is not the case. In fact, the more irritating or foul smelling the gas (ammonia), the normal human reaction is to escape the area and thereby reduce exposure. Thus, with true noxious exposures, the patient is often trapped or rendered unconscious by the agent or by the accident that caused its release. It is therefore imperative that the physician examine the patient for signs of trauma, blood loss, or other internal injury at the time of initial assessment. Conversely, gases that are odorless and colorless (oxygen, carbon monoxide, methane) often cause more injury because exposure to them is sustained as a result of the inability to detect them.

The dose and duration of exposure are important factors in causation. Even if the concentration of an agent is low, should the duration of exposure be long enough, severe injury may occur. The converse is also true. For example, sudden exposure to a concentration of 1 percent carbon monoxide (10,000 parts per million) leads to immediate loss of consciousness and is lethal in less than 5 minutes. Exposure to 0.1 percent carbon monoxide (1,000 PPM) can be tolerated for up to several hours depending on the patient's underlying state of health.[3] This observation points up an important general principle, i.e., that preexisting disease alters the response to, or extent of, inhalation injury. Both children and adults with high metabolic rates have an increased minute ventilation and therefore have an increased exposure to an injurious agent. Individuals with heart disease or anemia are less able to tolerate any injury that reduces oxygen supply (asphyxiants), delivery (carbon monoxide), or tissue utilization (cyanide). Thus, the healthier the individual, the better able or longer he will be able to tolerate any given exposure.

The absorption of the chemical or gas onto particulate matter serves to prolong the contact of the agent with the lung or upper respiratory tract. Such absorption allows the agent to travel deeper into the lung, possibly retarding its clearance and resulting in more contact time with the airway or alveolus.

Finally, the physical form of a noxious agent can vary. Although the terms defined in Table 41-1 often are used interchangeably in the description of an injurious agent, remember that each form has a distinct property that will modify exposure, dose delivered, and dose retained.

TYPES OF INHALATION INJURY

Inhalation of gases and chemicals typically causes four different types of injury. They are (1) asphyxiation, (2) systemic toxicity, (3) immunologic damage, and (4) mucosal and alveolar damage. Asphyxiation has several com-

TABLE 41-1 Physical Form of Inhaled Agents

Gas:	A completely elastic fluid that does not become liquid or solid at ordinary temperature
Vapor:	A completely elastic fluid near its temperature of liquification
Fume:	Fine (<0.05 μm) particulate material resembling a gas but condensing to a solid at room temperature
Smoke:	Fume with droplets
Mist:	Tiny liquid droplets condensed about a solid nucleus

ponents and is typified by the injury sustained by smoke inhalation in fires. Systemic toxicity has been designated "metal fume fever." The third broad category of occupational asthma represents immunologic injury to the lung. The final category of diffuse mucosal and alveolar damage most often is associated with the inhalation of noxious gases and chemicals. The remainder of the chapter discusses examples of these four general categories, with emphasis on the first and last, as they are most frequently encountered in clinical practice.

ASPHYXIATION

Asphyxiation can occur in several ways. First, there can be a fall in the fractional concentration of inspired oxygen (FIO_2) either by replacement by another gas or by consumption of the ambient oxygen. Second, there can be alteration in oxygen carriage by the blood and therefore inadequate delivery to the tissue. Lastly, there can be interference with the utilization of oxygen by poisoning at the cellular level.

Normally the FIO_2 is about 0.21; any fall results in hypoxemia and, if severe enough, anoxia and death. The simplest way to produce a fall in FIO_2 is to replace ambient oxygen by another gas. These gases, often referred to as simple asphyxiants, include carbon dioxide, methane, and ethane, which cause no chemical or cellular injury themselves, but if present in high enough concentrations replace the ambient oxygen, resulting in suffocation and death. Sudden loss of consciousness and death occur when the FIO_2 equals or is less than 0.06.[4] Any gas, even those that cause cellular injury, can, in addition, cause asphyxiation by lowered FIO_2 if the leak occurs in an enclosed space and the victim is unable to escape.

Fire, the most frequently encountered of all causes of inhalation lung injury, also results in a fall in FIO_2. A reduced ambient FIO_2 can be caused by consumption of oxygen by the fire itself. When a room "bursts into flame" it does so by consuming the available oxygen to support the combustion. The resultant drop in FIO_2 can lead to hypoxemia and death regardless of the associated burns.

There are about 7,000 deaths in the United States per year due to the effects of smoke and hot air on the lungs.[5,6] Ten to 35 percent of all burn patients sustain some form of lung injury.[5] It was once widely held that facial burns were a reliable sign of lower respiratory tract injury from a fire. More recent studies suggest that, in fact, the opposite is true. Over 80 percent have no evidence of facial burns, with less than 50 and 15 percent experiencing hoarseness or singed nasal hairs, respectively.[7] Some investigators advocate flexible fiberoptic bronchoscopy for the detection of airways injury in the lower respiratory tract.[6,8] However, pulmonary function studies, [33]Xenon lung scan, and bronchoscopy all are unreliable ways to predict which injuries will progress to respiratory failure or death.[5,8] In addition, the systemic damage caused by carbon monoxide or cyanide poisoning (frequently associated with smoke inhalation from fires) does not correlate with airways injury.

Direct thermal injury to the lower respiratory tract occurs infrequently. The upper airways do a remarkable job of cooling and conditioning air before it reaches the intrathoracic airways and alveoli, even in the presence of pharyngeal burns. Only steam, because of its greater heat-carrying capacity, causes direct thermal injury to lower airways. This type of lower tract injury seems to be proportional to the extent and depth of the concomitant body surface burns.[5]

Chemical asphyxiants generated in the smoke and absorbed via the lungs result in alterations in oxygen carriage by the blood and cellular poisoning. These chemical asphyxiants are frequent causes of death in fires.

Carbon monoxide (CO) poisoning occurs in 50 to 70 percent of all fire victims with or without body burns.[4] CO, which has 200 to 250 times the affinity of O_2 for hemoglobin, binds reversibly to this molecule. Even in low concentrations it thus significantly reduces the O_2 carrying capacity of the blood. In addition, carboxyhemoglobin (COHb) shifts the oxyhemoglobin dissociation curve to the left, thereby impairing the release of any remaining O_2 to the tissues. This combined effect leads to a greater degree of tissue hypoxemia than an equivalent reduction of either FIO_2 or hemoglobin concentration would.[3] Significant CO exposure can also arise from automobile exhaust (any combustion engine), improperly vented furnaces and water heaters, and paint strippers containing methylene chloride, especially if encountered in enclosed spaces.[9]

The extent and severity of CO exposure is determined by the measurement of COHb saturation. Symptoms are related to the COHb saturation (Table 41-2). Remember that smokers and those living in large, smog-ridden cities can have chronic elevation of COHb, at times approaching the moderate range found in acute exposures.

Patients with acute CO poisoning present with a wide variety of symptoms. Dizziness and headache are prominent early symptoms, but the patient may present in coma. Patients with underlying cardiac disease may present with anginal pain or arrhythmias signifying cardiac hypoxia. Not surprisingly, there are usually few pulmonary symptoms unless the lung has been injured by other components of fire and smoke. This phenomenon occurs because the arterial partial pressure of oxygen (PaO_2) in pure CO poisoning usually is normal. Therefore, the carotid body, which senses a reduced PaO_2, is not stimulated and thus, tachypnea does not result. Only when tissue hypoxia results in metabolic (lactic) acidosis does tachypnea occur. Thus the arterial

TABLE 41-2 Symptoms Related to Various Levels of
Carboxyhemoglobin in the Blood

	Carboxyhemoglobin Saturation (COHb %)	Symptom*
Mild	1–15	None†, headache
Moderate	16–20	Headache
	20–40	Severe headache, nausea, vomiting, loss of coordination, loss of consciousness
Severe	40–60	Seizures, coma
	>60	Coma, death

* Symptoms do not always progress in an orderly fashion. Patients with underlying cardiorespiratory or metabolic disease or children may experience more severe symptoms at lower COHb %.
† These COHb levels can be found routinely in cigarette smokers.

blood gas level in CO poisoning initially can be normal, and it should not be relied on in assessing the severity of CO exposure.

In about 5 percent of fires, especially those in which polyurethane, nylon, or acrylic polymers are burned, hydrogen cyanide (HCN) may cause chemical asphyxiation. Cyanide combines directly with the cytochrome complex in the mitochondria and blocks the final step in oxidative phosphorylation, thereby preventing oxygen utilization by the cell.[1] The symptoms of HCN poisoning may be indistinguishable from CO intoxication. HCN poisoning must be suspected based on the knowledge of what materials were burning and in the presence of metabolic acidosis that persists in the face of falling COHb saturation.[7]

SYSTEMIC TOXICITY

Systemic effects of agents inhaled by the lung are relatively uncommon clinical problems. Most of these illnesses are related to specific occupations, and it is unusual for the practicing physician to see them outside of the workplace setting. These clinical problems are typified by the entities known as metal fume fever and polymer fume fever.

Metal fume fever is a result of inhalation of fumes of certain metals with low melting points. These metals are usually zinc, copper, and magnesium, but toxicity also can result from exposure to cadmium, iron, manganese, nickel, selenium, tin, and antimony fumes. These fumes often are found in industries utilizing welding; the welding process forms tiny particles of the oxides of these metals, which appear to be the specific injurious agents. Particle size seems to be the most important factor in determining toxicity.[10] Oxidized particles of less than 1.5 microns (usually 0.02 to 0.25 microns) come in contact with the alveolar wall and are thought to be chemotactic to polymorphonuclear leukocytes.[10] The chain of events brought on by the influx of leukocytes results in a typical presentation. Thirst and a metallic taste in the mouth occur 4 to 8 hours after exposure. Fever, rigors, myalgias, headache, and weakness follow 2 to 6 hours later. The symptoms often are suggestive of a pneumonia, but despite the lung being the portal of entry for these particles, the chest roentgenogram is usually normal. Laboratory testing usually reveals a leukocytosis. The symptoms resolve over the course of the next day or day and a half. Symptoms are recurrent for each new exposure, but tolerance develops after repeated exposures over a short period of time. The tolerance is short-lived, however, and typically symptoms recur upon returning to work after a weekend off. This reaction does not seem to be immunologically mediated, and there are no diagnostic tests to determine exposure; history and symptoms are the diagnostic criteria.

A similar syndrome has been noted upon exposure to polymer fumes; Teflon (polytetrafluoroethylene) is the common offending agent. Again, attacks are repetitive without evidence of sensitization to polymer and without evidence of injury to the lung itself. Other metal fumes, mercury, vanadium, and osmium among the more prominent, can cause systemic symptoms. In contrast to metal and polymer fume fever, they can cause direct airways or parenchymal lung injury.[10]

IMMUNOLOGIC INJURY

Lung injury that is immunologically mediated encompasses the large group of diseases known as occupational asthma. This topic is too broad to cover in detail, but two key issues are worth emphasizing. The first issue is the controversy over whether the offending agents are truly antigenic, i.e., the airways reactivity is on an immunologic basis, or whether the asthma is purely an irritative phenomenon with resultant nonspecific bronchospasm. Agents such as platinum salts, trimetalic anhydride (TMA), and toluene diisocyanate (TDI) appear to be immunologically mediated with detectable levels of immunoglobulin E (IgE) in serum.[10,11] Other agents probably cause occupational asthma by direct irritation of the airways. Formaldehyde is the best example of an agent that causes wheeze, cough, and dyspnea by a nonimmunologic mechanism.[12,13] To complicate matters further, lung injury from agents such as TDI may result from both irritative and immunologic mechanisms.[11]

The second issue of controversy is the specificity of circulating antibody in the diagnosis of occupational asthma. Often evidence of an immunologic reaction cannot be detected. Even when present, it may merely indicate exposure and not be the cause of the airways disease.[11,14,15] Thus, even when testing is available, it is not always useful in confirming the diagnosis.

Whether an irritative or immunologic cause is operative, occupational asthma is treated the same as any other type of asthma. Avoidance of the agent coupled with the use of bronchodilators, steroids, and mast cell stabilizers (cromolyn sodium) are indicated to control both chronic and acute symptoms.

MUCOSAL AND ALVEOLAR DAMAGE

Damage to the airway mucosa, either localized or diffuse, or to the alveolar surface is the most common type of inhalation injury. Other than asphyxiation, this type of injury is most often associated with noxious or toxic gas or fume exposure. When injury is primarily localized to the airways, an obstructive picture is usually seen with airways symptoms being prominent. When the injury is primarily at the level of the alveoli, the clinical picture is one of respiratory impairment or failure with diffuse infiltrate, stiff lungs, and hypoxemia, that is, an adult respiratory distress syndrome (ARDS) pattern.

The agents most often associated with these types of injury are listed in Table 41-3. The extent of injury from these agents is dependent on four factors. The first factor is their physical and chemical properties. The most important of these properties is solubility. The more soluble the gas, the easier it dissolves in, and is absorbed by, the upper respiratory tract, thus leading to the sensation of the gas being noxious (ammonia, chlorine, sulfur dioxide). The resulting injury is to the nasopharyngeal, bronchial, or bronchiolar mucosa. Gases of lesser solubility (oxides of nitrogen, phosgene, ozone) can penetrate deeper into the lung before detection and therefore predispose to alveolar injury. Concentration of the gas is the second most important factor.

TABLE 41-3   Common Agents That Cause Mucosal or Alveolar Damage

Agent	Tissue Injury Caused By
Oxygen, ozone (O_2, O_3)	Superoxide radicals, singlet oxygen
Ammonia (NH_3)	Ammonia hydroxide
Chlorine (Cl_2)	Hydrochloric acid, oxygen radical
Hydrogen chloride (CHl)	Hydrochloric acid
Oxides of nitrogen (NO, NO_2, N_2O_4)	Nitric acid, nitrates, nitrites
Phosgene ($COCl_2$)	Hydrochloric acid
Sulfur dioxide (SO_2)	Sulfurous acid

Clearly, injury can occur rapidly in the presence of a high gas concentration, but prolonged exposure to lower concentrations, especially if the gas is poorly soluble, can lead to injuries of similar severity. Thus, duration of exposure becomes the third most important factor. Here not only time but gas density is important. If a patient loses consciousness during an industrial accident and falls to the floor, more injury will occur if exposure is to a gas that is denser than air (chlorine). Fourth, minute ventilation is important in modulating the extent of injury in these exposures. The greater the minute ventilation, the more gas will be in contact with the respiratory system and thus the greater potential for injury.

The interaction of these factors produces injury at many levels of the respiratory tract. Thus, bronchitis and alveolar injury (ARDS) can occur in one individual, while upper airways obstruction and bronchospasm might predominate in another exposed to the same gas but under different circumstances. Typically, sulfur dioxide, which is a more soluble gas, causes severe upper respiratory tract and tracheal irritation with mucosal edema and sloughing, thus resulting in upper airway obstruction.[1,10] In severe exposures, irreversible bronchiolitis obliterans may occur. On the other hand, the oxides of nitrogen, which are less soluble, cause only minor upper respiratory irritation, but ARDS may ensue within the first 24 hours. If ARDS resolves, or in milder exposures where ARDS does not develop, a picture of bronchiolitis obliterans may appear in 2 to 4 weeks and may be fatal.[1,10]

Symptoms following exposure to any of the agents listed in Table 41-3 initially may be minimal. Choking and cough are prominent with few abnormalities on physical examination or chest roentgenogram. In the following hours to days, however, oropharyngeal edema, exudative bronchitis, and ARDS may ensue with all their attendant complications (hypoxemia, atelectasis, secondary infections). In 1 to 4 weeks, improvement begins despite the persistence of some cough and wheeze. Recovery may be complete following this period, though the issue of chronic disease remains a matter of debate.[10] Finally, recall that oxygen itself is a toxic gas when used in high concentrations, and therefore it needs to be used with caution in the treatment of these patients.[16]

THERAPY OF INHALATION INJURY

As with most occupational or environmental lung diseases, the best form of therapy in inhalation injury is prevention. Workers dealing with any of the agents mentioned should work in well-ventilated areas and avoid use in closed spaces. Safety procedures and proper protective equipment should be mandatory at all times. Individuals should avoid working without a co-worker(s) having knowledge of their activity and whereabouts. Of great importance is the rescuer's knowledge of potential injury to themselves. All too often a courageous co-worker or neighbor rushes headlong into the fume-filled room or burning house only to meet the same fate as the victim he is trying to save. This type of heroism should be avoided.

Specific therapy or antidotes for inhalation injury are few. The therapy of asphyxiants, primarily carbon monoxide, however, has been well worked out. Oxygen should be given immediately, as it displaces the CO from the hemoglobin molecule. The half-life of COHb is approximately 5 hours while breathing room air (FIO_2 = 0.21). This half-life can be reduced to approximately 80 minutes by inspiring 100 percent O_2 (FIO_2 = 1) and to about 30 minutes when 100 percent O_2 is inspired at three atmospheres pressure (hyperbaric oxygen). Hyperbaric therapy not only disassociates COHb more rapidly, but dissolves enough O_2 in the plasma to supply tissue needs without hemoglobin.[9] In addition, hyperbaric oxygen may reduce the chronic neurologic sequel of CO poisoning.[9,17] Unfortunately, hyperbaric chambers are not accessible to the majority of practicing physicians.

In cyanide poisoning caused by fires, attempts can be made to compete with the cyanide for the cytochrome oxidase system. This can be accomplished by administering 330 mg (10 ml) of 10 percent sodium nitrate by slow intravenous push followed immediately by 12.5 g (50 ml) of 25 percent sodium thiosulfate. The sodium nitrate combines with hemoglobin to form methemoglobin, which in turn binds the cyanide to form cyanmethemoglobin. This latter compound then reacts with the administered thiosulfate to form thiocyanate, which is not toxic.[1,10] This therapy, which may be repeated as needed, is not without risks as the methemoglobin created can impair O_2 transport itself.

Most of the therapy for inhalation injury is supportive. Prompt removal from the agent and washing of the skin is mandatory. Close observation of those not unconscious or in immediate respiratory distress is mandatory. For those overcome by smoke or fumes, establishment and maintenance of an airway and adequate oxygenation and ventilation along with cardiovascular support are essential as with any critically ill patient.

Bronchodilators should be used if wheezing is present. However, steroids have no use in inhalation injury unless the patient has an occupational asthma syndrome. Because the lung has such a large surface area and either rapidly absorbs or neutralizes the inhaled agent, bronchoalveolar lavage to remove the injurious agent is of no benefit in reducing injury. Finally, antibiotics should not be used prophylactically, but only if there is evidence of aspiration pneumonia or if secondary infection develops in the hospitalized patient being treated for inhalation injury.

References

1. Schwartz DA. Acute inhalation injury. State Art Rev Occup Med 1987; 2:297–318.
2. Summer W, Haponik E. Inhalation of irritant gases. Clin Chest Med 1981; 2:273–287.
3. Stewart RD. The effects of carbon monoxide on humans. Annu Rev Pharmacol 1975; 15:409–423.
4. Terrill JB, Montgomery RR, Reinhardt CF. Toxic gases from fires. Science 1978; 200:1343–1347.
5. Cahalane M, Demling RH. Early respiratory abnormalities from smoke inhalation. JAMA 1984; 251:771–773.
6. Trunkey DD. Inhalation injury. Surg Clin North Am 1978; 58:1133–1140.
7. Cohen MA, Guzzardi LJ. Inhalation of products of combustion. Ann Emerg Med 1983; 12:628–632.
8. Robinson L, Miller RN. Smoke inhalation injuries. Am J Otolaryngol 1986; 7:375–380.
9. Norkool DM, Kirkpatrick JN. Treatment of acute carbon monoxide poisoning with hyperbaric oxygen: a review of 115 cases. Ann Emerg Med 1985; 14:1168–1171.
10. Seaton A, Morgan WKC. Toxic gases and fumes. In: Morgan WKC, Seaton A. Occupational lung disease. 2nd ed. Philadelphia: WB Saunders, 1984: 609.
11. Seaton A. Occupational asthma. In: Morgan WKC, Seaton A. Occupational lung disease. 2nd ed. Philadelphia: WB Saunders, 1984: 498.
12. Bardana EJ. Formaldehyde: hypersensitivity and irritant reactions at work and in the home. Immunol Allergy Practice 1980; 2:60–72.
13. Frigas E, Filley WV, Reed CE. Bronchial challenge with formaldehyde gas: lack of bronchoconstriction in 13 patients suspected of having formaldehyde-induced asthma. Mayo Clin Proc 1984; 59:295–299.
14. Bernstein IL. Occupational asthma. Clin Chest Med 1981; 2:255–272.
15. Jones RN. Occupational asthma. Clin Chest Med 1984; 5:619–622.
16. Sicilian L, Fanburg BL. Oxygen toxicity. In: Parrillo JE, ed. Current therapy in critical care medicine. Toronto: BC Decker, 1987: 192.
17. Myers RA, Snyder SK, Emhoff TA. Subacute sequelae of carbon monoxide poisoning. Ann Emerg Med 1985; 14:1163–1167.

HEMATOLOGIC DISEASE AND CANCER

42 | ANEMIA

FREDERICK R. ARONSON, M.D.

Anemia may result from any of a wide variety of underlying disorders and nearly always requires further evaluation because it provides an objective sign of underlying disease. Early diagnostic evaluation is particularly important because, in many cases, prompt diagnosis may have a major effect on clinical outcome. For example, early carcinoma of the colon may present with anemia caused by iron deficiency. However, early evaluation is not always pursued because anemia is an extremely common clinical finding. The recent National Health and Nutrition Examination Survey estimates that approximately 3.8 percent of all noninstitutionalized Americans are anemic, and other studies indicate that approximately one in four medical inpatients are anemic.[1,2] Although iron deficiency or chronic disease account for many of these cases, any of a broad spectrum of other underlying diseases are present in the remainder. Furthermore, in many cases anemia develops as a consequence of the combined effects of several disorders. An orderly approach to diagnosis is therefore essential if the clinician is to avoid either inadequate or excessive evaluation and treatment. This chapter presents a logical approach to the evaluation of the anemic patient that emphasizes the use of readily available clinical and laboratory information to narrow the scope of the differential diagnosis. In addition, the major issues relevant to the clinical management of anemia are discussed.

INITIAL CONSIDERATIONS

Is the Patient Anemic?

Whether clinically suspected or incidentally noted, the evaluation of anemia begins with a laboratory measurement that indicates an abnormally low concentration of hemoglobin and/or an abnormally low packed red cell volume (hematocrit) in a sample of the patient's blood. Before proceeding with additional diagnostic or therapeutic maneuvers, the clinician must first determine whether the abnormal laboratory result correctly indicates that the patient is anemic. Although the critical importance of this step is readily apparent, it is not always a part of the process of evaluation in practice.

To address the question of whether or not a patient is anemic requires an understanding of the definition of anemia. Anemia is best defined as an absolute reduction in the total circulating red cell mass.[3,4] Aside from acute blood loss, such a reduction is accompanied by an increase in plasma volume such that blood volume remains constant. A reduction in the mass of circulating red cells, or anemia, is therefore most readily detected as a decrease in the concentration of hemoglobin or red cells in the blood.

Isolated Expansion of Plasma Volume

The hemoglobin and hematocrit, however, also decrease when plasma volume expands in the absence of an associated increase in the circulating red cell mass. This occurs routinely during the third trimester of pregnancy, in marathon runners and other endurance athletes,[5] in patients with massive splenomegaly,[6] in renal failure patients who are overhydrated, in some patients with an IgM paraprotein, and occasionally in hypoalbuminemic patients shortly after lying down. In these instances it may be difficult to equate the concentration of hemoglobin or red cells with the total red cell mass. Direct measurement of the red cell mass by use of radiolabeled red cells may therefore be necessary to differentiate between simple expansion of plasma volume and actual anemia, which also occurs in all of these settings.

The Definition of Normal

A second aspect of determining whether a patient is anemic relates to the definition of the normal range of the hemoglobin concentration and of the hematocrit. Normal values are derived empirically from the distribution of these measurements in a healthy reference population.[7,8] Consequently, the definition of what is abnormal depends both on the degree of deviation below the population mean that is considered abnormal and on the composition of the reference population. Given that the lower limit of normal for the population is assigned in an arbitrary fashion, it follows that some patients with normal values are actually anemic while some patients with values below normal are, in fact, not anemic.

In attempting to determine whether the hematocrit of an individual patient indicates that the patient is anemic, the clinician must avoid rigidly equating the range of normal for the population with the normal range of the patient. Rather, population-based values should be used by the clinician to estimate the likelihood that the patient is anemic: the lower the hematocrit, the greater the likelihood that the patient truly is anemic. When available, previous measurements of a patient's hematocrit provide a better standard for comparison than do population norms. Decreases of 10 percent or more from previous values are likely to be significant.

In addition, any of a variety of technical errors occasionally results in spuriously low measurements of the hemoglobin and hematocrit and may lead to an unnecessary anemia work-up. Unexpected or sudden drops in the hematocrit should therefore be verified with a repeat measurement in a new blood sample.

Recognizing the Problem

Despite these considerations, the failure to recognize, evaluate, and treat anemia is a much more prevalent problem in practice than is the over-recognition of 'anemia' in patients who are not truly anemic. A recent study from Oklahoma[2] found that anemia went completely unrecognized in 25 percent of patients with anemia on a medical service. Furthermore, even when recognized, anemia was neither evaluated nor treated in an additional 20 percent of cases. According to the authors, poor understanding of the definition of anemia and of the clinical implications of ignoring its presence, as well as simple lack of attention to laboratory reports of abnormal red cell indices or morphology, were at the root of the problem in their institution.

CLINICAL EVALUATION

Once recognized, anemia is evaluated in the same organized fashion used in approaching any complex clinical problem. Although it may seem obvious, it cannot be overemphasized that this process begins with the history and physical examination and then proceeds with selected laboratory testing. The evaluation of anemia all too often begins with a barrage of laboratory testing, perhaps because anemia is usually first recognized when laboratory test results are found to be abnormal. Although such an approach may be considered expeditious, more often than not it leads to confusion and frustration when the results fail to indicate the diagnosis. As with most complex clinical problems, laboratory results are most informative when considered in the context of information obtained from the history and physical examination.

History

Our approach to the evaluation of the anemic patient begins with an attempt to answer the five questions listed in Table 42-1. In addition to providing information regarding the nature, duration, and severity of the patient's symptoms, the history is the primary source of information needed to answer several of the questions listed in the table. Having discussed the first question, we will proceed under the assumption that the patient is anemic. Because anemia is often the result of the combined effects of several underlying disorders, *each* of these questions should be reviewed carefully to avoid the pitfall of identifying one contributing cause while missing one or several others.

Inherited Disorders

The history is often useful in approaching the question of whether anemia is congenital or acquired. This issue should not be overlooked because the differential diagnosis of the inherited disorders that result in anemia is quite different from that of the disorders that result in acquired anemia. A past or family history of anemia, of splenectomy, of refusal as a blood donor, or of treatment with iron, B_{12}, or folate should be actively sought and, when present, suggest the possibility that the disorder is congenital. Furthermore, because the frequency of several of the heritable anemias varies markedly in different ethnic groups, a brief exploration of the patient's ancestry is often helpful. Sickle cell disease,[9,10] the thalassemias,[11] glucose-6-phosphate dehydrogenase[12] and other enzyme deficiencies,[13] and hereditary spherocytosis and elliptocytosis[14] account for the vast majority of the inherited anemias. When anemia is caused by one of these disorders, the primary mechanism is either chronic or episodic hemolysis, and prominent red cell morphologic abnormalities are usually present on either routine blood smear preparations or on special

TABLE 42-1 Evaluating Anemia

Is the patient anemic?
Is the anemia congenital or acquired?
Has the patient been exposed to drugs or toxins?
Is there evidence of blood loss or hemolysis?
Is there evidence of systemic or chronic inflammatory disease?

preparations designed to reveal Heinz bodies or sickle cells. For a variety of reasons, however, these disorders do not uniformly result in either anemia or abnormal red cell morphology in other family members. The presence of one of these disorders in the patient, therefore, cannot be excluded by the absence of a positive family history.

Drugs and Toxins

A history of exposure to certain drugs or toxins may provide important clues to the cause of anemia. Special care must often be given to detecting these exposures because over-the-counter medications and environmental toxins are frequently overlooked by patients. Drugs may result in anemia when they suppress bone marrow function, when they provoke either immune or oxidative hemolysis, or when they cause or promote blood loss; prominent examples are listed in Table 42-2. Drug-induced oxidative hemolysis occurs almost exclusively in individuals with glucose-6-phosphate dehydrogenase deficiency. Because of the complexity of the various interactions between drugs and hematopoiesis, the clinician should review suspect drugs on an individual basis by consulting the prescribing information provided in the package insert or by consulting one of the major texts listed in the references of this chapter.[3,4]

Alcohol and its metabolites directly suppress erythropoiesis and antagonize the action of folate. Furthermore, excessive alcohol consumption frequently is associated with a diet poor in folates, with both chronic and acute gastrointestinal blood loss, and with decreased red cell survival (a consequence of the altered red cell membrane lipid composition and hypersplenism that may accompany liver disease). All of these mechanisms should be considered when attempting to determine the cause of anemia in patients who abuse alcohol.[15,16]

Although it rarely presents with isolated anemia, lead intoxication interferes with a variety of red cell enzyme systems required for hemoglobin synthesis and results in either micro- or normocytic anemia with prominent basophilic stippling of the red cells and ringed sideroblasts in the bone marrow. A blood lead level should be obtained whenever lead intoxication is suspected.

Blood Loss and Hemolysis

Bleeding and hemolysis often occur episodically and may not be active at the time of evaluation. Therefore, the history is particularly important in considering whether these processes are contributing to the development of anemia. In addition to a detailed menstrual history, an attempt should be made to determine whether the patient has noted epistaxis, hemoptysis, hematemesis, hematuria, or melanotic or bloody stool. Diagnostic and therapeutic phlebotomy, unreplaced surgical blood loss, and hemodialysis should not be overlooked as potential sources of significant blood loss. Symptoms such as pica (craving to eat dirt, clay, ice, or laundry starch) or sore tongue and signs such as koilonychia (spooned nails), glossitis, or angular stomatitis suggest iron deficiency attributable to chronic blood loss. A history of jaundice or

TABLE 42-2   Drugs That May Result in Anemia*

Drugs that may interfere with red cell production
   By inducing marrow suppression or aplasia
      Alcohol
      Antineoplastic drugs
      Antithyroid drugs
      Antibiotics
      Oral hypoglycemic agents
      Phenylbutazone
      Azidothymidine (AZT)
   By interfering with B_{12}, folate, or iron absorption or utilization
      Nitrous oxide
      Anticonvulsant drugs
      Antineoplastic drugs
      Isoniazid, cycloserine

Drugs capable of promoting hemolysis
   Immune-mediated
      Penicillins
      Quinine
      Alphamethyldopa
      Procainamide
   Mechanical
      Mitomycin C
   Oxidative
      Antimalarials
      Sulfa drugs
      Nalidixic acid
      Nitrofurantoin

Drugs that may produce or promote blood loss
   Aspirin
   Alcohol
   Nonsteroidal anti-inflammatory agents
   Corticosteroids
   Anticoagulants

* This table is intended as a review of the mechanisms by which drugs *may* aggravate or produce anemia. It includes only the most important categories and agents and should not be considered to be exhaustively complete. See text.

hepatitis, gallstones or cholecystectomy, splenectomy, or episodes of dark or cola-colored urine should prompt consideration of the various hemolytic disorders outlined in Table 42–3.

TABLE 42–3   Classification of the
Hemolytic Disorders

Intrinsic to red cell
    Congenital
        Hemoglobinopathy
            sickle-cell disease
            thalassemia
        Membrane abnormality
            hereditary spherocytosis
            hereditary elliptocytosis
        Enzymopathy
            glucose-6-phosphate dehydrogenase deficiency
            pyruvate kinase deficiency
            others
    Acquired
        Paroxysmal nocturnal hemoglobinuria

Extrinsic to red cell
    Immune-mediated (microspherocytes)
        Warm-reactive antibodies (Coombs' positive)
            Autoimmune
            Drug-induced
            Lymphoproliferative disease
        Cold-reactive antibodies
            Paroxysmal cold hemoglobinuria
                Chronic idiopathic
                Acute transient (after viral illness)
                Syphilis
            Cold agglutinins
                Polyclonal (titer less than 1:1,000)
                    Mycoplasma
                    Epstein-Barr virus
                Monoclonal (titer greater than 1:1,000)
                    Chronic idiopathic
                    Lymphoproliferative disease
    Traumatic (schistocytes)
        Macroangiopathic
            Valvular heart disease
            Marching, bongo playing, and so on

Table continues on following page

Table 42-2 *(Continued)*

Microangiopathic
    Disseminated intravascular coagulation
    Vasculitis
    Peripartum
    Malignant hypertension
    Giant cavernous hemangioma (Kasabach-Merritt
      syndrome)
    Hemolytic uremic syndrome
    Thrombotic thrombocytopenic purpura
    Severe diabetic vascular disease
Infective
    Malaria
    Babesiosis
    Clostridial sepsis
Environmental
    Burns
    Copper intoxication
    Snake or spider bites
Hypersplenism

Past Medical and Surgical History

An attempt to identify the various chronic or systemic disorders that may result in anemia begins with a careful history and physical examination. The major disease categories to be considered are neoplasia,[17] chronic renal disease,[18] chronic liver disease, endocrine disorders,[19] chronic infection, and chronic inflammatory disorders such as rheumatoid arthritis, ulcerative colitis, and Crohn's disease. In addition, a remote history of ulcer disease or bowel surgery may be forgotten by the patient and, if present, sometimes provides an important clue to identifying the source of iron, B_{12}, or folate deficiency.

Physical Examination

A number of findings on physical examination may be helpful to direct the clinician's attention to the cause of anemia. A careful rectal and pelvic examination, in particular, should not be overlooked in the evaluation of the anemic patient. In addition to performing a thorough general physical examination, particular attention should be paid to the findings listed in Table 42–4.

LABORATORY INVESTIGATION

The list of laboratory tests that may be indicated during the evaluation of the anemic patient is as diverse as the various underlying disorders that result in anemia.[20] As discussed previously, a logical approach to the selection of tests appropriate to a given patient is essential if the laboratory is expected to assist, rather than confound, the process of evaluation. The approach presented here uses the information provided by the results of a limited panel of preliminary tests in conjunction with the information obtained from the history and physical examination to direct a subsequent round of investigations directed at establishing the diagnosis.

TABLE 42-4 Physical Examination Findings Associated with Anemia

Findings	Associated Anemia
Pallor, tachypnea, tachycardia, postural hypotension	Acute blood loss
Green-tinged pallor, koilonychia, glossitis, angular stomatitis, blood in stool	Iron deficiency
Fever, cachexia, signs attributable to neoplasia, chronic infection, rheumatoid arthritis, ulcerative colitis, Crohn's disease, or other inflammatory disorders	Chronic disease
Lemon-yellow pallor, vitiligo, glossitis, diminished vibration and position sense, dementia	B_{12} deficiency
Pallor, glossitis, signs of malabsorption, alcohol abuse, pregnancy, exfoliative dermatitis, absence of neurologic findings of B_{12} deficiency	Folate deficiency
Bradycardia, narrow pulse pressure, hypothermia, cool coarse dry skin, sallow pallor, reduced scalp and body hair, nonpitting edema of face, hands, and extremities, goiter, husky voice, slow speech, poor hearing, poor memory, peripheral neuropathy, "hung-up" reflexes	Hypothyroidism
Jaundice, icterus, spider angiomata, gynecomastia, hemorrhoids, encephalopathy	Liver disease
Sallow pallor, excoriations, uremic frost, pericardial rub, peripheral neuropathy, proximal myopathy	Chronic renal disease
Gingival lead line, abdominal tenderness, peripheral neuropathy	Lead poisoning
Fever, segmented conjunctival capillaries, retinal neovascularization, hepatomegaly, cholecystitis, bone tenderness, leg ulcers, stroke	Sickle cell disease
Jaundice, boney abnormalities, hepatosplenomegaly, cholecystitis, leg ulcers	Thalassemias
Ecchymoses, bone tenderness, encephalopathy, peripheral neuropathy	Multiple myeloma
Fever, pallor, petechiae, ecchymoses	Aplastic anemia
Fever, pallor, petechiae, ecchymoses, adenopathy, sternal tenderness, splenomegaly	Leukemia, myelodysplasia, or myeloproliferative syndrome

Initial Studies

The initial laboratory evaluation of the anemic patient should always include a careful review of the complete blood count and the peripheral blood smear, a determination of the reticulocyte count, and an examination of at least one stool sample for the presence of occult blood.

Complete Blood Count

In addition to providing a measure of the concentration of hemoglobin and red cells in the blood, the complete blood count includes a determination of the mean corpuscular volume (MCV) of the red cells, a total and differential white cell count, and a platelet count.

The MCV is widely used in the classification of anemia and often provides a useful first approach to narrowing the scope of the differential diagnosis. A review of the classification of the causes of anemia based on the MCV (Table 42–5), however, quickly reveals some important limitations of focusing exclusively on this parameter. In particular, the MCV is of minimal value in distinguishing between the two most common causes of anemia, chronic disease and iron deficiency.

The total and differential white cell count and the platelet count must also be reviewed when investigating anemia. Leukopenia and/or thrombocytopenia in conjunction with anemia (bi- or pancytopenia) strongly suggests the presence of either a primary or a secondary disorder of the bone marrow, megaloblastic anemia, or hypersplenism and should lead to a prompt investigation of these possibilities, beginning with the blood smear. Oval macrocytes and hypersegmented neutrophils suggest megaloblastic anemia, and their absence in patients with bicytopenia or pancytopenia should be evaluated with a bone marrow aspirate and biopsy. Hypersplenism is likely when cytopenias and splenomegaly are present with a cellular marrow that shows normal maturation of all precursors.

TABLE 42-5   Classification of the Causes of Anemia Based on MCV

Microcytic anemia (MCV less than 80 fl)
  Iron deficiency
  Thalassemia
  Chronic disease
  Sideroblastic anemia
    Lead
    Alcohol
    Antineoplastic drugs
    Pyridoxine-responsive
    Hereditary

Normocytic
  Chronic disease
  Early iron deficiency
  Sickle cell disease
  Recent blood loss
  Hemolysis
  Liver disease
  Renal disease
  Hypothyroidism
  Adrenal insufficiency
  Marrow disorders
    Aplasia
    Dysplasia
    Fibrosis
    Neoplasia
      Leukemia
      Lymphoma
      Myeloma
      Metastatic

Macrocytic (MCV greater than 100 fl)
  Megaloblastic
    Vitamin B_{12} deficiency
    Folate deficiency
    Antineoplastic drugs
    Hereditary
  Nonmegaloblastic
    Reticulocytosis
    Alcohol
    Liver disease
    Hypothyroidism
    Marrow disorders (see Normocytic,
      Marrow disorders)

The Peripheral Blood Smear

Examination of the blood smear should be directed toward identifying the features listed in Table 42-6. When present, a number of these abnormalities immediately suggest the associated diagnoses listed in the table. Furthermore, the absence of some of these findings provides strong negative evidence that is useful in excluding the disorder in question from further consideration.

TABLE 42-6   Peripheral Blood Smear Findings in the Diagnosis of Anemia

Findings	Associated Anemia
Oval macrocytes, hypersegmented neutrophils	Megaloblastic anemia
Schistocytes (fragmented red cells)	Traumatic hemolysis
Microspherocytes	Immune-mediated hemolysis, hereditary spherocytosis
Elliptocytes (more than 25%)	Hereditary elliptocytosis
Target cells	Liver disease, thalassemia, other hemoglobinopathies
Coarse basophilic stippling of red cells	Thalassemia, lead intoxication
Sickle cells	Sickle cell disease and variants
Microcytic, hypochromic red cells and small numbers of elliptocytes	Iron deficiency
Nucleated red cells	Intense marrow stimulation after hemorrhage or hypoxia or postsplenectomy
Nucleated red cells and immature granulocytes	Marrow infiltration by tumor, granuloma, infection, or lipid storage disease
Nucleated red cells, immature granulocytes, and teardrop-shaped red cells	Myelofibrosis
Rouleaux	Myeloma or macroglobulinemia
Agglutinated red cells	Cold agglutinin disease, generally monoclonal
Parasites	Malaria, babesiosis, trypanosomiasis

The Reticulocyte Count

When corrected for the degree of anemia, an increased reticulocyte count provides immediate insight into the mechanism of anemia. Correction of the reticulocyte count for the degree of anemia is necessary because the reported value almost always refers to the percentage of reticulocytes relative to the number of red cells counted. In the presence of anemia, when the red cell count is decreased, the percentage of reticulocytes is increased simply because the denominator in this fraction is decreased. Of the several techniques used to correct for the degree of anemia, the most straightforward is to simply multiply the reported reticulocyte count by the patient's hematocrit divided by 45 (an arbitrarily selected value of the normal hematocrit); normal values range from 1 to 2 percent. Corrected values greater than 5 percent that persist in the absence of an increasing hematocrit imply the presence of either hemolysis or ongoing blood loss. The absence of reticulocytosis, however, does not exclude these possibilities because an additional disorder that interferes with a normal marrow response to anemia may also be present. Corrected values of less than 0.5 percent in association with significant anemia strongly suggest aplasia of the marrow that should be evaluated with marrow aspiration and biopsy.[21]

Stool Occult Blood

Testing of stool for the presence of occult blood must not be omitted from the evaluation of the anemic patient. The value of this simple procedure is widely recognized in the detection of a variety of gastrointestinal lesions. Because bleeding often occurs episodically, however, multiple samples obtained over 1 to 2 weeks should be tested before concluding that gastrointestinal bleeding is not present.[22] Other sources of false-negative testing include the ingestion of vitamin C supplements and the use of outdated testing reagents. False-positive test results can be produced by the ingestion of large amounts of cherries, tomatoes, or red meats.

Additional Laboratory Testing

After a careful history and physical examination have been completed and initial test results have been reviewed, further laboratory investigation usually is required to establish the cause(s) of anemia. Ideally, each component of this phase of the evaluation is selected to test specific hypotheses generated during the initial evaluation.

Iron Studies

Iron studies should be performed early in the evaluation of most patients with anemia because iron deficiency is common and because its presence indicates the need to identify a source of blood loss. Iron studies, however, are not indicated in the presence of significant reticulocytosis because this finding reliably indicates the presence of adequate iron stores. Furthermore, because the results of these tests are altered during the acute phase response, iron studies do not accurately reflect the patient's iron stores in the presence of fever or of acute infection and are not helpful in the evaluation of anemia under these circumstances.

Thyroid, Renal, and Liver Function Tests

Tests of thyroid, renal, and liver function also should be obtained in the evaluation of most patients with anemia. They need not be performed when the cause of anemia is clearly identified from the results of other studies. Even then, the clinician should consider obtaining tests to exclude hypothyroidism since subtle features of hypothyroidism are easily missed. For example, this diagnosis should be considered in anemic women with abnormal menses, particularly if suspected iron deficiency anemia does not respond to iron supplements, since menometrorrhagia may occur as a consequence of hypothyroidism.

The creatinine clearance should be estimated in the evaluation of normocytic anemia of uncertain etiology. Anemia caused by chronic renal disease is usually proportional to the degree of renal insufficiency. Because other causes of anemia occur frequently in patients with chronic renal failure, their presence should be carefully excluded before attributing anemia to renal disease.

When chronic liver disease is suspected, the serum albumin concentration and the prothrombin time should be determined along with the direct and indirect bilirubin, the lactic dehydrogenase (LDH), the alkaline phosphatase, and the transaminases. It is unlikely that anemia is a result of liver disease if all of these tests are normal. In addition to detection of liver disease, elevations of the indirect bilirubin and the LDH are useful indicators of hemolysis and ineffective erythropoiesis. When liver disease is present, mild to moderate anemia may develop as a consequence of shortened red cell survival. In these cases, examination of the blood smear usually reveals target cells or burr cells. Other potentially correctable causes of anemia, such as folate deficiency, blood loss, or hypersplenism, should be sought before attributing anemia to liver disease per se.

Tests for Hemolysis

Anemia caused by decreased red cell survival (hemolysis) may be suspected on the basis of the history, physical examination, or initial laboratory evaluation. Before attempting to establish a diagnosis of one of the disorders listed in Table 42–3, evidence of hemolysis should be sought by determination of the levels of the indirect serum bilirubin, the LDH, and the haptoglobin. Although the presence of reticulocytosis suggests that hemolysis (or blood loss) is present, the absence of reticulocytosis cannot be considered evidence against hemolysis because other processes may prevent a normal marrow response to anemia.[23] Both intravascular and, to a lesser degree, extravascular (reticuloendothelial) destruction of red cells result in increases in the levels of the indirect bilirubin and the LDH and decreases in the haptoglobin level. Although recent transfusion or resolving hematoma also may alter the haptoglobin and the bilirubin, the LDH is not affected by these factors. When the results of these tests are confounded by other processes, the free hemoglobin level of the plasma may also be helpful in documenting ongoing intravascular hemolysis. In addition, red cell survival may be measured directly by using isotopic techniques such as the [51]chromium red cell survival test. In cases where an episode of hemolysis is believed to have occurred and subsided before an evaluation could begin, a sample of urine sediment from a freshly voided specimen should be stained for iron and promptly examined for the presence of hemosiderin-containing renal tubular cells. In contrast to the aforementioned blood tests, these cells may be observed in the urine for up to 14 days following episodes of intravascular or severe extravascular hemolysis.

Once the presence of hemolysis has been established, further evaluation to determine the cause of hemolysis is best directed by the features of the history, the findings on physical examination, and a review of the blood smear (see Table 42–3). For example, a Coombs' test should be used to establish the presence of warm antibody-mediated hemolysis, hemoglobin electrophoresis should be performed if the presence of an abnormal hemoglobin is suspected, and osmotic fragility should be evaluated when hereditary spherocytosis is suspect.

Tests for B_{12} and Folate Deficiency

When present, any of the previously noted findings from the history, the physical examination, or the initial laboratory evaluation that suggest the presence of B_{12} or folate deficiency should be confirmed by direct measurement. Although this covers a wide variety of possibilities, it should be recalled that untreated megaloblastic anemia is almost always accompanied by the characteristic presence of hypersegmented neutrophils and oval macrocytes on the peripheral blood smear. In the absence of these or of the particular neurologic features of B_{12} deficiency, the diagnostic yield of measuring B_{12} and folate levels is low. On the other hand, an elevated MCV should not be relied on as a clinical screen for the presence of B_{12} or folate deficiency.[24,25] Macrocytosis may be absent in the presence of megaloblastic hematopoiesis as a result of concomitant iron deficiency, thalassemia, infection, inflammation, or renal disease.

When megaloblastic hematopoiesis is recognized, however, B_{12} and folate levels should be measured to define which deficiency is present.[26] An understanding of the limitations of these measurements is important because diagnostic errors in these patients may result in unacceptable morbidity. Serum folate levels, for example, can be unreliable for the detection of folate deficiency because truly low serum folate levels frequently normalize as a consequence of improved diet soon after hospital admission. In the absence of transfusion, red cell folate levels are not subject to rapid alterations, but they are frequently low in the presence of primary B_{12} deficiency and thus may lead to the inappropriate treatment of B_{12} deficiency with folate. If this occurs, irreversible neurologic damage attributable to untreated B_{12} deficiency may develop, even though the anemia and signs of megaloblastic hematopoiesis resolve. Some measure of caution is therefore appropriate in the interpretation of the results of either of these tests for folate deficiency. Fortunately, current assays of serum B_{12} are generally quite sensitive for the detection of B_{12} deficiency when it is present. Because these assays are designed for maximum sensitivity, however, falsely low levels of B_{12} are also occasionally reported. This occurs primarily in the presence of folate deficiency, transcobalamin I deficiency, multiple myeloma, pregnancy, or oral contraceptive use. When necessary, measurement of the urinary excretion of methylmalonic acid (MMA) can definitively resolve this issue because MMA excretion is increased in B_{12} deficiency, but not in folate deficiency.

Bone Marrow Examination

The presence of bi- or pancytopenia, profound reticulocytopenia, leukoerythroblastosis (circulating immature myeloid and erythroid precursors), or a suspicion of multiple myeloma should be evaluated with bone marrow biopsy and aspiration. Bone marrow examination also is useful in the evaluation of anemia to definitively determine the status of iron stores, to confirm the presence of megaloblastosis, to evaluate combined nutritional deficiency states, or to investigate moderate or severe anemia of uncertain cause.

SELECTED CAUSES OF ANEMIA

The two most common causes of anemia, chronic disease and iron deficiency, as well as the anemia of chronic renal disease and of megaloblastic anemia are of sufficient importance to the clinician to merit additional brief discussion in this review.

The Anemia of Chronic Disease

Most neoplasms and virtually all of the chronic inflammatory and infectious disorders result in a syndrome widely known as 'the anemia of chronic disease'.[27] Although the name may suggest that this syndrome occurs in any of a vast array of chronic diseases, this diagnosis should only be considered in association with an inflammatory, infectious, or neoplastic process. Furthermore, because other causes of anemia are frequently present in these settings, the anemia of chronic disease should be considered as a diagnosis of exclusion to avoid missing other less readily apparent causes of anemia.

The syndrome is characterized by moderate anemia (hematocrit rarely less than 25 percent), normocytic or slightly microcytic red cells, normal or slightly increased numbers of reticulocytes, decreased concentrations of both serum iron and the iron-binding protein transferrin, and an increased serum ferritin. The latter two features are particularly useful in distinguishing the anemia of chronic disease from that of iron deficiency, which also occurs in a number of these settings.[28,29] In contrast to the anemia of chronic disease, the serum transferrin increases and the ferritin decreases in iron deficiency.[30,31] Furthermore, iron deficiency results in anisocytosis (variation in the size of the red cells), which is not generally present in the anemia of chronic disease. The width of the red cell size distribution (RDW), now included in the results of most automated cell counters, provides an objective quantification of anisocytosis and thus may also be helpful in this differential diagnosis.[32,33] The RDW is increased in the presence of iron deficiency and is usually normal in the anemia of chronic disease. These contrasts are less apparent, however, when both iron deficiency and the anemia of chronic disease are present simultaneously. In these cases, only the absence of iron in a sample of bone marrow or an increase in the hematocrit with a trial of iron therapy definitively indicates the presence of iron deficiency. In the absence of high fever or cardiopulmonary disease, the anemia of chronic disease rarely is symptomatic, and transfusions generally are unnecessary.

Iron Deficiency Anemia

When severe, anemia caused by iron deficiency is easily recognized. Hypochromic and microcytic red cells, decreased serum iron and ferritin levels, and increased serum transferrin levels (iron-binding capacity) usually are present in such cases. Not infrequently, one or several of these classic features are absent and establishing the diagnosis may be more challenging.[28-31] A serum ferritin of less than 12 μg per liter, however, is a reliable indicator of the presence of iron deficiency even in patients with liver disease or chronic inflammation.[34] When iron deficiency is suspected and blood iron studies are inconclusive, the status of the patient's iron stores should be evaluated either with an examination of the marrow for stainable iron or with a therapeutic trial of oral iron supplements.

Once recognized, the proper management of iron deficiency anemia includes not only treatment with iron supplements,[35] but also a search for the source of the deficiency (blood loss) and careful follow-up to insure that treatment completely corrects the problem. Most often, iron deficiency occurs as a consequence of any of a great variety of gastrointestinal lesions. Other causes of iron deficiency are listed in Table 42-7. Oral iron supplements should

TABLE 42-7   Causes of Iron Deficiency Other Than Gastrointestinal Blood Loss

Pregnancy, lactation, and delivery
Blood donation
Medical phlebotomy
Dietary insufficiency: in infants*, adolescents, menstruating women, and strict vegetarians
Genitourinary losses: menstrual bleeding; uterine, cervical, or vaginal lesions; renal, ureteral, or bladder lesions; chronic intravascular hemolysis; hemodialysis
Malabsorption: after gastric or small bowel surgery* or in malabsorption syndromes* (celiac disease, food allergy, others)
Pulmonary losses: idiopathic pulmonary hemosiderosis or chronic hemoptysis of any etiology
Self-induced phlebotomy

* Gastrointestinal blood loss also frequently contributes.

be administered for at least 6 months in order to correct both the anemia and the depleted body iron stores. Failure of the anemia to respond completely to iron therapy within 2 months implies either continued blood loss, non-compliance with therapy, impaired ability to absorb iron as a consequence of gastric and/or small bowel pathology, or an incorrect or incomplete initial diagnosis.

The Anemia of Chronic Renal Disease

The results of recent trials of recombinant erythropoietin in the treatment of the anemia of end-stage renal disease provide striking evidence that the major cause of this anemia is erythropoietin deficiency.[36] Other factors may contribute to the development of anemia in this setting.[18] These include iron deficiency attributable to both hemodialysis-associated and gastrointestinal blood loss, dietary or dialysis-induced folate deficiency, aluminum toxicity, hyperparathyroidism, decreased red cell survival, and perhaps nondialyzable uremic inhibitors of erythropoiesis. In addition, hemolysis may occur in these patients as a consequence of improper hemodialysis if blood is exposed to formaldehyde, heat, or hypotonic media. Aside from the possible use of erythropoietin, the management of anemia in patients with chronic renal disease begins, as in other settings, with an attempt to correct any reversible causes of anemia that are present. Androgens or periodic transfusion may be needed when other measures are inadequate and treatment is required.

Megaloblastic Anemia

Once megaloblastic anemia has been recognized[37] and the results of serum B_{12} and folate tests indicate which deficiency is present, treatment should be instituted[35] and a cause of the deficiency identified. Gluten-sensitive enteropathy or tropical sprue should be suspected if both vitamins are simultaneously deficient. When B_{12} deficiency is present, pernicious anemia is the most likely cause and can be documented by demonstration of the presence of anti-intrinsic factor antibodies or by performance of a Schilling test that corrects with exogenously administered intrinsic factor. Folate deficiency occurs as a consequence of any or several of the following: dietary insufficiency; nutritional malabsorption caused by drugs, enteritis, enteropathy, or gastric or jejunal resection; or the increased nutritional requirements of infancy, pregnancy, chronic hemolytic disease, malignancy (also attributable to poor diet), or chronic exfoliative dermatitis. In patients who drink alcoholic beverages on a regular basis, poor diet, ethanol-induced interruption of the enterohepatic circulation of folates, and a direct antifolate action of ethanol frequently lead to significant folate deficiency, even though beer contains high levels of folate. When features of megaloblastic hematopoiesis are identified, but B_{12} and folate levels are not decreased, a primary bone marrow disorder such as myelodysplasia[38] or marrow dysfunction caused by drug or toxic exposure should be considered by a review of the history and by examination of bone marrow aspirate and biopsy specimens.

MANAGEMENT

The optimal management of the anemic patient must include efforts directed not only at treating the symptoms attributable to anemia itself, but also at correcting the cause(s) of the anemia insofar as that may be possible. In virtually all cases, treatment of the underlying disorder is ultimately of much greater significance to the patient's welfare than are measures such as transfusion or replacement of depleted iron stores. Such measures can be expected to correct anemia only transiently and may adversely affect the patient's prognosis by delaying necessary treatment of the underlying disease. With this caveat in mind, however, it is appropriate to consider those aspects of management related to the correction of anemia per se.

Transfusion

The transfusion of packed red cells to correct anemia is indicated if the patient is symptomatic or if anemia threatens damage to the brain, heart, or other organs. Common symptoms attributable to severe anemia include exertional dyspnea and other forms of exercise intolerance, headache, dizziness, faintness, profound fatigue, angina pectoris, and claudication. There is a great deal of individual variation with regard to which symptoms predominate. When anemia develops over a prolonged period, as is often the case, these problems generally do not develop until the hemoglobin falls below 7 g per deciliter unless there is coexisting pulmonary or cardiovascular disease. In any case, when transfusion is contemplated it should be regarded as a potentially morbid therapeutic option. This concept has been made tragically clear in recent years with the appearance of the acquired immunodeficiency syndrome. In addition to the human immunodeficiency virus,[39] each transfusion carries a definite risk of transmitting the agent of non-A, non-B hepatitis,[40] the hepatitis B virus,[41] the hepatitis A virus,[42] the cytomegalovirus, the Epstein-Barr virus, and a host of other pathogens. Although screening tests are helpful in reducing these risks, it must be clear that even the best of screening procedures do not make transfusion a risk-free therapy. In addition, because plasma volume expands and cardiac output increases in response to chronic anemia, transfusion carries a risk of precipitating acute pulmonary edema and death. Other important complications of transfusion include hemolytic, febrile, and allergic transfusion reactions and the eventual development of body iron overload. In view of the various risks of transfusion as well as the need to conserve the limited resources of the nation's blood supply, the practices of transfusion based on arbitrarily selected values of the hematocrit, transfusion to increase intravascular volume, and prophylactic transfusion before surgery are to be condemned.

Synthetic Red Cell Substitutes

Synthetic red cell substitutes may someday offer an alternative to red cell transfusion in the management of severe anemia. However, a recent clinical study evaluating the use of an oxygen-carrying perfluorochemical emulsion in individuals with religious objections to transfusion demonstrated that the treatment was unnecessary in moderately severe anemia and ineffective in severe anemia.[43] Although intriguing, the use of synthetic red cell substitutes in the management of anemia must be considered experimental at this time.

Hormonal Therapy

The effects of pharmacologic doses of androgens on erythropoiesis may be useful in the treatment of anemia in selected clinical settings. Androgens such as oxymetholone and fluoxymesterone have been used for a number of years to stimulate erythropoiesis in patients with anemia caused by diminished production of red cells. These compounds are sometimes able to induce clinically significant increases in red cell production both by increasing the production of erythropoietin and by enhancing the effects of erythropoietin on the marrow. Beneficial effects have been observed in patients with idiopathic myelofibrosis, myelodysplasia, aplastic anemia, paroxysmal nocturnal hemoglobinuria, and the anemia of chronic renal disease.[3,4] Unfortunately, however, their clinical use is frequently limited by the development of unacceptable side effects such as cholestatic hepatitis, virilization, or salt and water retention.

The recent cloning and expression of the human gene for erythropoietin will likely have important clinical implications for the management of a number of disorders that result in anemia. Although it is probably too early to be overly enthusiastic, recombinantly-produced human erythropoietin has recently demonstrated impressive efficacy without significant toxicity in patients with the anemia of end-stage renal disease.[36] Furthermore, the apparent beneficial effect of this treatment on several patients with transfusion-induced body iron overload suggests another useful effect of erythropoietin therapy. Although it remains to be seen, this novel therapy may well have more widespread applications in the management of other anemias and in the treatment of iron overload.

Splenectomy

Splenectomy is sometimes effective in the management of anemia attributable to the increased destruction of red cells by the spleen. This surgery should be considered in children and young adults with hereditary spherocytosis because it markedly reduces the risk of gallstones and severe anemia caused by aplastic or hemolytic crisis.[4] Splenectomy may be warranted in patients with immune-mediated hemolytic anemia refractory to tolerable doses of corticosteroids and, occasionally, in other settings where the spleen plays an important role in the development of anemia and other therapeutic options are deemed unacceptable. In patients with myeloid metaplasia, however, some consideration should be given to the possibility that extramedullary splenic hematopoiesis is as beneficial to the patient as hypersplenism is detrimental. Furthermore, even with presently available pneumococcal and meningococcal vaccines, splenectomy results in a life-long increased risk of overwhelming infection by encapsulated bacteria.

References

1. Dallman PR, Yip R, Johnson C. Prevalence and causes of anemia in the United States, 1976 to 1980. Am J Clin Nutr 1984; 39:437–445.
2. Self KG, Conrady MM, Eichner ER. Failure to diagnose anemia in medical inpatients: Is the traditional diagnosis of anemia a dying art? Am J Med 1986; 81:786–790.
3. Wintrobe MM, Lee GR, Boggs DR, Bithell TC, Foerster J, Athens JW, Lukens JN, eds. Clinical hematology. 8th ed. Philadelphia: Lea & Febiger, 1981.
4. Williams WJ, Beutler E, Erslev AJ, Lichtman MA, eds. Hematology. 3rd ed. New York: McGraw-Hill, 1983.
5. Editorial. "Anaemia" in athletes. Lancet 1985; i:1490–1491.
6. Hess CE, Ayers CR, Sandusky WR, Carpenter MA, Wetzel RA, Mahler DN. Mechanism of dilutional anemia in massive splenomegaly. Blood 1976; 47:629–644.

7. Yip R, Schwartz S, Deinard AS. Hematocrit values in white, black, and American Indian children with comparable iron status: Evidence to support uniform diagnostic criteria for anemia among all races. Am J Dis Child 1984; 138:824–827.

8. Yip R, Johnson C, Dallman PR. Age-related changes in laboratory values used in the diagnosis of anemia and iron deficiency. Am J Clin Nutr 1984; 39:427–436.

9. Dean J, Schechter AN. Sickle-cell anemia: Molecular and cellular bases of therapeutic approaches. N Engl J Med 1978; 299:752–763, 804–811, 863–870.

10. Ballas SK, Lewis CN, Noone AM, Krasnow SH, Kamarulzaman E, Burke ER. Clinical, hematological, and biochemical features of Hb SC disease. Am J Hematol 1982; 13:37–51.

11. Orkin SH, Nathan DG. The thalassemias. N Engl J Med 1976; 295:710–715.

12. Desforges JF. Genetic implications of G-6-PD deficiency. N Engl J Med 1976; 294:1438–1440.

13. Miwa S, Fujii H. Molecular aspects of erythroenzymopathies associated with hereditary hemolytic anemia. Am J Hematol 1985; 19:293–305.

14. Palek J, Lux SE. Red cell membrane skeletal defects in hereditary and acquired hemolytic anemias. Semin Hematol 1983; 20:189–224.

15. Colman N, Herbert V. Hematologic complications of alcoholism: Overview. Semin Hematol 1980; 17:164–176.

16. Larkin EC, Watson-Williams EJ. Alcohol and the blood. Med Clin North Am 1984; 68:105–120.

17. Doll DC, Weiss RB. Neoplasia and the erythron. J Clin Oncol 1985; 3:429–446.

18. Eschbach JW, Adamson JW. Anemia of end-stage renal disease (ESRD). Kidney Int 1985; 28:1–5.

19. Tudhope GR. Endocrine diseases. Clin Haematol 1972; 1:475–506.

20. Wallerstein RO. Role of the laboratory in the diagnosis of anemia. JAMA 1976; 236:490–493.

21. Camitta BM, Storb R, Thomas ED. Aplastic anemia: Pathogenesis, diagnosis, treatment, and prognosis. N Engl J Med 1982; 306:645–652, 712–718.

22. Niv Y. Positive Hemoccult tests and colonoscopic results (letter). Ann Intern Med 1986; 105:470–472.

23. Conley CL, Lippman SM, Ness PM, Petz LD, Branch DR, Gallagher MT. Autoimmune hemolytic anemia with reticulocytopenia and erythroid marrow. N Engl J Med 1982; 306:281–286.

24. Spivak JL. Masked megaloblastic anemia. Arch Intern Med 1982; 142:2111–2114.

25. Green R, Kuhl W, Jacobson R, Johnson C, Carmel R, Beutler E. Masking of macrocytosis by alpha-thalassemia in blacks with pernicious anemia. N Engl J Med 1982; 307:1322–1325.

26. Lindenbaum J. Status of testing in the diagnosis of megaloblastic anemia. Blood 1983; 61:624–627.

27. Bentley DP. Anaemia and chronic disease. Clin Haematol 1982; 11:465–479.

28. Finch CA, Huebers H. Perspectives in iron metabolism. N Engl J Med 1982; 306:1520–1528.

29. Patterson C, Turpie ID, Benger AM. Assessment of iron stores in anemic geriatric patients. J Am Geriatr Soc 1985; 33:764–767.

30. Cook JD. Clinical evaluation of iron deficiency. Semin Hematol 1982; 19:6–18.

31. Lanzkowsky P. Problems in diagnosis of iron deficiency anemia. Pediatr Ann 1985; 14:618–636.

32. Bessman JD, Gilmer R, Gardner FH. Improved classification of anemias by MCV and RDW. Am J Clin Pathol 1983; 80:322–326.

33. Flynn MM, Reppun TS, Bhagavan NV. Limitations of red blood cell distribution width (RDW) in evaluation of microcytosis. Am J Clin Pathol 1986; 85:445–449.

34. Witte DL, Kraemer DF, Johnson GF, Dick FR, Hamilton H. Prediction of bone marrow iron findings from tests performed on peripheral blood. Am J Clin Pathol 1986; 85:202–206.

35. Crosby WH. Overtreating the deficiency anemias. Arch Intern Med 1986; 146:779.

36. Eschbach JW, Egrie JC, Downing MR, Browne JK, Adamson JW. Correction of the anemia of end-stage renal disease with recombinant human erythropoietin; results of a combined phase I and II clinical trial. N Engl J Med 1987; 316:73–78.

37. Herbert V. Megaloblastic anemias. Lab Invest 1985; 52:3–19.

38. Bennett JM, Catovsky D, Daniel MT, Flandrin G, Galton DAG, Gralnick HR, Sultan C. Proposals for the classification of the myelodysplastic syndromes. Br J Haematol 1982; 51:189–199.

39. Ward JW, Deppe DA, Samson S, Perkins H, Holland P, Fernando L, Feorino PM, Thompson P, Kleinman S, Allen JR. Risk of human immunodeficiency virus infection from blood donors who later developed the acquired immunodeficiency syndrome. Ann Intern Med 1987; 106:61–62.

40. Koziol DE, Holland PV, Alling DW, Melpolder JC, Solomon RE, Purcell RH, Hudson LM, Shoup FJ, Krakauer H, Alter HJ. Antibody to hepatitis B core antigen as a paradoxical marker for non-A, non-B hepatitis agents in donated blood. Ann Intern Med 1986; 104:488–495.

41. Haugen RK. Hepatitis after the transfusion of frozen red cells and washed red cells. N Engl J Med 1979; 301:393–395.

42. Gocke DJ. Hepatitis A revisited. Ann Intern Med 1986; 105:960–961.

43. Gould SA, Rosen AL, Sehgal LR, Sehgal HL, Langdale LA, Krause LM, Rice CL, Chamberlin WH, Moss GS. Fluosol-DA as a red-cell substitute in acute anemia. N Engl J Med 1986; 314:1653–1656.

43 | AN APPROACH TO THE BLEEDING PATIENT

CHRISTOPHER D. HILLYER, M.D.
KENNETH B. MILLER, M.D.

The evaluation of a patient with a bleeding disorder is simplified by having a solid grasp of blood vessel, platelet, and coagulation physiology. Clinically, one should ascertain the location, spontaneity, extent, and timing of any current, prior, or familial bleeding. A detailed medication history is also vital because several common therapeutic agents such as aspirin, and non-steroidal anti-inflammatory drugs (NSAID) (Table 43–1 and 43–2) may interfere with platelet function. It may also provide insight into underlying illnesses that can be associated with bleeding such as lupus and renal failure. In the laboratory, screening tests are a useful start in the investigation of the bleeding patient and may be followed by more specialized and diagnostic tests. Before describing the clinical manifestations and laboratory perturbations of the different bleeding disorders, we will briefly review normal hemostasis.

Hemostasis may be divided into two separate, though related, phases: (1) primary hemostasis, in which there is rapid occlusion of a vascular lesion by a platelet plug, and (2) secondary hemostasis, which results in the formation of a stable fibrin clot. Disruption of vascular endothelium results in immediate vasoconstriction, which is both intrinsic to the vessel and secondary to the release of humoral factors. These normal factors also modulate platelet adherence and promote platelet aggregation, thus fostering formation of the platelet

TABLE 43–1 Common Medications Associated With Platelet Dysfunction

Agent	Action	Effect
Aspirin	Irreversible acetylation of platelet cyclo-oxygenase (for full life of the platelet)	Increased BT, blocks platelet aggregation
Dipyridamole	Inhibits platelet phosphodiesterase	No change in BT
NSAID	Reversible inhibitor of cyclo-oxygenase (within 24–48 hours)	Alters platelet aggregation, often without affecting the BT

BT = Bleeding time

TABLE 43-2   Common Drugs That Inhibit Platelet Function

Anti-inflammatory agents (indomethacin, ibuprofen, naproxen, etc.)
Antihistamines (diphenhydramine)
Aspirin
Caffeine
Clofibrate
Corticosteroids
Dextrans
Dipyridamole
Ethanol
Furosemide
Penicillins (penicillin G, ampicillin, ticarcillin, some cephalosporins)
Procaine
Propranolol
Phenothiazines
Phentolamine
Tricyclic antidepressants

plug. Once this plug forms, the secondary phase of hemostasis begins by factor activation through the coagulation cascade, ultimately resulting in a stable fibrin clot overlying and strengthening the initial platelet plug. Factor activation via the coagulation cascade requires a series of enzymatic reactions depicted in Figure 43-1. Central to the coagulation cascade is the activation of Factor X, which converts prothrombin to thrombin; thrombin, in turn, cleaves fibrinogen to fibrin. The end result is the formation of an interlinked, insoluble fibrin clot and cessation of bleeding. Factor X can be activated by either the intrinsic pathway, generally measured by the partial thromboplastin time (PTT), or by the extrinsic pathway, measured by the prothrombin time (PT).

Clotting factors are made predominately in the liver. Factor VIII is also made by endothelial cells. In the hepatocyte, vitamin K is required for the synthesis of prothrombin and Factors VII, IX, and X. These "vitamin K-dependent" clotting factors contain a unique amino acid residue called gamma-carboxyglutamic acid.

Finally, regulation of hemostasis occurs via the fibrinolytic pathway, which is mediated by the proteolytic enzyme plasmin, and results in dissolution and remodeling of the fibrin clot. The proteolysis of fibrin by plasmin produces debris designated "fibrin split products" (FSP); these low-molecular-weight proteins are important in hemostatic regulation, inhibit the action of thrombin on fibrinogen, and interfere with platelet activation.

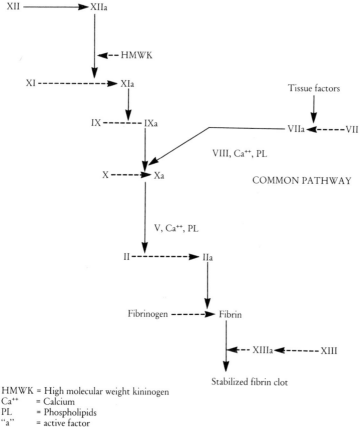

Figure 43-1 The clotting cascade.

Patients with an abnormality of a soluble coagulation factor (e.g., hemophilia) form a normal platelet plug and therefore have normal primary hemostasis. Individuals with vascular or platelet abnormalities (e.g., vasculitis or thrombocytopathy) have a defect in primary hemostasis, but are able to form a normal fibrin clot. Coagulation studies help to determine whether a primary or a secondary hemostatic abnormality is present. The interpretation of these studies is complicated, however, by the close nexus between the two phases and the overlap found in diseases that affect both phases of hemostasis.

Four readily available tests are useful in the initial evaluation of the bleeding patient: (1) bleeding time (BT), (2) platelet count, (3) prothrombin time (PT), and (4) partial thromboplastin time (PTT) (Table 43-3).

A platelet count of less than 50,000 per mm^3 is associated with an increased risk of post-traumatic bleeding, while a platelet count of less than 20,000 per mm^3 may be associated with spontaneous bruising and petechiae. There is a linear correlation between the platelet count, the bleeding time, and the risk of spontaneous bleeding, provided there is not concomitant platelet dysfunction.

The bleeding time reflects platelet adherence and intrinsic platelet function and is prolonged in disorders that affect platelets (but is normal when defects are in the soluble coagulation cascade). The bleeding time, while the best test to evaluate the primary phase of coagulation, requires careful performance for reliable results. Best results are obtained when a 1 cm longitudinal

TABLE 43-3   Tests Used in Evaluation of Bleeding Patients

Test	Normal	Pathway	Abnormality
Partial thromboplastin time (PTT)	25–40 s	Intrinsic	Hemophilia, von Willebrand's disease, factor deficiency (VIII, IX, XII), circulating anticoagulant, DIC
Prothrombin time (PT)	8–12 s	Extrinsic	Warfarin therapy, vitamin K deficiency, liver disease, DIC
Bleeding time (BT)	4–9 min	Primary hemostasis, intrinsic platelet function	Platelet disorders, von Willebrand's disease, thrombocytopenia
Thrombin time (TT)	10–15 s	Fibrinogen fibrin	Dysfibrinogenemias, DIC with FSP, hypofibrinogenemia, heparin

incision is made by a spring-loaded blade and performed by a limited number of trained technologists.

The prothrombin time and partial thromboplastin time screen defects in the coagulation cascade. Prolonged test times imply an abnormality in either the intrinsic or the extrinsic pathway, as already noted.

Specialized clotting tests are often required to further define the hemostatic abnormality and include thrombin time (TT), reptilase time, Stypven time, fibrinogen and fibrin split product measurement, intrinsic platelet function tests, and the ristocetin cofactor assay. The thrombin time is prolonged in the presence of heparin, fibrin split products, or abnormal or low serum fibrinogen. If the thrombin time is prolonged, a reptilase time should be performed. The reptilase time is *not* prolonged in the presence of heparin and is therefore helpful in evaluation of a patient with a prolonged PTT when a heparin effect is questioned. The Stypven time directly measures the activation of Factor X and is independent of Factor VII activation. The ristocetin cofactor assay is most useful in the evaluation of von Willebrand's disease.

With this review as background information, we can now turn to an analysis of the major hereditary and acquired coagulation defects and quantitative and qualitative platelet disorders.

HEREDITARY COAGULATION DISORDERS

The most commonly inherited disorders of coagulation are hemophilia A, hemophilia B, and von Willebrand's disease.[1] While inherited hypofibrinogenemias and quantitative and qualitative abnormalities of Factors V, VII, XII, and XIII have been described, these are rare and beyond the scope of this text.[2]

The diagnosis of hemophilia A (Factor VIII deficiency) should be suspected in any male with a hemarthrosis or in men with abnormal PTTs and family histories of bleeding. Hemophilia A, a sex-linked recessive disease that affects more than 15,000 males in the United States, has serious associated morbidity and mortality. Up to 15 percent of the cases may be sporadic, and rare cases occur in females. The defect in hemophilia A is a mutation in the q28 region of the X chromosome that results in failure to make functional Factor VIII. Laboratory tests reveal a prolonged PTT and a low Factor VIII level and activity that are diagnostic of classic hemophilia. The PT and bleeding time are normal. The frequency and severity of the bleeding is directly related to the Factor VIII measurements. Severe hemophiliacs have a Factor VIII activity of less than 1 percent and often bleed in infancy; moderate hemophiliacs have activities between 1 and 5 percent; individuals with levels greater than 5 percent generally have mild disease and seldom spontaneously bleed.[3]

Patients with moderate to severe hemophilia have a variety of life-long bleeding problems related to soft-tissue and intra-articular bleeding, while mucosal bleeding is rare. The most notable problem is hemarthrosis, which commonly involves the knees and other large joints. A hemarthrosis is a painful, tender, and swollen joint with blood in the intracapsular space. Over time, repeated hemarthroses lead to severe degenerative joint disease. Spontaneous soft-tissue bleeding may occur, but is rarely severe. Retroperitoneal bleeding can produce a syndrome mimicking an acute abdomen. Intracranial bleeding is a serious situation. Any patient with hemophilia who suffers head trauma requires immediate evaluation and prophylactic Factor VIII admistration.

In general, patients with mild hemophilia have little serious bleeding. These patients may be asymptomatic and may only be diagnosed during adulthood. The mild hemophiliac, however, can develop serious bleeding after significant trauma or surgery and may require treatment and proof of its efficacy prior to surgical or dental procedures.

Therapy for hemophilia A historically required the infusion of cryo-precipitate and, later, Factor VIII concentrates. This practice, however, was complicated by the transmission of infectious hepatitis and human immuno-deficiency virus (HIV). Recently, monoclonal-purified, virus-inactivated Factor VIII has become available. This agent is not associated with the transmission of infection, but is extremely expensive. Factor VIII products may be self-administered on an outpatient basis at the first sign of a bleeding event. If started early, hemarthroses may be controlled with one infusion of 7 to 15 units of Factor VIII per kilogram with an additional dose after 12 to 24 hours if there is evidence of continued bleeding. Restoration of normal hemostasis after serious bleeding usually requires a Factor VIII level of 30 to 50 percent. Therapy must be continued for several days after cessation of bleeding and for at least 10 days after surgery. Some authorities have suggested maintenance levels under 20 percent, but this remains controversial. The use of epsilon aminocaproic acid (4 g every 4 hours) decreases the amount of Factor VIII required after dental surgery.

In patients with mild to moderate hemophilia A, DDAVP, the synthetic vasopressin analog, is an important therapeutic alternative. DDAVP administered intravenously causes an increase in circulating Factor VIII by releasing endothelial stores. An intravenous dose of 0.3 μg per kilogram often raises the level of Factor VIII fourfold for 6 to 24 hours. This may be adequate in patients with mild disease, but it is rarely sufficient to prevent bleeding during minor surgery or trauma in those with severe disease. DDAVP is easily administered and lacks significant side effects.

As many as 10 to 15 percent of hemophilia patients do not have a rise in

Factor VIII level after adequate factor administration or develop renewed bleeding and lower factor levels some 5 to 8 days after starting factor infusion. This renewed bleeding is due to the presence or development of an antibody to Factor VIII, which inhibits its action. Two groups of patients have inhibitors: patients with a low, constant level of antibody that is not affected by antigenic stimulation (noninducible), and patients whose antibody titer rises dramatically following administration of Factor XIII (inducible). Patients with a noninducible inhibitor generally require a substantial increase in Factor VIII dosage. Patients with an inducible inhibitor may require extremely high doses of Factor VIII, immunoabsorption over a Staph-A column, infusion of procine-derived Factor VIII, or administration of activated clotting factors (FEIBA/Autoplex) that bypass Factor VIII in the clotting cascade. In some patients, bleeding is difficult to control by any means. Fortunately these patients are rare.

Hemophilia B, a sex-linked recessive disorder, is clinically identical to hemophilia A, though due to Factor IX deficiency. The pattern of standard coagulation test abnormalities is identical to hemophilia A, but the Factor IX activity is low. Logically, treatment of hemophilia B requires the infusion of Factor IX concentrate.

The final common hereditary coagulation disorder is von Willebrand's disease, an autosomally transmitted defect that affects males and females equally. As with the clotting factor disorders, the defect may be qualitative or quantitative. Von Willebrand's Factor (vWF), a large-molecular-weight multimeric protein, circulates as the Factor VIII carrier protein. VWF binds both to the disrupted endothelial surface at the site of vessel injury and to the platelet surface membrane, thereby allowing platelet adherence. In the absence of a normal vWF, platelets cannot bind to ruptured vascular endothelium and bleeding ensues.

The clinical manifestations of von Willebrand's disease are variable, but usually include some form of mucous membrane bleeding. Patients may have a long history of recurrent nose bleeds, easy bruising, or menorrhagia. Spontaneous hemarthroses are extremely rare. Interestingly, there is a tendency for the severity of many of the symptoms to decrease with age. Because the history in patients with von Willebrand's disease is difficult to interpret, all patients with prolonged postsurgical bleeding or with a history of excessive bruising after mild trauma should be evaluated for this disorder.

More than three subtypes of von Willebrand's disease have been described, depending on the specific vWF abnormality. Type I patients have a quantitative decrease in vWF. Type II patients have qualitative abnormalities, including abnormal assembly of multimeric vWF or abnormalities that lead to rapid vWF clearance. Type III is the absolute absence of vWF, and patients present with severe bleeding at a young age.

Laboratory tests obtained in patients with suspected von Willebrand's disease are listed in Table 43-4. Because von Willebrand's factor is required for platelet adherence, patients have a prolonged BT. Since vWF is the Factor VIII carrier protein, affected patients have reduced levels of Factor VIII and thus the PTT is prolonged. Platelet adhesion studies and the ristocetin agglutination tests are abnormal, while intrinsic platelet aggregation (platelet-platelet binding) tests are normal.

Treatment of von Willebrand's disease requires the replacement of the missing or abnormal vWF. DDAVP may raise the level of vWF by releasing endothelial stores and is best used in mild Type I disease after a test dose insures adequate improvement in the BT.[4] A rare subtype of Type II is associated with DDAVP-induced thrombocytopenia. Tachyphylaxis to DDAVP occurs over time. Further, the response to DDAVP is quite variable. Emergency replacement of vWF is most easily accomplished by the twice daily infusion of cryoprecipitate, a plasma fraction rich in both Factor VIII and vWF. For severe bleeding, surgery, or before parturition, cryoprecipitate should be given every 12 hours with a goal of a BT less than 5 minutes. Factor VIII concentrates have no role in the therapy of von Willebrand's disease.

ACQUIRED COAGULATION DISORDERS

Acquired coagulation disorders may be segregated into four categories: (1) disorders of decreased factor production, (2) disorders of increased factor destruction, (3) circulating factor inhibitors, and (4) factor dilution secondary to massive transfusion. Any one of these defects can cause severe bleeding. The PT and/or PTT are prolonged while the BT is usually normal.

Vitamin K deficiency, the most common of the acquired coagulation disorders, results in decreased factor production because Factors II, VII, IX, X, protein C, and protein S all require vitamin K for their terminal activation.

TABLE 43-4 Bleeding Tests in von Willebrand's Disease

Abnormal	Normal
BT	PT, TT
PTT	Intrinsic platelet tests
Platelet adhesion	
Ristocetin cofactor assay	
Ristocetin agglutination	
VWF antigen	
VIII activity and antigen	

Decreased vitamin K levels are found in patients receiving warfarin or some beta-lactam antibiotics and in those with intestinal malabsorption. The beta-lactam antibiotics interfere with vitamin K metabolism and reduce gut flora, which synthesizes vitamin K. Acute and chronically ill patients with poor oral intake, especially those taking antibiotics, are at high risk for the development of vitamin K deficiency and subsequent severe bleeding.

Therapy is aimed at replacing vitamin K. All patients suspected of vitamin K deficiency should receive vitamin K 10 mg subcutaneously daily for 3 days while changes in the PT are monitored; most deficiencies correct in 12 to 18 hours. If a patient is seriously bleeding, the administration of FFP immediately replaces the needed clotting factors. The short half-life of factors in FFP allows only transitory improvement and incurs the risks of blood product infusion. Patients requiring warfarin are of special concern because administration of vitamin K to correct an excessively prolonged PT may make future anticoagulation difficult. These patients may best be treated by FFP therapy or observation.

In severe liver disease, vitamin K-dependent factors are not synthesized. Because all clotting proteins are made in the liver, both the PT and PTT are prolonged. In addition, patients with severe liver disease may be thrombocytopenic from accompanying hypersplenism and may have increased fibrinolysis and dysfibrinogenemia. While vitamin K is an important initial treatment, few patients respond. In general, the prognosis of patients with liver disease and impairment of clotting factor synthesis is poor. During episodes of bleeding, attempts to correct the clotting factor deficiency in severe liver disease require large quantities of FFP.[5] In early liver disease, fibrinogen levels are increased. In late and severe hepatic disease, fibrinogen levels fall and cryoprecipitate also is required to control bleeding.

Acquired coagulation defects secondary to increased factor destruction include disseminated intravascular coagulopathy (DIC), rattlesnake toxin effects, and amyloid. DIC, by far the most common, is the consumption of coagulation factors during intravascular coagulation. Bleeding in DIC is due to factor depletion and secondary fibrinolysis.

The diagnosis of DIC is suggested by a pattern of laboratory results that includes an elevation in PT, PTT and thrombin times, thrombocytopenia, and the presence of fibrin split products. The peripheral blood smear allows documentation of microangiopathic hemolytic changes, including fragmented erythrocytes and thrombocytopenia. DIC usually results from a systemic disease, and treatment must be aimed at the underlying disorder (Table 43-5). The release of procoagulant substances may initiate DIC and occurs with amniotic fluid embolism, snake bite, malignancy, tissue injury, and the contact of blood with abnormal surfaces. Infection, burns, and extracorporeal circulation devices also may cause DIC.

TABLE 43-5 Disorders Associated With DIC

Sepsis*
Malignancy*
Surgery*
Liver disease*
Heat stroke
Burns
Obstetric complications*
  (amniotic, placental, tissue emboli)
Trauma*
Promyelocytic leukemia
Acute intravascular hemolysis
Systemic lupus erythematosus
Transfusion reaction

*Over 50 disorders have been associated with the development of DIC. Those indicated by an asterisk account for 80 percent of the clinically important causes of DIC.

Acute treatment of the bleeding patient with DIC is aimed at replacing the consumed clotting factors. Patients should receive platelets, FFP, and cryoprecipitate with measurement of coagulation parameters and fibrinogen levels. Most importantly, therapy must be directed at the underlying disease to interrupt the cause for consumptive coagulopathy.[6] The use of heparin to inhibit coagulation remains controversial and is recommended only when thrombosis complicates the DK.

Circulating inhibitors of specific coagulation factors also may cause severe bleeding. Factor inhibition is secondary to an antibody directed against a specific factor, most often Factor VIII or X. These antibodies may occur in conjunction with autoimmune diseases such as systemic lupus erythematosus or rheumatoid arthritis. Antibodies against vWF also have been described in acquired von Willebrand's disease. Inhibitors are measured in Bethesda Units (BU), a measure of concentration. In nonhemophiliacs, an inhibitor level greater than 15 BU is associated with major hemorrhage, while bleeding with an inhibitor level less than 10 BU is usually minor. Interestingly, these often elderly patients can present with spontaneous soft-tissue bleeding but rarely with hemarthrosis. Acute therapy may be ineffective and expensive and includes very high Factor VIII dosing, porcine Factor VIII, exchange transfusion, therapeutic plasmapheresis, or activated procoagulant complex. Recently, intravenous immunoglobulin has been shown to be effective in a dose of 1 g per kilogram per day for 2 days for acquired von Willebrand's disease.

In 5 to 10 percent of patients with active systemic lupus erythematosus (SLE), the PTT often is prolonged in vitro due to an antibody toward the test-dependent phospholipid. These "lupus anticoagulants," often seen in patients without SLE, represent an important cause of a prolonged PTT in asymptomatic individuals. A one-to-one mixture of FFP with patient plasma fails to correct the abnormality. Lupus anticoagulants do not selectively inactivate any of the clotting factors and rarely interfere with hemostasis in vivo. Paradoxically, these patients have a 30 percent incidence of thrombosis.[7]

Finally, transfusion of large quantities of blood and colloid can result in a dilutional coagulopathy because these replacement products do not contain significant amounts of coagulation factors. Though guidelines may lead to a false sense of security, generally 2 units of FFP may be required for every 10 units of packed red cells administered, and cryoprecipitate is given to correct a measured fibrinogen deficiency. Close monitoring of the PT, PTT, and platelet count is required to avoid overlooking a concomitant consumptive coagulopathy. In addition, most patients will develop dilutional thrombocytopenia after 10 to 20 units of banked blood have been transfused. It is difficult to discern the role of dilutional coagulopathy from that of platelet consumption either during bleeding and/or clotting or secondary to consumption. Patients with pure dilutional thrombocytopenia require platelet infusion only for continued bleeding or noticeable capillary oozing.

QUANTITATIVE PLATELET DISORDERS

Bleeding may result from either low platelet numbers or poor platelet function. There are many rare platelet disorders that cause significant bleeding, and the reader is referred to specialized texts for additional information.

Thrombocytopenic patients with platelet counts above 50,000 per mm^3 rarely bleed. Spontaneous and potentially lethal bleeding is rarely seen above 20,000 platelets per mm^3. Unexpectedly low platelet counts should be verified by direct visualization of the peripheral smear in order to rule out platelet clumping.

Abnormalities in platelet production can be due to congenital megakaryocytic hypoplasia, marrow infiltration due to granuloma or tumor, aplastic anemia, or toxic and/or immunologic bone marrow damage. Drug-induced thrombocytopenia can occur from either bone marrow toxicity or peripheral platelet destruction. A drug may be a direct platelet toxin or may act as a hapten. Quinine and quinidine are most commonly associated with thrombocytopenia, as well as heparin, gold, methyldopa, and sulfa-containing medications. Alcohol abuse often is implicated in bone marrow suppression, and it may be accompanied by folate deficiency and hypersplenism; severe bleeding rarely is seen without coexisting liver disease. The platelet count usually returns to normal within 1 to 2 weeks after cessation of alcohol use. Thiazide diuretics may produce a mild thrombocytopenia that is reversible with discontinuation of the causative drug.

Drug-induced thrombocytopenia is often paroxysmal, and severe bleeding may ensue. In life-threatening cases, we recommend the administration of platelets even though the infused platelets have a short half-life and may not be effective. The use of steroids is controversial. Bone marrow recovery usually occurs within 1 to 2 weeks after cessation of the medication.

Idiopathic thrombocytopenic purpura (ITP), an immune mediated thrombocytopenia purpura unrelated to drugs, occurs in acute and chronic forms and is a relatively common disorder. Antiplatelet antibodies often are implicated, though they may not be detected.

Acute ITP may be seen in any age group, but is more common in children, especially after viral infection. With the exception of petechiae and purpura, the children appear well and hepatosplenomegaly is rare. The platelet count is low and additional clotting tests are normal. Acute ITP generally has a favorable outcome, and over 80 percent of patients recover spontaneously. The remainder have chronic ITP and require long-term corticosteroids, maintenance immunoglobulin, or splenectomy. Of concern are the 1 to 2 percent of acute ITP patients at risk for intracranial bleeding. Recent data suggest that 500 to 1,000 mg per kilogram per day of intravenous immunoglobulin is a reliable means of raising the platelet count.[8] A combination of intravenous immunoglobulin and steroids appears to be becoming a mainstay of therapy (though smaller doses may be as efficacious) and should certainly be used in high-risk patients. Adults presenting with acute ITP require steroids. If clinical bleeding develops, intravenous immunoglobulin (400 mg per kilogram daily for 4 days) will often raise the platelet count rapidly and is clearly indicated.

Chronic ITP, predominantly an adult disease, may present acutely, but often is insidious and has no relation to viral illness. Patients are usually treated with steroids, and those patients who are refractory require splenectomy. Occasionally, patients respond to anabolic steroids such as danazol or to long-term immunosuppressive therapy. Chronic ITP may occur in a primary form or may be seen in association with chronic lymphocytic leukemia, lymphoma, or SLE. Recently, immunoabsorption by staphylococcal protein A column has resulted in a rise in platelet count in a limited number of patients with acute and chronic ITP.[9]

Thrombotic thrombocytopenic purpura (TTP), a rare syndrome seen predominantly in women, is associated with low platelet counts, purpura, anemia, atypical neurologic findings, fever, and renal insufficiency. The anemia is a microangiopathic hemolytic anemia with schistocytes and reticulocytes seen on peripheral blood smear. Arteriolar occlusion may be responsible for renal dysfunction. Neurologic signs include headache, psychosis, and coma. TTP remains a severe disease with a mortality rate exceeding 60 percent. Therapy must include plasma infusion or plasma exchange (with plasma as the replacement fluid) and should include the concomitant administration of corticosteroids.

The hemolytic-uremic syndrome (HUS) is a disorder of children with a Coombs'-negative microangiopathic hemolytic anemia related to TTP. In HUS, by definition, there are no neurologic findings. Renal dialysis is the primary supportive therapy; the role of plasmapheresis remains unclear.

QUALITATIVE PLATELET DISORDERS

Despite an adequate number of platelets, abnormalities in platelet function can result in bleeding. Abnormal laboratory tests include abnormal agglutination with ristocetin, epinephrine, or adenosine diphosphate (ADP). These disorders occur in both hereditary and acquired forms. Platelet dysfunction frequently occurs after consumption acetylation of platelet cyclooxygenase that lasts the life of the platelet (10 days). Platelet administration thus may be required if there is severe bleeding and a prolonged BT.

Uremia is associated with mucous membrane, gastrointestinal, and skin bleeding. The cause of this bleeding is primarily due to extrinsic platelet dysfunction that increases as uncleared metabolites accumulate. The BT is often markedly abnormal as are specialized platelet function tests. Dialysis will partially correct the abnormal platelet function. Recently, DDAVP has been shown to correct the coagulopathy of uremia. The mechanism of action of DDAVP in these patients is unclear, but may relate to the release of vWF from the vascular endothelium. The use of cryoprecipitate is controversial.

References

1. Bachmann F. Diagnostic approach to mild bleeding disorders. Semin Hematol 1980; 17:292–305.
2. Thompson AR, Harker LA. Manual of hemostasis and thrombosis. 3rd ed. Philadelphia: FA Davis, 1983.
3. Gill FM. Congenital bleeding disorders: hemophilia and von Willebrand's disease. Med Clin North Am 1984; 68:601–615.
4. Mannucci PM. Desmopressin: a nontransfusional form of treatment for congenital and acquired bleeding disorders. Blood 1988; 57:1449–1455.
5. NIH Consensus Conference. Fresh frozen plasma: indications and risks. JAMA 1985; 253:201–203.
6. Merskey C. DIC: identification and management. Hosp Pract 1982; 17:83–94.
7. Lechner K, Pabinger-Fashing I. Lupus anticoagulants and thrombosis. A study of 25 cases and a review of the literature 1985; 15:254–262.
8. Imbach P, Wagner HP, Berchtold W, et al. Intravenous immunoglobulin versus oral corticosteroids in acute immune thrombocytopenic purpura in childhood. Lancet 1985; 2:464–468.
9. Guthrie TH, Oral A. Immune thrombocytopenic purpura: A pilot study of staphylococcal protein A immunomodulation in refractory patients. Semin Hematol 1989; 26:3–9.

44 | LEUKOCYTOSIS

KENNETH B. MILLER, M.D.

Leukocytosis, an elevation of the white blood cell count (WBC), is one of the most common problems in clinical medicine. Leukocytosis can reflect an acute infection, inflammation, exposure to a noxious agent, malignant disease, or even a benign physiologic response.

The normal range for the absolute leukocyte and differential count is presented in Table 44-1. In the normal adult, approximately 55 to 70 percent of the circulating leukocytes are neutrophilic granulocytes, 20 to 40 percent are lymphocytes, and the remaining 1 to 8 percent are monocytes and eosinophils.[1] Basophils are not usually seen during a 100-cell differential count. Lymphocytes are divided based on their functional and phenotypic markers, i.e., T cell, B cell, NK cell, and so on. A discussion of the changes in the proportion of lymphocyte subsets and their significance is beyond the scope of this chapter.

Approximately 100 billion granulocytes and monocytes are produced in the bone marrow and released into the peripheral circulation each day. In the peripheral circulation, neutrophils are evenly divided into a circulating and a marginal pool. The peripheral WBC reflects the cells in circulating pools, while cells adherent to the vascular endothelium of the microcirculation are part of the marginal pool. The average neutrophilic leukocyte circulates in the blood for approximately 12 hours and can move freely between these two pools. However, once the neutrophil leaves the marginal pool to enter the tissues, it cannot return. Lymphocytes, in contrast, can recirculate between the blood

TABLE 44-1 Normal Adult Leukocyte and Leukocyte Differential Counts

	Number (Cells/mm³)	%
Total leukocytes	4,100–10,900	
Neutrophils	2,266– 7,670	55–70%
Eosinophils	0– 492	0–1%
Monocytes	123– 804	1–8%
Basophils	0– 156	0%
Lymphocytes	832– 3,140	20–40%

and the peripheral lymphoid tissues. Granulocytes leave the marginal pool (demarginate) and enter the circulating pool in response to stimuli that alter blood flow through the microcirculation or that affect cell adhesion to the vascular endothelium. Demargination results in a shift in the normal equilibrium between the circulating and marginal pools and can result in a transient, but sometimes pronounced, leukocytosis.

In the bone marrow, granulocytic precursors are divided into two compartments: the myeloblasts, promyelocytes, and myelocytes in the mitotic compartment are capable of cell division, while the metamyelocytes, bands, and segmented neutrophils comprise the postmitotic (or maturation) compartment. The postmitotic compartment, containing twice the number of cells as the mitotic compartment, provides for the rapid release of mature granulocytes into the circulation. To provide a sustained granulocytosis, the bone marrow increases the rate and number of cells undergoing mitosis at each stage in the mitotic compartment. In the postmitotic compartment, the transit time can be accelerated and neutrophils released into the peripheral blood at the metamyelocyte or band stage. Neutrophil production and maturation are under the control of a number of different growth and colony-stimulating factors.

Lymphocytes are derived from a separate stem cell, then populate central lymphoid tissue. While granulocytes have a short life span, lymphocytes may survive as immunocompetent cells for the life of the individual. When exposed to the appropriate antigen or stimuli, lymphocytes transform, undergo activation, and divide. Lymphocyte proliferation and activation are under the control of a number of growth factors that are important in the immunoregulatory process.

EVALUATION

The evaluation of an elevated total WBC should start with a review of the peripheral smear by the physician. It is critical to determine whether the circulating leukocytes or lymphocytes are normal, mature cells typically found in the peripheral blood, or abnormal and suggestive of an underlying leukemia or malignant disease. Moreover, there are several distinctive morphologic features in the granulocytes that may provide important clues to the cause of the leukocytosis. For instance, the finding of Döhle's bodies, toxic granules, or vacuoles in the granulocytes is suggestive of an ongoing infection. Auer rods, malformed granules containing lysosomal enzymes, when present in immature granulocytes are diagnostic of acute myelogenous leukemia. Reviewing the peripheral smear also confirms the elevated WBC.

In most laboratories the WBC is determined by an electronic cell counter. While these counters generally provide reliable, reproducible, and accurate measurements of cell concentrations, there are possible sources for error. The WBC can be falsely elevated in the presence of circulating nucleated red blood cells (RBCs) or large abnormal platelets. Reviewing the peripheral smear also provides information on the other cellular elements. For instance, teardrop-shaped red blood cells are suggestive of myelofibrosis. The finding of circulating nucleated red blood cells and immature granulocytes, termed leukoerythroblastosis, is suspicious of a metastatic or infiltrative disease that involves the bone marrow. Atypical "activated" lymphocytes suggest a recent viral infection. Epstein-Barr virus infections result in transformed lymphocytes that may resemble lymphoblasts with irregular nuclei.

The differential count obtained from the peripheral smear is important in the evaluation of the leukocytosis. An elevated WBC should be designated by the name of the principal cell type, i.e., neutrophilic, eosinophilic, basophilic, lymphocytic, or moncytic leukocytosis.

The most common cause of a leukocytosis is an increase in the absolute neutrophil count (Table 44-2). A bacterial infection is the most common cause of a neutrophilic leukocytosis. The neutrophilia that accompanies a bacterial infection is usually associated with "a shift to the left" of the circulating granulocytes. A shift to the left refers to a relative increase in bands and metamyelocytes in the peripheral blood smear. Occasionally, neutrophilia may be the presenting or only sign of an occult infection. Chronic bacterial endocarditis, deep-seeded or partially treated abscesses, and chronic fungal infections should be considered in the differential diagnosis of an unexplained neutrophilia. As noted, the presence of Döhle's bodies or toxic granules in the granulocytes is further evidence of an ongoing infection. Qualitative disorders in neutrophil function do not result in an elevation of the peripheral neutrophil count.

Noninfectious causes of neutrophilia can reflect (1) a physiologic response, (2) a response to metabolic disorders or tissue necrosis, (3) part of an underlying hematologic disease, or (4) a response to the administration of a number of different drugs or chemicals.[2]

Physiologic causes of neutrophilia reflect changes in the distribution of the neutrophils between the circulating and marginal pools. Neutrophils demarginate in response to stress, strenuous exercise, epinephrine, and corticosteroids. Transient neutrophil counts as high as 22,000 per cubic millimeter can occur after a brief period of strenuous exercise. Moreover, the magnitude of the leukocytosis with exercise appears to depend primarily on the intensity of the activity, rather than on its duration. Pain, nausea, vomiting, and intense

TABLE 44-2   Causes of Neutrophilic Leukocytosis

Physiologic conditions	Exercise, pregnancy, ovulation, stress, cigarette smokers, nausea, vomiting
Infections	Bacterial, fungal, viral, parasitic
Hematologic disorders	Leukemia, myeloproliferative disorders, hemolytic anemias, hemorrhage
Inflammatory disorders	Rheumatoid arthritis, vasculitis, gout
Metabolic disorders	Uremia, diabetic acidosis, eclampsia
Tissue breakdown	Myocardial infarction, carcinoma
Cell necrosis	Lymphomas, Hodgkin's disease, brain tumors
Drugs	Steroids, epinephrine, lithium, digitalis

anxiety also may cause a transient neutrophilic leukocytosis in the absence of infection. A neutrophilia can occur during ovulation, reflecting an increase in the level of circulating 17–hydroxy-corticosteroids. Pregnancy may be associated with a neutrophilic leukocytosis in the 15,000 to 20,000 per cubic millimeter range; the neutrophilia increases as term approaches. The onset of labor rarely may be accompanied by a neutrophilic leukocytosis as high as 34,000 per cubic millimeter in the absence of an infection. However, the physician should be cognizant of the possibility that neutrophilia occurring during pregnancy also may signify a serious complication such as eclampsia, bleeding, or fetal distress.

Neutrophilia in the absence of an infection may be seen in cigarette smokers. Idiopathic neutrophilia, a sporadic familial disorder, is characterized by a chronic mild elevation of the neutrophil count (12,000 to 20,000 per cubic millimeter) without evidence of any underlying pathology. The elevated WBC is presumed to represent the normal range for these individuals.[3]

Although neutrophilia may be a physiologic response to a variety of stimuli, it is more commonly encountered as a reaction to an underlying disease process. Inflammation or tissue damage and necrosis can produce a markedly elevated leukocyte count. The finding of a leukocytosis may help differentiate a myocardial infarction with tissue necrosis from angina pectoris. Neutrophilia may occur with a number of collagen vascular diseases such as acute glomerulonephritis, serum sickness, and rheumatic fever. Metabolic disorders such as ketoacidosis, uremia, and eclampsia may produce prominent neutrophilia. A neutrophilic leukocytosis may accompany poisoning by a variety of chemicals and drugs including lead, mercury, digitalis, and benzene derivatives. Patients taking therapeutic doses of lithium or Tegretol may develop a chronic neutrophilia without evidence of toxicity or infection. In malignant diseases the neutrophilia may reflect tissue injury or inflammation. Metastatic cancer of the liver or bone marrow may present with a leukocyte count that, in some cases, may mimic a leukemia.

LEUKEMOID REACTION

A WBC of greater than 50,000 per cubic millimeter, with circulating immature myeloid cells mimicking a leukemia, is called a leukemoid reaction. The leukemoid reaction is characterized by a leukocytosis of a greater degree than would be expected with the underlying diseases, immature myeloid cells in the peripheral smear, and an abnormally high concentration of immature cells in the bone marrow. The leukemoid reaction must be differentiated from chronic myeloid leukemia (CML) and other myeloproliferative disorders (Table 44-3). The leukocyte alkaline phosphatase (LAP) score and cytogenetic testing are particularly helpful studies to differentiate CML from a leukemoid reaction.

The LAP is a cytochemical stain scored from 0 to +4 based on the intensity of the staining. One hundred cells are counted and the score of each of the cells is totaled. Therefore an LAP score may vary from 0 (no cells staining) to 400 (all cells staining). In stable phase CML, the LAP score is very low (0 to 5), while in the leukemoid reaction, the LAP score is high (100 to 400). However, the interpretation of an LAP score is difficult in certain clinical settings. In some patients with CML, the LAP score in fact may be elevated, thereby reflecting an intercurrent infection, pregnancy, or an inflammatory

TABLE 44-3   Evaluation of a Leukemoid Reaction

Test	Leukemoid Reaction	Chronic Myelogenous Leukemia
WBC	20,000–50,000/mm³	20,000–150,000/mm³
Basophil and eosinophil counts	Normal	Increased
Platelet count	Normal	Normal or Increased
Uric acid level	Normal	Increased
LAP	High (100–400)	Low (0–5)
Cytogenetics	Normal	Philadelphia chromosome (90%)
Spleen size	Normal	Enlarged
RBC morphology	Normal	Occasional nucleated RBCs seen

reaction. Therefore, while a 0 LAP score is diagnostic of CML, a mildly elevated LAP score does not exclude the diagnosis. In these settings it is essential to perform a bone marrow aspirate to search for the diagnostic cytogenetic marker of CML, the Philadelphia chromosome. The Philadelphia chromosome, a balanced cytogenetic translocation involving chromosomes 9 and 22 (t 9:22), reflects the rearrangement of a defined area on chromosome 22 (bcr region).

MYELOPROLIFERATIVE DISORDERS

When all other causes of neutrophilia have been excluded, consideration should be given to one of the other myeloproliferative disorders. Polycythemia vera is associated with an elevation of the RBC mass, thrombocytosis, and splenomegaly. The leukocytosis in polycythemia vera is often modest in contrast to the elevated hematocrit. In myelofibrosis and myeloid metaplasia, splenomegaly is prominent and the peripheral smear usually reveals teardrop-shaped RBCs and nucleated RBCs. However, early in the course of myelofibrosis or polycythemia vera, leukocytosis may be the presenting finding. The therapy of neutrophilia clearly depends on the underlying disease; an infection must be treated with the appropriate antibiotics; the specific inflammatory disease, acute injury, or tissue necrosis should be identified and treated. In myeloproliferative disorders, therapy should be directed towards the primary disease. In polycythemia vera, periodic phlebotomy may be required, followed by cytotoxic chemotherapy. In chronic myelogenous leukemia, there are a number of therapeutic options, depending on the age of the patient, the extent of the disease, and the presenting symptoms. Bone marrow transplantation, interferon, and chemotherapy represent possible therapies for patients with CML.[4]

LEUKEMIA

Patients with leukemia may present with a very high WBC. While a WBC of greater than 100,000 per cubic millimeter generally requires treatment, it is the absolute blast count that is most important. A circulating blast count of greater than 50,000 per cubic millimeter predisposes the patient to the signs and symptoms of leukostasis and requires urgent treatment. However, an elevated WBC composed mainly of mature neutrophils and rare myeloblasts (chronic phase CML) or mature lymphocytes (chronic lymphocytic leukemia) does not require emergency intervention. The treatment and prevention of leukostasis is aimed at rapidly lowering the WBC. Leukapheresis, hydroxy-urea, allopurinol, and adequate hydration are important components of the therapy of leukostasis.

EOSINOPHILIA

Eosinophils normally make up 3 percent of the circulating leukocytes and are derived from a separate bone marrow progenitor cell. Eosinophils are increased in certain allergic conditions and parasitic infections, thereby reflecting the release of material chemotactic for eosinophils from activated local tissue mast cells. Like the neutrophil, the eosinophil moves freely between a circulating and a marginal pool. Eosinophilia is diagnosed when the absolute blood eosinophil count is in excess of 500 per cubic millimeter. Eosinophils are increased in atopic and parasitic diseases, drug reactions, neoplastic conditions, and collagen vascular disorders. Table 44–4 lists the major causes of eosinophilia.

The most common cause for eosinophilia in hospitalized patients is a drug reaction. Allergic disorders and hypersensitivity states associated with parasitic infections are also common causes of eosinophilia. However, the mere presence of a parasitic infestation is not necessarily associated with an eosinophilia. The parasite must actually invade the host to cause an eosinophilia. *Strongyloides*, schistosomiasis, filariasis, *Toxocara*, and other tissue invasive helminths are most commonly associated with an eosinophilia. Trichinosis should be suspected in cases with muscle tenderness and weakness, prominent eosinophilia (20 to 70 percent), elevated muscle enzymes, and a normal sedimentation rate. Serologic testing, skin tests, or a muscle biopsy may be

TABLE 44–4 Causes of Eosinophilic Leukocytosis

Allergic conditions	Asthma, hay fever, insect bites, urticaria, drug reactions
Neoplastic diseases	Hodgkin's disease, polycythemia vera, metastatic carcinoma
Parasitic diseases	Trichinosis, visceral larva migrans, strongyloidiasis, filariasis
Collagen vasucular diseases	Polyarteritis nodosa, systemic lupus erythematosus
Pulmonary diseases	Löffler's syndrome, occupational lung disease
Infections	Aspergillosis, coccidioidomycosis, hypereosinophilic syndrome
Primary hormonal disorders	Adrenal insufficiency, hypothyroidism

necessary to confirm this diagnosis. Stool examination for ova and parasites should be part of the evaluation of all patients with an unexplained eosinophilia. Eosinophilia is seen in most types of allergic or hypersensitivity respiratory diseases including asthma, hay fever, and occupational lung disease. Allergic rhinitis and nasal polyps are a common cause of eosinophilia.

An extreme and persistent elevation of the eosinophilic count without a detectable cause is referred to as the hypereosinophilic syndrome. This disorder is defined by three criteria: (1) a persistent eosinophilia above 1,500 per cubic millimeter, (2) organ dysfunction secondary to infiltration with mature eosinophils, and (3) the absence of a known cause for the eosinophilia. The hypereosinophilic syndrome is a heterogenous group of disorders with a range of organ involvement from minor skin changes to life-threatening cardiovascular and neurologic complications. Patients may present with only endocardial fibrosis and a restrictive endomyocardiopathy. An endomyocardial biopsy may be required to demonstrate damage to the endothelium and the eosinophilic infiltrate. Patients with the hypereosinophilic syndrome are at risk for thrombotic events related to the endomyocardial disease and the development of mural thrombi.

The evaluation of eosinophilia should start with a thorough personal and family history, including details of all recent travel. Physical examination should focus on skin, pulmonary, and cardiac findings. Laboratory evaluation should include liver and renal functions studies, immunoglobulin E (IgE) levels, stools for ova and parasites, chest roentgenograms, and pulmonary function studies where appropriate. If these studies do not reveal the cause of the eosinophilia, markers for a possible myeloproliferative disorder, including an LAP score, a serum B_{12} level, and a bone marrow aspirate with chromosome analysis, may be helpful. If all tests fail to define an underlying cause of the eosinophilia, then the diagnosis of a hypereosinophilic syndrome should be considered.[5] Treatment of the eosinophilia depends on the underlying disease. Therapy of the hypereosinophilic syndrome is aimed at preventing the complications of progressive organ involvement and thromboembolic complications and includes the use of corticosteroids, cytotoxic chemotherapy, and anticoagulation.

BASOPHILIA

The basophil is the least numerous of the circulating leukocytes and a rare cause of leukocytosis.[6] The basophil matures in the bone marrow through stages similar to the other granulocytes. However, the fate of the basophil in the peripheral blood remains poorly understood. Basophilia is defined as a basophilic leukocyte count greater than 50 cells per cubic millimeter or persistently greater than 1 percent of the circulating leukocytes. Table 44–5 lists the most common causes of basophilia. Basophilia is associated with hypersensitivity states and myeloproliferative disorders. The finding of a persistent basophilia should alert one to the possibility of an evolving myeloproliferative disorder. In chronic myelogenous leukemia, for instance, basophilia is a common presenting finding. However, a persistent basophilia of greater than 15 percent is an ominous sign and often heralds the onset of terminal-blastic-accelerated-stage. Basophilia is seen in the other myeloproliferative disorders, including polycythemia vera and myelofibrosis, but does not have the same prognostic significance in these disorders.

MONOCYTOSIS

The monocyte spends only a short time in the peripheral circulation, but, unlike the neutrophil, continues to differentiate in the tissues to form a variety of mononuclear phagocytic cells that can survive for weeks to months. Monocytes have a ubiquitous role in inflammation and host defense.[7] Monocytosis is defined as greater than 750 monocytes per cubic millimeter. Neoplastic, immune, and chronic inflammatory or infectious diseases are the leading causes of monocytosis (Table 44–6). This condition is associated with a number of primary hematologic disorders, including hemolytic anemias, myelodysplastic syndromes, Hodgkin's disease, and acute leukemias.

From the clinical point of view, the association of monocytosis and malignant disease must be emphasized. An unexplained, persistent monocytosis with either a macrocytosis or low-grade anemia is suggestive of a myelodysplastic or myeloproliferative disorder. Monocytosis also is seen in a number of chronic infections, including tuberculosis, subacute bacterial endocarditis, secondary syphilis, and brucellosis. Cirrhosis of the liver from multiple causes may be associated with a relative but persistent monocytosis. The primary malignant monocytic disorders include acute monocytic leukemia and chronic myelomonocytic leukemia. These disorders are characterized by prominent gum and skin infiltrates with atypical monocytes.

TABLE 44–5   Causes of Basophilic Leukocytosis

Hematologic disorders	Myeloproliferative disorders, chronic myelogenous leukemia, polycythemia vera, pernicious anemia
Inflammatory disorders	Ulcerative colitis
Miscellaneous disorders	Hypersensitivity drug eruptions, myxedema

Monocytosis often appears during the recovery phase of viral or bacterial infections. Monocytes also are the first cells to reappear after agranulocytosis or chemotherapy-induced myelosuppression. Monocytosis may occur in the context of lipid storage diseases, including Gaucher's and Niemann-Pick disease. Collagen vascular disorders such as rheumatoid arthritis, systemic lupus erythematosus, and periarteritis nodosa may rarely present with a mild monocytosis.

As noted, monocytosis is usually associated with a chronic inflammatory disease. Tuberculosis, chronic liver disease, and partially treated subacute bacterial endocarditis are frequent, but often overlooked, causes for a persistent monocytosis. The combination of a monocytosis and a macrocytic anemia is suggestive of a myelodysplastic or myeloproliferative disorder. Moreover, the peripheral smear may reveal basophilic stippling of the RBCs and atypical neutrophils. A history of chemotherapy for a prior malignancy or of an occupational exposure to a known or possible carcinogen is important in planning the work-up.

All patients with an unexplained monocytosis and anemia should be thoroughly evaluated for a possible myelodysplastic syndrome. A bone marrow aspirate and biopsy may reveal ringed sideroblasts and dysplastic changes in the myeloid, erythroid, and megakaryocytic precursors. Therapy of the myelodysplastic syndromes is still far from satisfactory. Androgens, low doses of chemotherapy, and growth factors all have been tried with varying degrees of success. A myelodysplastic syndrome developing in a patient exposed to a known hematotoxin is a poor prognostic sign. These patients typically rapidly progress to an acute nonlymphatic leukemia that responds poorly to standard chemotherapy.

LYMPHOCYTOSIS

Lymphocytes make up 20 to 40 percent of peripheral blood leukocytes.[8] A lymphocytosis is defined as greater than 4,000 cells per cubic millimeter. The causes of a lymphocytosis are listed in Table 44-7. Viral infections are the most common causes of a transient lymphocytosis. Mumps, varicella, and cytomegalovirus (CMV) all are associated with a prominent lymphocytosis. Infectious mononucleosis typically produces a marked lymphocytosis in association with splenomegaly and lymphadenopathy. As previously noted, the lymphocytosis is characterized by many atypical and large reactive cells. Lymphocytosis is rare during acute bacterial infections, with the exception of pertussis in which the total WBC is usually between 20,000 to 50,000 per cubic millimeter with 60 percent or more lymphocytes. Most of the lymphocytes are of the small mature type with rare atypical reactive cells. Other infections associated with a

TABLE 44-6 Causes of Monocytosis

Infections	Tuberculosis, syphilis, brucellosis, leprosy, rickettsial disease, typhoid fever, subacute bacterial endocarditis
Neoplastic diseases	Hodgkin's disease, myelodysplastic syndrome, monocytic leukemias, histiocytic medullary reticulosis
Collagen vascular diseases	Rheumatoid arthritis, systemic lupus erythematosis, periarteritis nodosa
Chronic inflammatory disorders	Cirrhosis, ulcerative colitis, regional enteritis
Miscellaneous disorders	Sarcoidosis, drug reactions, lipid storage disorders, hemolytic anemia, recovery from myelosuppression and agranulocytosis

lymphocytosis include brucellosis and chronic tuberculosis. A relative lymphocytosis, usually in the presence of neutropenia, is seen in hyperthyroidism and in many drug reactions.

An increase in the number of mature lymphocytes in the absence of an intercurrent viral infection is one of the earliest signs of chronic lymphocytic leukemia. Chronic lymphocytic leukemia (CLL), one of the most common hematologic neoplasms, is characterized by the proliferation and accumulation of mature-appearing lymphocytes. In most cases the cells are of B-cell origin and, by definition, are derived from a single clone. When a patient presents with a total WBC of greater than 20,000 per cubic millimeter with 80 percent small lymphocytes, generalized lymphadenopathy, and splenomegaly, the diagnosis of CLL is obvious. However, a modest elevation of the lymphocyte count with a normal total WBC may be difficult to interpret. The diagnosis of CLL in the early stages relies on the demonstration of an expansion of a monoclonal population of cells expressing a single immunoglobulin chain. While B-cell CLL is the most common cause of an unexplained lymphocytosis

TABLE 44-7 Causes of Lymphocytosis

Acute infections	Infectious mononucleosis, pertussis, mumps, rubella, infectious hepatitis, CMV infection
Chronic infections	Brucellosis, tuberculosis, secondary syphilis
Hematopoietic disorders	Acute lymphocytic leukemia, chronic lymphocytic leukemia, lymphoma, T cell disorders
Metabolic disorders	Thyrotoxicosis

in an adult, the other lymphocytic neoplasms must be kept in mind as possible diagnoses. The leukemic phase of indolent lymphomas, prolymphocytic leukemia, and, rarely, hairy-cell leukemia may resemble CLL. The leukemias of differentiated T cells are becoming more widely recognized. Adult T-cell leukemia is endemic in certain regions in southwest Japan and in the Caribbean. This type of leukemia is associated with a unique human retrovirus—the human T-cell lymphotrophic virus (HTLV-1).[9] After a several-year incubation period, infection with the HTLV-I virus results in an acute, rapidly progressive, fatal T-cell lymphoproliferative disorder. The disease is characterized by large numbers of atypical-appearing circulating T lymphocytes, prominent skin lesions, hypercalcemia with lytic bone lesions, and peripheral lymphadenopathy.

Other T-cell disorders include Sézary syndrome and Tγ-cell disorders.[10] The Tγ-cells function as natural killer cells (NK cells), possess unique surface immune markers, and have characteristic prominent azurophilic granules. The Tγ-cell disorders usually have a chronic indolent course characterized by moderate splenomegaly; lymphocyte counts in the 5,000 to 40,000 per cubic millimeter range with prominent large granular lymphocytes (LGL cells); neutropenia; and evidence of abnormal immunoregulation. This disorder is probably a neoplastic variant of chronic lymphocytic leukemia of the T cell type, although considering its chronic course and lack of a rapidly proliferating clone, many prefer the name "chronic T-cell lymphocytosis with neutropenia". T-cell receptor studies, however, have demonstrated the clonal nature of the T cell in most of these patients.

The evaluation of lymphocytosis should start with a review of the peripheral smear. As noted, the appearance of many atypical "reactive" lymphocytes suggest an ongoing viral illness. The presence of many circulating large granular lymphocytes suggests a T-cell disorder, and small mature-appearing lymphocytes suggest chronic lymphocytic leukemia. The use of surface markers or T-cell receptor studies are helpful in defining the clonal nature of the lymphocytes in selected cases. The use of immunofluorescent stains for surface immunoglobulins may be necessary when the clinical evidence for the diagnosis of CLL is equivocal. Serologic studies may help in the diagnosis of an active or resolving viral illness. Many of the special viral titers are now available at selected laboratories or regional centers.

Therapy of a lymphocytic disorder clearly depends on the underlying cell population. In CLL or one of its variants, the choice of therapy depends on the stage of the disease, the age of the patient, the symptoms, and other associated medical conditions.

References

1. Shapiro MF, Greenfield S. The complete blood count. Ann Intern Med 1987; 106:65–74.
2. Malech HL, Gallin JI. Neutrophils in human diseases. N Engl J Med 1987; 317:687–694.
3. Herring WB, Smith LG, Walke RJ, Harion JC. Hereditary neutrophilia. Am J Med 1974; 56:729–738.
4. Champlin R, Gale RP, Foon KA, Golde DW. Chronic leukemias: oncogenes, chromosomes, and advances in therapy. Ann Intern Med 1986; 104:671–688.
5. Fauci AS, Harley JB, Roberts WC, Ferrans VJ, Gralnick HR, Bjornson BH. The idiopathic hypereosinophilic syndrome: clinical, pathophysiologic, and therapeutic considerations. Ann Intern Med 1982; 97:78–92.
6. Dvorak HF, Dvorak AM. Basophilic leukocytes: structure, function and role in disease. Clin Haematol 1974; 4:651–684.
7. Johnston RB. Monocytes and macrophages. N Engl J Med 1988; 318:747–752.
8. Chanarin I, Harrisingh D, Tidmarsh E, Skacel PO. Significance of lymphocytosis in adults. Lancet 1984; 2:897–899.
9. Broder S, Bunn PA Jr, Jaffe ES, et al. T-cell lymphoproliferative syndrome associated with human T-cell leukemia/lymphoma virus. Ann Intern Med 1984; 100:543–565.
10. Newland AC, Catousky D, Linch D, et al. Chronic T-cell lymphocytosis: a review of 21 cases. Br J Haematol 1984; 58:433–446.

45 | LYMPHADENOPATHY

RICHARD A. RUDDERS, M.D.

Enlarged lymph nodes are a common clinical sign that requires further evaluation. The potentially malignant nature of adenopathy necessitates that the diagnostic work-up be selective and proceed in an expeditious manner. As a general rule the older the patient and the larger the lymph node, the greater the likelihood that a neoplasm is present. The definitive diagnostic test in many cases is a lymph node biopsy. It is important that a pathologist experienced in lymph node pathology participate in the evaluation. Incorrect diagnosis that results from inadequately prepared or processed biopsy material or from inexperience is unfortunately all too common in this difficult area of pathology.

NORMAL LYMPH NODE ANATOMY

Organized lymphoid tissue consists of a network of lymph nodes, liver, spleen, bone marrow, Waldeyer's ring (refers to lymphatic tissue in the oropharynx), and Peyer's patches in the gut. Blood and lymph are vehicles that provide traffic between these way stations. There are numerous other deposits of lymphoid tissue scattered in almost every organ, but they are not termed lymph nodes because of their lack of strict anatomic organization and structure. Lymph nodes are distributed peripherally and centrally, with the largest bulk of nodal tissue being found in the midline in the thorax and abdomen. The amount of nodal tissue declines as one moves peripherally. This is an important point because the patient usually detects enlargement of peripheral nodes, for instance in the neck, axilla, or groin, and often the great bulk of node enlargement is hidden and not obvious clinically.

HOW BIG IS BIG?

The most important initial clinical decision to be made is whether or not to call lymph nodes enlarged. Lymph nodes less than 0.5 cm in diameter (barely palpable) are not a cause of concern. This is particularly true in the younger patient who is likely to have enlarged neck nodes related to respiratory infections. There is, however, no guarantee that small nodes are benign, and they must be viewed in the context of the entire picture. For instance, an individual with multiple small nodes and abnormal blood counts may have a serious underlying disease, while a child with multiple small nodes may be entirely normal. Another potentially confusing problem relates to groin nodes. Individuals of all ages are likely to have palpable groin nodes. If the nodes are small they are likely to be normal. The larger the nodes, the greater the cause for concern. Lymph nodes greater than 2 to 3 cm in diameter, particularly when multiple, have a high risk of malignancy in any age group and in any location and should be evaluated promptly. One cannot emphasize too strongly that there is a fine line between the urgent need to evaluate significantly enlarged nodes and the inadvisability of needlessly subjecting individuals to expensive and morbid diagnostic procedures.

WHY DO LYMPH NODES ENLARGE?

Lymph nodes are organized collections of lymphoid tissue and consist of several types of immunocompetent cells such as lymphocytes and macrophages. There are three major causes of lymph node enlargement: lymphadenitis, lymphadenopathy, and neoplasia (Table 45-1). Lymphadenitis is the normal physiologic response to an inflammatory (infectious) stimulus that can be either regional or systemic. In some cases the inflammatory agent is not readily identified (e.g., benign reactive hyperplasia), but in many cases a clear relationship to a viral or bacterial agent can be defined. Prominent generalized adenopathy may be a feature of mononucleosis, cytomegalovirus, and toxoplasmosis infections.

Lymphadenopathies consist of a diverse group of diseases. Many, such as systemic lupus erythematosus and other collagen diseases, are associated with immunologic hyperfunction, which leads to node enlargement. Any systemic disorder associated with hyperfunction or abnormal function of the lymphoid system can be associated with adenopathy. Lymphadenopathy may be prominent in the case of drug reactions, such as those related to phenytoin. The adenopathy in such cases waxes and wanes with the activity of the underlying disease.

The most important cause of adenopathy from the therapeutic standpoint is neoplasia.[1] This is particularly the case in recent years, since a great many of the primary neoplasms of lymph nodes, namely lymphoma and leukemia, are potentially curable. It is essential to identify as quickly as possible individuals with neoplasms that are curable in order to ensure the highest likelihood of therapeutic success. Non-Hodgkin's lymphoma and Hodgkin's disease are two such examples (Figure 45-1). Metastatic tumors also may cause lymph node enlargement. Although this may be a less favorable situation,

TABLE 45-1 Selected Causes of Adenopathy

Lymphadenitis

  Benign reactive hyperplasia

  Viral diseases
    Infectious mononucleosis
    Varicella zoster
    Cytomegalovirus
    Vaccina measles

  Bacterial diseases
    Bacterial
    Tuberculosis
    Leprosy
    Syphilis

  Other
    Toxoplasmosis
    Cat scratch disease
    Lymphagranuloma venerium

Lymphadenopathy

  Systemic lupus erythematosus

  Rheumatoid arthritis

  Sjögren's syndrome

  Drug reactions

  Reactions to chemicals and tumor products

  Sarcoidosis

Neoplasia

  Hematopoietic
    Non-Hodgkin's lymphoma
    Hodgkin's disease
    Chronic leukemia
    Acute leukemia

  Nonhematopoietic
    Lung cancer
    Breast cancer
    Melanoma
    Nasopharyngeal carcinoma
    Soft tissue sarcoma
    Seminoma

regional metastases from an occult primary cancer such as breast, oropharynx, or melanoma are important to identify, since in many cases cure or extended remission with appropriate treatment is possible.

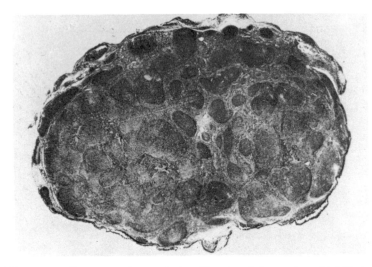

Figure 45-1 Low power microscopic view of lymph node from patient with follicular (nodular) non-Hodgkin's lymphoma. The lymphoma nodules can be seen clearly at this magnification.

CLINICAL CLUES TO THE CAUSES OF ADENOPATHY

In the clinical evaluation a number of important clues help decide whether further evaluation is mandatory. As stated, age is an important variable that influences our level of concern. The older the patient with significant adenopathy, the more likely the presence of serious illness. The distribution of nodes is an important clue. Nodes in a single area suggest the possibility of a local cause, whereas generalized nodes suggest a systemic process. In either case distribution does not distinguish benign from malignant enlargement. Another important characteristic to appreciate is the consistency of the nodes. If the nodes are extremely firm and matted, a neoplastic process is suggested. If they are discrete, painful, and particularly if they are regional, an infectious cause is suggested. Again, this is not an absolute sign, since more than one neck node from a suspected abscessed tooth has proved to be a metastasis from an oropharyngeal carcinoma. Since it is common for tumors to infarct, pain may be produced in the node, thereby mimicking inflammation.

One cannot overemphasize the value of the clinical history in this type of evaluation. The rate of progression of the adenopathy, the presence of pain, and the association with another illness, either chronic or acute, are vitally important clues. One should also pay particular attention to drug ingestion and to exposure to animals to rule out toxoplasmosis, cat scratch disease, and the like.

Based on these considerations, one must make an initial decision regarding further evaluation. If the adenopathy appears to be the result of a benign self-limited problem, no further studies are indicated. However, I would urge that all patients have at least one follow-up examination to confirm that the adenopathy is benign and is not progressive. If an infectious agent, particularly a virus, is suspected then further evaluation should include appropriate cultures and serum viral antibody titers. No further evaluation is necessary if the suspected infection is proven, although again a follow-up examination is advisable. Most individuals seen in the office, particularly younger individuals with a definable infectious illness, require no further evaluation other than careful follow-up. But what of the patient with significant adenopathy that is progressive and not infectious in origin? In such cases the next step is biopsy.

LYMPH NODE BIOPSY

There is considerable confusion on the subject of lymph node biopsy. There are two types of biopsies: needle aspiration biopsy and incisional or excisional biopsy.[2] Needle biopsies should be discouraged as the initial diagnostic biopsy. A needle biopsy provides material for culture and cytology, but the sample size is small, the ability to distinguish benign from malignant is moderate, and if a malignancy is present subclassification is very difficult. For these reasons we prefer an excisional biopsy of readily accessible nodes.

In certain circumstances enlarged nodes may be present in the thorax or abdomen, thus making biopsy more problematic. Although computed tomography (CT) or ultrasonography can be helpful in guiding a biopsy, more often than not an excisional biopsy is necessary. It is a matter of clinical judgment as to when a thoracotomy or laparotomy should be done to establish a diagnosis. Often other more accessible areas, such as the bone marrow, are biopsied first in order to avoid surgery to diagnose leukemia or lymphoma. Most patients with central adenopathy require an excisional biopsy even after exhausting noninvasive maneuvers.

One cannot stress too much the importance of proper handling of the biopsy material. Material should be sent to the pathology laboratory fresh in sterile saline, not fixed in formalin. This ensures that lymphocyte marker studies, immunocytochemistry, and cultures can be done on the material. These tests are not possible with formalin-fixed material. Close collaboration with the pathologist is needed in order to ensure that maximum information is obtained from each biopsy and that an accurate diagnosis can be made. Lymph node pathology can be extremely difficult, and good preparation of material is vitally important to improve diagnostic accuracy (Table 45–2).

OTHER DIAGNOSTIC TESTS

CT Scanning

CT scanning is the best study to evaluate the size of lymph nodes since it can detect nodes as small as 0.5 to 1.0 cm in diameter with reasonable accuracy and it is noninvasive.[3] CT scans of the chest and abdomen have become a routine part of the evaluation of all patients with neoplastic adenopathy (Figure 45–2). Based on these findings patients with lymphoma, for example, can be placed into a stage and the correct treatment modality chosen. Patients with non-neoplastic adenopathy documented by biopsy rarely require further evaluation.

Pedal Lymphangiography

Pedal lymphangiography delineates the size and characteristics of pelvic and low retroperitoneal nodes. The use of this diagnostic study has declined with the widespread availablity of CT scanning. However, there are selected situations where lymphangiography may be useful (Figure 45–3). This particularly is the case in patients with lymphomas that have equivocal CT scan findings in the abdomen. The disadvantage of this type of study is that it is invasive and potentially morbid, particularly in older individuals. Dye allergy and pulmonary disease are contraindications to this type of study.[4]

TABLE 45–2   Studies Performed on Lymph Node Biopsies

Study	Comment
Light microscopy	H & E stain
Immunocytochemistry	Fluorescent labelled antibodies
Surface marker studies	Flow cytometry
Electron microscopy	In selected cases
Culture and special stains	In selected cases

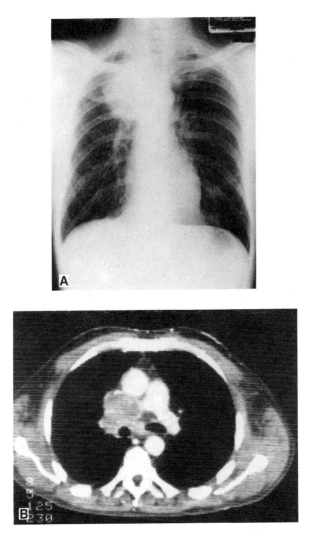

Figure 45-2 *A.* Chest x-ray of patient with large right sided mediastinal and paratracheal mass. *B.* CT scan of the chest of the same patient with delineation of the mass, which is comprised of lymph nodes subsequently shown to be lung cancer.

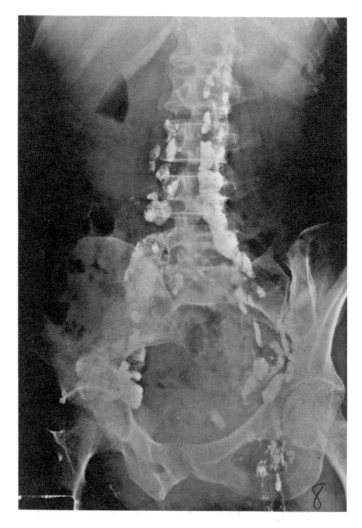

Figure 45-3   Lymphangiogram from patient with Hodgkin's disease. Lymph nodes on the right are enlarged and have a foamy appearance. Lymph nodes on the left are normal, for comparison.

Gallium Scanning

Gallium scanning is a noninvasive study that can provide information about the presence of disease in multiple anatomic sites. Gallium is taken up by neoplastic lymphoid tissue and by certain solid tumors, such as melanoma. Gallium also localizes in abscesses. If lymph nodes are enlarged and also take up gallium, they are likely to be neoplastic. The converse is not true, however, since many tumors do not avidly bind gallium. Therefore, a negative gallium scan does not necessarily rule out neoplastic lymphadenopathy. Numerous studies have shown a significant false positive and false negative rate in hematologic malignancies. thus, gallium scans are performed now only in selected situations.

DIFFICULT PREMALIGNANT LESIONS

There are a number of instances where the cause of the adenopathy is obscure and/or its biologic significance is not clear. Many such lesions fall into the category of premalignancy. Many cases of lymphadenopathy in this group regress spontaneously or remain stable for long periods of time. Many, however, evolve into frank malignancy, usually a non-Hodgkin's lymphoma.

Atypical Lymphoid Hyperplasia

Individuals with atypical lymphoid hyperplasia present with adenopathy that is often generalized and that may either persist or wax and wane. When a node is biopsied, the pathologist is unable to state that it is benign or malignant since atypical features that are disturbing are present in the node. Such changes may be cellular atypia, capsular spillage, or architectural distortion. In our experience many such individuals progress to frank malignant lymphoma over a period of time. It is not clear whether the original biopsy could have represented a sampling error in some of these cases, but in other cases a clear evolution to lymphoma can be documented. Lymphocyte phenotype analysis of the nodal tissue has been illuminating, since such studies often define a malignant clone of lymphocytes. Restricted expression of surface membrane immunoglobulin has been most useful in defining a malignant proliferation of B lymphocytes (Table 45–3).

TABLE 45-3   Surface Marker Studies of Lymph
Node Cells

Antibody	Cell Lineage (Specificity)
OKT3	Pan T
OKT4	T helper
OKT8	T suppressor
Leu 1	Pan T
HLA-DR	T, B
Ig*	B
B1	B
CALLA	Precursor cell

OKT series – Ortho diagnostics
Leu series – Becton-Dickinson
CALLA – common ALL antigen

* Ig = surface immunoglobulin

Angioimmunoblastic Lymphadenopathy

Patients with this disease present with lymphadenopathy and a host of associated immunologic abnormalities. The cause of the syndrome is not clear, but it most likely represents an abnormal immune response to an undefined antigen and associated faulty immunoregulation. Although one-third of these patients remit spontaneously, one-third die of progressive disease while the remainder progress to frank malignant lymphoma. The lymph node biopsy is characteristic and displays a pleomorphic lymphoid infiltrate, extensive necrosis, and neovascularization (Figure 45–4). A definitive diagnosis of lymphoma usually cannot be made at this stage. Because of the varied outcome, most patients are not treated aggressively with chemotherapy unless they progress to frank lymphoma.

Abnormal Immune Responses

A number of patients present with adenopathy that is neither atypical hyperplasia nor classic immunoblastic lymphadenopathy. Such cases have been lumped into a separate category termed abnormal immune response.[5] Again, in our experience this may be considered a potentially premalignant lesion since many patients progress to frank lymphoma and/or have a progressive and fatal disease. This is an extremely difficult group of patients to evaluate since no

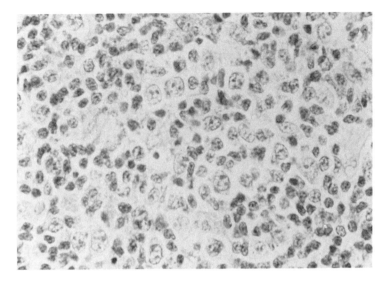

Figure 45-4 High power microscopic view of cervical lymph node biopsy from patient with angioimmunoblastic lymphadenopathy. Note large immunoblasts with prominent nuclei.

definitive malignancy is present. As with atypical hyperplasia, lymphocyte phenotyping has been helpful in defining malignant subpopulations of lymphocytes.

Acquired Immunodeficiency Syndrome (AIDS)

This retrovirus related disease often presents with generalized adenopathy in its early stages.[6] This lymphadenopathic phase is a precursor to full blown AIDS and to the potential development of frank malignant lymphoma. HIV may be cultured from the lymph nodes in these cases. The histologic picture in the lymph node is that of an abnormal immune response and is not frankly neoplastic. It is not known what proportion of patients with lymphadenopathy will progress to full blown AIDS or how many have reversible findings. Again, lymphocyte phenotyping of the lymph nodes has been helpful in defining the abnormality since there is usually total T cell depression and a reduction in T helper cells, thereby causing a reversed T helper:T suppressor ratio. It is also unknown whether treatment with antiviral agents or with chemotherapy will abort the development of AIDS in individuals with lymphadenopathy syndrome.

References

1. Rosenberg SA. Lymphosarcoma: a review of 1269 cases. Medicine 1961; 40:31–84.
2. Ioachim HL, ed. Lymph node biopsy. Philadelphia: JB Lippincott, 1982.
3. Mass AA, ed. Computed tomography of the body. Philadelphia: WB Saunders, 1983.
4. Cabanillas F. Comparison of lymphangiograms and gallium scans in the non-Hodgkin's lymphomas. Cancer 1977; 39:85–88.
5. Lukes RJ. Immunologic approach to non-Hodgkin's lymphomas and related leukemias. Analysis of the results of multiparameter studies of 425 cases. Semin Hematol 1978; 15:322–351.
6. NIH Conference. Acquired immunodeficiency syndrome: epidemiologic, clinical, immunologic and therapeutic considerations. Ann Intern Med 1984; 100:92–106.

46 | CANCER SCREENING

HARRY KIMBALL, M.D.
KENNETH B. MILLER, M.D.

Cancer-related check ups—the tests, procedures, and counseling related to the prevention and early detection of cancer—have enormous medical, social, and economic implications. To be accepted by physicians and patients, cancer screening should adhere to the following basic principles.

1. The cancer being screened for should be an important health problem for the individual and/or the community.
2. A screening test should be available that is reliable, acceptable to patients, ideally risk-free, and inexpensive.
3. The natural history of the disease should be well understood and should have a recognizable early or asymptomatic stage.
4. There should be an acceptable, practical, and effective form of therapy available for patients found to have an early cancer. Screening for a disease with no effective therapy offers only a diagnosis and is of questionable value.
5. Screening and early treatment of the cancer should be proven to favourably influence the survival time and/or quality of life for the patients.

There are several kinds of bias that characterize early detection programs and that may affect the interpretation of results. "Lead-time bias" refers to the fact that a disease found by screening has a longer course, or natural history, simply because of its earlier discovery. The longer survival of the screened patient therefore may be independent of whether or not any benefit resulted from having discovered the cancer early. "Length bias" refers to the fact that cancers with an inherently slower growth rate, and thus a relatively more favorable outlook, are disproportionately detected. The longer the preclinical duration of the disease, the stronger is this length bias. Patient self-selection bias is obvious; people who select or seek out screening programs may take better care of themselves and may be healthier than those who do not. Finally, overdiagnosis or erroneous diagnosis can affect the interpretation of results of screening—when is a cancer a cancer? When dealing with early, limited disease, some patients who are diagnosed as having a cancer may in fact not have a malignancy. Patients without a true cancer obviously have a more improved outcome than patients with cancer.

Screening tests must also address the issues of sensitivity, specificity, and predictive value. Sensitivity is the likelihood of the test being positive when the disease is present; specificity is the likelihood of the test being negative when the disease is absent. The reciprocal of specificity is referred to as the false positive rate. Predictive value is the proportion of patients with positive tests who have the disease in question. The predictive value of a test is what most concerns the physician.

The predictive value of a test is critically dependent not only on the specificity of the test but also on prevalence of the disease in the population being screened. For example, if a population of 100,000 were screened for a disease with a 2 percent prevalence (which would make the disease a very common one) and if sensitivity and specificity of the test was 95 percent, there would be a total of 6,800 positive tests (Fig. 46–1). However, only 1,900 would be true positives, e.g., positive tests in patients who have the disease. In this example the positive predictive value is defined as:

$$\frac{\text{true positives}}{\text{true} + \text{false positive}},$$

$$\frac{1,900}{1,900 + 4,900} = 28\%.$$

Therefore when one screens large numbers of patients even for a common disease with a very specific test, the positive predictive value is still low. This problem is further magnified when the disease is less common and the population is very large.

Cancer detection in the asymptomatic patient has focused on five diseases: breast, colon, cervical, uterine, and lung cancer. The American Cancer Society has recently updated its recommendations regarding these cancers (Table 46–1).

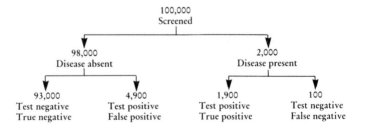

Figure 46-1 Screening test: the predictive value is dependent on the prevalence of the disease and the sensitivity of the test.

TABLE 46–1 Summary of American Cancer Society Recommendations
For The Early Detection of Cancer in Asymptomatic People

	Population		
Test or Procedure	*Sex*	*Age*	*Frequency*
Sigmoidoscopy	M and F	Over 50	After two negative examinations 1 year apart, perform every 3–5 years
Stool guaiac slide test	M and F	Over 50	Every year
Digital rectal examination	M and F	Over 40	Every year
Papanicolaou's test	F	20–65 Under 20 if sexually active	After 2 negative examinations 1 year apart, perform at least every 3 years
Pelvic examination	F	At menopause	At menopause
Breast self-examination	F	Over 20	Every month
Breast physical examination	F	20–40 Over 40	Every 3 years Every year
Mammography	F	35–40 41–40 Over 50	Baseline Every 1–2 years Yearly
Chest x-ray			Not recommended
Sputum cytology			Not recommended
Health Counseling and Cancer	M and F M and F	Over 20 Over 40	Every 3 years Every year

BREAST CANCER

Breast cancer is a common disease that carries a heavy burden of emotional and physical suffering. Breast cancer occurs in more than 100,000 women each year and kills 36,000 women yearly. One in 10 women will be affected sometime during their lifetime. The risk factors for breast cancer include a positive family history, particularly in mother or sisters, previous breast cancer, increasing age, obesity, and perhaps drinking more than three alcoholic drinks a week. Not having children, having children late, and early menarche also are associated with higher risk for breast cancer. Exercise and a diet low in saturated and animal-derived fat may possibly lower the risk for breast cancer.

There are three ways of finding breast cancer at an early stage: (1) breast self-examination, (2) physical examination of the breast by a trained clinician, and (3) mammography. In clinical practice, however, only about half of all cancers of the breast are detected at a stage in which the cancer is small and has not spread to regional lymph nodes. The prognosis is critically dependent on the extent of the disease at the time of diagnosis.

Breast self-examination has been recommended by health care providers for many years. Self-examination has recently been the subject of review by the World Health Organization and the United States Preventative Services Task Force.[1] The task force concluded that the sensitivity and specificity of self-examination is quite low (20 to 30 percent) compared with mammography and physical examination of the breast by a physician. While the task force did not recommend abandoning self examination of the breast, serious questions were raised about its usefulness. The World Health Organization concluded that "there is insufficient evidence that breast self-examination as applied to date is effective in reducing mortality from breast cancer...although there is equally insufficient evidence to change them (guidelines) where they exist". In calling for additional research on breast self-examination, both organizations noted that the problem with breast self-examination was not evidence for the lack of effect of breast self-examination, but lack of evidence. We agree with these findings, but continue to recommend breast self-examination for all female patients. We suggest to our patients that the breast self-examination should be performed at the same time each month, preferably after each menstrual period, and any new masses should be reported to their physicians.

Screening for breast cancer by mammography has been the principal focus of a number of studies over the last decade. The sensitivity of the mammogram examination is about 80 to 90 percent and it is age dependent; in young women with dense breasts, lesions are more difficult to locate and define. Specificity is approximately 15 to 25 percent, i.e., about one of every four or five mammographic lesions found prove to be malignant. Radiation exposure is low with the newer mammographic technology, averaging six one-hundredths of a rad, which is about the same as two chest x-rays.

Studies of breast cancer screening by mammography began in the late 1960s. The Health Insurance Plan (HIP) of New York enrolled some 31,000 women aged 40 to 64 in a prospective breast cancer screening study.[2] These women were screened by a combination of yearly physical examinations of the breast and mammograms. The control group consisted of a matched group of 31,000 women from the same prepaid medical group plan who received their usual medical care. Ten years after this study was initiated, the mortality rate in the screened group was 30 percent less than that of the nonscreened group. At 18 years, the difference between screened and nonscreened women was 21 percent. A significant difference applied only to women over the age of 50. There was no significant reduction in breast cancer deaths in the HIP study for women under the age of 50 at the time of diagnosis.

When this information became available, the American Cancer Society and the National Cancer Institute jointly sponsored a large study known as the

Breast Cancer Detection Demonstration Project (BCDDP).[3] The project started in 1974 and ended in 1981. Twenty-nine sites around the country were selected and a total of 283,000 women were enrolled. The age range was between 35 and 74 years with a median age of 50. The woman were younger than those screened in the HIP study. All women were screened with a combination of physical examination and mammography. The BCDDP was organized as a demonstration project and not as a research study. There was no control population and the asymptomatic women were self-selected. Moreover, in this study there was an overrepresentation of women at higher risk for breast cancer as compared with the general population, a bias also found in the HIP study.

Over a million mammograms were performed in the BCDDP study. After 10 years, 4,485 breast cancers were found; 3,557 (80 percent) were discovered by the screening process. Fifty-nine percent of the noninfiltrating tumors and 53 percent of small (<1.0 cm) cancers were found only by mammography (Table 46–2). Forty-two percent of all cancers were found only by mammography; of note, 20 percent of patients with breast cancer were found to have positive nodes at surgery in this study. This low percentage of nodal involvement compares with approximately 53 percent of patients in studies of breast cancer not detected by screening programs. At 5 and 10 years, the survival rates in this study were 88 and 79 percent respectively.

There has been a great deal of controversy regarding the BCDDP data base; the study was not controlled and the women were self-selected. However, despite these limitations the data clearly demonstrated the effectiveness of mammography in detecting early stage breast cancer. These data, along with

TABLE 46–2   Breast Cancer Detection Demonstration Project (All Ages)

		Infiltrating			
	Non infiltrating	< 1.0 cm	> 1.0 cm	Not Specified	Total
Mammogram only	461	195	631	194	1481
Physical examination	43	31	161	73	308
Mammogram and physical examination	258	135	1038	252	1683
Unknown	20	10	41	14	85
Total	782	371	1871	533	3557
	(22%)	(10%)	(53%)	(15%)	
Positive nodes at surgery	15	53	547	84	699 (19.7%)

Adapted from: Baker LH. Breast cancer detection demonstration project: five year summary report. CA 1982; 32:194.

similar studies that have been done in Sweden and Utrecht, the Netherlands, demonstrated that yearly screening with mammography results in finding more breast cancers that are smaller and at a more favorable stage for surgical intervention.[3,4] Mortality, while not an end-point in both studies, was favorably affected.

Given the findings of these studies, which concluded in the late 1970s, the American Cancer Society developed very strong recommendations regarding breast cancer screening with mammography. The recommendations include:

1. A baseline mammogram on all women between the ages of 30 and 40;
2. Mammograms every 1 to 2 years for all women between the ages of 41 and 50; and
3. Mammograms every year after the age of 50.

Recently there has been controversy about routine mammograms between the critical ages of 40 and 50 years. The benefits of mammography after the age of 50 are well documented, but for the younger age group the evidence is still inconclusive. The incidence of breast cancer is considerably lower below the age of 50 and, as noted, mammograms are more difficult to interpret in this age group. At present there is simply no consensus among experts whether mammograms should be done as a screening test in this age group.[5] Performing mammograms on asymptomatic women between the ages of 40 and 49 at 1 to 2 year intervals as recommended by the American Cancer Society is not cost effective and has not yet been proven in long-running studies to result in lower mortality. In the HIP study at 18 years there was a difference of only six deaths in screened versus nonscreened patients under the age of 50. Moreover, the American College of Physicians, the Canadian Task Force on the Periodic Health Examination, the American College of Obstetricians and Gynecologists, and a screening committee of the International Union Against Cancer do not recommend mammography for women under the age of 50 years.[6] Given the lack of consensus, our approach is to provide patients with the evidence and let them make up their own minds. We tell patients under 50 years of age that the mammogram carries a very low risk for harm, but the chance of finding a lesion is likewise low. We believe this to be the best approach at this time. On the other hand, we strongly recommend annual mammograms for patients in this age group with one of the known risk factors.

For women over the age of 50 years, we agree with the recommendations of the American Cancer Society and recommend yearly mammography.

How well are physicians following these recommendations? The American Cancer Society did a survey and found that in 1985 only 9 percent of physicians were recommending screening mammograms. More recently, 34 to 40 percent of physicians recommend at least one mammogram after age 50.[7]

COLON CANCER

Colon cancer affects 138,000 people each year and accounts for 60,000 deaths annually. Risk factors include previous colon cancer, familial polyposis, villous or adenomatous polyps, and ulcerative colitis. Favorable influences may include low dietary fat and a high fiber diet. The polyp–neoplasia sequence for the genesis of carcinoma of the colon is now well accepted. This refers to the concept that most colon cancer arises from preexisting villous or adenomatous polyps. Malignant transformation of these polyps occurs over a prolonged period of time — on the order of several years or longer — thus providing an opportunity for early diagnosis at the time when the disease is localized. The screening tests available for colon cancer include digital rectal examination, stool blood testing, and sigmoidoscopy.

Cancer of the colon has seemingly migrated away from the rectum and toward the cecum. Despite this fact and the limitations of digital examination of the rectum, this test continues to be part of our routine examination. There are no studies specifically evaluating the digital examination as a screening test for colon cancer. However, we feel that this examination should continue to be performed.

Testing the stool for the presence of blood is likewise well entrenched, but, in contrast to the digital examination, has been the subject of several large controlled studies. In two ongoing controlled studies from New York and Minnesota, a total of 67,000 patients aged 50 or over were enrolled for prospective screening with guaiac-impregnated Hemoccult cards.[8,9] Approximately 2 percent of the population screened had a positive stool guaiac, and of these, 8 to 12 percent were found to have a colon cancer; 30 percent had polyps, but in the majority (50 to 60 percent) no specific cause was found. Sixty-five percent of the patients with colon cancer had an early stage, Dukes' stage A — no extension of the cancer through the bowel wall or to regional lymph nodes. This percentage is higher than one would expect to find in a non-screened population. These data, however, are subject to length and lead-time biases.

False positive examination with stool guaiac testing remains a significant problem. Agents or foods that can cause a false positive guaiac stool test are noted in Table 46–3. Since approximately half of the patients with positive stool guaiac tests have no demonstrable pathology, many persons without disease undergo the cost, discomfort, and anxiety of endoscopy or barium contrast studies to evaluate the positive Hemoccult test.

Not withstanding these facts, the American Cancer Society and the Canadian Task Force on the periodic health examination have endorsed the use of screening by means of the stool guaiac test on a yearly basis after the age of 50. The U.S. Preventative Services Task Force while noting that the results from uncontrolled trials suggest "a potential benefit from occult blood screen-

TABLE 46–3   Substances That Interfere With The Stool Guaiac Test

May produce a false positive test
    Rare red meat, broccoli, cantaloupe, cauliflower, red radish, horseradish, parsnips, artichoke, zucchini, iron medication

May produce a false negative test
    Vitamin C, prolonged storage of sample

ing, the high proportion of false-positive test results with unavoidable attendant risks, together with problems of patient compliance, mandate caution in the development of any recommendations." In summary, they conclude that there is insufficient evidence to endorse the routine use of occult blood screening. The task force suggested that patients should be informed concerning the uncertainties in the screening test and allowed to participate in the decision. We agree with the finding of the task force and accept the limitation of the stool guaiac test but continue to recommend the stool guaiac test on a yearly basis after the age of 50.

The issue of routine sigmoidoscopy is more controversial. Adenomatous and villous polyps are the precursors for cancer of the colon, but the rate of malignant degeneration is low, on the order of less than 1 percent. When flexible sigmoidoscopy to 65 cm is performed, approximately 10 percent. of asymptomatic people over the age of 50 are found to have adenomatous polyps. These polyps are frequently multiple, and on colonoscopy, up to 35 percent have synchronous lesions beyond 65 cm. This last observation has given rise to the recommendation that the discovery of one polyp on a screening sigmoidoscopy must be followed by colonoscopic examination of the entire colon. The benefit of proctosigmoidoscopic screening was suggested by the Preventive Medicine Institute–Strang Clinic study in New York City.[10,11,12] More than 26,000 asymptomatic patients underwent a total of 47,091 rigid sigmoidoscopic examinations. Fifty-eight cancers were detected, i.e., one out of every 450 patients screened. Eighty-one percent of the cancers detected were in the early stage, and at 15 years follow-up 90 percent of these patients are still alive. In a study in Minnesota, now 25 years old and involving 18,158 patients over the age of 45 years, it has been shown that screening with a 25-cm rigid scope and removal of rectal polyps resulted in a lower than expected incidence of colon cancer.[9] By inference then, flexible sigmoidoscopy with its greater ability to examine the colon should be even more effective than rigid 25-cm sigmoidoscopy. Since 50 to 60 percent of colon cancers are accessible to the 60-cm flexible instrument, the development of colon cancer may be prevented by removing antecedent "premalignant adenomas".

The Minnesota and the New York studies were uncontrolled and therefore subject to the previously discussed biases. However, considering the number of individuals studied, the long follow-up, and the noted effects on survival and cancer rates, the observed effects must be due at least in part to the screening procedures.

The American Cancer Society, the National Cancer Institute, and others recommend a digital rectal examination to detect colorectal cancer for all persons aged 40 and over. To date, only the American Cancer Society of the major advisory groups has recommended that sigmoidoscopy be done on a regular screening program. They recommend that all persons over the age of 50 have a sigmoidoscopy performed every 3 to 5 years after two negative studies 1 year apart.

The U.S. Preventative Services Task Force recently evaluated the use of screening sigmoidoscopy. They concluded that there is insufficient evidence from controlled trials to either recommend or not recommend the use of sigmoidoscopy as a screening test in populations with no known risk.[13] They recommend colonoscopy for high risk patients so as to evaluate the entire colon. We agree with the finding of the U.S. Preventative Services Task Force and explain to our low risk patients that there are insufficient data to support the routine screening of all patients with sigmoidoscopy. We discuss with patients the recommendations of the American Cancer Society and allow them to participate in the decision. However, all patients with a family history of familial polyposis coli or a first degree relative with colorectal cancer are encouraged to have periodic colonoscopy.

CANCER OF THE CERVIX

Invasive cancer of the cervix occurs in about 13,000 women annually in the United States and is responsible for 7,000 cancer-related deaths. Survival rates, as for most cancers, are dependent on the stage of the disease when it is detected. The 5-year survival for carcinoma of the cervix in situ in virtually 100 percent, while for advanced disease it is 45 percent.

The Pap test for screening for cancer of the cervix is accepted by most women and their physicians. There are, however, no prospective controlled studies evaluating the use of the Pap test. All evidence supporting the use of this test is indirect and is based on projections from what is known of the natural history of the disease. Carcinoma of the cervix in situ is thought to precede invasive carcinoma. The in situ carcinoma presumably persists for a long time in a detectable but not invasive stage. This concept, however, has been questioned in some studies. Peterson in 1956 followed but did not treat women with in situ carcinoma of the cervix. One-half of the patients regressed spontaneously within the first year, and at 10 years follow-up, only 30 percent of the patients developed invasive carcinoma.[14] Moreover, the duration of the carcinoma in situ stage may last on the order of three decades. Christopherson, evaluating a large screening program, found the average duration of carcinoma in situ to be about 22 years.[15] Other studies have also confirmed that in situ carcinoma of the cervix detected by the Pap smear is preceded by a very long in situ stage.[16] The finding and interpretation of cervical dysplasia is also controversial. From multiple studies it is clear that not all cases of dysplasia progress to carcinoma in situ and not all cases of carcinoma in situ progress to invasive cancer.[17] In fact, in a number of serial studies, the incidence of carcinoma in situ was much greater than the known incidence of invasive carcinoma.

The Pap test has a number of real and potential technical problems. The test interpretation can vary greatly among different laboratories. The test is easy to perform but difficult to read. In one representative study, the referring diagnosis was questioned in one-third of the specimens reviewed by a panel of expert pathologists.[18] Moreover, abnormal cells may not appear on the slide. In a study evaluating dysplasia of the cervix, 50 percent of the slides showed a discrepancy on two slides taken at the same time from the same woman.[19]

Despite the limitations of the Pap test, it remains an important screening test. A number of large epidemiologic studies clearly have demonstrated that the use of the Pap test has contributed to the reduction of mortality from cervical cancer. In August 1987, the American Cancer Society held a workshop to reexamine the scientific data about Pap smears and cervical cancer. That report recommended that all women who are or who have been sexually active or who are over the age of 18 years have an annual Pap test and pelvic examination.[20] After a woman has had three or more consecutive normal annual examinations, the test may be performed "less frequently at the discretion of her physician". This recommendation attempts to address the uncertainty about the optimal frequency of screening and the likelihood that cervical cancer may be related to a sexually transmitted agent, perhaps a papilloma virus. The new guidelines do not place an upper age limit on testing for cervical cancer. Other groups now have similar recommendations, including the National Cancer Institute, the American Medical Association, and the American College of Obstetricians and Gynecologists. In contrast, programs in England and Canada still recommend a Pap smear every 3 years from age 18 until age 35 in sexually active women, and then every 5 years until age 60. Despite the difficulties associated with the Pap smear, we agree with the recommendations of the American Cancer Society.

CANCER OF THE UTERUS

Carcinoma of the endometrium, the most common malignancy of the female genital tract, comprises about 13 percent of all malignant tumors in women. Over 34,000 cases are diagnosed annually, and cancer of the endometrium accounts for 3,000 cancer-related deaths. The prevalence of carcinoma of the endometrium has increased steadily over the last 20 years thus reflecting the increased life span of women and perhaps the decreased likelihood of cervical cancer. Endometrial cancer is most common in postmenopausal women. High-risk patients include women with a history of infertility, obesity, failure of ovulation, abnormal uterine bleeding, and a prior history of prolonged administration of exogenous hormones.

Endometrial aspiration and biopsy has been recommended as a screening test. In a screening study of endometrial carcinoma in asymptomatic women using endometrial aspiration, eight cancers were found in 1,280 women.[21] Seven of the eight had one or more risk factors for endometrial cancer. The role of endometrial aspiration or biopsy in asymptomatic patients without one of the previously noted risk factors remains unclear. The American Cancer Society recommends that every woman at the time of menopause have a pelvic examination and that high-risk women have an endometrial tissue sample examined. Despite these recommendations, less than 2 percent of all women have undergone this screening test. At this time we recommend that only high-risk women should consider an endometrial aspiration. We do not recommend the routine use of this screening test. However, women should be informed about the importance of promptly reporting any postmenopausal bleeding to their physician.

CANCER OF THE LUNG

Cancer of the lung is the most common lethal cancer in men and the second leading cause of cancer deaths in women 35 to 74 years old. Over 150,000 new cases are diagnosed annually with 139,000 cancer-related deaths. The age-adjusted cancer deaths for lung cancer is doubling approximately every 15 years. Despite advances in the use of radiation therapy, surgery, and chemotherapy, the overall 5-year survival for lung cancer remains in the 8 to 10 percent range.

A number of large studies have evaluated the efficacy of screening x-rays and sputum cytology in detecting early lung cancer. The Philadelphia Pulmonary Neoplasm Research Project screened 6,136 male volunteers over the age of 45 with chest x-rays and questionnaires every 6 months.[22] The 5-year survival for lung cancers detected in this uncontrolled study was 7 percent, a number similar to the nonscreened national average. The Veterans Administration study screened 14,607 men at high risk for developing lung cancer with chest x-rays and sputum cytology every 6 months for 3 years. Two hundred cancers of the lung were diagnosed, but only 26 were resectable, and only three of the patients resected survived for greater than 3 years.[23] Again, this study was not controlled, but these data failed to demonstrate a significant benefit of screening x-rays and sputum cytologies even in this high-risk population.

Randomized prospective studies conducted by John Hopkins, the Mayo Foundation, Memorial Sloan Kettering Cancer Center, and the University of Cincinnati have used chest x-rays and sputum cytologies for men who smoked more than one pack of cigarettes a day.[23,24,25] While the details of the studies were slightly different at the four institutions, the results were similar and disappointing. The overall 5-year survival was less than 15 percent. These data indicate that, even in an intensively screened population, few patients had cancer detected in a curable stage. Overall, the mortality from lung cancer was the same in the screened and in the control nonscreened group.

Given the data, we believe that at this time there is no proven benefit to routine screening of patients for lung cancer with chest x-rays or sputum cytology. The physician's primary role in preventing lung cancer is to educate patients regarding the many risks associated with smoking and to strongly encourage patients who do smoke to stop. The American Cancer Society does not recommend screening x-rays or sputum cytologies.

ROLE OF TUMOR MARKERS

A number of "tumor" markers have been developed in the last decade that are useful in the management of patients with known cancer. These markers include carcinoembryonic antigen (CEA) for patients with colon, breast, pancreatic, and ovarian cancer; alpha-fetoprotein (AFP) for liver and germ cell tumors; prostatic acid phosphatase for prostate cancer; and CA 125 for ovarian cancer. None of these markers is specific enough to be used as a screening test for cancer, and we do not recommend their use as screening tests.

References

1. Self-examination in the early detection of breast cancer. WHO, Geneva 1983.
2. Habbema JDF, van Oortmarssen GJ, van Putten DJ, et al. Age-specific reduction in breast cancer mortality by screening: an analysis of the results of the Health Insurance Plan of Greater New York. J NCI 1986; 77:317.
3. Baker LH. Breast cancer detection demonstration project: five year summary report. Cancer 1982; 32:194.
4. Tabar L, Fagerberg CJG, Gad A, et al. Reduction in mortality from breast cancer after mass screening with mammography. Lancet 1985; 1:829.

5. Eddy DM, Hasselblad V, McGivney W, et al. The value of mammography screening in women under age 50 years. JAMA 1988; 259:1512–1529.

6. Day NE, Baines CJ, Chamberlain J, et al. UICC project on screening for cancer: report of the workshop on screening for breast cancer. Int J Cancer 1986; 38:303–308.

7. National Cancer Institute. Cancer control objectives for the nation: 1985–2000. Bethesda, Maryland: US Department of Health and Human Services, 1986. DHHS publication no. (NIH) 86-2880. (NCI monograph no. 2).

8. Winawer SJ, Fleisher M, Baldwin M, et al. Current status of fecal occult blood testing in screening for colorectal cancer. CA 1982; 32:100–102.

9. Gilbertsen VA, McHugh R, Schuman L, et al. The earlier detection of colorectal cancer: a preliminary report of the results of the Occult Blood Study. Cancer 1980; 45:2899.

10. Knight K, Fielding JE, Battista RN. Occult blood screening for colorectal cancer. JAMA 1989; 261:587.

11. Hertz RE, Deddish MR, Day E. Value of periodic examination in detecting cancer of the rectum and colon. Postgrad Med 1960; 27:290–294.

12. Dales LG, Fredman GD, Ramcharan S, et al. Multiphasic checkup evaluation study. 3. Outpatient clinic utilization, hospitalization, and mortality experience after seven years. Prev Med 1973; 2:221.

13. Selby J, Friedman G. Sigmoidoscopy in the periodic health examination of asymptomatic adults. JAMA 1989; 261:595.

14. Petersen O. Spontaneous course of cervical pre-cancerous conditions. Am J Obstet Gynecol 1956; 72:1063–1071.

15. Christopherson WM, Parker JE. Microinvasive carcinoma of the uterine cervix. A clinical-pathological study. Cancer 1964; 17:1123–1131.

16. Barron BA, Richart RM. Statistical model of the natural history of cervical carcinoma. II. Estimates of the transition time from dysplasia to carcinoma in situ. J Natl Cancer Inst 1970; 45:1025–1030.

17. Kashigarian M, Dunn JE. The duration of intraepithelial and preclinical squamous cell carcinoma of the uterus cervix. Am J Epidemiol 1970; 92:221–222.

18. Kern WH, Zivolich MR. The accuracy and consistency of the cytologic classification of squamous lesions of the uterine cervix. Acta Cytol 1977; 21:519–523.

19. Brudnell M, Cox BS, Taylor CW. The management of dysplasia, carcinoma in situ and microcarcinoma of the cervix. J Obstet Gynaecol Br Comm 1973; 80:673–679.

20. Fink DJ. Change in American Cancer Society Guidelines for Detection of Cervical Cancer. CA:A Cancer Journal For Clinicians 1988; 38(2):27–129.

21. Koss LG, Schreiberk, Oberlander SG, et al. Screening of asymptomatic women for endometrial cancer. CA:A Cancer Journal For Clinicians 1981; 31(6):301–317.

22. Weiss W, Boucot KE, Cooper DA. The Philadelphia pulmonary neoplasm research project. Survival factors in bronchogenic carcinoma. JAMA 1973; 216:2119–2123.

23. Grzybowski S, Coy P. Early diagnosis of carcinoma of lung: simultaneous screening with chest x-ray and sputum cytology. Cancer 1970; 25:113–120.

24. Melamed M, Flehinger B, Miller D, et al. Preliminary report of the lung cancer detection program in New York. Cancer 1977; 39:369–382.

25. Martini N. Results of the Memorial Sloan-Kettering lung project. Recent Results Cancer Res 1982; 82:174–178.

47 | ADJUVANT TREATMENT OF CANCER

RICHARD A. RUDDERS, M.D.

As new cancer treatments are developed, strategies to optimize the results of these treatments follow. Predicated on persuasive theoretical and practical arguments, so-called adjuvant treatment is such a strategy. In oncologic practice we now are usually able to remove the bulk of a given tumor with one of several modalities. The residual disease (both metastatic and microscopic), however, is a major cause of treatment failure leading to overt recurrence of cancer and death. Since the total tumor burden is often quite small after an initial attempt at curative treatment, there is an opportunity to successfully eradicate any residual tumor, even though there is distant spread. Use of a variety of treatment modalities to eradicate residual disease is the guiding principle of adjuvant treatment. Before discussing some specific examples of adjuvant therapy, I will review some fundamental concepts regarding adjuvant therapy. This background information will aid the clinician in analyzing newly published data on adjuvant cancer therapy and in answering a common question: Should I have additional treatment after my operation?

ADJUVANT TREATMENT—A DEFINITION

Broadly speaking, the term 'adjuvant' signifies something in addition to or added. With respect to cancer treatment, adjuvant therapy is any form of specific therapy given in addition to a primary mode of treatment, again, with the intent of improving outcome. Such a definition has no restriction in terms of type, mode of administration, or duration, as long as the intent is to improve results without jeopardizing the result of the primary therapy. Thus, adjuvant cancer treatment may be chemotherapy, radiation therapy, surgery, or any other modality deemed suitable. In contrast, the use of a second mode of treatment that is directed at bulk tumor as part of primary therapy, strictly speaking, should be classified as 'combined modality' treatment, rather than adjuvant treatment.

BASIC PRINCIPLES

Historically, the rationale for adjuvant treatment was closely tied to prevailing concepts of tumor cell kinetics. From animal and in vitro model

520

systems, early investigators recognized that anticancer interventions were more successful when tumor burdens were small and when treatments were given in maximum doses.[1] It then was reasoned that treatment would more likely be successful in situations where minimal tumor burden existed. We now know that, with increasing tumor size and proliferation, the degree of tumor heterogeneity also increases (through mutational events), thereby setting the stage for resistance to treatment.[2] Both of these factors, sheer tumor bulk and cellular resistance, tend to defeat therapeutic maneuvers. Ideally, then, to optimize outcome, treatment should be given as early as possible in the course of the disease when tumor bulk is small and cellular resistance is minimal. This concept remains the foundation for adjuvant therapy.

Given this foundation, what remains is to define the proper setting in which to use adjuvant therapy. Historically, adjuvant therapy was employed following surgical removal of a tumor in situations where there remained a high rate of recurrence or relapse. In such instances, tumor progression was primarily due to growth of occult micrometastases at distant sites that were present prior to surgery. It was argued and demonstrated that postoperative chemotherapy could eradicate these microscopic foci of disease. One classic adjuvant treatment protocol, therefore, would be systemic treatment, such as chemotherapy, after primary resection of a tumor. This concept logically can be extended to include any situation where primary therapy may not suffice and additional treatment may add benefit.

Adjuvant treatment need not be chemotherapy, but may be radiation therapy, a so-called biologic response modifier (see subsequently), or surgery. Furthermore, a regional approach may be warranted, rather than a systemic approach, if a specific site of micrometastases constitutes the greatest liability in terms of future recurrence and morbidity. An example of such a regional approach is regional infusion of the liver with 5-fluorouracil following primary resection for colon cancer in patients at high risk for hepatic recurrence.

It seems obvious that to choose a form of adjuvant therapy that is not likely to be successful is counterproductive. Unfortunately this is often done with the best of intentions. In an effort to spare the patient morbidity from an additional treatment, a drug regimen that is ineffective is employed. A basic principle of adjuvant chemotherapy is: if the drug is not an effective treatment in a nonadjuvant setting, don't use it in an adjuvant setting. This argument does not apply, however, to substances classified as biologic response modifiers. Biologic response modifiers are geared to work optimally in patients with low tumor burdens and may have little or no demonstrable activity when tumor burdens are high.

Cancer treatment to a considerable extent remains empiric, and certain aspects of strategies such as adjuvant treatment remain hard to define. One such dilemma relates to the duration of treatment. Since by definition no visible tumor exists, how does one gauge the adequacy of adjuvant chemotherapy? Empiric observations, long-term follow-up, and, occasionally, the use of tumor markers are the only methods. Anything less assures no likelihood of obtaining useful information. Clearly, careful planning in implementing adjuvant treatment is necessary.

THE DESIGN OF AN ADJUVANT TREATMENT

Except in some specific settings (see subsequently), adjuvant therapy remains largely experimental. Adjuvant therapy therefore is ideally given in the context of a clinical trial using a well-defined protocol. I believe that ad hoc or random treatment of patients with adjuvant therapy should not be carried out without a protocol. In general, an adjuvant therapy study requires a sizable number of patients and a long follow-up to be statistically valid. The foundation of a well-designed study of adjuvant therapy is the principle of randomization. Patients are assigned randomly to one of several treatment options. A simple adjuvant study randomizes patients between a primary treatment option only and a primary treatment plus adjuvant treatment option. In this way, the single variable in the system is the adjuvant therapy. When a large enough patient sample is entered and sufficient time has elapsed, the effect of the adjuvant treatment can be quantified by comparing the responses in the experimental group to the relapses in the control group. More complicated studies that ask several questions at once can be designed. Although this approach may be appealing because it appears quicker and more cost-effective, more complicated studies are more difficult to analyze and the results more difficult to interpret.

The goal of all adjuvant treatment is to increase disease-free survival and ultimately to cure. This means that, for a given cohort of patients, the number of patients that remain free of any evidence of tumor following therapy is statistically significantly increased compared to a control population (Fig. 47-1). If such a cohort is followed long enough, disease-free survival of sufficient duration becomes equivalent to cure. The accuracy of judging cure varies with the natural history of each tumor. Certain tumors recur early, and survival without relapse for more than 2 years predicts a high cure rate. Other tumors may recur late and many years must elapse before a cure is assured. The usual presentation of cure rates as 5-year survivals is therefore arbitrary, and cure rates must be evaluated in the context of individual tumors.

Although less desirable, an increase in total patient survival or in delay of relapse (Fig. 47-2), even if cure is not achieved, may be the most a given adjuvant treatment can accomplish. This effect, although less than hoped for, may be highly desirable, depending on the magnitude of the increase in survival

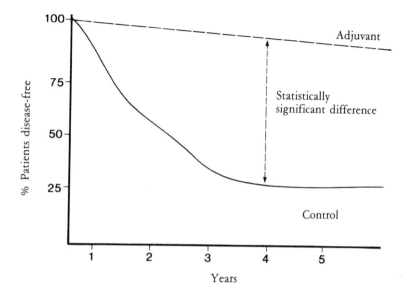

Figure 47-1 Prolongation of disease-free survival for adjuvant group versus control group.

relative to the cost; the latter must be measured both in true cost and in terms of toxicity of the treatment and of side effects suffered by the patient. The more successful the treatment, the higher the therapeutic index. The lower the therapeutic index, the more toxicity and less benefit, and survival curves with and without adjuvant therapy will be comparable (Fig. 47-3).

The clinician should know the common pitfalls in interpreting the results of adjuvant therapy trials. The most common error is to draw a hasty conclusion from preliminary data, i.e., after too little time has elapsed. Early prolongation of disease-free survival may be meaningless in terms of cure if relapse is merely delayed (see Fig. 47-2). Projecting a marked increase in disease-free survival or in cure rate based on preliminary data is a common practice in studies of adjuvant treatment and should be discouraged. More often than not, a totally different picture emerges when the data mature. If the cure rate is not increased, a new approach may be necessary. However, if a lesser but still desirable effect occurs, such as prolongation of total survival or delay of relapse, modification of the original treatment may be indicated as the next step.

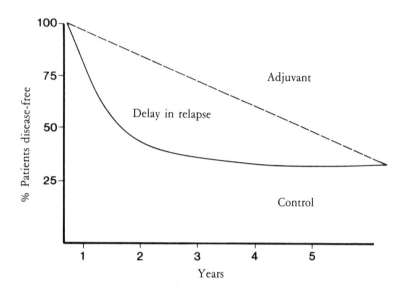

Figure 47-2 Delay in relapse for adjuvant group versus control group. Disease-free survival after 5 years becomes similar.

Judging the benefit of any treatment is difficult, but particularly so when toxic treatments with low therapeutic indices are used. The benefits of adjuvant treatment must be carefully weighed against the cost in terms of both acute and delayed side effects.

SPECIFIC EXAMPLES OF ADJUVANT THERAPIES

Several specific examples of current adjuvant therapies are listed in Table 47-1. The list is in no way intended to be comprehensive, but serves to illustrate several common tumor types considered amenable to adjuvant treatment. The competent consultant must be aware of these examples and of the various approaches to adjuvant treatment they exemplify.

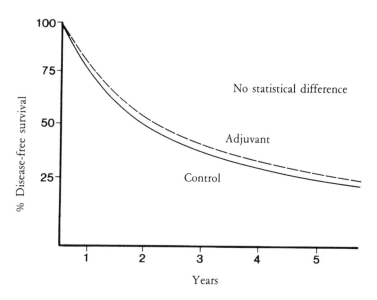

Figure 47-3 No difference in disease-free survival between adjuvant and control groups.

Breast Cancer—An Adjuvant Success Story

More has been written about the adjuvant therapy of surgically resectable breast cancer than perhaps any other cancer.[3,4] Breast cancer is an important tumor for several reasons. First, it is extremely common and is the leading cause of cancer death in women. Second, adjuvant therapy in breast cancer clearly works! The studies of adjuvant therapy have been numerous, international, well controlled, and carefully done. Adjuvant chemotherapy with a number of different combination regimens, usually given for 6 months in the postoperative period, clearly prolongs disease-free survival for certain well-defined subsets of patients (Fig. 47-4). This effect has been demonstrated in axillary node-positive patients who fall into two broad categories: premenopausal patients treated with chemotherapy and postmenopausal patients treated with hormonal therapy (tamoxifen). Current trials are aimed at defining these broad categories of response according to hormone receptor status. To date it is unknown whether the premenopausal group will show benefit from hormonal therapy or whether the postmenopausal group will benefit

TABLE 47-1 Specific Adjuvant Therapies

Type of Cancer	Patient Characteristics	Therapy	Outcome
Breast*	Postsurgical resection Stage 1 Premenopausal		
	Receptor +	Hormonal therapy	Unknown
	Receptor −	Chemotherapy	Unknown
	Postmenopausal		
	Receptor +	Hormonal therapy	Unknown
	Receptor −	Chemotherapy	Unknown
	Stage II Premenopausal		
	Receptor +	Chemotherapy	Unknown
	Receptor −	Chemotherapy	Increase DFS
	Postmenopausal		
	Receptor +	Hormonal/chemotherapy	Increase DFS
	Receptor −	Chemotherapy	Unknown
Colorectal	Postsurgical resection, Duke's stage B, C	Chemotherapy, portal vein infusion chemotherapy	Unknown Unknown
Pancreas Stomach	Postsurgical, resectable	Systemic chemotherapy, Intraperitoneal chemotherapy	Unknown Unknown
Lung Small Cell	Postchemotherapy, induction Postchemotherapy, induction	Radiation to primary site and CNS Surgical excision primary site	Unknown Unknown
Lung Non-Small Cell	Postsurgical resection of primary site	Irradiation, chemotherapy	Unknown
Melanoma	Postsurgical resection of primary site Stage II	Chemotherapy, BRM, i.e., interferon	Unknown Unknown
Sarcoma Osteogenic*	Preoperative	Chemotherapy	Increase in limb salvage, possible increase in DFS
Testicular*	Postsurgical Stage II retroperitoneal node dissection no choriocarcinoma	Chemotherapy	Increase in cure

TABLE 47-1 (Continued)

Type of Cancer	Patient Characteristics	Therapy	Outcome
Lymphoma*	Large cell stages I & II	Radiotherapy/ chemotherapy	Increase in cure
		Chemotherapy/ radiotherapy	Unknown
	Burkitt's lymphoblastic	CNS radiation and/or chemotherapy	Unknown
	All types advanced disease	High-dose chemotherapy, radiation, bone marrow salvage	Unknown
Leukemia*	All	CNS radiation and/or chemotherapy	Increase in cure
Renal Cell	Postsurgical, local extrarenal extension	Interferon or other BRM	Unknown
Head and Neck Cancer, Squamous	Postsurgical resection of primary site	Chemotherapy	Unknown

*Tumors in which adjuvant therapy has a well-documented effect. BRM = biologic response modifier; DFS = disease-free survival; ALL = acute lymphoblastic leukemia; CNS = central nervous system.

from chemotherapy.[5] Although some studies of adjuvant therapy in patients with breast cancer have been ongoing for as long as 12 years, it is still too early to tell whether the cure rate has been significantly affected by this treatment or whether the major effect is delay of relapse (see Fig. 47–2). Since breast cancer is notorious for late recurrences, sufficient time must elapse in a large cohort of patients to definitively answer this question.

As with any therapy, the potential benefits of adjuvant chemotherapy for breast cancer must be weighed against the risks of treatment. The short-term effects of chemotherapy are well defined and vary with the type of drugs used and the duration of treatment. Tolerance of drug therapy for 6 months (the usual duration of treatment) is highly variable, potentially morbid, but rarely fatal. We are just now in a position to evaluate the potential long-term effects. I believe that the greatest concern is the development of second malignancies, particularly leukemia, although sterilization is also an important issue. The incidence of leukemia is definitely increased, particularly in patients treated with the alkylating agent melphalan. The incidence, however, is in the range of only 1 percent at 10 years. An increase in leukemia in patients treated with cyclophosphamide, the other alkylating agent in common use, has not been reported.

Fortunately the acute toxic adverse effects of hormonal therapy with tamoxifen, the agent most commonly used, have been few. Little is known

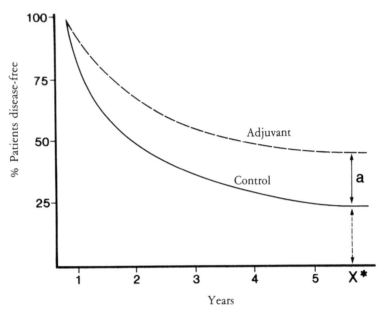

* The difference in disease-free survival (a) in various trials,
depending on the follow-up interval (×), is 10 to 25%.

Figure 47-4   Effect of adjuvant chemotherapy in node-positive breast cancer. Magnitude of benefit varies in different clinical trials.

about the potential long-term carcinogenic effects of chronic tamoxifen use (2 to 5 years). The possible effect on endocrine-sensitive tumors, such as endometrial cancer, remains to be defined.

Overall, the adjuvant story in breast cancer has been a successful one. This experience serves as a model for the development of similar strategies in other tumors.

Other Tumors—Potential Success Stories

Adjuvant therapy has had a clear cut impact on either survival or cure in patients with other types of cancer (Table 47–1). Unfortunately many of these tumors are uncommon. Some results have been so exciting, however, that the potential to apply these principles to other more common tumors is an important spin-off from these experimental studies. Certain subsets of patients with testicular cancer, non-Hodgkin's lymphoma, sarcomas, and acute leukemia benefit from adjuvant treatment.[6] For instance, aggressive treatment of testicular cancer has resulted in a substantial increase in cure rate. In the case of osteogenic sarcoma, chemotherapy treatment may alleviate the need for radical amputation.

PROSPECTS FOR THE FUTURE

As previously stated, I believe adjuvant treatment of cancer is in large part an experimental approach. Except for the instances noted herein, I do not consider it standard treatment. Rather, patients should be encouraged to enter into clinical trials, obviously after giving consent. The future of adjuvant therapy looks bright. As newer treatments are developed, the patient with a small body burden of tumor is a favorable testing ground for adjuvant treatment. A partially effective treatment in patients with 'bulk disease' may be highly effective in the patient with only microscopic disease. The recent development of an exciting new class of compounds referred to as biologic response modifiers (antibodies, cytokines, immunomodulators) is an extremely interesting and promising approach with applicability especially to patients with low tumor burden. In future years, these compounds may prove to be invaluable in salvaging patients at high risk for recurrence of cancer.

References

1. Skipper HE, Schnabel FM Jr, Wilcox WS. Experimental evaluation of potential anticancer agents. XII. On the criteria and kinetics associated with the "curability" of experimental leukemia. Cancer Chemother Rep 1950; 54:431–450.
2. Goldie JH, Coldman AJ. Quantitative model for multiple levels of drug resistance in clinical tumors. Cancer Treat Rep 1983; 67(10):923–931.
3. Adjuvant therapy of breast cancer. JAMA 1985; 254:3461–3463.
4. Henderson IC. Adjuvant systemic therapy for early breast cancer. Curr Probl Cancer 1987; 2:125–207.
5. Adjuvant therapy for breast cancer. N Engl J Med 1988; 318:443–444.
6. Salmon SE, ed. Adjuvant therapy of cancer V. Orlando, FL: Grune & Stratton, 1988.

48 | PIGMENTED SKIN LESIONS

FRANCIS RENNA, M.D.

Pigmented skin lesions are important because they suggest a melanocytic neoplasm, the most worrisome being cutaneous melanoma. They derive their color from the melanocytic pigment, melanin, which, depending on its amount and location within the skin, may produce the colors brown, black, or their shades—tan, dark brown, blue-black, and gray. Every clinician knows that melanoma is one of the most treacherous of all cancers because it can spread internally and cause death after arising from a seemingly external, superficial, and usually friendly outpost of our bodies, our skin. The appearance of a single fatality from melanoma, especially in a young, productive, and otherwise healthy person, can cause widespread concern, even panic, in a community. Many individuals will then call their own physicians asking if they have to worry about their own pigmented lesions. By knowing the early signs of melanoma and its precursors and by teaching them to our patients, we can help allay their fears and reduce the risk of fatal disease when these lesions do appear.

The incidence of melanoma is increasing faster than any other human cancer,[1] largely because of increased unprotected sun exposure. In 1985, there were 22,000 melanomas diagnosed, a doubling compared to 1979[2]; the lifetime risk of a white child developing melanoma in 1985 was about one in 150.[3] At the current rate of increase, the risk is predicted to be one in 100 by the year 2000,[4] underscoring the need for greater sun protection and correction of other emerging risk factors, such as thinning of the earth's ozone layer.

Fortunately the prognosis for patients with melanoma is improving. In the 1940s, the 5-year survival from melanoma was 40 percent, while in the 1980s it rose to 85 percent for clinical Stage I (localized, primary skin tumor).[2] Credit for this improved outlook is due to the earlier recognition of melanoma when it is thinner and less apt to have metastasized. No effective treatment for metastatic melanoma currently exists. Further reduction in the incidence and fatality rate from melanoma has come from the recognition of its precursor lesions: congenital melanocytic nevi, lentigo maligna, acral-mucosal pigmented lesions, and the dysplastic nevus—the most recently described and most important precursor of melanoma based on its incidence and tendency for malignant change.[3]

Given these facts, our ability to diagnose melanoma early and to recognize its precursors becomes of paramount importance. Use of this knowledge should result in a reduction of the overall death rate from melanoma to less than 5 percent.[5] My emphasis in this chapter is to review the early signs of melanoma and its precursors and to distinguish them from benign pigmented growths.

Potentially dangerous pigmented growths can be diagnosed only if we look for them. Examination of the entire skin for pigmented lesions, including hidden sites (scalp, genital, perineal, perianal, and mucous membranes), should be part of every physical examination. Such examination requires the naked eye aided by the use of a hand magnifier (5x to 10x power) and oblique (side) lighting, the latter to distinguish slightly elevated (possible early melanoma) from macular (flat) benign or precancerous pigmented lesions.

CLINICAL GUIDELINES

Microscopic cellular dysplasia and malignant change in melanocytes translate into a macroscopic "disorderly" change that can be detected with the naked eye. The most important observation for early detection of a dangerous pigmented lesion is its disorderly appearance. Regardless of the examiner's familiarity with the various pigmented skin lesions, observation of the degree of disorderliness— reflected in four physical features (in order of their importance: color, border, surface topography, and size)—will reliably distinguish benign from malignant melanocytic lesions and their precursors.

The presence of disorderliness in any one of these four features means that the lesion should be removed, size and location permitting, by an excision of the entire lesion. Microscopic thickness can then be determined, which directly relates to prognosis and the need for regional lymph node removal. The five-year survival for clinical Stage I melanoma based on tumor thickness in millimeters is: less than or equal to 0.85 mm, 99 percent; 0.85 to 1.69 mm, 94 percent; 1.70 to 3.64 mm, 78 percent; and greater than or equal to 3.65 mm, 42 percent survival.[2]

The four physical features that define a pigmented lesion's potential for melanoma are as follows.

Color. Color is the most important of the four features. Benign pigmented lesions have a uniform brown or tan color or a regular pattern of colors (stippled). Early melanoma, especially superficial spreading and lentigo maligna melanoma, has haphazard or variegated shades of brown (tan, medium, and dark brown) mixed with red (representing focal sites of inflammation and secondary vasodilation), white (focal regressed or amelanocytic melanocytes), blue (due to the scattering of incident light), and black or shades of black, i.e., blue-black, blue-gray, and purple. Black, or its shades, is the most ominous color and is an important exception to the requirement for variegated color. When black occurs uniformly as the only color, it signals the potential presence of nodular melanoma, which invades early in its biologic life and carries the worst prognosis of all melanomas. Hence the dictum that any uniformly black or shades of black lesion, unless diagnosable by some other objective criterion (e.g., a small traumatic hematoma that can be evacuated by needle aspiration) demands removal for definitive histologic diagnosis. While many black lesions turn out to be benign, e.g., seborrheic keratoses, small hemangiomas, and the blue nevus (a benign nevus whose deep dermal component appears blue because of reflected and scattered light), the possibility of missing a nodular melanoma at a more curable stage justifies their removal.

Border. Benign pigmented lesions are symmetrical and have a uniformly round or oval shape. Early melanomas, especially superficial spreading and lentigo maligna melanomas, have irregular borders. Superficial spreading melanoma has a horizontal, noninvasive growth phase, providing an opportunity for cure by early diagnosis. Lentigo maligna melanoma also has a delayed invasive phase and arises within a precursor lesion, lentigo maligna, which may be present for up to 25 years as a mottled-brown macule on sun-exposed skin prior to the emergence of melanoma within its borders. Superficial spreading melanoma, the most common and easily recognizable form, has the most dramatic irregularity to the border, often appearing jaggedly irregular, asymmetrical, with one or more notches or protrusions along its edge. Nodular melanoma is an exception in that it usually has a uniform round or oval margin and sometimes appears large and polypoid in shape. Polypoid nodular melanoma may be pink with small islands of brown or black at the periphery; it often is the most rapidly growing melanoma, arising over a period of months.

Surface. Benign pigmented nevi have a uniformly elevated surface. If multiple elevations are present they are similar in size and shape and are symmetrically placed (cobblestone-like pattern). Early melanoma demonstrates an asymmetrically placed elevation, often with darker color within the elevation or an irregular arrangement of multiple elevations. Nodular melanoma presents as a solitary elevation from its onset.

Size. Size alone is the least reliable indicator for melanoma. Remember that most early melanomas are greater than 6 mm, while most benign nevi are less than 6 mm in diameter. Lentigo maligna melanoma may be quite large, 3 to 6 cm, while superficial spreading melanoma is usually 2.5 cm or less in diameter. Of course, melanomas can be less than 6 mm. Hence, reliance on size alone will miss smaller melanomas that demonstrate other suspicious features. Relative size is important, because any pigmented lesion that is clearly larger than the surrounding majority catches the physician's or patient's eye as marching out-of-step compared to the others. If other diagnostic features are present, the lesion should be removed. The absence of definitely worrisome physical, chronologic, or subjective features allows the lesion to be monitored for the development of such changes. Alternatively, the lesion could be removed if the patient or physician continue to worry about it. In fact, I believe that one criterion for removing any pigmented lesion is the presence of concern on the patient's part, which may prompt a visit to the physician. Asking a patient "not to worry" about a lesion if in fact he or she is worried about it burdens the patient and abrogates the physician's responsibility to provide peace of mind to the patient. Since surgical excision of most pigmented lesions is easily done with low risk, it should always be discussed as a way of achieving ultimate peace of mind, so that the patient will not be embarrassed or afraid of choosing removal (Table 48–1).

The diagnosis of dangerous pigmented lesions also is aided by the history and symptomatology. The most telling historical early warning signs are a change in color or size in a preexisting melanocytic nevus or the appearance of a new pigmented lesion, often noted by the patient, spouse, or friend. A personal or family history of melanoma or dysplastic nevi should heighten the surveillance and suspicion regarding other existing or new pigmented lesions. The

TABLE 48–1   Clinical Features of Several Pigmented Skin Lesions

	Common Nevi	Dysplastic Nevi	Cutaneous Melanoma
Overview	Orderly, regular, and symmetric	Orderly or disorderly, symmetric or asymmetric	Disorderly, irregular, asymmetric
Color	Uniform shades of brown	Regular or irregular mixture of browns, often pink, rarely black	Haphazard pattern of any mixture of brown, black, blue, gray, white, pink, or red. Uniform black, blue, or blue-black suggests nodular melanoma.
Border	Regular, well-demarcated, round, or oval	Regular, round, oval, or irregular with less severe notching. Edge may fade into surrounding skin.	Jaggedly irregular, may have a large notch
Surface	Uniform; if multiple elevations, similar size and shape and symmetrically placed (cobblestone-like)	Regular, symmetric, or irregular, asymmetric, single or multiple elevations	Asymmetrically placed single or multiple, different-sized elevations
Size	Usually less than 6 mm	Usually greater than 6 mm. Can be diagnosed when smaller.	Usually greater than 6 mm. Can be diagnosed when smaller.

presence of symptoms without obvious cause, e.g., friction, trauma, or sunburn, especially within one of many pigmented lesions in the absence of other physical signs, could reflect an early malignant change.

Features that may deceive physicians into discounting the presence of melanoma include the absence of symptoms. The physical changes described so far usually occur in the absence of symptoms. Likewise, the presence or absence of hair within a lesion has no bearing on its being benign or malignant. The duration of a pigmented lesion is helpful only if it has recently appeared. A long duration does not exclude a dangerous lesion, because often patients are not aware of subtle, gradual changes in lesions they have come to take for granted.

To summarize, disorderliness in color, surface, border, or size, a uniform black or blue-black color, or any change in size, shape, surface, or color within a pigmented lesion (which marks it as marching out-of-step compared to others), especially a change in color toward black, warrants definitive diagnosis by surgical removal and histologic studies. Less reliable but often important are the appearance of unprovoked and unremitting symptoms within a pigmented lesion or a patient's unremitting worry over such a lesion.

COMMON BENIGN PIGMENTED LESIONS

Seborrheic Keratosis

Seborrheic keratosis, a common flat-topped plaque ranging in size from a few millimeters to several centimeters, often is uniformly colored with shades of brown or even black. It represents a benign proliferation of epidermal cells (keratinocytes) that retain the ability to form keratin (scale). The pattern of growth is outward, above the plane of the surrounding skin, providing their "stuck-on" appearance and their ability to be flicked or scraped off without penetrating the dermis. Seborrheic keratoses have a cobblestone or wart-like surface of many uniform, small-sized, closely set symmetrical elevations. Older lesions are obviously covered by flat scales (hyperkeratotic) that may not be readily visible in early lesions unless the edge is scraped. The border is well demarcated and slightly pedunculated (tucked in where it meets the skin) or square-shouldered on cross section. They appear anywhere, but are most common on the trunk, chest, and neck.

The thickened nature of seborrheic keratoses allows for the accumulation of the normal cellular complement of melanin such that grossly they are pigmented. The pattern of color may be asymmetrical and irregular and may be associated with irregular, well-demarcated margins; therefore they can be confused with melanoma. A round or oval seborrheic keratosis with uniform black or blue-black color may be confused with nodular melanoma. The presence of hyperkeratotic scales throughout the lesion and the stuck-on appearance are important clinical signs arguing against melanoma, which normally is not a keratinizing tumor. It may be difficult to detect scales, and moreover, the color and pattern as well as the irregular margin may be so suggestive of melanoma that histologic examination is necessary.

Lentigines

Lentigo refers to any small brown macule composed of an increased number of normal melanocytes. Three types of lentigines are recognized: simple lentigo, solar lentigo, and lentigo maligna. Freckles are also brown macules that occur on sun-exposed skin, but histologically they may not show an increased number of melanocytes.[6] A simple lentigo is small, about 1.5 mm, may be the first stage of the common acquired mole beginning in childhood, is well demarcated, and is round with a uniform brown or dark brown color. Occasionally a simple lentigo is a dark brown color with smooth or regularly finely jagged edges. It appears anywhere on the skin.

A solar lentigo, a benign melanocytic hyperplasia present on sun-exposed skin especially of the face, chest, and dorsum of hands, is erroneously referred to as a "liver spot" instead of a "sun spot". A solar lentigo often is larger than a simple lentigo and ranges from a few millimeters to several centimeters. It often has an irregular border, but as long as it is not black, lacks islands of darker and lighter shades of brown, white, or gray, and has no component elevated (oblique lighting often is required), then lentigo maligna (a macule with shades of brown or black — see subsequently) and lentigo maligna melanoma (elevated darkly pigmented islands appearing against a macular, mottled brown background) need not be considered.

Common Acquired Nevomelanocytic Nevi (Common Nevi)

Common nevi are round or oval, well demarcated with a smooth border, tan to dark brown and occasionally black, with varying degrees of elevation from macular to dome-shaped papules, most often up to 5 mm in size. Common nevi represent accumulations of nevus cells (immature melanocytes that have not completed their migration from the neural crest to the epidermis as mature melanocytes) at different anatomic levels within the skin. Accumulations at the dermoepidermal junction appear as flat or slightly raised brown to dark brown lesions called junctional nevi. If the nevus cells are within both the superficial dermis and the dermoepidermal junction, the lesion is more raised, may include hair, and is called a compound nevus. If the nevus cells are only in the deeper dermis, the lesion is called a dermal nevus and may have a smooth or rough surface and contain coarse hairs.

All of these nevi are easily recognized as benign pigmented lesions because of their overall orderly appearance, regular borders and surfaces, and regular shades of brown.

Junctional nevi usually arise in childhood or around puberty, but occasionally appear later in life. Since their appearance after the age of 40 is uncommon, their appearance beyond this age demands that they be followed closely for possible evolution into dysplastic nevi or melanoma.[4] Before the age of 40, junctional nevi also may evolve into compound or intradermal nevi, becoming more raised and larger and retaining their orderly appearance. If these changes arouse physician or patient concern, especially if they appear disorderly, removal is in order. Normal changes in common nevi are apt to occur during growth spurts in toddlers, just before or during puberty, or during pregnancy. However, all nevi should change together. Any one nevus marching out-of-step, changing in size, border, surface, or color at any time in life, warrants removal.

Several other criteria in addition to visible change within a nevus argue for removal. A nevus that is continually irritated may assume symptoms and size and color changes that can be confused with those of an early melanoma. Nevi in hidden sites, especially if darkly colored or if there is a personal or family history of dysplastic nevi or melanoma, should be removed since they are difficult to monitor.

I urge clinicians to make special note of darkly pigmented or irregularly marginated lesions on acral sites, especially palms, soles, and toewebs, because these pigmented lesions have a higher risk for malignant change that is more biologically aggressive, thus leading to earlier metastasis. Although the more darkly pigmented races normally have darkly pigmented nevi, their occurrence on the palms and soles carries the same hazard. In a white person, pigmented lesions involving the nailfolds, which manifest as a longitudinal brown pigmented streak within the nailplate, as well as pigmented conjunctival lesions warrant biopsy; these lesions are uncommon and carry a greater malignant potential. Darkly pigmented people have a higher incidence of benign nail-associated and conjunctival pigmented lesions, so that their lesions are biopsied or removed on an individual basis, according to whether there has been a recent change in a longstanding lesion, an appearance of a new lesion, or a personal and/or family history of melanoma or its precursors.[6]

MELANOMA PRECURSORS

Lentigo Maligna

Lentigo maligna is a macular hyperplasia of atypical melanocytes along the epidermal basement membrane. The color is variegated with shades of brown to black occurring together with an irregular border. Often there are colors that suggest focal regression: white, blue-gray, pink, or, more rarely, no color (amelanosis). Size varies from a few millimeters to several centimeters, and these lesions appear mostly on sun-damaged skin on the head, neck, and upper extremities, usually around the age of 50 to 60 years.[6] Lentigo maligna grows slowly; about 30 percent eventually develop focal invasive melanoma (lentigo maligna melanoma) after a long latent period (5 to 50 years).[2] Invasion manifests as a small, slightly or obviously raised segment, usually of darker color, within the macular background. Any macular, mottled brown to dark brown lesion, even in the absence of black, on the face, neck, or upper extremities in an elderly patient should be biopsied from the darkest portion. If it is a lentigo maligna, the entire lesion should be excised if the site, size, and patient's condition allow. Lentigo maligna seldom causes symptoms and, because of its long duration and slow change, may not worry or be noticed by the patient. Thus, although the patient may not bring it to my attention, I always look for lentigo maligna when examining an elderly patient.

Congenital Melanocytic Nevi (Congenital Nevi)

Congenital melanocytic nevi are present at birth or appear within the first 12 months of life and consist of nevus cells that are present deeper in the dermis than in common acquired nevi. In the absence of a reliable history, a congenital nevus should be suspected in a pigmented nevus greater than or equal to 1.5 cm[6]; at the same time the lesion will have none of the features of a dysplastic nevus (see later discussion of dysplastic nevi). They appear as round or oval raised lesions with a uniform brown or dark brown color and smooth regular borders. Frequently the surface is covered by papillomatous elevations that become more raised and irregular with time. Coarse long hairs are often present and may become darker and coarser in late childhood. More atypical congenital nevi have haphazard shades of brown, dark brown, black, and blue-black and may be poorly demarcated with or without irregular margins. Clearly these latter are worrisome and require removal when feasible.

Congenital nevi are arbitrarily subclassified as small if less than or equal to 1.5 cm in diameter, medium if 1.5 to 19.9 cm, and large if greater than or equal to 20 cm in diameter.[4] When large congenital nevi cover a major portion of the body, they are referred to as giant or great hairy nevi, which were the first congenital nevi to be associated with an increased risk for melanoma, the risk ranging from 2 to 40 percent.[7] Melanomas appear within giant congenital nevi early, often within the first 3 years of life, and are difficult to detect because of their dark color and rough surface as well as the often deep origin of the melanoma within these lesions. Hence, early full-thickness excision is recommended (after careful planning and discussion with the parents) after the first 6 months of life; before 6 months the risk of general anesthesia is too great.

There is controversy over the management of small and medium-sized congenital nevi, because there is no agreement over the degree of risk for melanoma in these lesions. I believe that the best estimate of risk is about 5 percent. Considering that small and medium-sized congenital nevi are responsible for up to 15 percent of melanomas and that they are present in 1 percent of newborns,[6] the projected number of melanomas that arise from them becomes a significant public health concern. Any congenital nevus that displays irregular size, shape, or color is best removed without delay. For nonworrisome-appearing small and medium-sized congenital nevi, the increased risk for melanoma begins just before puberty, increases through the teenage years, and then decreases. Since most parents, physicians, and children are uneasy about monitoring such lesions during these higher-risk years, I examine them yearly until the child is 8 to 10 years of age (patients and parents check them every 2 to 3 months), at which time I suggest that these congenital nevi be excised, barring problems with cosmetics and functional deficits. This is also a time when children are better able to tolerate local anesthesia and minor surgery.

Dysplastic Nevus

The dysplastic nevus is an acquired pigmented lesion consisting of intra-epidermal melanocytic dysplasia. Its special significance is that it is the most frequently occurring precursor for melanoma, appearing in 2 to 5 percent of white adults and occurring in both a familial and sporadic (nonfamilial) pattern.[8] Since it can be confused clinically with common nevi and melanoma, definitive diagnosis depends on histologic examination of the removed lesion.

Clinically, dysplastic nevi appear on any mucocutaneous surface and usually are larger than common nevi, from 6 to 12 mm in diameter. The surface is often macular with slightly to moderately elevated components. The border is often irregular and may be ill-defined, fading into the surrounding skin. The color is often variegated, tan to dark-brown, often with a prominent pink component. Dysplastic nevi are common on the sun-exposed trunk and extremities, but also on the sun-protected scalp, buttocks, breast, and genital skin. Unlike melanoma, there is usually the absence of black or its shades and an overall milder degree of disorderliness. The dysplastic nevus can be thought of as a "watered-down" melanoma, intermediate in appearance between common nevi and melanoma.

Three distinctive clinical variants of dysplastic nevus are recognized. The "fried egg" type has a central, normal-appearing, round or oval, tan or, as it regresses, paler and fleshier raised element associated with a slowly expanding macular halo of darker color; the halo represents the expanding area of atypical melanocytes. The "patterned" or "regularly irregular" dysplastic nevus is slightly raised with a regular speckling of darker brown against a paler brown or pink background. A change in the pattern, often the appearance of a darker brown or black element at an edge, heralds evolution towards melanoma and requires its entire removal. The "chaotic" or "irregularly irregular" dysplastic nevus is usually macular or barely elevated and has large areas of different colors occurring more haphazardly without a regular pattern. The border often is irregular, reflecting the different growth rates of the various subclones. This lesion often cannot be distinguished from superficial spreading, lentigo maligna, or acral-lentiginous melanoma and causes great concern until the histologic diagnosis is in hand.[9]

Dysplastic nevi may occur as a solitary lesion or as a group of a few lesions up to more than 100 in number. They begin around puberty and continue to appear throughout life; hence the need for lifelong surveillance.

In the familial, autosomal dominant form of dysplastic nevus, if two or more family members have had melanoma, the risk of melanoma for any other family member with dysplastic nevi is 100 percent by age 76.[6] The lifetime risk for melanoma in people with sporadically occurring dysplastic nevi or familial dysplastic nevi associated with one or no melanoma is estimated at 5 to 10 percent.[4]

Often the family history regarding dysplastic nevi is not known, or if dysplastic nevi are present in the family, melanoma may not yet have developed. Therefore, the risk for melanoma in a single person or family cannot be accurately determined at the outset. It is, therefore, best that all first-degree relatives of people with dysplastic nevi be examined for their presence. In the setting of dysplastic nevi, melanoma most often arises within a dysplastic nevus, but may also arise de novo in normal-appearing skin. Hence, the entire skin, not just the dysplastic nevi, needs to be watched.

Current knowledge regarding the dysplastic nevus dictates a prudent step-wise plan for the management of patients with these melanoma precursors as well as of their blood relatives. First, after examination of the entire skin, the diagnosis should be confirmed by excising one to three of the most atypical-appearing dysplastic nevi. The pathologist also will grade the degree of dysplasia, aiding the decision for future removals based on clinical correlation with the degree of histologic dysplasia. Also, dysplastic-appearing nevi should be removed if located in hidden sites, if they are changing or have an extremely atypical appearance, or if the patient is on immunosuppressive medications or has Hodgkin's disease. Second, remaining dysplastic nevi can be mapped or photographed to detect changes or new lesions. Third, the patient should perform self-examinations every 4 to 6 weeks looking for changes in one of the four features or for new lesions. Fourth, the patient should have physician examinations at a frequency that reflects the degree of risk for melanoma. If there is a positive personal or family history of melanoma, examinations are done every 3 to 6 months, while if the personal and family histories are negative for melanoma, examinations can be 6 months to yearly. Fifth, blood relatives of people with dysplastic nevi and/or melanoma also need to be examined. Children within the kindred who have multiple common acquired nevi should be checked carefully just before and during puberty and yearly throughout the teen years for the evolution of dysplastic nevi. Pregnancy and the use of oral contraceptives or estrogen should increase the frequency of the surveillance program, although any added risk for melanoma related to these hormonal changes is not presently clear. If there have been two or more melanomas within the family, *all* blood relatives should be examined once, children by 10 years of age and then yearly to age 20 if no dysplastic nevi are found. For people with one or more dysplastic nevi and no personal or family history of melanoma, only *first-degree* relatives beyond puberty need to be checked once and then followed only if dysplastic nevi are found. Sixth, all patients with dysplastic nevi should minimize ultraviolet light exposure and use high-potency sun protection (#15 sun protection factor) with protective clothing when outdoors.[6] For patients and physicians alike, it is encouraging to remember that melanomas detected as part of a dysplastic nevus surveillance program have been removed at a nearly 100 percent curable stage (Table 48–2).[5]

MELANOMA

Any pigmented lesion that appears disorderly; that is manifested by an irregular color pattern consisting of shades of brown mixed with red, white, or blue, or by the presence of black or its shades; or that has an irregular border or surface topography is a suspect for melanoma and should be removed for definitive diagnosis. Other warning signs for melanoma occurring within pigmented lesions are

1. Size greater than 6 mm,
2. Any change in color or shape,
3. Unprovoked, nonremitting symptoms,

TABLE 48-2   Management of Patients with Dysplastic Nevi

1. Examine the entire skin, including hidden areas.

2. Review the family history for the presence of dysplastic nevi and melanoma.

3. Excise 1–3 of the most atypical appearing dysplastic nevi for definitive histologic diagnosis and grading of dysplasia.

4. Examine all first-degree relatives for the presence of dysplastic nevi or melanoma.

5. Instruct all affected individuals how to recognize dysplastic nevi and melanoma and in the technique of self-examination, to be done at 4–6 week intervals.*

6. Map or photograph the patient's lesions.

7. Regular physician examinations for life. If there is a personal or family history of melanoma, examinations are done every 3–6 months. If there is no personal or family history of melanoma, examinations are done 6 months to yearly. Children who are first-degree relatives of people with dysplastic nevi or melanoma should be checked just before and during puberty and throughout the teen years for the evolution of dysplastic nevi and melanoma.

8. Discourage the use of oral contraceptives and other estrogen-containing drugs.

9. Avoid unprotected ultraviolet light exposure. Use sunscreens and sun-protective clothing.

10. Excise any nevi undergoing suspicious changes.

---

* A patient's guide, *Dysplastic Nevi and Malignant Melanoma*, is available from The Skin Cancer Foundation, Box 561, NY, NY, 10156.

Adapted from Rhodes AR. Neoplasms: benign neoplasias, hyperplasias, and dysplasias of melanocytes. In: Fitzpatrick TB, Eisen AZ, Wolff K, et al, eds. Dermatology in general medicine. 3rd ed. New York: McGraw-Hill, 1987:877.

4. New pigmented lesions after age 40,
5. Any precursor lesions: lentigo maligna, congenital nevus, acral-mucosal lesions, and dysplastic nevi, and
6. Pigmented lesions in hidden sites.

Since early melanoma is often curable and later melanoma often is not, patients should be instructed to perform regular self-examinations, and physicians should check the skin during routine examinations, more often if there is a personal history of melanoma or one of its precursors or a family history of melanoma or dysplastic nevi. Examination should include the entire skin including hidden sites. With greater awareness and detection of early dangerous pigmented lesions, the death rate from melanoma should decrease to less than 5 percent.

References

1. Bale SJ, Dracopoli ND, Tucker MA, et al. Mapping the gene for hereditary cutaneous malignant melanoma-dysplastic nevus to chromosome 1p. N Engl J Med 1989; 21:1367–1372.

2. Sober AJ, Rhodes AR, Mihm MC, et al. Neoplasms: malignant melanoma. In: Fitzpatrick TB, Eisen AZ, Wolff K, et al, eds. Dermatology in general medicine. 3rd ed. New York: McGraw-Hill, 1987:947.

3. Rhodes AR, Weinstock MA, Fitzpatrick TB, et al. Risk factors for cutaneous melanoma: a practical method of recognizing predisposed individuals. JAMA 1987; 258:3146–3154.

4. Friedman RJ, Rigel DS, Kopf AW. Early detection of malignant melanoma: the role of physical examination and self-examination of the skin. CA 1985; 35:130–151.

5. Clark WH. The dysplastic nevus syndrome. Arch Dermatol 1988; 124:1207–1210.

6. Rhodes AR. Neoplasms: benign neoplasias, hyperplasias, and dysplasias of melanocytes. In: Fitzpatrick TB, Eisen AZ, Wolff K, et al, eds. Dermatology in general medicine. 3rd ed. New York: McGraw-Hill, 1987:877.

7. Duray PH. Congenital nevomelanocytic nevi, a review of the clinical challenge. Current Concepts in Skin Disorders, Fall 1986:5–11.

8. Fitzpatrick TB, Rhodes AR, Sober AJ. Prevention of melanoma by recognition of its precursors (editorial). N Engl J Med 1985; 312:115–116.

9. McLean DI. Dysplastic nevus, take it or leave it? Int J Dermatol 1988; 27:238–239.

49 | PARANEOPLASTIC SYNDROMES

LARRY NATHANSON, M.D.
JAN ROTHMAN, M.D.

A paraneoplastic syndrome may be defined as a constellation of findings in an organ remote from a primary cancer, findings not resulting from the space-occupying tumor per se. In some syndromes the cause is the production by the tumor of a clearly identified physiologically active substance (Table 49-1). In other cases we can only conjecture about the mechanistic relationship between the underlying malignancy and the paraneoplastic syndrome. Because all clinical abnormalities in a cancer patient may not be causally related to a paraneoplastic syndrome, we must identify criteria that justify such a causal linkage. These criteria include:

1. Association of the syndrome with the presence of an actively growing tumor,
2. Identification of excess amounts of a factor in circulation, which decline with the removal of tumor,
3. Identification of excess amounts of the factor within tumor cells,
4. An arteriovenous gradient of the factor across the tumor bed,
5. Production of the factor by tumor cells in vitro, and
6. Identification of messenger ribonucleic acid (mRNA) in tumor cells specific for factor synthesis using a complementary deoxyribonucleic acid (complementary DNA) hybridization (northern blot) technique.

We estimate that a paraneoplastic syndrome will be present at the time of diagnosis in 7 to 10 percent of patients with malignancy. As many as half of all patients with malignancy, however, manifest an organ-specific paraneoplastic syndrome sometime during the course of their illness.[1] Furthermore, if one includes metabolic paraneoplastic manifestations such as anorexia, cachexia, anemia of chronic disease, or fever, virtually all cancer patients experience a paraneoplastic manifestation. Firstly, paraneoplastic manifestations may herald the onset of malignancy and, in fact, may lead to its diagnosis. Secondly, alleviation of a symptomatic manifestation often significantly improves the quality of life for the patient, even if the tumor is incurable. Thirdly, paraneoplastic manifestations may be misinterpreted as evidence of metastatic disease and deter the clinician from the pursuit of potentially curative treatment. Fourthly, some of the humeral factors produced by tumors may serve as

TABLE 49-1 Established and Putative Humoral Factors in Paraneoplastic Syndromes

Clinical Syndrome	Tumors	Factors
Metabolic syndromes		
Cachexia	Many	CACH, TNF
Fever	Hodgkin's disease, lymphoma, hypernephroma, others	IL-1, PGE, EP
Night sweats	Many	? IL-1, PGE, EP
Endocrine syndromes		
Hypercalcemia	Squamous carcinomas	PHRP, TGF
Hypercalcemia	Myeloma	OAF, LYT, TNF, IL-1
Hypercalcemia	Adult T-cell lymphoma	1,25-DHVD
Inappropriate ADH (hyponatremia)	Small cell carcinoma of lung, others	AVP, ? ANF
Cushing syndrome	Small cell carcinoma of lung, others	CRF, POMC, ACTH
Hypoglycemia	Retroperitoneal sarcomas, others	SM, ILGF
Acromegaly	Pancreatic, carcinoid	GH, GHRF
Hyperthyroidism (choriocarcinoma)	Trophoblastic	? hCG
Hypophosphatemic osteomalacia	Mesenchymal tumors	?
Connective tissue syndromes		
Dermatomyositis	Breast, lung, ovary, others	?
Hypertrophic pulmonary osteoarthropathy	Lung, intrathoracic	? TAF, ANG
Gynecomastia	Lung, germ cell	? hCG, FSH

Hematologic syndromes		
Erythrocytosis	Hypernephroma, cerebellar hemangioblastoma	EPO
Leukemoid reaction	Many	? G-CSF, GM-CSF
Pure RBC aplasia	Thymoma	? ANTI-EPO
Migratory thrombophlebitis	Pancreas, lung, other	?
Gastrointestinal syndromes		
Carcinoid syndrome	Carcinoid	5-HT, BRAD, HIS, CAL, 5-OHT
Hepatopathy syndrome	Hypernephroma, schwannoma	?
Dermatologic syndromes		
Acanthosis nigricans	GI adenocarcinoma, other	? MSH

PHRP = parathyroid hormone-related protein
TGF = transforming growth factor-alpha
PGE = prostaglandins
IL-1 = interleukin-1
EP = endogenous pyrogen
TNF = tumor necrosis factor
CACH = cachectin
LYT = lymphotoxin (or TNF-β)
OAF = osteoclast activating factor
1,25-DHVD = 1,25-dihydroxyvitamin D$_3$
AVP = arginine vasopressin
ACTH = adrenocorticotropic hormone
CRF = corticotropin releasing factor
POMC = proopiomelanocortin
SM = somatomedin
ILGF = insulin-like growth factor
hCG = human chorionic gonadotropin

FSH = follicle-stimulating hormone
GH = growth hormone
ANF = atrial natriuretic factor
GHRF = growth hormone releasing factor
ANG = angiogenin
TAF = tumor angiogenic factor
EPO = erythropoietin
ANTI-EPO = anti-erythropoietin
G-CSF = granulocyte-colony stimulating factor
GM-CSF = granulocyte/macrophage-colony stimulating factor
BRAD = Bradykinin
SER = serotonin
5-HT = 5-hydroxytryptamine
CAL = calcitonin
HIS = histamine
5-OHT = 5-hydroxytryptophan
MSH = melanocyte stimulating hormone

markers for tumor growth (and thus for the efficacy of treatment). Lastly, these manifestations may give us insight into the basic biology, or even pathogenesis, of certain malignancies.

The spectrum of paraneoplastic syndromes is extensive.[2,3] It includes the almost ubiquitous presence of general or metabolic manifestations, such as anorexia, cachexia, fever, chronic anemia, as well as specific target organ syndromes. Like Gaul, the more specific paraneoplastic syndromes can be divided into three parts. Approximately one-third are due to tumor production of a physiologically active humeral factor. Another third are manifest by abnormalities in the skin, the connective tissue, or the neuromuscular system. The final third of these syndromes reside within the hematologic, immunologic, vascular, or gastrointestinal domains.

Ectopic hormonal syndromes have an adverse prognostic significance. Patients with such syndromes are more likely to have extensive or visceral metastatic disease than limited disease, and tend to have a three- to four-month shorter median survival time than do patients without such syndromes. Conversely, presumably because of their more rapid proliferative rate, these tumors are somewhat more likely to regress when treated with chemotherapy.[4]

Note that this chapter does not include reference to neoplastic endocrine syndromes that are not strictly ectopic with reference to primary organ site. Thus, for example, pancreatic islet cell carcinoma with production of insulin, glucagon, gastrin, or vasoactive intestinal peptide (highly treatable with streptozotocin), or multiple endocrine adenoma syndrome, are not mentioned.

METABOLIC SYNDROMES

Cachexia

One of the most ubiquitous manifestations of cancer is the cachexia syndrome. This syndrome includes anorexia, a relative or absolute decline in nutrient intake, and resultant weight loss and asthenia. Compared to starved individuals, there is a relative hypermetabolic state (increased basal metabolic rate). There is wasting of lean body mass, often in excess of adipose tissue, and mild hyperglycemia. We have known for years that, after glucose loading, there is a delayed removal of radiolabeled glucose from the blood of cancer patients compared to normal subjects. This impaired utilization of glucose may be accompanied by the presence of lipemic serum with an increased level of very low-density lipoprotein (VLDL).

The possible causes of anorexia in malignant disease include alteration in taste or smell, production of lactate, ketones, or tumor toxins (which may have a direct effect on the CNS appetite center), or psychological depression. The recent identification of cachectin (tumor necrosis factor) in cancer patients with the cachexia syndrome suggests the possibility that tumors may stimulate increased synthesis or release of this factor from the macrophages that usually produce it. Cachectin or other humeral factors may result in inhibition of lipoprotein lipase and of a variety of enzymes responsible for glucose uptake in muscle or liver, and may mediate the observed defects of carbohydrate or lipid metabolism. Although the treatment of this syndrome is generally ineffective, the use of high-dose megestrol (400 to 800 mg daily), anabolic steroids, or glucose plus insulin has been employed. We do not generally recommend such treatment, however, because enteral or parenteral hyperalimentation in the absence of an effective anticancer therapy is of little value. An increased supply of nutrients to the tumor cell as well as to the normal cell may, in fact, have a deleterious effect on patient survival.

Fever

Fever may accompany cancer (in the absence of infection or other inciting cause) and parallel its clinical course, particularly in lymphoma, Hodgkin's disease, hypernephroma, or metastatic hepatic tumors. Although there is no simple pathognomonic sign of fever of cancer origin, frequently such patients lack the rigors, malaise, and anorexia that bacterial or inflammatory fever confer. The mechanism of tumor fever is not well understood, but presumably is related to direct or indirect production of Interleukin-1 (IL-1; endogenous pyrogen) by tumor cells. Tumor cells also may secrete tumor necrosis factor (cachectin), which in turn may act directly on the hypothalamic temperature center, thereby resulting in release of prostaglandins and producing fever. Such fever usually disappears with effective antitumor treatment. If effective treatment is unavailable, we use standard antipyretics such as acetaminophen, aspirin, and/or indomethacin.

Night Sweats

Night sweats are a fairly common manifestation of Hodgkin's disease and traditionally occur in lymphomas or myeloproliferative disease. Such sweats must be distinguished from those due to infections, such as tuberculosis, and are best treated with antipyretics. Their etiology appears to be similar to that of tumor fever.

Anemia of Chronic Disease

Anemia accompanying malignancy is an extremely common occurrence. Differentiating between the anemia of chronic disease and anemias due to myelophthisis factor deficiency (iron deficiency with bleeding, or nutritional deficiency such as B_{12} or folate), microangiopathic hemolytic anemia, or marrow suppression due to cancer therapy may be difficult. Anemias of mixed etiology are common, e.g., iron deficiency due to blood loss together with anemia of chronic disease, or microcytic anemias like beta-thalassemia and iron deficiency. Details about anemia with malignancy may be found in Chapter 42: *Anemia*.

Tumor Lysis Syndrome

Treatment of lymphoid, myeloid, and occasionally solid tumors can be accompanied by an extremely rapid lysis of cancer cells with a consequent release of a variety of intracellular metabolites. Hyperuricemia, hyperphosphatemia with hypocalcemia, lactic acidosis, azotemia, renal failure, cardiac arrhythmias, and even death may result. This syndrome usually has an onset within 12 to 48 hours of chemotherapy and requires emergent treatment. The use of prophylactic hydration, allopurinol, and, later, diuresis to accompany chemotherapy is critical. During the course of the illness, correction of electrolyte abnormalities is essential. In the event of severe renal failure, temporary peritoneal or hemodialysis may be the only effective therapeutic approach.

Nephropathy

Nephropathy with renal insufficiency including nephrotic syndrome and membranous glomerulonephritis may occur in patients with cancer. Leaving aside direct tumor invasion of the kidney, the most common cause of nephropathy is tubular damage as seen in myeloma, Waldenström's macroglobulinemia, chronic lymphocytic leukemia, and non-Hodgkin's lymphoma. This is primarily due to excretion of light chains, serum hyperviscosity, hypercalcemia, and hyperuricemia. In addition, deposition of light chains in the kidneys may result in amyloidosis. Renal infection or nephrotoxicity from chemotherapeutic agents are other causes of renal insufficiency. Minimal change disease is a mild form of nephrotic syndrome most often seen in Hodgkin's disease, possibly due to circulating proteases. This process may improve with successful treatment of the underlying malignancy or with steroids. Some cases of paraneoplastic nephropathy are presumably the result of development of immune complexes involving a variety of tumor products, including anticarci-noembryonic antigen antibody, antiferritin antibody, or the like. Treatment is that of the specific nephropathy irrespective of cause.

ENDOCRINE SYNDROMES[5,6]

Hypercalcemia

Hypercalcemia probably is the most common paraneoplastic syndrome in cancer patients and occurs in as many as 5 percent of all patients sometime during the course of their illness. This syndrome encompasses a variety of probable mechanisms and can best be categorized from an etiologic point of view. We believe that separation of patients with hypercalcemia into those with and those without detectable bone metastases is often artificial. Metastatic deposits of tumor in bone may produce hypercalcemia by the production of locally active humeral factors similar to those seen in patients without metastases. In addition, microscopic bone metastases may escape detection in patients thought to have localized disease. A better etiologic classification recently has been proposed by G.R. Mundy, who has suggested that three types of hypercalcemia may be distinguished. Type I includes patients with carcinomas of lung (especially squamous carcinoma), head and neck, kidney, and ovary with or without metastatic disease. An increase in bone calcium release, renal tubular calcium absorption, and nephrogenous cyclic adenosine monophosphate (AMP), and a decrease in 1,25-dihydroxyvitamin D_3 (1,25-DHVD) and gut calcium absorption are seen in these patients. Tumor production of factors that bind to parathyroid hormone (PTH) receptors or that stimulate osteoclasts seem responsible for this syndrome. These factors may include growth factors (e.g., transforming growth factor-alpha) or peptides that have some sequence homology to PTH, but they are not immunoreactive to anti-PTH antibody such as parathyroid hormone-related protein. Type II hypercalcemia is epitomized by myeloma where local humeral factors such as osteoclast activating factor (OAF) or lymphotoxin (beta-tumor necrosis factor) stimulate bone resorption. These factors act together with decreased glomerular filtration and impaired renal calcium excretion to produce hypercalcemia. Type III hypercalcemia is exemplified by adult T-cell lymphoma-leukemia, (human T-cell leukemia virus [HTLV-1] disease). Here, it appears that the tumor produces or stimulates production of 1,25-dihydroxyvitamin D_3, resulting in increased bone resorption and gut absorption of calcium.

The differential diagnosis of malignant hypercalcemia and hyperparathyroidism is summarized in Table 49–2. Whereas hypercalcemia of cancer is often of brief duration and rapid onset, hyperparathyroidism more commonly is

TABLE 49-2 Distinguishing Between Primary Hyperparathyroidism and Humeral Hypercalcemia of Malignancy

	Primary Hyperparathyroidism	Humeral Hypercalcemia of Malignancy
History	Fluctuating, slowly progressive	Brief, rapidly progressive
Clinical manifestations	Renal calculi Pancreatitis Peptic ulcer disease	Weight loss, symptoms of tumor
Laboratory findings		
IPTH (RIA)	N or ↑	N or ↓
1,25-DHVD	N or ↑	N or ↓
Serum calcium	High normal or ↑	Usually >14 mg/dl
Serum chloride	High (>102 mmol/L)	Low
Steroid suppression of serum Ca+	Rare	Variable

IPTH = immunoreactive parathyroid hormone
RIA = radioimmunoassay
1,25-DHVD = 1,25-Dihydroxyvitamin D_3

slowly progressive. Pancreatitis and renal calculi are rare in hypercalcemia of cancer, but levels of calcium above 14 mg per deciliter are common. Serum phosphate is usually decreased in hyperparathyroidism, but not in cancer. Serum chloride concentration is often low in cancer, but usually high in hyperparathyroidism. Steroid treatment is rarely effective in hyperparathyroidism.

Clinical manifestations of hypercalcemia are ubiquitous and include neurologic manifestations such as itching, fatigue, muscle weakness, hyporeflexia, lethargy, stupor, and coma; renal manifestations including polyuria, polydypsia, and renal insufficiency; gastrointestinal manifestations including anorexia, nausea, vomiting, constipation, abdominal pain; and cardiovascular manifestations with hypertension and arrhythmias. Treatment of these syndromes involves aggressive rehydration with normal saline and the use of a variety of drugs that inhibit resorption of calcium from bone. These include mithramycin (25 μg per kilogram), oral phosphate or diphosphonates (may produce diarrhea), corticosteroids (especially in myeloma), or calcitonin. Diuretics such as furosemide further promote calciuria, but should never be used until the hypercalcemic patient is first adequately hydrated. The use of edetic acid (EDTA) or of hemodialysis is a last therapeutic resort.

Syndrome of Inappropriate Antidiuretic Hormone Secretion (SIADH)

This syndrome is characterized by serum hypo-osmolality and concentrated urine (i.e., the urine is not maximally dilute despite systemic hypo-osmolality; Table 49–3). It must be distinguished from other causes of hyponatremia, adrenal and renal insufficiency (Table 49–4). Arginine vasopressin (antidiuretic hormone [ADH]) inappropriately secreted by the tumor results in excessive water resorption in the collecting tubule and consequent hyponatremia (assuming continued ingestion of solute-free water). Serum sodium levels in the order of 125 mEq per liter, plasma osmolality around 260 mOsm per kilogram, and urinary osmolalities over 400 to 600 mOsm per kilogram are commonly seen. Small cell carcinoma of the lung (SCCL) is far and away the most common cause of this syndrome, although it may occur in other tumor types including bronchial carcinoid, pancreatic, duodenal, and laryngeal carcinomas, and even in lymphomas. Because SIADH may declare itself before other clinical manifestations of SCCL, otherwise unexplained SIADH justifies a work-up including fiberoptic bronchoscopy and computed tomographic (CT) scanning of the chest and abdomen, even in the absence of an abnormal chest x-ray. Neurophysins (vasopressin or oxytocin) may also be clinical markers of neoplastic progression. Certain drugs including vincristine and cyclophosphamide may mimic this syndrome. Treatment is primarily that of water restriction to less than 500 ml in 24 hours. The goal is to raise the serum sodium concentration to 125 to 130 mEq per liter, not to make the serum sodium normal. In the face of severe hyponatremia, the use of additional therapies, including demeclocycline (a nontoxic tetracycline analog that blocks ADH activity in the renal tubule), may be useful. In addition, hypertonic saline infusion and furosemide (simultaneously raising serum sodium and preventing salt retention) may be helpful.

TABLE 49–3   Diagnostic Features of SIADH

Serum hyponatremia (usually <125 mm/L) and hypo-osmolality (usually <270 mOsm/kg)

Urine osmolality greater (usually >400 mOsm/kg) than appropriate for the degree of systemic hypotonicity

Urinary sodium excretion >20 mEq

Absence of volume contraction

Normal renal, adrenal, and thyroid function

TABLE 49-4 Differential Diagnosis of SIADH

Malignant tumors

CNS disorders
  CNS Infection
  Head trauma
  Space occupying lesions
  Vasculitis
  Acute intermittent porphyria
  Guillain-Barré syndrome

Pulmonary infection

Drugs
  Morphine
  Nicotine
  Vincristine
  Cyclophosphamide
  Chlorpropramide
  Ethanol

Idiopathic causes

Ectopic Cushing's Syndrome

One of the earliest reported and best understood ectopic hormone syndromes is that of ectopic Cushing's syndrome. The syndrome usually presents with a rapid onset and is, therefore, rarely accompanied by "moon facies", cutaneous striae, or truncal obesity. Osteoporosis, renal stones, or other common clinical manifestations of Cushing's disease are seen even less frequently. Hypertension, glucose intolerance, and pigmentation, however, are often seen in ectopic Cushing's syndrome. Clues to the etiology of this syndrome are found in the equal distribution of males and females with ectopic Cushing's syndrome (compared to the predominance of females with Cushing's disease), and the average age of patients is in the fifties, as opposed to the early thirties in Cushing's disease.

Proopiomelanocortin, or "big ACTH", is synthesized by a variety of tumors. A 241-amino acid glycoprotein, it contains the peptide sequences for various hormones including ACTH, MSH, beta-lipoprotein, beta-endorphin, and metenkephalin. The clinical expression of the syndrome depends on the pattern of cleavage of the precursor molecule into various subunits. Thus, MSH may result in skin pigmentation, and beta-endorphin with its morphine-like activity may be responsible for the high pain threshold seen in certain cancer patients. The production by tumor cells of CRF, which acts on the pituitary and results in ACTH release, may be an etiologic mechanism in some patients. Plasma ACTH levels greater than 200 pg per milliliter, cortisol levels greater than 40 mEq per deciliter, the loss of diurnal cortisol variation (between 8:00 AM and 6:00 PM), and a loss of cortisol suppression with dexamethasone 2 mg every 6 hours are all highly suggestive of ectopic ACTH syndrome in patients with cancer (Table 49–5). Severe hypokalemic alkalosis (saline resistant) is common in ectopic ACTH syndrome. The primary treatment of the syndrome is treatment of the underlying malignancy, whether it be SCCL (the most common tumor) or a variety of other tumors including pancreatic tumors, thymic tumors, medullary carcinoma of the thyroid, or carcinoid. In addition, adrenal steroid biosynthesis may be inhibited by the use of aminoglutethimide, metyrapone, mitotane (op'DDD), or a combination of aminoglutethimide and metyrapone. In any case, replacement steroids must be used together with any of these treatments to prevent adrenal insufficiency.

Rare Ectopic Hormone Syndromes

A variety of rare ectopic hormone syndromes occur in cancer. Severe hypoglycemia is most commonly associated with mesenchymal and retroperitoneal fibrosarcomas, mesotheliomas, leiomyosarcomas, or hemangiopericytomas. Hepatomas, adrenal cortical carcinomas, carcinomas of the gastroin-

TABLE 49–5   Distinguishing Between Ectopic ACTH Syndrome and ACTH Secreting Pituitary Tumors

	Ectopic ACTH Syndrome	ACTH Secreting Pituitary Tumors
Distribution	Men=women; median age 55	Predominantly women; median age 30
Natural history	Short duration, correlates with aggressiveness of tumor	Chronic, more indolent
Major clinical features	Weight loss, frequent hyperpigmentation	Truncal obesity, buffalo hump, moon facies, cutaneous striae
Laboratory findings		
Hypokalemic alkalosis	Common	Rare
Plasma ACTH	High, usually >200 pg/ml	High normal or moderately raised
High-dose dexamethasone ($8 mg/m^2 \times 2$ days)	No suppression	Suppressed

testinal tract, or lymphomas rarely produce this syndrome. The hypoglycemia is mediated by tumor production of peptides with insulin-like biological activity, i.e., somatomedins. A member of the insulin-like growth factor (ILGF) family has also been identified in some tumors, but its functional activity is unclear. Some tumors may utilize excessive amounts of glucose, produce tryptophan metabolites that interfere with gluconeogenesis, or induce hypoglycemia secondary to liver parenchymal destruction. Other than effective therapy of the tumor, there is little treatment available for this syndrome. Continuous enteral or parenteral alimentation or corticosteroid therapy may be tried.

Another rare ectopic syndrome, oncogenic osteomalacia, is characterized by hypophosphatemia, normal serum calcium, inappropriately suppressed 1,25-dihydroxyvitamin D_3, and osteomalacia. The urinary excretion of phosphorus is increased. This syndrome is associated with benign and malignant mesenchymal tumors including giant cell tumors, osteomas, sclerosing hemangiomas, and, occasionally, carcinomas such as those of the prostate. The mechanisms are poorly understood and the treatment is that of the underlying tumor.

Hyperthyroidism, manifest by typical laboratory values (after exclusion of intrinsic disease of the thyroid), has been reported in trophoblastic tumors including choriocarcinoma and hydatidiform mole. The production by these tumors of human chorionic gonadotrophin (hCG), which has a common alpha chain with thyroid stimulating hormone (TSH) and which appears to have a TSH-like effect, may be responsible. Treatment is that of the underlying tumor.

Reports of adult acromegaly associated with pancreatic and carcinoid tumors have recently appeared. In these patients, growth hormone releasing factor (GHRF), as well as growth hormone (GH) itself, may be responsible. Laboratory findings include failure of suppression of elevated growth hormone levels by glucose. As with other rare ectopic hormone syndromes, its treatment is that of the underlying tumor.

CONNECTIVE TISSUE SYNDROMES

Dermatomyositis

Dermatomyositis has long been associated with malignancies and even may antedate the diagnosis of tumor. The most common underlying tumors have included those of breast, lung, ovary, stomach, colon, and uterus. The gradual appearance of weakness and pain, more severe in proximal than distal muscle groups, together with erythematous and violaceous induration of the skin, particularly of the trunk, is typical. Laboratory evidence of inflammatory change with elevated sedimentation rate, creatine kinase, and aldolase may also occur. This syndrome is common in some tumor types that occur exclusively or predominantly in the male (lung, stomach, colon, nasopharynx, and prostate). Thus, a male over the age of 50 with new onset dermatomyositis has about a 50 percent chance of having an underlying malignancy. In such a patient, a careful history and physical examination, routine chemistry and acid phosphatase levels, chest roentgenography, possibly a thoracic CT scan, an abdominal CT scan, and, if indicated, further gastrointestinal work-up are justified. Electromyography and biopsy of the affected muscles may confirm the diagnosis. Treatment, other than that of the underlying malignancy, includes the use of a variety of anti-inflammatory agents and steroids.

Hypertrophic Pulmonary Osteoarthropathy (HPO)

Clubbing of the fingers or toes and periosteal elevation and calcification in the long bones, especially of the distal lower extremities (periostitis), with or without arthralgia and arthritis, comprise the major features of this syndrome. Rarely, pachydermoperiostosis (hypertrophy of connective tissues often with leonine appearance of the facies) may occur. Clubbing is characterized by increased ballottability of the nail bed against the distal phalanx, as well as by loss of the nail angle (the normal slight upward angulation of the base of the nail compared to the distal phalanx of the digit). The distal lower extremities may be painful and tender, and polyarthritis with joint deformity simulating that of rheumatoid arthritis may be noted. The osteoarthropathy may antedate tumor diagnosis and thus herald underlying malignancy. Tumors associated with this syndrome include primarily lung cancer or any other intrathoracic tumor, such as esophageal carcinoma. It is particularly associated with adenocarcinomas, occasionally with mesothelioma, and rarely with carcinoid or melanoma. Abnormal radioisotope uptake may be seen on bone scan. The etiology of this syndrome, which is accompanied by a proliferation of connective tissue in the vessels of the nail bed, is possibly due to some angiogenic and osteoblastic stimulatory factor, perhaps a growth factor. Its treatment is that of the underlying tumor, together with the use of analgesics and anti-inflammatory agents, including indomethacin.

Gynecomastia has been reported alone or in association with HPO. This is usually bilateral and must include palpable enlargement of glandular tissue in a retroareolar distribution, not just adipose deposits in the breast area. Follicle-stimulating hormone (FSH) produced by tumor may be detectable. One should exclude an undifferentiated thoracic germ cell tumor that produces hCG as a cause of gynecomastia.

HEMATOLOGIC SYNDROMES

Anemia

Anemias are discussed under the heading Metabolic Syndromes and in Chapter 42: *Anemia*.

Erythrocytosis

Expansion of the red cell mass, as opposed to expansion of multiple hematopoietic progenitor cell lines as in polycythemia vera, is an uncommon but well-described syndrome. Erythrocytosis occurs primarily in patients with hypernephroma, cerebellar hemangioblastoma, ovarian cancer, adrenal cortical carcinoma, and hepatoma. It may also occasionally complicate benign conditions of the kidney, including renal cysts, and uterine fibroids, presumably due to tumor cell production or stimulation of excess renal production of erythropoietin (EPO). This complication must be distinguished from secondary polycythemia due to stimulation of EPO production by systemic hypoxia, as is the case with erythrocytosis of chronic smoking. Treatment is that of the underlying disease and phlebotomy is rarely indicated.

Leukemoid Reactions

Leukemoid reaction, a syndrome of relative and/or absolute granulocytosis (over 20,000 cells per cubic millimeter), accompanies many tumors. This syndrome may occur with or without accompanying fever and laboratory findings of elevated leukocyte alkaline phosphatase. Colony stimulating factors (perhaps G-CSF or GM-CSF) produced by tumors and resulting in selective bone marrow granulocyte precursor proliferation may be responsible.

Pure Red Cell Aplasia

A rare complication of thymoma is the accompanying syndrome of pure red cell bone marrow aplasia. This syndrome is presumably the result of production by the tumor of an "anti-erythropoietin", although this substance has never been precisely defined. Successful excision of the primary tumor may result in remission of the syndrome.

Nonbacterial Thrombotic Endocarditis

This constellation of findings is characterized by deposition of sterile fibrin on cardiac valves including mitral, aortic, or, rarely, tricuspid valves. This deposition is often accompanied by mild scarring of the valve and may proceed to the development of extensive thrombotic vegetations. Venous thrombosis and/or clinical thrombophlebitis occur in about one-half of these patients, and pulmonary emboli are common. Arterial embolization and infarction occur most commonly in the brain, spleen, kidneys, and heart, but also may involve the extremities or abdominal viscera. The patients are afebrile and have negative blood cultures; usually murmurs are inconspicuous or absent. The most common underlying tumors are those of the pancreas, stomach, and lung. Other gastrointestinal or urogenital malignancies, however, may trigger the syndrome. Acute treatment of accompanying disseminated intravascular coagulopathy may be indicated, but treatment of the underlying malignancy is the most effective approach to this process.

Migratory Thrombophlebitis (Trousseau's Syndrome)

Thrombophlebitis often heralds underlying malignancies, usually of the lung, pancreas, or other mucin-producing gastrointestinal sites. The clinical features of this syndrome include multiple episodes of thrombophlebitis (often involving superficial veins) in different sites of the body. Moreover, the involvement of upper extremity veins, an uncommon site for thrombophlebitis in the absence of invasive procedures, helps to diagnose this process.

Coagulopathies and Idiopathic Thrombocytopenic Purpura-Like Syndromes

These syndromes are discussed in Chapter 43: *An Approach to the Bleeding Patient.*

GASTROINTESTINAL SYNDROMES

Carcinoid Syndromes

Carcinoid tumors, small round cell tumors thought to be of Kulchitsky cell origin, are found predominantly in the gastrointestinal tract and bronchus of the lung. When benign, they most commonly occur in the appendix and are not associated with the characteristic carcinoid syndrome. When malignant, they occur most frequently in the ileum and occasionally in the rectum, duodenum, stomach, and/or in association with Meckel's diverticulum. Midgut carcinoids are characteristically argentaffin and argyrophil (silver stain) positive and predominantly produce hydroxytryptamine (serotonin) plus bradykinin as secretory products. The "classical carcinoid" syndrome consists of an erythematous flush frequently spreading up over the head and neck, diarrhea, bronchospasm, and occasionally right-sided cardiac valvular and endocardial lesions. The foregut carcinoid tumors (bronchus, stomach, and pancreas) may be associated with the production of 5-hydroxytryptophan as well as histamine and are often associated with a bright red flush on eating, which is prolonged and accompanied by facial edema and hypotension. Occasionally, peptic ulcer, Cushing's syndrome, and multiple endocrine adenomas (MEA I) may be associated with this entity. Hindgut (rectal) carcinoids, even when malignant, are not associated with carcinoid syndrome. In addition to the characteristic histopathologic appearance of the tumor, the detection of elevated levels of hydroxyindoleacetic acid in the urine, greater than 25 mg daily, is diagnostic. This syndrome, much more common in patients with hepatic metastases, may be the most important symptomatic accompaniment of an indolent underlying malignancy. Treatment of carcinoid syndrome has been markedly improved by the use of somatostatin, usually given in a dose of 150 μg three times daily subcutaneously. This treatment usually will satifactorily control the symptoms of carcinoid syndrome, and even has been associated with objective regression of tumor in the liver and elsewhere. Treatment of the underlying malignancy, usually with a combination of 5-fluorouracil, Adriamycin, and/or streptozotocin, may produce regression of the syndrome and/or underlying malignancy.

Malabsorption Syndromes

Malabsorption can be seen in any diffuse infiltrative disease of the bowel, most commonly in gastrointestinal lymphoma. Occasionally these patients present with preexisting celiac sprue. Certain tumors also may be associated with secretory enteropathy in which electrolytes (as in villous adenoma) or proteins are excreted into the bowel, thus resulting in malnutrition. Malabsorption occasionally may be associated with diffuse gastric malignancies (linitis plastica).

Hepatopathy Syndromes

Abnormalities of liver function in the absence of hepatic metastases have been associated with hypernephroma and malignant schwannoma. Early melanoma may be associated with the syndrome of increased radionuclide uptake in the reticuloendothelial system of the spleen and splenomegaly. True hypersplenism does not appear to accompany this process. These syndromes appear to respond to appropriate treatment of the primary malignancy and should not be confused with visceral metastases since these patients may still be amenable to curative therapy.

CUTANEOUS SYNDROMES

Acanthosis Nigricans

Acanthosis nigricans is a lesion usually located in the axilla, intertrigo, or periareolar area of the breast. The typical changes of lichenification, hyperkeratosis, and hyperpigmentation are present. Associated tumors include gastrointestinal adenocarcinomas, prostate cancer, or melanoma. This association must be distinguished from a type of acanthosis that is congenital or associated with drugs such as corticosteroids. Tumor production of MSH or a variant thereof has been reported as a cause of this process.

Erythema Gyratum Repens

Erythema gyratum repens is a skin lesion with an irregular serpiginous erythematous margin and central scaling and pruritus. It has been seen in carcinomas of the esophagus, breast, and lung.

Necrolytic Migratory Erythema

Necrolytic migratory erythema occurs only in glucagonoma, a type of islet cell carcinoma of the pancreas. Gyrate and circinate areas of blistering and erythema may occur in the extremities, with or without stomatitis. Treatment of these latter two conditions, which are almost always associated with malignancy, is usually ineffective.

NEUROPATHIES

Approximately 17 percent of cancer patients are noted to have neurologic complications on admission to the hospital. True neurologic paraneoplastic syndromes account for a small minority of these patients and can be diagnosed only after metastatic disease, toxic metabolic abnormalities, infection, vascular events, and complications of therapy have been excluded. A brief description of some of the more common paraneoplastic neuropathies is presented herein. Note that progressive multifocal leukoencephalopathy has been excluded from these syndromes because of its presumed viral etiology.[7]

Central Nervous System Syndromes

Subacute cerebellar degeneration presents with ataxia, incoordination, dysarthria, and personality changes. Pyramidal tract signs may be present. Loss of Betz cells through the cerebellar and cerebral cortex may result in dementia. The most common associated malignancy is bronchogenic carcinoma.

Amyotrophic lateral sclerosis-like syndrome is seen occasionally with Hodgkin's disease. It is manifest by ophthalmoplegia, ocular palsy, involuntary movements, muscle weakness, wasting, and sensory impairment.

Peripheral Nerve Syndromes

Sensory neuropathy with distal sensory loss and diminished deep tendon reflexes, but with normal strength and normal motor nerve conduction, is one of the more common neuropathies. This syndrome often antedates the diagnosis of cancer that is most commonly of pulmonary origin. These neuropathies must be differentiated from peripheral neuropathy of vincristine, Platinol, hexamethylmelamine, and other drugs and are rarely responsive to any type of treatment.

Motor neuropathies, often with insidious onset and without a sensory component, are most frequently seen in lymphoma patients. This subacute process may exacerbate and remit, but overall is usually progressive. Its etiology is not known and treatment is ineffective.

Mixed neuropathies with both sensory and motor components may occur; orthostatic hypotension, increased CSF fluid protein, and pleocytosis are frequently present.

Eaton-Lambert syndrome has some of the clinical characteristics of myasthenia gravis with muscle weakness and fatigue, especially in the pelvic girdle and thighs (Table 49–6). However, ocular and facial muscle involvement is

TABLE 49-6   Features of Myasthenia Gravis and Eaton-Lambert Syndrome

	Myasthenia Gravis	*Eaton-Lambert Syndrome*
Associated tumor	Thymoma >90%	SCCL
Natural history	Chronic waxing and waning	Progressive, associated with underlying tumor
Major clinical features	Extraocular and bulbar muscle weakness	Fatigue, proximal muscle weakness
Exercise induced muscle contractility	Decreased	Temporarily improved
Mechanism	Antibody-mediated postsynaptic disorder	Impaired presynaptic release of acetylcholine
Response to anti-cholinesterase treatment	High	None

significantly less frequent than is the case in myasthenia gravis. Exercise and muscle stimulation show gradual strengthening of muscle twitch, the opposite of that observed in true myasthenia. SCCL is the primary underlying neoplasm. Occasionally responses are seen with guanidine, but edrophonium chloride (anticholinesterase) is usually ineffective. The most effective therapy is that of the underlying tumor.

References

1. Nathanson L. Remote effects of cancer on the host. In: Horton J, Hill GJ, eds. Clinical oncology. Philadelphia: WB Saunders 1977:49.
2. Bunn PA, Minna JD. Paraneoplastic syndromes. In: DeVita VT, Hellman S, Rosenberg SA, eds. Cancer, principles and practice of oncology. 2nd ed. Philadelphia: JB Lippincott, 1985:1797.
3. Ihde D. Paraneoplastic syndromes. Hosp Pract 1987; 22(4):79–98.
4. Markman M. Response of paraneoplastic syndromes to antineoplastic therapy. West J Med 1986; 144:580–585.
5. Mundy GR. Ectopic hormonal syndromes in neoplastic disease. Hosp Pract 1987; 22(4):113–128.
6. Kohler PC, Trump DL. Ectopic hormone syndromes. Cancer Invest 1986; 4(6): 543–554.
7. Chad DA, Recht LD. Neurological paraneoplastic syndromes. Cancer Invest 1988; 6(1):67–82.

50 | SPLENOMEGALY

FREDERICK R. ARONSON, M.D.
RICHARD A. RUDDERS, M.D.

Splenomegaly occurs in association with a wide spectrum of underlying disorders. Some are benign and self-limited, others are malignant and may be fatal despite treatment. The cause of splenomegaly can be dificult to determine because of the great variety of diseases that may result in splenomegaly and because many of these disorders are rare. However, common causes of splenic enlargement vary significantly in different age groups as well as in different parts of the world. Knowledge of these factors can therefore help narrow the list of likely causes in a particular patient. In conjunction with the history, a careful physical examination and selected laboratory tests focus the differential diagnosis and suggest appropriate areas for additional investigation. Management of the patient with splenomegaly depends primarily on the underlying disease. In some cases, simple observation is appropriate; in others, exploratory laparotomy or cytotoxic chemotherapy is indicated. Clearly, no one management strategy is best in all cases.

This chapter provides a brief description of the characteristics of normal and enlarged spleens and of some of the diagnostic tests used to evaluate suspected splenomegaly. The differential diagnosis and the principles of management of splenomegaly are then reviewed.

THE NORMAL SPLEEN

The spleen is situated under the left hemidiaphragm and posterolaterally within the abdominal cavity. It is surrounded entirely by peritoneum that forms a visceral capsule and attaches the spleen to the stomach by the gastrolienal ligament. The body wall attachments are to the diaphragm and to the left kidney via the phrenicolienal and the lienorenal ligaments, respectively.

Normal spleen size averages 150 g, with a range of 100 to 250 g. Spleen size varies to a greater extent between individuals than in the same individual over time. Although the size of the spleen often decreases to as little as 50 g after age 70, the cause of this change is uncertain and splenic function is generally preserved.

THE ENLARGED SPLEEN

Splenomegaly more often than not represents an important clue to potentially serious underlying disease, particularly in older patients, and indicates the need for additional diagnostic evaluation. Occasionally, however, a clearly palpable spleen is detected in the absence of any demonstrable underlying disease. The majority of such cases occur in infants and in children and are believed to be caused by the generalized lymphatic hypertrophy that accompanies the immune response to the viral infections that are prevalent in this age group. Most cases of splenomegaly of undetermined cause in young adults are also probably attributable to unrecognized viral infection because modest splenic enlargement may persist for weeks following viral infection. In one study, 58 (2.6 percent) of 2,200 freshmen entering Dartmouth College in the 1960s had palpable spleens that could not be attributed to body habitus or to associated disease. Although splenomegaly persisted in many of these students for several years, they had no greater prevalence of illness after 10 years of follow-up than students without splenomegaly.[1]

Symptoms

Rapid enlargement or parenchymal infarction of the spleen usually results in left upper quadrant pain or tenderness. Parenchymal infarction caused by local thrombosis is an important cause of splenic pain that occurs periodically in children with sickle cell disease and occasionally in patients with myeloproliferative disorders, Hodgkin's disease, acute leukemia, or vasculitis. Painful splenic infarcts occur, perhaps even more frequently, because of thromboemboli or septic emboli of cardiac origin.[2] Rapid splenic enlargement with capsular stretching and pain, a relatively uncommon problem, occurs primarily in patients with acute infection, aggressive lymphoma, or traumatic subcapsular or intraparenchymal hemorrhage. In these and other clinical settings when rapid enlargement does occur, the patient is at risk for splenic rupture, a potentially life-threatening event.[3] Pain and signs of an acute abdomen are usually, but not invariably, present if rupture occurs. Pain referred to the left shoulder occurs when the diaphragmatic surface of the spleen becomes inflamed. This is an ominous symptom that should not be ignored, because it indicates that the patient is at risk for splenic rupture.

Splenic enlargement more often proceeds slowly and produces few, if any, symptoms. The likelihood of experiencing ill-defined symptoms, such as early satiety, bloating, fullness, and swelling or asymmetry of the abdomen, increases as spleen size increases, although patients with chronically enlarged spleens often experience none of these symptoms. The disorders most frequently associated with massive splenomegaly, but minimal if any symptoms, are vascular congestion,[4] the myeloproliferative diseases,[5-7] the indolent lymphoproliferative diseases,[8,9] sarcoidosis, [10] Gaucher's disease,[11] and cystic lesions of the spleen.[12-14]

Physical Findings

Palpation is the most sensitive technique for demonstrating splenic enlargement by physical examination.[15] Increases of as little as 40 percent above normal size can be detected using this technique. The enlarged spleen is first palpable beneath the left lateral costal margin as a tip that descends with inspiration. As the spleen enlarges, its tip descends inferiorly and to the right just beneath the anterior abdominal wall. With progressive enlargement, the spleen becomes palpable as a mass that extends along a diagonal from the left upper quadrant towards and, in cases of massive enlargement, into the right lower quadrant.

Not all enlarged spleens are palpable, however. Obesity, ascites, or surgical scars of the abdomen decrease the sensitivity of the physical examination for the detection of splenomegaly. Local tenderness and other causes of limited patient cooperation also tend to interfere with the abdominal examination. Even with the patient in the right lateral decubitus position and with careful bimanual palpation, the spleen may be up to twice its normal size, yet remain undetectable. Extremely large spleens may also be missed if the examiner fails to search the entire path of enlargement, from the extreme right lower quadrant to the left costal margin, for the characteristic lower edge.

In addition, not all left upper quadrant masses are attributable to enlarged spleens. When a structure adjacent to the spleen becomes palpable, it may simulate splenomegaly.[16] The most common example of this is enlargement of the left lobe of the liver. However, gastric or colonic tumors, cysts or tumors of the pancreas, left ovary, left kidney, or adrenal gland, metastatic carcinoma, or hematomas or tumors of the structures of the anterior abdominal wall may also be misinterpreted as splenomegaly. In addition, a marked flattening of the left hemidiaphragm, a subphrenic abscess, or other processes that produce a mass effect occasionally displace a normal spleen to within reach of the examiner's hand.

Several findings on physical examination are useful in distinguishing splenomegaly from other left upper quadrant masses. Movement of the inferior margin, or tip, of the spleen downward with inspiration is probably the best known of these findings. The presence of an inferior edge, but no palpable superior edge, is another characteristic finding when the mass in question is caused by splenomegaly. In addition, a single indentation in the lower medial margin — the splenic notch — is often apparent on gentle palpation in patients with moderately enlarged spleens. Care must be taken, however, not to confuse the splenic notch with a polycystic left kidney, which may produce a left upper quadrant mass with a "notch." In these cases, the presence of a superior margin and the relative lack of movement with respiration suggest that the mass in question is not an enlarged spleen.

IMAGING TECHNIQUES

When there is a question about the nature of a left upper quadrant mass or when splenomegaly is suspected, but not clearly present on examination, one or more of several radiologic imaging techniques should be used to confirm the examiner's impressions and to search for associated findings. Computerized axial tomographic (CT) scanning, radionuclide scintigraphic scanning, ultrasound imaging, and plain roentgenography may all be of use in the initial or the serial evaluation of patients with suspected splenomegaly.

Plain Roentgenography

Given the frequent clinical use of plain chest and abdominal x-rays, it is not surprising that unsuspected splenomegaly is sometimes first detected by these studies.[17] Plain x-rays in conjunction with the physical examination are often adequate for the serial evaluation of patients with splenomegaly, especially when they provide a clear definition of the splenic outline. In addition, this technique offers the obvious advantages of wide availability, minimal patient risk, and modest expense. The clinician must remain cautious when interpreting these studies, however, because of their limited sensitivity and specificity in detecting and evaluating left upper quadrant masses.

Ultrasound

Ultrasound imaging is essentially without risk to the patient and is usually accurate in measuring spleen size and detecting the presence of cystic structures. This modality is particularly useful to assess the parenchymal texture of an enlarged spleen and to guide needle aspiration in the rare case where this procedure is indicated.[18] However, high quality studies are difficult to obtain in some patients for technical reasons, and these problems occasionally limit the usefulness of this technique in the evaluation of patients with splenomegaly.

Scintigraphic Scans

The [99m]technetium sulfur colloid liver-spleen scan, widely used to image functional splenic tissue, is most useful in the evaluation of spleen size and function and in the detection of accessory splenic tissue.[19,20] In addition, the liver-spleen scan is sometimes useful diagnostically, such as when increased marrow uptake of isotope is seen in patients with hepatic cirrhosis and congestive splenomegaly. Scintigraphic scans performed after the infusion of blood cells that are labeled with various radioisotopes are sometimes used in cytopenic patients with suspected hypersplenism in an effort to predict patient response to splenectomy. Although this approach is theoretically attractive and has research applications, it is not sufficiently accurate to be recommended for routine clinical use at present.[21,22] As with all noninvasive tests, the liver-spleen scan cannot be used reliably to either document or exclude splenic involvement by tumors, particularly infiltrative lesions, since both false-positive and false-negative results are fairly common.

Computerized Tomographic Scans

Computerized axial tomography offers a number of advantages in the evaluation of patients with a newly discovered left upper quadrant mass. It is the most accurate of the noninvasive techniques in the assessment of the size and parenchymal consistency of the spleen and other abdominal viscera and is the only noninvasive method capable of evaluating intra-abdominal lymph nodes above the level of the renal bed.[23,24] Furthermore, a single CT scan is often preferable to a series of other noninvasive tests because it provides information about most of the abdominal viscera and spaces. Limitations of CT scans include the production of artifacts by patient movement, by surgical clips, or by other metallic foreign bodies, and the relative disadvantages of greater patient radiation exposure and higher cost than other techniques. These problems will likely be improved by the development of more sophisticated machines.

DIFFERENTIAL DIAGNOSIS

Table 50–1 lists the wide variety of disorders that may be associated with splenomegaly. As with other clinical findings caused by a wide spectrum of underlying disorders, establishment of the correct diagnosis is the critical first step in determining the optimal management of the patient with splenomegaly. To accomplish this, the clinician first prepares a differential diagnosis

TABLE 50-1   Causes of Splenomegaly

Infectious Causes
  Infectious mononucleosis
  Endocarditis
  Human immunodeficiency
    virus (HIV) infection
  Abscess
  Salmonella infection
  Brucellosis
  Mycobacterial infection

  Spirochetal infection
  Rickettsial infection
  Psittacosis
  Histoplasmosis
  Tularemia
  Listeriosis
  Toxocariasis
  Malaria and other tropical
    diseases

Hematological Causes
  Lymphoproliferative Disorders
    Chronic lymphocytic leukemia
    Hodgkin's disease
    Non-Hodgkin's lymphoma
    Waldenström's macroglobulinemia
    Heavy-chain disease
    Angioimmunoblastic lymphadenopathy
    Acute lymphocytic leukemia
  Myeloproliferative Disorders
    Chronic myelogenous leukemia
    Polycythemia vera
    Myeloid metaplasia
    Essential thrombocythemia
    Chronic myelomonocytic leukemia
    Acute myelogenous leukemia
  Red Cell Disorders
    Hereditary spherocytosis
    Thalassemia
    Hemoglobin SC
    Other hemoglobinopathy or hemolytic syndrome
  Others
    Histiocytosis
    Systemic mastocytosis
    Malignant hypereosinophilic syndrome

Immune Causes
  Collagen-vascular Diseases
    Rheumatoid arthritis
    Systemic lupus erythematosus
    Behçet's syndrome
  Granulomatous Diseases
    Sarcoidosis
    Crohn's disease
    Berylliosis
  Hypersensitivity Reaction
    Diphenylhydantoin

Endocrine Causes
  Hyperthyroidism

Table continues on following page

TABLE 50-1 *(Continued)*

Infiltrative Causes
    Lipoidosis
        Gaucher's disease
        Niemann-Pick disease
        Hyperlipidemias
    Amyloidosis

Congestive Causes
    Hepatic cirrhosis (Banti's syndrome)
    Splenic or portal venous thrombosis
    Congestive heart failure (rarely)

Tumors and/or Cysts
    Tumors
        Metastatic (melanoma, carcinoma of the lung, breast, pancreas)
        Locally invasive (carcinoma of the pancreas, left kidney, stomach)
        Primary (see Hematologic causes)
    Cysts
        Epithelial
        Lymphangiomatous
        Post-traumatic

Unknown Etiology
    Idiopathic non-tropical (Dacie's syndrome)
    Chronic renal failure patients on hemodialysis
    Idiopathic portal hypertension

---

based on the patient's history, the findings on physical examination, and the results of preliminary laboratory tests, and then uses additional tests to both establish the correct diagnosis and exclude the incorrect diagnoses in the differential.[17,25,26] The ability to construct a differential diagnosis and to select the tests necessary to establish a diagnosis requires a knowledge of the epidemiology and the clinical features of the various disorders listed in Table 50-1. Although a detailed discussion of all these disorders is beyond the scope of this chapter, the following comments should be helpful in most cases encountered in practice today.

Infectious Diseases

Splenomegaly occurs in a large number of infectious diseases (Table 50-2). Many of these diseases, however, are uncommon in the United States. For example, malaria,[27] the tropical splenomegaly syndrome,[28,29] schistosomiasis,[30] and various other tropical infections can usually be excluded from the differential diagnosis in the absence of an appropriate history of exposure.

the United States are found almost exclusively in patients who are infected as a consequence of a well-defined exposure. Splenic abscess occurs almost exclusively in patients with congenital or acquired immunodeficiency, including that caused by treatment with chemotherapy or steroids, and in patients with disseminated infections or with various other serious illnesses. Splenic abscess is notably uncommon in patients with AIDS.[36] Other examples include tularemia after contact with infected rabbit meat or brucellosis in patients employed as meat packers. Thus, in most cases, these disorders can be excluded from further consideration on the basis of the history.

The mononucleosis syndrome of malaise, fever, adenopathy, and splenomegaly with circulating atypical lymphocytes occurs in patients of all ages and is caused by a variety of infectious, immune, and neoplastic disorders. This syndrome occurs most commonly in adolescents as a consequence of infection by the Epstein-Barr virus.[37] In the elderly, splenomegaly may be a prominent feature of the chronic subacute form of disseminated tuberculosis that occurs with recrudescent infection and may present with a mononucleosis-like syndrome.[38] Cytomegalovirus infection may resemble infectious mononucleosis; however, splenomegaly is uncommon in this syndrome, in toxoplasmosis, in other leptospiral diseases with the rare exception of pretibial (Fort Bragg) fever, and in the mononucleosis-like syndromes that occasionally accompany infection by adenovirus, herpes simplex type II, rubella, varicella-zoster, and other unidentified agents. In cases where the clinical course or the results of serologic tests are not consistent with a viral cause of infectious mononucleosis, the clinician should give careful consideration to other diseases that may resemble mononucleosis, such as bacterial endocarditis, lymphoproliferative disease, collagen vascular disease, or an atypical form of one of the infections listed in Table 50–2.

A number of disorders that may result in splenomegaly typically present with other, more prominent, features. The differential diagnosis in these patients, therefore, is not based solely on the isolated finding of an enlarged spleen, but, rather, is suggested by the presence of the characteristic associated features. For example, fever, rash, headache, and myalgia coupled with a recent history of a tick bite should lead to the consideration of Rocky Mountain spotted fever,[39] typhus, or Colorado tick fever. Fever, gastrointestinal symptoms, rash, and splenomegaly are typical of the typhoid and paratyphoid forms of *Salmonella* infection. Disseminated infection with obvious multisystem disease is present in most patients who have splenomegaly caused by histoplasmosis or toxocariasis and in neonates with listeriosis, toxoplasmosis, rubella, syphilis, or cytomegalovirus disease. Lymphadenopathy is present in many patients with infection or neoplastic disease, and thus there is a great deal of overlap in the differential diagnosis of patients with these findings. Patients with a number of noninfectious causes of splenomegaly, such as lupus, rheumatoid arthritis,[40] thalassemia major,[41] amyloidosis,[42,43] Behçet's syndrome,[44] the histiocytoses,[45] systemic mastocytosis,[46] the hypereosinophilic syndromes,[47,48] and the granulomatous disorders, generally present with other more prominent clinical features that should suggest the correct diagnosis.

In contrast, infectious mononucleosis, subacute bacterial endocarditis, the lymphoproliferative and myeloproliferative disorders, some red cell disorders, brucellosis, early rickettsial infection, disseminated tuberculosis, the lipoidoses, and others sometimes present with splenomegaly and either nonspecific or absent associated features.[49] Blood cultures, careful examination of the peripheral blood and bone marrow, and serologic tests are often required in these cases to establish a diagnosis.

Hematological Disorders

Abnormalities of the blood counts, blood smear, bone marrow, lymph nodes, or serum proteins typically are present in patients with splenomegaly caused by hematological disease.

Patients with chronic hemolysis usually develop mild to moderate splenomegaly. Hemolysis may be caused by either a congenital red cell disorder, such as hereditary spherocytosis[50] or thalassemia,[41] or any of a variety of acquired disorders. Establishment of a diagnosis of one of these disorders begins by demonstrating active hemolysis and then depends on a systematic search for a specific cause of hemolysis.

The myeloproliferative disorders are usually discovered in older patients and may present with asymptomatic splenomegaly. Polycythemia vera, myelofibrosis with myeloid metaplasia, essential thrombocythemia, and chronic myelogenous leukemia are generally easily recognized by their characteristic clinical and peripheral blood features.[5-7] Bone marrow examination is usually necessary, however, to establish the diagnosis of either acute leukemia[51] or chronic myelomonocytic leukemia,[52] a myelodysplastic or preleukemic disease that is associated with splenomegaly.

Splenomegaly is often present in patients with chronic lymphocytic leukemia, Waldenström's macroglobulinemia, or heavy-chain disease.[8] In contrast, splenomegaly is only rarely a prominent feature or a diagnostic clue in patients with acute lymphocytic leukemia, Hodgkin's disease, or one of the non-Hodgkin's lymphomas.[53] Hairy-cell leukemia, although relatively uncommon, should be considered in elderly patients with mild pancytopenia, splenomegaly, and recurrent infections.[9] The finding of tartrate-resistant, acid phosphatase-positive lymphocytes in peripheral blood or bone marrow strongly suggests a diagnosis of hairy-cell leukemia. To establish the diagnosis of any of the lymphoproliferative diseases nearly always requires careful examination of the peripheral blood, the bone marrow, and lymph node biopsy, and may require electrophoresis of serum and/or urine proteins.

Congestive Disorders

Vascular congestion is frequently the cause of chronic splenomegaly in adults. Hepatic cirrhosis, primarily caused by alcohol abuse and/or chronic hepatitis, is the most common cause of portal hypertension in the United States that results in splenic congestion and enlargement.[4] Disorders that result in portal or splenic vein thrombosis, such as pancreatitis, local tumor or aneurysm, and, occasionally, severe congestive heart failure, may also result in this syndrome.[54] Most patients with congestive splenomegaly have variable cytopenias (hypersplenism) attributable to splenic sequestration of blood cells, and show signs of either chronic liver disease or portal hypertension. Splenectomy may be indicated in the management of variceal bleeding in these patients, but is rarely required to manage hypersplenism.[21,22]

Lipid Storage Diseases

Although severe forms of the lipoidoses often present in childhood, variant forms may present with splenomegaly in any age group. Gaucher's and Niemann-Pick disease are autosomal recessive disorders characterized by the accumulation in macrophages of glucocerebroside or of sphingomyelin and ceroid, respectively.[12,55] Examination of marrow or other biopsy material in these cases usually reveals Gaucher's cells or the foam cells typical of Niemann-Pick disease. Assays of white blood cells or cultured fibroblasts for glucocerebrosidase or sphingomylinase activity can be used to confirm these diagnoses.

MANAGEMENT

Since splenomegaly is most often associated with another disease, usually systemic, it is not surprising that management is directed primarily at the underlying disorder. The splenomegaly that occurs secondary to most infectious, congestive, hyperimmune, and infiltrative disorders does not require treatment per se. Treatment of the underlying disease or observation usually suffices.

On the other hand, interventions directed at the spleen may be required in patients with splenomegaly caused by neoplastic diseases, particularly if symptoms are severe. Systemic chemotherapy and/or local radiotherapy may be useful in alleviating symptoms. More often, however, splenomegaly is seen in the context of widespread disease; in these cases treatment is, and should be, systemic, rather than directed solely at the spleen.

The acute splenomegaly associated with infectious disease, particularly infectious mononucleosis, may lead to splenic rupture. Patients who develop this catastrophic life-threatening event should be evaluated promptly for exploratory laparotomy.[3,49] Early splenectomy is also indicated in the rare patient with a splenic abscess.[36]

The clinician may need to consider surgical removal of the spleen because of peripheral blood cytopenias attributable to hypersplenism.[21] For example, splenectomy may be necessary if blood counts are severely depressed because of congestive splenomegaly or if blood cytopenias accompany infiltrative diseases of the spleen. In such cases, the blood counts often improve, and bleeding and infectious complications resolve following surgery. The decision to remove a spleen for hypersplenism must be weighed carefully, however, since the splenectomy may fail if bone marrow compromise is also contributing to the peripheral cytopenias.[22] In addition, the surgical risk of splenectomy and the risk of postoperative infection are often relatively high in these patients.[22,56] Splenectomy is occasionally required to manage hemolytic anemia when other treatments fail. Splenic irradiation may also be effective when splenectomy is indicated but cannot be performed safely.[57] Finally, splenectomy is indicated in the management of some patients with congenital defects of the red cell membrane, such as hereditary spherocytosis or elliptocytosis, and in some patients with Gaucher's disease.[58,59]

CONCLUSION

Splenomegaly is associated with a host of diseases. Attention to certain clues, however, frequently narrows the differential diagnosis to the more likely causes. When evaluating any patient with suspected splenomegaly, the clinician should ask the following questions:

1. Is the spleen really enlarged?
2. What is the age (Table 50–3) and geographic background of the patient?
3. Is the enlargement acute or chronic?
4 What are the pertinent findings from the history, physical examination, blood smear, and routine laboratory tests?

Additional diagnostic tests should then be selected to investigate the most likely diagnoses based on this information. In the vast majority of cases a diagnosis can be established on the basis of a careful history and physical examination combined with appropriate laboratory and imaging studies. Although bone marrow or lymph node biopsy may be required to diagnose hematological or neoplastic disease, laparotomy and splenectomy are rarely

TABLE 50-3   Common Causes of Splenomegaly in the United States (by Age)

Infants and Children
  Red cell disorder, including sickle cell disease
  Infection, especially in the newborn as part of the
      TORCH (TOxoplasmosis, Rubella, Cytomegalovirus,
      Herpes simplex) syndrome
  Trauma
  Hematological and/or neoplastic disease
  Lipoidosis
  Congestive disorder

Adolescents
  Infectious mononucleosis, usually due to Epstein-Barr
      virus
  Other infection
  Hodgkin's disease, non-Hodgkin's lymphoma, leukemia
  Other hematological disorders
  Collagen-vascular or other immune disorder
  Lipoidosis

Adults
  Congestive disorder
  Myeloproliferative disorder
  Lymphoproliferative disorder
  Infection
  Red cell disorder
  Immune disorder
  Amyloidosis
  Lipoidosis

necessary. Likewise, splenic biopsy is indicated to establish a diagnosis only rarely, particularly in view of the potential hazards of splenic aspiration. The management of patients with splenomegaly is based, to a large extent, on the underlying disease. The therapeutic approach varies from observation alone to treatment of the underlying condition. Occasionally, enlarged spleens are so symptomatic that they have to be surgically removed or irradiated, but this is not often necessary.

References

1. Ebaugh FG, McIntyre OR. Palpable spleens: ten-year follow-up. Ann Intern Med 1979; 90:130–131.
2. O'Keefe JH Jr, Holmes DR Jr, Schaff HV, Sheedy PF, Edwards WD. Thromboembolic splenic infarction. Mayo Clin Proc 1986; 61:967–972.
3. Peters RM, Gordon LA. Nonsurgical treatment of splenic hemorrhage in an adult with infectious mononucleosis. Am J Med 1986; 80:123–125.
4. Okuda K, Kono K, Ohnishi K, Kimura K, Omata M, Koen H, et al. Clinical study

of eighty-six cases of idiopathic portal hypertension and comparison with cirrhosis with splenomegaly. Gastroenterology 1984; 86:600–610.

5. Koeffler HP, Golde DW. Chonic myelogenous leukemia — new concepts. N Engl J Med 1981; 304:1201–1209, 1269–1274.

6. Laszlo J. Myeloproliferative disorders: myelofibrosis, myelosclerosis, extramedullary hematopoiesis, undifferentiated, and hemorrhagic thrombocythemia. Semin Hematol 1975; 12:409–432.

7. Adamson JW, Fialkow PJ, Murphy S, Prchal JF, Steinmann L. Polycythemia vera: stem-cell and probable clonal origin of the disease. N Engl J Med 1976; 295:913–916.

8. Gale RP, Foon KA. Chronic lymphocytic leukemia: recent advances in biology and treatment. Ann Intern Med 1985; 103:101–120.

9. Cheson BD, Martin A. Clinical trials in hairy cell leukemia: current status and future directions. Ann Intern Med 1987; 106:871–878.

10. Peter SA. Massive splenomegaly as the presenting manifestation of sarcoidosis. J Natl Med Assoc 1986; 78:243–244.

11. Beaudet AL. Gaucher's disease. N Engl J Med 1987; 316:619–621.

12. Dawes LG, Malangoni MA. Cystic masses of the spleen. Am Surg 1986; 52:333–336.

13. Pistoia F, Markowitz SK. Splenic lymphangiomatosis: CT diagnosis. AJR 1988; 150:121–122.

14. Tada T, Wakabayashi T, Kishimoto H. Peliosis of the spleen. Am J Clin Pathol 1983; 79:708–713.

15. Sullivan S, Williams R. Reliability of clinical techniques for detecting splenic enlargement. Br Med J 1976; 2:1043–1044.

16. Noseda A, Bellens R, Gansbeke DV, Gangji D. Rectus sheath hematoma mimicking acute splenic disease. Am J Gastroenterol 1983; 78:566–568.

17. Rosenthal DS, Harris NL. Case records of the Massachusetts General Hospital (Case 48-1985). N Engl J Med 1985; 313:1405–1412.

18. Solbiati L, Bossi MC, Bellotti E, et al. Focal lesions in the spleen: sonographic patterns and guided biopsy. AJR 1983; 140:59–65.

19. Larson SM, Tuell SH, Moores KD, Nelp WB. Dimensions of the normal adult spleen scan and prediction of spleen weight. J Nucl Med 1971; 12:123–126.

20. Zhang B, Lewis SM. Use of radionuclide scanning to estimate spleen size in vivo. J Clin Pathol 1987; 40:508–511.

21. Coon WW. Splenectomy for splenomegaly and secondary hypersplenism. World J Surg 1985; 9:437–443.

22. Wilson RE, Rosenthal DS, Moloney WC, Osteen RT. Splenectomy for myeloproliferative disorders. World J Surg 1985; 9:431–436.

23. Heymsfield SB, Fulenwider T, Nordlinger B, Barlow R, Sones P, Kutner M. Accurate measurement of liver, kidney, and spleen volume and mass by computerized axial tomography. Ann Intern Med 1979; 90:185–187.

24. Gilbert T, Castellino RA. Critical review: the spleen in Hodgkin's disease: diagnostic value of CT. Invest Radiol 1986; 21:437–439.

25. Eichner ER, Whitfield CL. Splenomegaly: an algorithmic approach to diagnosis. JAMA 1981; 246:2858–2861.

26. Schnipper LE, Harris NL. Case records of the Massachusetts General Hospital (Case 15-1982). N Engl J Med 1982; 306:918–925.

27. Rosse WF. The spleen as a filter. N Engl J Med 1987; 317:704–706.

28. Hoffman SL, Piessens WF, Ratiwayanto S, Hussein PR, Kurniawan L, Piessens PW, Campbell JR, Marwoto HA. Reduction of suppressor T lymphocytes in the tropical splenomegaly syndrome. N Engl J Med 1984; 310:337-341.

29. DeCock KM, Lucas SB, Rees PH, Hodgen AN, Jupp RA, Slavin B. Obscure splenomegaly in the tropics that is not the tropical splenomegaly syndrome. Br Med J 1983; 287:1347-1348.

30. DeCock KM. Hepatosplenic schistosomiasis: a clinical review. Gut 1986; 27:734-745.

31. Von Reyn CF, Levy BS, Arbeit RD, Friedland G, Crumpacker CS. Infective endocarditis: an analysis based on strict case definitions. Ann Intern Med 1981; 94:505-518.

32. Laufer D, Lew PD, Oberhansli I, Cox JN, Longson M. Chronic Q fever endocarditis with massive splenomegaly in childhood. J Pediatr 1986; 108:535-539.

33. Abrams DI, Lewis BJ, Beckstead JH, Conrad CA, Drew WL. Persistent diffuse lymphadenopathy in homosexual men: endpoint or prodrome? Ann Intern Med 1984; 100:801-808.

34. Cooper DA, Gold J, Maclean P, Donovan B, Finlayson R, Barnes TG, et al. Acute AIDS retrovirus infection: definition of a clinical illness associated with seroconversion. Lancet 1985; i:537-540.

35. Smith R. Liver-spleen scintigraphy in patients with acquired immunodeficiency syndrome. AJR 1985; 145:1201-1204.

36. Nelken N, Ignatius J, Skinner M, Christensen N. Changing clinical spectrum of splenic abscess: a multicenter study and review of the literature. Am J Surg 1987; 154:27-34.

37. Evans AS, Niederman JC, McCollum RW. Seroepidemiologic studies of infectious mononucleosis with EB virus. N Engl J Med 1968; 279:1121-1127.

38. Glassroth J, Robins AG, Snider DE. Tuberculosis in the 1980s. N Engl J Med 1980; 302:1441-1450.

39. Turner RC, Chaplinski TJ, Adams HG. Rocky mountain spotted fever presenting as thrombotic thrombocytopenic purpura. Am J Med 1986; 81:153-157.

40. Thorne C, Urowitz MB. Long-term outcome in Felty's syndrome. Ann Rheum Dis 1982; 41:486-489.

41. Orkin SH, Nathan DG. The thalassemias. N Engl J Med 1976; 295:710-714.

42. Kyle RA, Greipp PR. Amyloidosis (AL): clinical and laboratory features in 229 cases. Mayo Clin Proc 1983; 58:665-673.

43. Gertz MA, Kyle RA, Greipp PR. Hyposplenism in primary systemic amyloidosis. Ann Intern Med 1983; 98:475-477.

44. Chajek T, Fainaru M. Behçet's disease: report of 41 cases and a review of the literature. Medicine 1975; 54:179-188.

45. Deuel T, Pikul F. Clinicopathologic conference: fever, pancytopenia, renal insufficiency, and death in a 22-year-old man. Am J Med 1987; 82:787-795.

46. Roth J, Brudler O, Henze E. Functional asplenia in malignant mastocytosis. J Nucl Med 1985; 26:1149-1152.

47. Alfaham MA, Ferguson SD, Sihra B, Davies J. The idiopathic hypereosinophilic syndrome. Arch Dis Child 1987; 62:601-613.

48. Wynn SR, Sachs MI, Keating MU, Ostrom NK, Kadota RP, O'Connell EJ,

Smithson WA. Idiopathic hypereosinophilic syndrome in a 5½-month-old infant. J Pediatr 1987; 111:94–97.

49. Patel JM, Rizzolo E, Hinshaw JR. Spontaneous subscapular splenic hematoma as the only clinical manifestation of infectious mononucleosis. JAMA 1982; 247:3243–3244.

50. Croom RD, McMillan CW, Orringer EP, Sheldon GF. Hereditary spherocytosis: recent experience and current concepts of pathophysiology. Ann Surg 1986; 203:34–39.

51. Bennet JM, Catovsky D, Daniel MT, Flandrin G, Galton DAG, Gralnick HR, Sultan C. Proposals for the classification of the acute leukemias. Br J Haematol 1976; 33:451–458.

52. Bennet JM, Catovsky D, Daniel MT, Flandrin G, Galton DAG, Gralnick HR, Sultan C. Proposals for the classification of the myelodysplastic syndromes. Br J Haematol 1982; 51:189–199.

53. Spier CM, Kjeldsberg CR, Eyre HJ, Behm FG. Malignant lymphoma with primary presentation in the spleen. Arch Pathol Lab Med 1985; 109:1076–1080.

54. Moossa AR, Gadd MA. Isolated splenic vein thrombosis. World J Surg 1985; 9:384–390.

55. Dawson PJ, Dawson G. Adult Niemann-Pick disease with sea-blue histiocytes in the spleen. Hum Pathol 1982; 13:1115–1120.

56. Gelfand JA, Grabbe JP. Case records of the Massachusetts General Hospital (Case 0-1983). N Engl J Med 1983; 308:1212–1218.

57. Markus H, Forfar JC. Splenic irradiation in treating warm autoimmune haemolytic anaemia. Br Med J 1986; 293:839–840.

58. Agre P, Asimos A, Casella JF, McMillan C. Inheritance pattern and clinical response to splenectomy as a reflection of erythrocyte spectrin deficiency in hereditary spherocytosis. N Engl J Med 1986; 315:1579–1583.

59. Hobbs JR, Jones KH, Shaw PJ, Lindsay I, Hancock M. Beneficial effect of pre-transplant splenectomy of displacement bone marrow transplantation for Gaucher's syndrome. Lancet 1987; i:1111–1115.

CHRONIC DISEASE

51 | THE PATIENT WITH PAIN

JENNIFER DALEY, M.D.
JOHN T. HARRINGTON, M.D.

Pain is one of the most common reasons why patients seek a physician.[1] Difficult to define, Promethean in its guises, and challenging to treat, pain has two major components. First, pain is the perception in the central nervous system (CNS) of a pathophysiologic stimulus often severe enough to cause tissue injury. The objective signal is transmitted through complex neural pathways from the site of injury through the spinal column to the brain. The second crucial component of pain is the emotional and affective response of the injured person to the injury and pain. It is this second component (denoted as suffering in this chapter), influenced by the severity, significance, and time course of the injury, that makes the definition, diagnosis, and treatment of pain difficult in many instances.[2]

On a temporal basis, pain can be considered either acute (minutes to several days) or chronic (months to years). Although it is not difficult to define and distinguish the classic syndromes of acute pain, it is less easy to define the syndrome of chronic pain. Patients experiencing acute pain can usually describe the characteristics of the pain accurately; i.e., they can relate the onset, character, radiation, and timing of the pain. If patients are in acute pain, they show signs of autonomic discharge with diaphoresis, tachycardia, and pallor. The psychological reaction of the patient to acute pain is usually appropriate. Both pain (the first component) and suffering (the second component) can be relieved by identification and treatment of the underlying cause of the acute pain and by the provision of adequate analgesia. For example, patients with the severe pain of renal colic, an acute myocardial infarction, or an acute fracture are usually diagnosed readily and adequate analgesic therapy instituted in a short time.

The syndromes of chronic pain are more difficult to define; on a temporal basis, patients with chronic pain may have intermittent or unremitting complaints for months to years.[3,4] The longer the patient has suffered with the pain, the more difficult it becomes to characterize the pain accurately and reliably. The patient's report of the character, timing, and quality of chronic pain is often contradictory, vague, and uncertain. The patient's report of the pain usually does not conform to the classic acute pain syndromes. In addition, chronic pain is poorly relieved by the therapies used in acute pain. Thus, the physician is often led to the conclusion that the patient is consciously or unconsciously manufacturing the symptom of pain or exaggerating the severity of both the pain and the resulting disability. All too often, the physician and the patient end their professional relationship on an unpleasant note—the patient angry and frustrated, feeling the physician has been insensitive to his pain; the physician skeptical about the authenticity and the magnitude of the patient's pain and suffering.

This chapter describes our approach to patients with both acute and chronic pain. The first section discusses the general diagnostic approach to any patient with pain. In the subsequent sections, we describe the approach to the treatment of acute pain and the evaluation and management of the patient with chronic pain.

DIAGNOSIS OF THE PATIENT WITH PAIN

Diagnosis of the patient with pain begins with a meticulous medical history and careful physical examination. The importance of a detailed review of the patient's medical records cannot be over emphasized. The patient should be asked to bring medical records from other physicians to the first visit. In patients who have had chronic pain syndromes for many years, have seen numerous physicians, and have had extensive previous diagnostic evaluations, review of the medical record can seem like a burdensome and unnecessary task. The record, however, almost always reveals critical information about the extent of prior evaluations and the patient's physical and emotional response to attempts to diagnose and relieve the pain. Careful review of prior evaluations can also save both the patient and the physician from unnecessarily repeating previous studies.

The history should focus on a detailed and accurate description of the pain. What is the nature of the pain? Where does the pain arise and where is it distributed? When does the pain occur and in relation to what events? What are the factors that make the pain worse? What are the factors that make the pain better? What diagnostic efforts have been made to determine the cause of the pain? What therapies have been attempted and with what degree of success? A complete medical history is critical and special emphasis should be placed on ascertaining if the patient has any chronic illnesses that are strongly associated with pain (e.g., rheumatoid arthritis or metastatic cancer with bony involvement).

An equally important and often neglected part of the medical history of the patient with pain is a careful psychiatric history. The psychiatric history should focus on any signs or symptoms of depression. Particular attention should be paid to the presence of any vegetative signs of depression and the presence of sleep disorders. The patient should be questioned carefully about the extent to which pain inhibits or interferes with the patient's home, work, and sexual life. In patients with longstanding chronic pain, some symptoms of depression are appropriate reactions to the longstanding and debilitating nature of the problem. The physician should specifically inquire how the patient's behavior during pain affects his relationships with his family, friends, and co-workers and how those around him respond to the patient's pain and suffering.

The physical examination should be complete and thorough and should include a detailed neurologic examination. First, the physician should direct his attention to the site of pain, thereby assessing any abnormality or inflammation. Second, if the patient has reported any radiation of pain, the areas of radiation should be inspected. Regardless of whether the patient has reported radiation of pain, the physician should then thoroughly inspect the segmental dermatomes associated with the area of pain. For example, a patient complaining of persistent arm or shoulder pain may have involvement of the neural plexus by a Pancoast tumor, even in the absence of other neurologic signs. Finally, the physician should be aware of the common patterns of referred pain. Referred pain is pain perceived at a site distant from the actual source of injury, usually in some visceral organ. Commonly, referred pain is experienced by the patient in the cutaneous distribution of the segmental dermatome from which the visceral organ arises. Familiar examples of referred pain are the pain of an acute myocardial infarction experienced as pain radiating down the left arm or into the jaw, or the pain of renal colic experienced as groin or testicular pain.

Laboratory examination should be directed to the local area of pain as well as to the related areas of dermatome distribution, or referred pain. In the patient with acute pain, appropriate studies should be instituted immediately. In the patient with chronic pain who does not present with an acute emergency, it is mandatory to review the extent and quality of previous evaluations prior to embarking on extensive additional and perhaps repetitive laboratory testing.

TREATMENT OF THE PATIENT WITH ACUTE PAIN

Appropriate treatment of the patient with acute pain requires identification of the etiology of the pain and treatment of the underlying cause. Space precludes the description of the causes and treatments of all the acute pain syndromes here. The general management of the patient with acute pain will be outlined with special attention to the management of pain of the terminally ill.

An informed patient and a compassionate physician who takes time to explain the course of the patient's illness to the patient and his family and friends can significantly reduce the agitation, turmoil, and confusion that often accompany the patient in acute pain. Too often an afterthought in evaluating the patient with acute pain, communication and empathy can often prevent further acceleration of cycles of pain. However, in the patient with severe acute pain, patient education, reassurance, and the institution of appropriate therapy for the underlying disorder are usually insufficient to alleviate acute pain. Many physicians are reluctant to prescribe narcotic analgesics to patients with severe acute pain for fear of addicting them to narcotics. This fear is unfounded in patients with acute pain.

Several general principles should be remembered in treating acute pain. Analgesic therapy should be instituted promptly unless cardinal manifestations of the underlying disorder would be obscured by analgesic therapy (e.g., acute right lower quadrant pain in which appendicitis or visceral perforation is suspected). Analgesic therapy should be prescribed at frequent, regular intervals around the clock; the patient should have the right to refuse analgesic medication, but should be encouraged to accept prescribed medication for minor pain rather than waiting until pain becomes severe. Solid evidence exists that demonstrates that relying on a patient's requests for pain medication results in larger total doses of analgesic medication to control wide swings in intensity of pain and burdens the patient with deciding "when the pain is too much to bear." For these reasons, "when necessary" (PRN) pain medication dosing schedules in patients with severe acute pain should be avoided. Narcotic analgesics should never be given in combination with each other. Frequently, a combination of a non-narcotic analgesic such as phenothiazine (chlorpromazine 25 to 50 mg four times a day) and a narcotic analgesic achieves greater pain control and reduces the overall amount of narcotics administered, since the effects of these two separate classes of drugs are synergistic.

Analgesic agents, drugs that diminish pain without causing loss of consciousness, fall into three main categories: non-narcotic analgesics used in the treatment of mild pain, narcotic analgesics used for moderate pain, and narcotic analgesics used both parenterally and orally for severe pain (Table 51–1).

TABLE 51-1 Some Commonly Prescribed Analgesic Medications Used in Patients with Acute Pain

Drug	Usual Starting Dose	
	Oral	SC or IM
Non-narcotic analgesics for mild to moderate pain		
Aspirin	600 mg q3 to 4h	
Ibuprofen	200 to 600 mg q6h	
Acetaminophen	650 mg q6h	
Narcotic and narcotic antagonists for moderate to severe pain		
Codeine	15 to 30 mg q4 to 6h	
Oxycodone	5 mg q4 to 6h	
Meperidine	50 to 100 mg q3 to 4h	75 mg q3 to 4h
Narcotic and narcotic antagonists for severe pain		
Morphine	30 to 60 mg q3 to 4h	5 to 10 mg q3 to 4h
Levorphanol	2 to 4 mg q3 to 4h	1 to 2 mg q3 to 4h
Methadone	5 to 10 mg q8 to 12h	2.5 to 5.0 mg q8 to 12h
Hydromorphone	2.5 to 5 mg q4 to 6h	1 to 2 mg q4 to 6h

The physician should be intimately familiar with the dosing schedules, side effects, and drug interactions of two or three drugs of the hundreds available in each category. In patients with mild to moderate pain, drugs should be combined and rapidly added in a stepwise fashion until satisfactory pain control has been achieved. Aspirin (600 mg PO every 3 to 4 hours), acetaminophen (650 mg PO every 3 to 4 hours), or a nonsteroidal anti-inflammatory agent such as ibuprofen (400 mg every 6 hours) are good agents to initiate the treatment of mild pain. Both aspirin and nonsteroidal anti-inflammatory agents cause gastrointestinal irritation and bleeding and are contraindicated in patients with active gastrointestinal hemorrhage or peptic ulcer disease. These agents can be combined with acetaminophen for some improvement in mild pain. If anxiety plays a substantial role in the patient with mild pain, a mild benzodiazepam such as diazepam (5 to 10 mg PO twice a day) can be added, but these agents have little role in the relief of pain apart from reducing anxiety. In pain that is unresponsive to these agents, narcotic analgesics with a low likelihood of causing addiction such as codeine (15 to 30 mg every 4 to 6 hours) or oxycodone (5 mg every 4 to 6 hours) can be added. These agents are generally well tolerated, but do cause nausea, vomiting, constipation, and drowsiness, especially in large doses.

As already described, in the patient with acute pain narcotic analgesics are often under utilized by physicians fearful of the drugs' potential for addiction and their side effects in spite of their potent ability to relieve severe pain. Only rarely do patients hospitalized with severe acute pain of an organic etiology become addicted to narcotic analgesics. The most common side effects of narcotic analgesics used in the short-term management of hospitalized patients with acute severe pain are constipation and somnolence. Constipation can be prevented and managed by beginning a bowel care program when narcotics are first prescribed; somnolence can be managed by a reduction in the doses of narcotic analgesics and more frequent administration, or by use of another narcotic agent. Used in the long term for the management of severe pain, narcotic analgesics induce both tolerance and physical dependence. Tolerance to narcotics means that larger and larger doses are required to achieve analgesia; physical dependence means that patients treated for long periods of time must have the drug gradually discontinued if the drug is withdrawn. Virtually all the narcotic analgesics can be administered parenterally as well as orally with varying potencies and duration of action. Morphine (2 to 5 mg IM or SC), for example, has good parenteral effectiveness and a relatively long duration of action (4 to 5 hours) compared with parenteral meperidine (75 mg IM), which has a brief duration of action (3 to 4 hours). Narcotics with good oral efficacy include levorphanol (2 to 4 mg; duration of action 4 to 6 hours) and methadone (10 to 20 mg PO; duration of action 3 to 10 hours). Again, physicians should familiarize themselves with the characteristics of one or two parenterally and orally effective narcotic analgesics; narcotic analgesics should never be used in combination.

MANAGEMENT OF THE PATIENT WITH TERMINAL ILLNESS

In the patient with a terminal illness (defined as illness likely to cause death within 1 year) experiencing severe pain, pain control should be one of the central features in management.[5,6,7] The goal of management is indefinite pain control. Analgesics should be given on a regular dosing schedule for patients with continuous pain; PRN dosing schedules should be avoided. For terminally ill patients who can tolerate oral medication, levorphanol (2 mg every 3 to 4 hours) or methadone (10 to 20 mg every 4 hours) are recommended. Several side effects of these medications should be anticipated. First, constipation is a universal side effect of these medications; a bowel care regimen that includes stool softeners, laxatives, and dietary bulk should be prescribed from the outset to avoid obstipation. Secondly, drug tolerance and the requirement for increasing doses during the first few weeks of therapy should be expected. Bedtime doses of pain medication should be increased two- to three-fold in order to avoid the patient's waking with pain. Finally, patients experiencing sedation and somnolence with increasing doses of narcotic analgesics can take oral dextroamphetamine (5 to 20 mg daily in a single AM dose) to counter the sedative effects of the narcotic analgesics. The physician should *not* be concerned about addiction and habituation to these drugs when caring for patients with a terminal illness.

MANAGEMENT OF THE PATIENT WITH CHRONIC PAIN

Patients with chronic pain syndromes present for consultation with a physician, usually having seen several other specialists and having had extensive evaluations and, often, surgery. The diagnostic approach outlined previously should be followed carefully. We find it helpful when evaluating patients with chronic pain to keep in mind four major kinds of chronic pain syndromes. While there is often overlap among these types of pain syndromes even in the same patient, they are nevertheless helpful in the structuring of a treatment plan.

First, patients with chronic organic diseases can suffer bouts of pain as part of their disease. Patients with rheumatoid arthritis, osteoarthritis, or sickle cell anemia may have intermittent periods of moderate to severe pain. Second, patients may have chronic pain from some injury to the central or peripheral nervous system that causes dysesthesia and causalgia. Patients with peripheral neuritis, postherpetic neuralgia, and phantom limb pain after amputation are examples of patients with this kind of pain. Third, patients may have chronic pain initially caused by acute injury or trauma, but that persists long after the original injury has healed, because of its psychological significance for the patient. Such psychological pain should be treated with a combination of physical treatment and psychiatric care that addresses the psychological dimensions of the patient's pain. Fourth, patients have chronic pain as a manifestation of primary psychiatric or psychological disturbances in the absence of any known structural or physiologic abnormality. Patients with hypochondriasis, psychotic depression, and schizophrenia are examples of these disorders.

The management of patients with chronic pain syndromes usually involves multiple different modalities and collaboration with other specialists.[8] In each hospital it is helpful if a pain committee or consortium (staffed by Medicine, Neurology, Psychiatry, Rehabilitation, and Social Service) is available. The general principles of management are similar to those for treating acute pain. Treatment should be the least complicated means of effectively reducing pain and suffering; every effort should be taken to insure that the patient is pain free with a minimum of side effects. The initiation of therapy should be prompt in those patients not previously treated since breaking the pain cycle early may prevent the development of psychological pain behavior.

Although the management of chronic pain should be the least complicated, effective regimen, multiple different modalities should be used together since many of the different therapies are synergistic.

Evaluation by a psychiatrist is imperative in patients in whom a psychogenic component to their pain syndrome is suspected. When managing patients with both physical and psychological components of the pain syndrome, a good working relationship between the mental health therapist and the internist facilitates caring for the patient and may prevent unnecessary procedures and diagnostic testing. In patients whose pain is a manifestation of primary psychiatric disease, diagnosis and treatment require extended evaluation by a psychiatrist. The internist's role is to reassure the patient that no structural abnormality exists, to discourage repeated unnecessary evaluations, and to prevent unwarranted surgery. This often is a frustrating experience for both patient and physician.

The pharmacologic management of patients with chronic pain syndromes includes several different classes of drugs. Narcotics *should be avoided* in patients with chronic pain syndromes since these drugs have only limited efficacy, and the potential for tolerance and habituation is high in these patients. Antidepressants deserve a trial in almost all patients with chronic pain who have not responded to other interventions. Low doses of amitriptyline (25 to 75 mg at bedtime) have mild analgesic properties and are often helpful in alleviating the pain of chronic radiculopathy. Most chronic pain patients who have not responded to treatment deserve a supervised trial of antidepressants at levels used to treat major depression before any invasive treatments are considered. Drugs such as amitriptyline (150 to 250 mg at bedtime) or desipramine (75 to 125 mg at bedtime) should be tried; none of the antidepressants has been reported to be superior to any other in the treatment of chronic pain patients, and drug choice is empirical. In patients with chronic pain in whom anxiety is an important feature, antipsychotic agents in small doses (e.g., haloperidol 1 to 2 mg three times a day) may be effective in controlling both pain and anxiety. In patients with chronic pain secondary to injuries to the central or peripheral nervous system, such as postherpetic neuralgia or phantom limb syndrome, anticonvulsants may be helpful. Carbamazepine (300 to 1,200 mg daily), phenytoin (300 mg daily), or clonazepam (1 to 3 mg daily) should be tried.

Nonpharmacologic therapy of chronic pain syndromes includes numerous different techniques. Nondestructive procedures should be tried first, and the choice of therapies should be dictated both by the cause of the patient's pain and the skill and experience of the physician in providing some of these techniques. For patients with intractable or severe pain syndromes, multidisciplinary pain clinics provide consultation and treatment from teams of physicians experienced in treating chronic pain.[9] Noninvasive techniques that attempt to increase central pain inhibitory stimuli include hypnosis, biofeedback, and relaxation training. Hypnosis is more successful in the alleviation of acute rather than chronic pain. Biofeedback trains patients to control tension by teaching techniques to change physiologic parameters. Relaxation training, which involves progressive muscle relaxation, has become a popular and often successful adjunct to other therapies used in managing chronic pain.

Several neurologic techniques are available to interrupt the transmission of pain from peripheral nerves to the CNS. Some of these techniques attempt to stimulate large afferent nerve fibers that inhibit the transmission of signals along A-delta and smaller type C pain fibers.[10] Simply rubbing the skin around a painful area excites these large afferent fibers and reduces pain. Battery powered transcutaneous nerve stimulators (TENS) are available that apply continuous or intermittent stimuli to areas of injury to reduce pain. These stimulators are helpful in the management of phantom limb pain, chronic radiculopathies, and other peripheral nerve injuries. Acupuncture, introduced from Chinese medical practice, has been advocated for use in the management of chronic pain. Needles, placed into the skin, often at sites remote from the pain, provide stimulation when twirled or when an electrical impulse is applied through the needles. However, the mechanism of action and the effectiveness of acupuncture have not yet been definitively demonstrated in controlled trials. Peripheral nerve blocks, performed by anesthesiologists using injections of either anesthetic agents or neurolytic agents, can achieve short- and intermediate-term pain control. These techniques can also be used in ablating nerve root pain by injection into the subarachnoid space. These techniques should only be performed by physicians experienced in their use since the injection of neurolytic agents such as phenol into the spinal column can result in serious permanent damage.

Finally, a number of invasive neurosurgical procedures, including percutaneous spinothalamic cordotomy and cingulotomy—interruption of the cingulum bundle and its limb projections in the frontal lobe of the brain—have been used in the treatment of severe, intractable chronic pain that has not responded to any other therapies. Candidates for these neurosurgical procedures should have failed all other modalities and have had a full psychiatric evaluation that eliminates a psychogenic cause for the chronic pain.

References

1. Bonica JJ, Lindblom U, Iggo A, eds. Advances in pain research and therapy, Vol. 5. New York: Raven Press, 1983.
2. Sternbach R. Pain patients: traits and treatment. New York: Academic Press, 1974.

3. Rueler JB, Girard DE, Nardone DA. The chronic pain syndrome: misconceptions and management. Ann Intern Med 1980; 93:588–596.
4. Classification of chronic pain: descriptions of chronic pain syndromes and definitions of pain terms. Pain 1986; Suppl 3:S1–S225.
5. Health and Public Policy Committee, American College of Physicians. Drug therapy for severe, chronic pain in terminal illness. Ann Intern Med 1983; 99:870–873.
6. Foley KM. The treatment of cancer pain. N Engl J Med 1985; 313:84–95.
7. Payne R, Foley KM, eds. Cancer pain. Med Clin North Am 1987; 71:2.
8. Newburger PE, Sallan SE. Chronic pain: principles of management. J Pediatr 1981; 98:180–189.
9. Hallett EC, Pilowsky I. Response to treatment in multidisciplinary pain clinic. Pain 1982; 12:365–374.
10. Levine J. Pain and analgesia: the outlook for more rational treatment. Ann Intern Med 1984; 100:269–276.

52 | DIABETES

JENNIFER DALEY, M.D.
JOHN T. HARRINGTON, M.D.

Diabetes mellitus afflicts approximately 2.5 percent of Americans. In addition, another 3 percent of the population has glucose intolerance without overt diabetes. Patients with diabetes mellitus may exhibit physiologic and metabolic abnormalities of glucose metabolism as well as chronic diabetic syndromes that affect numerous end-organs. The common feature of all diabetic syndromes is abnormal glucose metabolism, characterized by the inability of the patient to dispose appropriately of a glucose load because of relative or absolute insulin deficiency. Protean in its clinical manifestations, diabetes mellitus ranges in severity from a mild glucose intolerance during the stress of an infection or surgery to marked glucose intolerance with retinopathy, nephropathy, and advanced, premature atherosclerosis. In this chapter, we briefly review the two major types of diabetes, insulin-dependent diabetes mellitus (IDDM), and non-insulin-dependent diabetes mellitus (NIDDM).[1] We then address in detail some of the more common questions for which we are consulted in our outpatient and inpatient practice.

OVERVIEW OF THE TWO MAJOR FORMS OF DIABETES MELLITUS

Most patients with diabetes fall into one of two general categories. Patients with classic insulin-dependent diabetes mellitus (IDDM) are also known as juvenile-onset, ketosis-prone, or Type I diabetics and constitute only 5 percent or so of all diabetics. Patients with non-insulin-dependent diabetes mellitus (NIDDM), the most commonly encountered diabetics, comprise 85 to 90 percent of all diabetics.[2] Other terms for NIDDM include maturity-onset diabetes, Type II, or stable diabetes. Insulin-dependent diabetes and non-insulin-dependent diabetes have distinctly different etiologies, patterns of inheritance, age of onset, and typical clinical characteristics (Table 52-1).

Insulin-dependent diabetics typically present between the ages of 10 and 17 with polydipsia, polyuria, rapid weight loss, occasionally a craving for sweets, and, not infrequently, acute diabetic ketoacidosis. The insulin-dependent diabetic develops an absolute lack of insulin secretion within 12 to 18 months of onset of disease. Genetic susceptibility to IDDM is transmitted

TABLE 52-1 Comparison of Insulin-Dependent Diabetes and Non-Insulin-
Dependent Diabetes

	Insulin-Dependent Diabetes	Non-Insulin Dependent Diabetes
Age at onset	Childhood or adolesence 7–18 years	Mid-life 45–85 years
Symptoms at onset	Polydipsia, polyuria, weight loss, acute ketoacidosis	Polydipsia, polyuria, weight gain
Pathophysiology	Absolute lack of insulin from pancreatic beta cell destruction	Decrease in pancreatic beta cell function Peripheral insulin resistance
Etiology	Autoimmune beta cell destruction, genetic susceptibility, ? induced by viral infection	? Genetic susceptibility
Treatment	Diet Insulin	Weight loss Diet Sulfonylureas Insulin
Ketoacidosis	Yes	No
Hyperosmolar states	No	Yes

on chromosome 6 near the major histocompatibility complex; patients with this susceptibility appear to develop an autoimmune response, perhaps virally-induced, to the insulin-producing beta cells of the pancreas. Because of their absolute lack of insulin secretion, patients with insulin-dependent diabetes require insulin therapy throughout their lives. Major chronic diabetic complications occur frequently. These patients are at substantial risk for development of blindness, premature aggressive atherosclerosis, and renal failure 20 to 30 years after the onset of disease.

Non-insulin-dependent diabetes, a more heterogeneous disease, is characterized by impaired release of insulin from beta cells as well as peripheral tissue insensitivity to the action of insulin.[3] The typical non-insulin-dependent diabetic is a 40 to 60-year-old overweight individual who has recently gained 10 to 30 pounds. Polydipsia and polyuria are common symptoms in the non-insulin-dependent diabetic. Occasionally, the patient may have experienced some weight loss following the onset of polydipsia and polyuria. Other common symptoms include an increase in soft tissue infections, such as cellulitis or vulvovaginal candidiasis, that are refractory to therapy. Most non-insulin-dependent diabetics never experience ketoacidosis and present with clinical manifestations of hyperglycemia or with one of the major chronic diabetic syndromes, such as microangiopathic peripheral vascular disease of the lower extremities, peripheral neuropathy, and "silent" myocardial infarction. These diabetics do not require insulin except during periods of stress (e.g., surgery, infection, acute myocardial infarction) and are best managed with a combination of diet, weight loss, and oral hypoglycemic agents.

Rarely, diabetes mellitus is caused by other problems or diseases, such as pancreatic resection for pancreatic pseudocyst or for carcinoma of the pancreas, severe pancreatic trauma, or infiltrative diseases such as hemochromatosis. Diabetes mellitus also may be found in association with other endocrine diseases that alter glucose homeostasis, such as Cushing's syndrome or pheochromocytoma.

DIAGNOSIS OF DIABETES MELLITUS

In our experience, a formal glucose tolerance test is rarely indicated to make the diagnosis of diabetes mellitus. Most insulin-dependent diabetics present with polydipsia and polyuria attributable to the marked hyperglycemia and glucosuria. In patients with ketoacidosis, the patient may complain of nausea or vomiting or may present with alterations in mental status and abdominal pain. The asymptomatic non-insulin-dependent diabetic is most often detected by routine screening during an annual check-up. Although most multichannel screening is done in the fasting state, a screening blood glucose level is best obtained 2 hours after eating a large breakfast. Blood glucose levels of less than 120 mg per deciliter (2 hours post cibum) eliminate the presence of diabetes. A fasting blood glucose of greater than 140 mg per deciliter is diagnostic of diabetes.

Infrequently, we are asked to pursue the diagnosis of diabetes in a patient with a normal fasting blood glucose level and some clinical syndrome suggestive of occult diabetes mellitus (e.g., lower extremity microvascular ulcers). In these cases, a formal oral glucose tolerance test (75 to 100 g of glucose) may be indicated. The patient should have an oral intake of more than 200 g of carbohydrate daily for 3 days prior to the glucose tolerance test. Unstressed healthy individuals should have a blood glucose level below 110 mg per deciliter before glucose ingestion; blood glucose levels should be less than 160 mg per deciliter at 1 hour and less than 120 mg per deciliter at 3 hours. These criteria reflect normal glucose tolerance for young and middle age patients. Glucose tolerance decreases with age; a 1 hour value of 180 mg per deciliter and a 2 hour value of 150 mg per deciliter is normal for patients over the age of 70. Patients whose values are greater than the upper limits of normal, but who do not have symptomatic hyperglycemia, are designated as having impaired glucose tolerance. Glucose tolerance can be affected by stress, anxiety, infection, hypokalemia, and prior fasting or carbohydrate deprivation. The results of any formal glucose tolerance test should be interpreted in the light of these factors.

INITIATING AND MONITORING THERAPY IN THE NONACUTE DIABETIC

By definition, insulin-dependent diabetics require therapy with insulin and diet. Occasionally in the insulin-dependent diabetic, a brief "honeymoon" of 3 to 18 months occurs after the initial episode of hyperglycemia. During this interval the patient may require little or no insulin, but ultimately the beta pancreatic cells cease functioning and the patient requires insulin. Many non-insulin-dependent diabetics, the vast majority of whom are overweight, can be treated by diet alone. Many non-insulin-diabetics who are motivated to lose weight can achieve good control of their serum glucose with a weight loss of as little as 10 to 15 pounds. If not, oral hypoglycemic agents are available. New-onset non-insulin-dependent diabetics who have lost a considerable amount of weight or in whom ketonuria is noted initially require therapy with insulin.

Diet

Dietary therapy is the *cornerstone* of the treatment of all diabetics.[4] The principles of dietary management for the non-insulin-dependent diabetic are the same as for an insulin-dependent diabetic. Obese diabetics should be instructed in a reducing regimen. Weight loss of as little as 10 to 15 pounds may lead to a marked improvement in the control of blood glucose levels and the symptoms of hyperglycemia in the obese non-insulin-dependent diabetic. Caloric requirements for all diabetics must be determined by the level of daily activity. All diabetics require a meal schedule of three meals a day at fixed times as well as midafternoon and bedtime snacks. General dietary recommendations include a well-balanced diet that avoids concentrated sweets and beverages and that is high in polyunsaturated fats, rather than saturated animal fats. Caloric intake should be balanced so that 40 percent of the daily kilocalories allowed are in the noon meal and afternoon snack, 40 percent are in the dinner meal and bedtime snack, and 20 percent of the daily kilocalories are at breakfast. A careful dietary history should be obtained from all diabetics to accommodate the patient's food preferences, activity levels, and eating habits. Extensive patient education by a trained dietician or nurse practitioner familiar with the principles of diabetic dietary management is extremely helpful in promoting patient education and compliance. Principles of diabetic dietary management, exchangeable food lists, and meal planning guides are available from the American Diabetes Association.

Insulin

A number of insulin preparations are available for use in the treatment of insulin-dependent diabetics and non-insulin-dependent diabetics who require insulin therapy.[5] The use of single-component or single-peak insulin from both pork and beef reduces the induction of antibody-related insulin resistance as does the use of the recently introduced human insulin (Humulin), a product of recombinant DNA technology.

Insulin regimens must be tailored to the individual patient's exercise level, caloric intake, and metabolic requirements. The goal of insulin therapy is to mimic a normal physiologic pattern of insulin secretion in response to diet and to exercise. Many diabetics require only a single injection of long-acting insulin in the morning prior to breakfast. However, diabetics who have had the disease for several years, especially those with insulin-dependent diabetes, require the addition of a small dose of regular (short-acting) insulin to intermediate or long-acting insulin before breakfast and a second injection of an intermediate-acting insulin before dinner. This "split-dose" regimen better mimics the normal physiologic pattern of insulin secretion.

One of the recent advances in the management of the diabetic patient (particularly those requiring split-dose insulin regimens) is the availability of blood glucose self-monitoring techniques. Physicians and patients have previously relied on urine testing to assess the adequacy of blood glucose control, but urinary levels do not always accurately reflect blood glucose levels. The use of blood glucose monitors (reflectometer) by the patient has made the adjustment of insulin dosages much more accurate. When insulin doses are being adjusted initially or in response to a change in a diabetic's lifestyle, blood glucose levels can be monitored before each meal, at bedtime, and, occasionally, in the middle of the night if hypoglycemia is suspected.

The major complication of insulin therapy is hypoglycemia.[6] Minor hypoglycemic reactions, characterized by mood changes or by difficulty in mentation, may be followed by hunger and signs of sympathetic overactivity with sweating, tachycardia, and anxiety. Treatment is the administration of oral carbohydrate, such as candy or fruit juice. Severe hypoglycemic reactions include unconsciousness and convulsions. Subcutaneous or intramuscular glucagon (1 mg) can be given by the patient, if conscious, or by family members. Hypoglycemia that occurs in an emergency room or office setting can be treated intravenously with 1 mg of glucagon or by the intravenous injection of 50 percent glucose (25 g). The major physiologic reaction to hypoglycemia is a rebound hyperglycemia known as the Somogyi effect.

Patients who experience nocturnal hypoglycemia may have rebound hyperglycemia in the morning with elevated blood sugars and glycosuria. Physicians and patients unfamiliar with the Somogyi effect may unknowingly increase insulin to "cover" the rebound hyperglycemia, thus increasing the nocturnal hypoglycemia. Nocturnal hypoglycemia may be documented by obtaining a 3 AM blood sugar; the treatment of early morning rebound hyperglycemia is a reduction of the insulin dose. A gradual decrease of insulin activity in the early morning hours may also result in morning hyperglycemia. This "dawn" phenomenon is not preceded by hypoglycemia and again can be distinguished from the Somogyi effect by obtaining a 3 AM blood glucose.

Oral Hypoglycemic Agents

Oral hypoglycemic agents (sulfonylureas) stimulate the secretion of insulin from the pancreas and increase the number of peripheral insulin receptors.[7,8,9] Because sulfonylureas work by increasing pancreatic secretion of insulin, they are not indicated in the treatment of insulin-dependent diabetics who no longer produce insulin endogenously. Treatment of non-insulin-dependent diabetics with sulfonylureas has been controversial since 1970 when the University Group Diabetes Program (UGDP) reported a higher incidence of sudden death among diabetics treated with tolbutamide than among those treated with insulin or placebo. Re-examination of this issue in recent years has indicated treatment with sulfonylureas can be beneficial in some patients. Non-insulin-dependent diabetics in midlife, either of normal weight or moderately obese, respond best to treatment with oral hypoglycemic agents. In contrast, non-insulin-dependent diabetics who are underweight respond better to treatment with insulin.

Oral hypoglycemic agents always should be used in conjunction with dietetic therapy and an exercise program. Obese non-insulin-dependent diabetics should be encouraged to lose weight because the efficacy of sulfonylureas is enhanced by even a moderate amount of weight loss. Six sulfonylureas are currently available for use in the United States. Tolbutamide, chlorpropamide, acetohexamide, and tolazamide are first generation sulfonylureas. The selection of one of these agents depends on several factors, including the patient's age, the use of other medications, and the presence of chronic liver or kidney disease. The drugs differ from each other in their duration of action and mechanism of drug elimination. Chlorpropamide (100 to 400 mg daily), for example, has a long duration of action (24 to 48 hours) and can be given on a once-a-day basis. Chlorpropamide is excreted unchanged by the kidneys and, therefore, is contraindicated in patients with chronic renal insufficiency. Patients receiving chlorpropamide should be monitored carefully for hypoglycemia (and hyponatremia as well). Tolbutamide (250 to 2,000 mg daily), the most commonly used hypoglycemic agent, has a shorter duration of action (6 to 12 hours) and must be given twice a day to achieve tight control of glucose levels. Tolbutamide is excreted by the liver.

Glipizide (2.5 to 30 mg daily) and glyburide (2.5 to 20 mg daily), two second generation sulfonylureas, have durations of action of 24 hours or more and can be given in single or divided doses. Occasionally, patients who have shown no response to first generation agents do respond to the second generation drugs. Drug interactions with all the sulfonylureas are common in patients taking thiazide diuretics, barbiturates, and anticoagulants such as warfarin; diabetics receiving these drugs with oral hypoglycemic agents should be carefully monitored and drug doses adjusted appropriately. Sulfonylureas are contraindicated in diabetics who are allergic to sulfa compounds and in the pregnant diabetic. Non-insulin-dependent diabetics with acute medical problems such as myocardial infarction or overwhelming infection usually require insulin therapy; oral hypoglycemic agents are of little value during the acute phases of these illnesses (Table 52-2).

TABLE 52-2   Oral Hypoglycemic Agents (Sulfonylureas)

Name	Daily Dose	Duration of Action
Chlorpropamide	100–500 mg in single dose	36 hours
Tolbutamide	0.25–3.0 g in divided dose	6–8 hours
Tolazamide	0.1–1.0 g in single or divided dose	24 hours
Acetohexamide	0.25–1.5 g in single or divided dose	12–18 hours
Glipizide	2.5–30 mg in single or divided dose	24 hours
Glyburide	2.5–20 mg in single or divided dose	24 hours

The Controversy Over Tight Metabolic Control

Debate still continues over how tightly diabetics should maintain control of their blood glucose levels. Tight metabolic control is felt to reduce or to prevent some of the complications of diabetes. Maintenance of tight metabolic control requires the diabetic to maintain the fasting blood glucose levels between 70 mg per deciliter and 125 mg per deciliter and to keep postprandial levels below 180 mg per deciliter. Maintenance of tight metabolic control requires frequent self-monitoring of blood glucose levels and multiple injections of insulin daily. The major side effect of maintaining tight control is frequent hypoglycemic reactions. Recent studies have strongly suggested that tight metabolic control over a long period of time decreases the progression of diabetic retinopathy, improves the diabetic's recovery rate from infection, and reduces the incidence of infection. The role of tight metabolic control in the prevention of the small vessel complications of diabetes and in diabetic renal disease has yet to be demonstrated.[10] We recommend maintaining blood glucose levels as close to normal as possible, particularly in the young insulin-dependent diabetic and in the non-insulin-dependent diabetic aged 40 to 55 at the onset of diabetes. These patients should be carefully monitored for hypoglycemic reactions. Older, non-insulin-dependent diabetics who have the onset of diabetes in the seventh or eighth decade do not require such vigorous control of blood glucose levels.

Hemoglobin A_1C, a glucose-conjugated hemoglobin in which approximately 7 percent of hemoglobin is combined with carbohydrate at the N-terminal of the beta chain, can be used to monitor the overall efficacy of glucose control.[11] Hemoglobin A_1C levels are helpful in the assessment of the average blood glucose level for the previous 4 weeks of insulin therapy and diabetes management. Hemoglobin A_1C levels are now routinely available through most commercial and clinical laboratories.

Insulin infusion pumps that deliver insulin continuously subcutaneously or intravenously have been used in recent years in insulin-dependent diabetics to achieve near normal glucose levels.[12] The patient receives a low dose continuous infusion of insulin and then increases insulin infusion in response to measured blood glucose levels or to meals. Diabetics with insulin infusion pumps measure blood glucose levels frequently and adjust their insulin requirements as necessary. Complications of the infusion pump include frequent episodes of hypoglycemia, occasional episodes of ketoacidosis, and infection at the site of the infusion. Failure of the battery-driven infusion pumps often results in episodes of ketoacidosis. Insulin infusion pumps are most appropriate for insulin-dependent diabetics who are highly motivated to control their blood glucose levels and are willing to measure their blood glucose levels frequently.[13]

DIABETIC EMERGENCIES

The acutely ill diabetic may develop acute diabetic emergencies in addition to hypoglycemic coma in diabetics treated with insulin or hypoglycemic agents. The first, diabetic ketoacidosis, is the result of insulin insufficiency. Fatty tissues, reacting as if in a prolonged fasting state, release free fatty acids, and the liver takes up circulating amino acids and free fatty acids, thereby generating maximal amounts of glucose and ketoacids. Plasma levels of glucose and ketoacids rise dramatically with resulting ketonuria and glucosuria. The osmotic load of glucose and ketones excreted in the urine leads to polyuria, intravascular volume depletion, ketoacidosis, and coma. Excessive lipolysis and the production of ketoacids is avoided in the non-insulin-dependent diabetic who still produces some insulin. However, if the patient becomes dehydrated in the face of profound hyperglycemia, intravascular volume depletion and hyperosmolarity occur. In the situation of the non-insulin-dependent diabetic, typically the elderly, the resultant diabetic crisis is hyperglycemic hyperosmolar coma.

Management of Diabetic Ketoacidosis

The primary concern in the management of a patient with acute diabetic ketoacidosis is the replacement of salt and water deficits,[14] although the underlying metabolic defect in diabetic ketoacidosis is insufficient insulin secretion. Patients with acute diabetic ketoacidosis present with hypovolemia, incipient or overt shock, dehydration, and Kussmaul's hyperventilation. Precipitating events include noncompliance with the prescribed regimen, poor patient education about the need to increase insulin dosages in the face of acute infection or stress, or the presence of previously unidentified sources of sepsis or infection, including cholecystitis, pneumonia, or urinary tract infection. Silent myocardial infarction also can precipitate diabetic ketoacidosis.

Management of diabetic ketoacidosis begins with a rapid assessment of the history and physical examination. Blood samples are obtained for the measurement of glucose, BUN, creatinine, electrolytes, and serum ketones, and urine samples are obtained for glucose and ketone measurements. At the same time these samples are being obtained, a large bore intravenous line should be inserted. The patient should have isotonic saline administered immediately, and unless the patient is in marked congestive heart failure or is anuric (unusual in the patient with diabetic ketoacidosis), the isotonic saline should be administered rapidly (approximately 10 ml per minute for the first hour). Average fluid deficits in patients with diabetic ketoacidosis are 4 to 6 L. One of the goals of prompt treatment should be the administration of approximately 1 L of normal saline per hour during each of the first 3 hours of therapy or until blood pressure has returned to normal. In addition to being severely volume depleted, patients with diabetic ketoacidosis are also profoundly total body potassium depleted owing to the accompanying metabolic acidosis and osmotic diuresis. The average potassium deficit is 300 mEq (range 200 to 600 mEq). In acidosis, potassium shifts from intracellular fluid to extracellular fluid, thereby producing hyperkalemia in spite of this total body potassium deficit. Potassium, in the form of potassium chloride or potassium phosphate, should be administered unless the serum potassium level is greater than 5.0 mEq per liter. Unless the patient has known renal insufficiency, 40 mEq of potassium should be given to the patient every hour until the deficit is repaired. We recommend administration of potassium chloride during the first hour and replacement with potassium phosphate during the second hour because diabetics also are typically phosphate depleted.

Patients with diabetic ketoacidosis also should have arterial blood gas measurements obtained on arrival in the emergency room. Once the arterial pH is known, consideration should be given to the administration of alkali. Although controversial, we recommend the administration of small amounts of sodium bicarbonate (1 ampule equals 50 mEq) in patients in whom the arterial pH is below 7.15 or in patients in whom the serum bicarbonate level is less than 8 mEq per liter. The goal of treatment with alkali is not to completely correct the acidemia, but to prevent further declines in pH and to return the arterial pH to approximately 7.2. Further administration of fluids, potassium, and insulin allows the metabolism of excess ketoacids from the blood and the restoration of serum bicarbonate to normal.

The mode of administration and the amount of insulin given to a patient in acute diabetic ketoacidosis also is the subject of some controversy. In recent years, the continuous intravenous infusion of insulin, by use of an initial bolus of regular insulin (0.2 units/kg) followed by a constant infusion of 0.1 units per kilogram per hour, has been advocated as both a safe and an easily controllable way of reducing blood glucose levels. Intravenous infusion assures a constant rate of delivery and a gradual decrease in levels of glucose and ketoacids. When the infusion of insulin is stopped, the patient should be given a subcutaneous injection of insulin to prevent rebound hyperglycemia and ketoacidosis. An effective response of blood glucose levels to the intravenous infusion of insulin is approximately a 10 to 15 percent decrease in blood glucose levels every hour. When blood glucose levels have fallen to the range of 200 to 300 mg per deciliter, glucose should be administered as a mixture of half normal saline and 5 percent dextrose in water to prevent hypoglycemia.

We cannot overemphasize the importance of constant observation of the patient in diabetic ketoacidosis and the use of a detailed flowchart that records the patient's clinical condition, vital signs, serum glucose, BUN, creatinine, electrolytes, arterial blood gases, infusion of intravenous fluids, potassium chloride and phosphate, sodium bicarbonate, and insulin. Patients with diabetic ketoacidosis should have a physician in attendance and be examined on an hourly basis with a review of their laboratory values and clinical condition. The typical patient with diabetic ketoacidosis stabilizes over a period of 3 to 8 hours. An intensive search for precipitating causes should be begun as soon as the patient is hemodynamically stable.

Hyperosmolar Coma

Patients with hyperosmolar hyperglycemic coma are typically elderly, non-insulin-dependent diabetics with severe intravascular volume depletion and an underlying acute stress such as pneumonia, urinary tract infection, stroke, or myocardial infarction, Blood glucose levels may range from 500 to 2,000 mg per deciliter. The goal of therapy is replacement of critical intravascular fluid and restoration of extracellular fluid volume. Initial treatment should be 2 L of isotonic saline infused over a period of 2 to 3 hours. Thereafter, hypotonic saline (1/2 normal saline) can be used if the patient remains significantly hyperosmolar. The patient's total body fluid deficit may be as much as 5 to 6 L. Volume replacement should take place expeditiously over the first few hours. Thereafter, volume replacement should be carried out more slowly. In elderly patients in whom fluid overload and congestive heart failure are concerns, careful monitoring of volume replacement may require the placement of a central venous catheter. Insulin requirements in hyperosmolar coma are generally quite small. In most patients, volume replacement with isotonic saline alone results in a prompt decrease in the blood glucose. Sometimes as little as 5 to 10 units of insulin administered subcutaneously results in a significant decrease in blood glucose levels. As in patients with diabetic ketoacidosis, potassium levels must be monitored and potassium replacement initiated if appropriate. A reduction in blood glucose levels to normal over 12 to 18 hours is the goal of therapy and avoids rapid shifts of fluid and glucose from extracellular to intracellular spaces.

END-ORGAN DIABETIC COMPLICATIONS

The acute metabolic complications of diabetes (e.g., hyperglycemia and hyperosmolarity) reverse with the administration of fluids and insulin over a period of hours to a few days. Physiologic changes from hyperglycemia, such as the glycosylation of hemoglobin, gradually reverse with the control of hyperglycemia. Chronic end-organ changes of diabetes are less clearly attributable to hypoinsulinemia. Also unclear is whether these changes are potentially reversible with the careful control of glucose levels. We will review the major diabetic complications and address areas in which there have been recent advances in diagnosis or therapy.[15]

Atherosclerosis

Atherosclerosis of large and medium sized vessels is much more common in diabetics who have had insulin-dependent diabetes for more than 20 years duration than in age and sex-matched controls. Diabetics are much more susceptible to myocardial infarction, peripheral vascular disease, and stroke. The management of these common complications does not differ significantly from patients without diabetes. The physician, however, should be aware that diabetics who suffer stroke, myocardial infarction, and the consequences of large vessel peripheral vascular disease have much higher levels of morbidity and mortality than patients without diabetes mellitus.

Microangiopathic changes of the capillaries of the eye, kidney, and skin are unique to diabetics. A growing body of evidence suggests that the extent and the severity of microangiopathy correlate with the extent and the duration of hyperglycemia. In addition to an increased incidence of cataracts and of glaucoma, diabetics develop exudative and proliferative retinopathy. Non-insulin-dependent diabetics more typically develop exudative diabetic retinopathy. Proliferative retinopathy develops in both insulin-dependent and non-insulin-dependent diabetics. Photocoagulation therapy can have dramatic results in diabetics with proliferative retinopathy, and both insulin-dependent and non-insulin-dependent diabetics should be seen annually by an ophthalmologist. The majority of insulin-dependent diabetics with diabetes for longer than 20 years also develop microangiopathic changes in the renal glomerulus. The diabetic typically develops end-stage renal failure within 3 to 5 years after the development of overt proteinuria. Many insulin-dependent diabetics with end-stage renal disease have been successfully treated with hemodialysis and renal transplantation. We suggest transplantation if at all possible.

Almost all diabetics develop some involvement of the nervous system within 5 to 10 years of the diagnosis of clinical diabetes. The most common form of neurologic involvement is a painful peripheral neuropathy, usually confined to the lower extremities and marked by painful paresthesias and nocturnal pain. Other manifestations of neurologic involvement include bladder dysfunction and autonomic nervous system involvement with delayed gastric emptying, malabsorption, impotence in males, and orthostatic hypotension. The treatment of the nervous system complications of diabetes is frustrating. Painful neuropathy of the lower extremities can be treated with amitriptyline (50 to 100 mg at bedtime) with some success.

PERIOPERATIVE MANAGEMENT OF THE DIABETIC PATIENT

Frequently, surgical colleagues request consultation about the management of the diabetic patient around the time of surgery. Control of hyperglycemia in the perioperative period decreases the chance of infection in the diabetic. Careful attention should be given to the maintenance of blood glucose levels under 200 mg per deciliter. Insulin-dependent diabetics should receive half their usual morning dose of insulin prior to anesthesia, and an infusion of 5 percent dextrose and water should be given throughout surgery. The balance of the morning insulin dose should be given after the procedure is completed, and blood glucose should be measured frequently in the 24 hours after surgery. We recommend obtaining a blood glucose level every 6 hours in the 24 hours after the surgery; elevations of blood sugar can be treated with appropriate intravenous doses of regular insulin. Once oral intake has been reinstituted, the patient's insulin can be adjusted for current metabolic needs, level of activity, and caloric intake.

THE MANAGEMENT OF THE PREGNANT DIABETIC

Insulin-dependent diabetics who become pregnant have a higher rate of fetal loss and of congenital abnormalities in the fetus and are more susceptible to eclampsia, hydramnios, and premature delivery.[16] Strict maintenance of glucose levels in the normal range during the course of pregnancy markedly reduces the incidence of these complications. The goal of therapy of the diabetic during pregnancy is to maintain glucose levels as close as possible to that of the nondiabetic pregnant woman. Normal glucose levels in pregnant nondiabetics vary with each trimester of pregnancy, and the pregnant diabetic should be managed by a physician who is experienced in the management of such patients. Insulin requirements may decrease in the first trimester of pregnancy. Blood glucose levels become more variable in the second trimester of pregnancy, and ketoacidosis should be avoided. Most pregnant diabetics need multiple split-dose injections and daily frequent blood glucose levels during their pregnancy; pregnant diabetics have been successfully treated with insulin infusion pumps. The primary goal of the treatment of the pregnant diabetic is to maintain the pregnancy until such a time as fetal lung maturity has been achieved. Physicians should keep in mind that insulin requirements drop markedly in the hours after delivery. Insulin dosages should be rapidly and greatly reduced to avoid hypoglycemia in the immediate postpartum period.

References

1. National Diabetes Data Group. Classification and diagnosis of diabetes mellitus and other categories of glucose intolerance. Diabetes 1979; 28:1039–1057.
2. Melton LJ, Palumbo PJ, Chu C. Incidence of diabetes mellitus by clinical type. Diabetes Care 1983; 6:75–86.
3. DeFronzo RA, Ferrannini E, Koivisto V. New concepts in the pathogenesis and treatment of non-insulin dependent diabetes. Am J Med 1983; 74:52–81.
4. American Diabetes Association. Principles of nutrition and dietary recommendations for individuals with diabetes mellitus: 1979. Diabetes 1979; 28:1027–1030.
5. Galloway JA. Insulin treatment for the early 80's: facts and questions about old and new insulins and their usage. Diabetes Care 1980; 3:615–622.
6. Galloway JA, deShozo RD. The clinical use of insulin and the complications of insulin therapy. In: Ellenberg M, Rifkin H, eds. Diabetes mellitus: theory and practice, 3rd ed. New Hyde Park, NY: Medical Examination Publishing, 1983:519.
7. Physician's guide to type II diabetes (NIDDM): diagnosis and treatment. New York: American Diabetes Association, 1984.
8. Lipson LG, Lipson M. The therapeutic approach to the obese maturity onset patient. Arch Intern Med 1984; 144:135–138.
9. Liu GC, Coulston AM, Lardinois CK. Moderate weight loss and sulfonylurea treatment of non-insulin dependent diabetes mellitus. Arch Intern Med 1985; 145:665–669.
10. The Kroc Collaborative Study Group. Blood glucose control and the evolution of diabetic retinopathy and albuminuria: a preliminary multicenter trial. N Engl J Med 1984; 311:365–372.
11. Bunn HF. Evaluation of glycosylated hemoglobin in diabetic patients. Diabetes 1981; 30:613–617.
12. Dupre J, Champion M, Rodger NW. Advances in insulin delivery in the management of diabetes mellitus. Clin Endocrinol Metab 1982; 11:525–548.
13. Mecklenburg RS, Benson EA, Benson JW Jr, et al. Long-term metabolic control with insulin pump therapy: report of experience with 127 patients. N Engl J Med 1985; 313:465–468.
14. Foster DW, McGarry JD. The metabolic derangements and treatment of diabetic ketoacidosis. N Engl J Med 1983; 309:159–169.
15. Watkins PA, ed. Long-term complications of diabetes. Clin Endocrinol Metab 1986; 15:4.
16. Freinkel N, Dooley SL, Metzger B. Care of the pregnant woman with insulin-dependent diabetes mellitus. N Engl J Med 1985; 313:96–101.

53 | HYPERTENSION

JENNIFER DALEY, M.D.
JOHN T. HARRINGTON, M.D.

Hypertension, the most significant risk factor for the development of cardiovascular disease and a leading cause of stroke, renal failure, and cardiac failure, affects sixty million Americans. Most patients with hypertension are evaluated and managed in office practices; the focus of this chapter, therefore, is on the ambulatory patient with hypertension. However, because a substantial minority of patients with newly diagnosed or poorly controlled hypertension is seen in hospital, the last section is devoted to the management of hypertension in the hospitalized patient.

HYPERTENSION IN THE OFFICE PRACTICE SETTING

Evaluation

Patients with hypertension arrive at the internist's office by a variety of routes. They may be referred by surgical or subspecialty medical colleagues, or they may be referred from community or work-related hypertension screening programs. Increasingly, patients who are aware through media campaigns of the long-term complications of untreated hypertension refer themselves for evaluation of hypertension.

Confirming the Presence of Hypertension

The first step in evaluating the patient with suspected hypertension is confirmation of the diagnosis and appropriate follow-up of single measurements of elevated pressure. Blood pressure should be measured on a bared arm with the patient seated comfortably. Systolic and diastolic blood pressures should be recorded; a minimum of two measurements should be taken at each visit and the average recorded. A large-size cuff must be used in obese individuals. Although there has been some controversy over the validity of casual blood pressure measurements, there is good evidence to regard such pressure measurements as an accurate representation of a patient's true blood pressure and as an accurate prediction of hypertensive complications. We do not use 24-hour blood pressure recordings routinely.

In adults the diagnosis of hypertension usually is confirmed when the average of at least two diastolic blood pressures on a minimum of two visits is

90 mm Hg or higher, or when the average of two or more systolic blood pressures is greater than 140 mm Hg. In fact, the World Health Organization (WHO) recommends three elevated blood pressure recordings over a 4-week period before making the diagnosis of hypertension.[1] The 1984 Joint National Committee on Detection, Evaluation, and Treatment of High Blood Pressure categorization of blood pressure is described in Table 53–1.[2] Recommendations for follow-up of elevated blood pressures are presented in Table 53–2. Patients whose diastolic blood pressures on repeat measurement are less than 85 mm Hg should have a blood pressure measurement repeated in 2 years; if the diastolic blood pressure is between 85 and 90 mm Hg, the blood pressure measurement should be repeated in 1 year, or sooner if the patient has an increased risk of developing further blood pressure elevations. Among the risk factors are a family history of hypertension or cardiovascular disease, obesity, black race, use of medications known to elevate blood pressure, or excessive alcohol consumption. Patients whose diastolic blood pressures are noted to be greater than 90 mm Hg on a subsequent measurement should be evaluated promptly.

Evaluation of the Patient with Confirmed Diastolic Hypertension

Three questions must be answered in the patient with confirmed diastolic hypertension.

Does the patient have evidence of end-organ damage from hypertension? Does the patient have additional risk factors for the development of cardiovascular disease?

TABLE 53–1 Classification of Blood Pressure

Range (mm Hg)	Category
Diastolic	
<85	Normal BP
85–89	High normal BP
90–104	Mild hypertension
105–114	Moderate hypertension
>115	Severe hypertension
Systolic (when diastolic BP <90)	
<140	Normal
140–159	Borderline isolated systolic hypertension
>160	Isolated systolic hypertension

From the 1984 Report of the Joint National Committee. Detection, evaluation, and treatment of high blood pressure. Arch Intern Med 1984; 144:1045–1057.

TABLE 53-2   Recommended Follow-Up for a Single Blood Pressure Measurement

Blood Pressure (mm Hg)	Follow-Up
Diastolic	
90–104	Confirm within 2 months
105–114	Evaluate or refer for evaluation within 2 weeks
>115	Evaluate or refer for evaluation immediately
Systolic (when diastolic BP <90)	
140–199	Confirm within 2 months
>200	Evaluate or refer for evaluation immediately

Adapted from The 1984 Report of the Joint National Committee. Detection, evaluation, and treatment of high blood pressure. Arch Intern Med 1984; 144:1045–1057.

Does the patient have any evidence for reversible or secondary causes of hypertension?

More than 90 to 95 percent of patients with diastolic hypertension have primary, or essential, hypertension. A detailed medical history, physical examination, and a few judicious laboratory tests usually exclude or detect reversible or secondary causes of hypertension and also provide information to answer the first two questions.

The medical history should document any previous history of hypertension and its treatment, the severity and complications of hypertension (cardiovascular, renal, or cerebrovascular disease), and, as well, any history of other cardiovascular risk factors (obesity, smoking, hyperlipidemia, diabetes mellitus). Careful attention should be paid to clues to secondary hypertension. A careful drug history should be taken, since the leading cause of reversible hypertension is the use of medications, both prescription and over-the-counter. The physician should ask specifically about the use of oral contraceptive agents, nonsteroidal anti-inflammatory agents, corticosteroids, nasal and oral decongestants, diet pills, and tricyclic antidepressants. Other relatively important causes of secondary hypertension include renovascular disease, renal parenchymal disease, coarctation of the aorta, and primary hyperaldosteronism. Hypertension is more rarely caused by Cushing's syndrome, pheochromocytoma, hypothyroidism, or hyperthyroidism. The patient should be questioned carefully about sources of stress in the home or workplace, and a record made of personal habits such as diet, excess sodium intake, weight gain, and alcohol or recreational drug use, that might have an impact on hypertension.

Physical examination of the hypertensive patient should focus on the search for end-organ damage and for clues to the presence of secondary hypertension. The examination should include the patient's weight, an examination of the fundi for evidence of hypertensive vascular changes, a neurologic examination, a detailed examination of the heart and lungs, an examination of the thyroid gland for evidence of enlargement, an examination of the abdomen for renal enlargement or abdominal bruits, and a vascular examination for evidence of peripheral vascular disease and coarctation of the aorta. Observation for the signs of Cushing's syndrome, hypothyroidism, hyperthyroidism, and pheochromocytoma also should be carried out.

Laboratory examination of the hypertensive patient has three purposes: (1) to exclude some of the secondary causes of hypertension, (2) to establish the presence or absence of other cardiovascular risk factors, and (3) to establish baseline values of the patient's biochemical profile that might be affected by antihypertensive therapy. Controversy exists over the costs and benefits of diagnostic tests in the evaluation of the hypertensive patient, but we believe that hemoglobin, hematocrit, serum potassium, serum creatinine or BUN, serum uric acid, fasting blood glucose, total and high density lipoprotein (HDL) cholesterol should be measured; complete urinalysis should be performed and an electrocardiogram (ECG) should be obtained. Further diagnostic evaluation must be tailored by the findings of significant end-organ damage, other cardiovascular risk factors, or possible secondary causes of hypertension found on initial evaluation.

Treatment

Involving the Patient in the Goals of Therapy

Once the presence of essential hypertension has been confirmed, the next critical step in the management of hypertension is to involve the patient in his own care. Patients need careful, detailed explanations of the asymptomatic nature of most hypertension, the extent of their hypertension, and the risks associated with untreated hypertension. Involvement of the patient in making decisions regarding appropriate, convenient, and flexible schedules of treatment and follow-up for hypertension engages the patient as an ally in the long-term management of this asymptomatic chronic illness. Patients and physicians need constant reinforcement that the goal of therapy of hypertension is the reduction of the likelihood of serious cardiovascular disease by the reduction of elevated blood pressure while maintaining the patient's life and work as free of significant side effects of therapy as possible.

Asymptomatic patients often ask, "Why do I need my blood pressure lowered?" In patients with moderate diastolic blood pressure (DBP 105 to 114 mm Hg) or severe (DBP >115 mm Hg) hypertension, good evidence exists that drug therapy can reduce cardiovascular mortality and morbidity.[3,4] Controversy exists whether treatment of mild hypertension (DBP 90 to 104 mm Hg) does reduce the incidence of end-organ damage.[5] We believe that all patients with sustained diastolic blood pressure greater than 100 mm Hg should be treated; usually we will treat patients with diastolic blood pressure levels greater than 95 mm Hg if other risk factors are present. We will return to this issue later. We will first discuss nondrug treatment and, subsequently, drug treatment of sustained diastolic hypertension.

Nonpharmacologic Therapy of Hypertension

Nonpharmacologic therapy of hypertension is being used as sole treatment for mild hypertension and as an adjunct in patients who also take antihypertensive medications. A variety of biofeedback and relaxation techniques have been shown to have a moderate sustained effect in the reduction of blood pressure in patients with mild hypertension.[6] These modalities have been used as initial steps in the management of patients with mild hypertension and no evidence of end-organ damages; however, these patients require frequent monitoring to assess the extent of blood pressure reduction and to anticipate the need for drug therapy if hypertension accelerates.

Obese hypertensive patients have been shown to have significant reductions in blood pressure with weight loss (approximately 2.3 mm Hg decrease in DBP per kilogram lost) independent of sodium restriction, and regardless of whether ideal body weight is achieved.[7] Moderate salt restriction (2 to 4 g daily sodium intake) may reduce blood pressure in some hypertensive patients, but this is not a universal phenomenon. Patients need to be monitored on an individual basis to assess their response to sodium restriction.[8] Reduction of unsaturated fat in the diet may reduce cardiovascular risk by lowering serum cholesterol, but has no antihypertensive effect. Similarly, hypertensive patients should be advised to avoid smoking to reduce further the risk of cardiovascular disease. Heavy or excessive alcohol use increases blood pressure in hypertensive patients and should be avoided.[9]

Drug Therapy of Hypertension: Stepped Care

The ultimate goal of antihypertensive therapy is the prevention of cardiovascular morbidity and mortality; stroke, renal insufficiency, hypertensive cardiomyopathy, atherosclerotic cardiovascular diasease, and peripheral vascular disease. More specifically, the strategic goal of treatment is to lower the diastolic blood pressure to 90 mm Hg or less in the absence of side effects.

The fundamental approach in the drug therapy of hypertension in the last two decades has been the "stepped care" approach.[2] The following discussion outlines our approach to treating hypertension, based heavily on the stepped care approach despite recent controversy about it.

Step 1. Initial therapy for hypertension is low or moderate doses of a thiazide diuretic or a beta-blocker. Single drug therapy with beta-blockers (e.g., atenolol 50 to 100 mg daily) is indicated in patients with concomitant symptomatic coronary artery disease and appears more successful in patients under 50 years of age.[10] Thiazide diuretics in low or moderate doses (up to 50 mg per day of hydrochlorothiazide) are suitable for elderly patients, patients with asthma or peripheral vascular disease, patients of black races, and other patients with volume dependent hypertension.[11] Drug dosages should be increased over several weeks until the blood pressure goal is achieved, maximum drug dose is reached, or side effects occur. We are skeptical regarding the potentially adverse cardiac risk of hypokalemia from diuretics and continue to use these agents frequently as step 1 agents.

Step 2. If adequate blood pressure control is not achieved with single drug therapy, two therapeutic possibilities exist. First, diuretic and beta-blocker therapy can be combined. Second, another adrenergic-inhibiting agent can be added to either thiazide diuretics or beta-blockers. Most of the adrenergic-inhibiting agents yield similar antihypertensive effects, especially when given with a diuretic.

If blood pressure is not adequately controlled on these regimens, several questions must be asked before progressing to another step. A careful review must be made for other factors that can result in poor blood pressure control. The patient should be questioned about suitability of, understanding of, and compliance with the drug regimen; a detailed drug history should be taken to look for drugs that may aggravate hypertension (*vide supra*). Reassessment of compliance with nonpharmacologic measures, in terms of excess sodium intake, weight gain, and excessive alcohol use, should be made. Lastly, a detailed review should be made of causes of secondary hypertension that may have emerged or been overlooked. This is especially true of patients with essential hypertension and atherosclerotic vascular disease whose hypertension may become suddenly refractory to an established regimen because of acquired atherosclerotic renovascular disease.

Step 3. If none of these reversible problems is discovered, several options are available. If the patient's regimen includes a diuretic and a beta-blocker, the addition of modest doses of an angiotensin converting enzyme inhibitor (e.g., captopril 37.5 to 75 mg per day), a vasodilator such as hydralazine 50 to 100 mg per day, or another adrenergic inhibitor (e.g., methyl dopa, in doses up to 1,000 mg per day) may bring the blood pressure under control. If therapy with a beta-blocker is contraindicated, then a diuretic can be combined with high doses of either a centrally acting or peripherally acting adrenergic inhibitor or with high doses of an angiotensin converting enzyme inhibitor (e.g., captopril 75 to 150 mg per day or enalapril 20 to 40 mg per day).

Step 4. If these steps are unsuccessful at achieving adequate blood pressure control, and if secondary causes of hypertension have been excluded, potent vasodilators such as minoxidil, 10 to 40 mg per day, and guanethidine, up to 100 mg per day, should be added.

Newer Drugs in the Treatment of Hypertension

In recent years two new classes of drugs have become available as potential antihypertensive agents: the angiotensin converting enzyme inhibitors and the calcium-channel blockers. Captopril and enalapril, previously approved for use as afterload reducing agents and as antihypertensive agents for severe hypertension, has recently been approved for use as a first or second line drugs for the treatment of mild high blood pressure in patients with normal renal function. Diltiazem and nifedipine also are potent vasodilators with known antihypertensive effects and are available for first or second line therapy of hypertension.

Special Situations

Mild Hypertension

There is no question that aggressive therapy of hypertension in patients with a diastolic blood pressure of greater than 100 to 105 mm Hg results in reduced cardiovascular morbidity and mortality. Several studies of treatment of patients with blood pressures ranging from 90 to 104 mm Hg have been carried out. Three major studies—the Oslo study[12], the Australian Management Committee study[13], and the Hypertension Detection and Follow-up Program (HDFP) of the National Heart, Lung, and Blood Institute[14]—demonstrated a significant reduction in stroke, heart failure and ventricular hypertrophy, and aortic dissection. The HDFP study also showed a significant decrease in cardiovascular morbidity and mortality from ischemic cardiac events. These studies confirm a decreased mortality in treated patients over the age of 50 years and in patients with diastolic blood pressures ranging from 95 to 104 mm Hg. As stated earlier, we believe that mild hypertension (DBP 95 to 104 mm Hg) merits drug therapy, especially if the patient has any evidence of end-organ damage or additional risk factors for cardiovascular disease.

Controversy still exists over appropriate therapy for patients with diastolic blood pressures ranging from 90 to 94 mm Hg in whom nonpharmacologic therapy has not reduced blood pressure adequately. Young patients with blood pressures in this range may be committed to many years of therapy with diuretics or beta-blockers; in these patients the long-term side effects of raising serum lipid levels may outweigh the benefits of lowering the blood pressure. Many physicians postpone treating younger patients with mild hypertension with drug therapy, preferring to continue nonpharmacologic treatment and to monitor blood pressure at frequent intervals. Physicians who elect to do so should have a clear follow-up plan for these patients; they should be informed about the possibility that they may require active drug therapy in the future.

Isolated Systolic Hypertension

Isolated systolic hypertension, predominantly a disease of the elderly, is defined as a systolic blood pressure greater than 160 mm Hg with a diastolic blood pressure less than 90 mm Hg. In general, the risk of stroke and cardiovascular events is greater in patients with isolated systolic hypertension, but it has never been clearly established that treatment of isolated systolic hypertension decreases these risks.[15] There are no clear cut guidelines for the therapy of isolated systolic hypertension, and evaluation and treatment must be tailored to the individual patient. Secondary causes of isolated systolic hypertension, including anemia, thyrotoxicosis, aortic regurgitation, and high output congestive heart failure, should be specifically sought and excluded. If treatment is deemed appropriate, the goal of treatment is to reduce the systolic blood pressure by 10 percent without precipitating serious side effects, especially orthostatic hypotension. The initial treatment of choice is diuretic therapy (e.g., hydrochlorothiazide 25 mg daily) which is usually effective without major side effects. Centrally acting adrenergic inhibitors or hydralazine can be added if diuretic therapy alone is not effective. Meticulous attention must be paid to the avoidance of symptomatic orthostasis since baroreceptor sensitivity is diminished in the elderly; the significant risk of orthostatic syncope should be seriously considered before any elderly patient is placed on medical therapy for isolated systolic hypertension.

Hypertension in Pregnancy

Hypertension in pregnancy usually results either from worsening of preexisting hypertension or from preeclampsia. Multigravida women in their 30s, with preexisting chronic hypertension, frequently develop an exacerbation of their hypertension in the second and third trimesters of pregnancy. Antihypertensive medications should be continued during pregnancy; thiazide diuretics, methyldopa, and hydralazine all have been used safely and effectively in the management of established hypertension during pregnancy. Beta-blockers have been used in pregnancy, but may contribute to low birth weight;

angiotensin converting enzyme inhibitors, reported to cause fetal death in some animal species, are contraindicated during pregnancy.

The syndrome of preeclampsia—edema, proteinuria, and blood pressures of 140/90 mm Hg or higher—is seen most commonly in young primagravida women. All the findings resolve completely with delivery of the fetus. Treatment consists of bedrest and judicious antihypertensive therapy. Though there is controversy regarding the use of diuretics, we and others have used them successfully for years. Hypertensive crisis in eclampsia is best treated by prevention, i.e., good prenatal care. Acute hypertension in eclampsia with diastolic blood pressures greater than 110 mm Hg can be treated with intramuscular or intravenous hydralazine.

Hypertension in Patients with Renal Parenchymal Disease

Most patients with renal parenchymal disease, especially glomerular disease, and sufficient renal impairment to reduce glomerular filtration by 50 percent, develop hypertension. This hypertension is in part secondary to the inability of the kidney to excrete sodium and the resultant salt retention and volume expansion. Therefore, an important part of therapy of hypertension in patients with renal insufficiency is the use of potent loop diuretics such as furosemide and ethacrynic acid. Doses up to 500 mg per day may be required, but one must be careful not to produce volume depletion and worsening azotemia by the excessive use of diuretics. Vasodilators and adrenergic inhibiting agents are often required in addition to the diuretics. Thiazide diuretics are ineffective in patients with serum creatinines greater than 2 to 3 mg per deciliter. Further aggressive therapy of uncontrolled hypertension in patients with chronic renal impairment by the use of minoxidil, clonidine, and captopril is critical in the maintenance of residual renal function.

HYPERTENSION IN THE HOSPITALIZED PATIENT

Management of the Stable Hypertensive Patient Undergoing Surgery

The basic assessment of the stable hypertensive patient prior to routine surgery is similar to that already outlined. A detailed history, a physical examination, and a review of laboratory tests including an ECG should reveal any significant cardiac events that might increase the patient's risk of anesthetic complications. In general, patients with diastolic blood pressures less than 110 mm Hg whose hypertensive medications are continued through surgery tolerate routine surgery without complication. If the diastolic blood pressure is greater than 110 mm Hg, any nonemergent surgery should be postponed until the hypertension is controlled.

Perioperative management of antihypertensive medications deserves some attention. Medications such as guanethidine, guanadrel, and monoamine oxidase inhibitors used in the treatment of depression should be replaced by other agents several weeks prior to surgery. All the alpha-adrenergic inhibiting agents, if withdrawn suddenly, can result in rebound hypertension. Therefore, patients should be continued on these agents perioperatively and placed on parenteral forms of alpha-adrenergic inhibitors, such as intravenous methyldopa 250 mg three or four times a day, if the patient is unable to take medication orally. Beta-blockers can be continued safely through surgery and do not need to be discontinued or tapered perioperatively.

The goal of the perioperative management of hypertension is to attain and to maintain blood pressure at its preoperative level, rather than to achieve perfect control. The hospital environment and perioperative period is accompanied by numerous medications, stress, pain, and physiologic changes that make it nearly impossible to tailor a hypertensive regimen to patients and their lives outside the hospital. We are often consulted to recommend therapy for patients initially noted to be hypertensive in the postoperative period. If the patient has mild to moderate hypertension and no acute end-organ changes requiring immediate therapy, we prefer to see the patient in the office within a week or two after surgery and to begin the process of confirming and evaluating hypertension once the patient has returned to his usual work and surroundings.

Management of Hypertensive Emergencies

Hypertensive emergencies include dissecting aortic aneurysm, acute left ventricular failure with pulmonary edema, intracranial hemorrhage, hypertensive encephalopathy, hypertension accompanying acute cardiac ischemia, and toxemia of pregnancy. Accelerated or malignant range hypertension may occur without devastating end-organ damage, but acute management of the blood pressure is required to ready the patient for any emergency surgery.

Patients with hypertensive crisis should be managed in an intensive care unit so that the blood pressure can be reduced rapidly to closer to normal range. We believe that the treatment of choice is the administration of intravenous sodium nitropresside (50 to 100 mg in 500 ml 5 percent dextrose in water (D_5W) at a rate of 0.5 to 1.0 μg per kilogram per minute initially to a maximum of 10 μg per kilogram per minute) under carefully monitored conditions. Rapid reduction in blood pressure levels may also be achieved by the use of 10 to 20 mg of sublingual or oral nifedipine (or intramuscular hydralazine) in situations where continuous invasive monitoring is not available.

Patients with malignant hypertension who require rapid control of their blood pressure in order to undergo emergency surgery can be managed with intravenous nitroprusside or sublingual nifedipine. Parenteral hydralazine can be used for less severely ill patients, but should be avoided in patients with cardiac disease because of reflex tachycardia. Labetalol also can be used intravenously to reduce blood pressure acutely over a matter of hours. Esmolol, a new beta-blocker released for control of supraventricular tachycardia, has been used intraoperatively to control hypertension rapidly; its half-life is only 9 minutes.

References

1. Buhler FR, Doyle AE, Epstein FH, et al. Guidelines for the treatment of mild hypertension: memorandum from WHO/ISH meeting. Bull WHO 1983; 6:53–56.
2. The 1984 Report of the Joint National Committee on Detection, Evaluation, and Treatment of High Blood Pressure. Arch Intern Med 1984; 144:1045–1057.
3. Veterans Administration Cooperative Study Group on Antihypertensive Agents. Effects of treatment on morbidity in hypertension: I. Result in patients with diastolic blood pressures averaging 115 through 129 mm Hg. JAMA 1967; 202:1028–1034.
4. Veterans Administration Cooperative Study Group on Antihypertensive Agents. Effects of treatment on morbidity in hypertension: II. Results in patients with diastolic blood pressures averaging 90 through 114 mm Hg. JAMA 1970; 213:1143–1152.
5. Narins RG. Nephrology forum: mild hypertension: a therapeutic dilemma. Kidney Int 1984; 26:881–894.
6. Engel BT, Glasgow MS, Garader KR. Behavioral treatment of high blood pressure: III. Follow-up results and treatment recommendations. Psychosom Med 1983; 45:23–29.
7. Reisin E, Abel R, Medan M, et al. Effect of weight loss without salt restriction on the reduction of blood pressure in overweight hypertension patients. N Engl J Med 1978; 298:1–6.
8. MacGregor GA, Best F, Cani J, et al. Double-blind randomized crossover trial of moderate sodium restriction in essential hypertension. Lancet 1982; 1:351–355.
9. Klatsky AL. The relationship of alcohol and the cardiovascular system. Annu Rev Nutr 1982; 2:51–71.
10. Buhler FR, Burkart F, Lutold BE, et al. Antihypertensive beta-blocking action as related to renin and age; a pharmacologic tool to identify pathogenetic mechanisms in essential hypertension. Am J Cardiol 1975; 37:653–669.
11. Moser M, Lunn J. Comparative effects of pindolol and hydrochlorothiazide in black hypertensive patients. Angiology 1981; 32:561–566.
12. Helgelund A. Treatment of mild hypertension: a five year controlled drug trial. Am J Med 1980; 69:725–732.
13. The Management Committee. The Australian therapeutic trial in mild hypertension. Lancet 1980; 1:1261–1267.

14. Hypertension Detection and Follow-up Program Cooperative Group. Five year findings of the hypertension detection and follow-up program I. Reduction in mortality of persons with high blood pressure, including mild hypertension; II. Mortality by race, sex and age; III. Reduction in stroke incidence among persons with high blood pressure. JAMA 1979; 242:2561–2562; JAMA 1979; 242:2572–2577; JAMA 1982; 247:633–638.
15. Gifford RW Jr. Isolated systolic hypertension in the elderly. JAMA 1982; 247:781–785.

54 | MEDICAL NONCOMPLIANCE

JENNIFER DALEY, M.D.
JOHN T. HARRINGTON, M.D.

WORKING WITH THE NONCOMPLIANT PATIENT

All physicians have struggled with patients who have difficulty in following a prescribed medical regimen. Such patients fail to keep scheduled appointments, fail to follow through on referrals or consultations, or, most commonly, do not adhere to a dietary or drug regimen. In this chapter, we will define compliance and discuss how the physician can identify the noncompliant patient, the reasons why patients may be noncompliant, and techniques for assisting patients in adhering to prescribed regimens.

DEFINING MEDICAL COMPLIANCE

Medical compliance conventionally has been defined as the degree to which a patient's behavior coincides with medical advice. The prescribed behavior may be taking medications, following a diet or a recommended life style (e.g., quitting smoking), or keeping scheduled appointments for tests, consultations, or follow-up. Patients who do not adhere to such advice or prescribed medical regimens are termed "noncompliant".[1] Some authors and physicians prefer the term "adherence". Although the term noncompliance is best considered nonjudgmental with respect to who bears the responsibility for the patient's behavior, some authors and physicians object to use of the term noncompliance on the grounds that blame is thus placed on the patient for failure to adhere to prescribed medical regimens.[2] These writers believe that use of the term compliance implies a paternalistic and authoritarian relationship in which an imbalance of power between the doctor and the patient exists—the doctor assuming an omniscient and dictatorial role in the relationship, with the patient dutifully following the physician's orders. These authors also believe that use of the term noncompliance implies a lack of mutual respect in the doctor-patient relationship and suggest that the term adherence be used in its stead. In this chapter we will use the terms compliance and adherence interchangeably.

A discussion of compliance does involve analyzing every aspect of the doctor-patient relationship that bears on the patient's ability to cooperate with the prescribed medical regimen. To achieve the optimal patient outcome, the ideal physician-patient relationship is one in which both the physician and the patient consent to a mutually agreed-upon plan that addresses the active medical problems. In the face of noncompliant behavior, both physician and patient ideally will avoid blaming each other and will take mutual responsibility for devising a suitable plan. Too often the search for the causes of noncompliance focuses exclusively on the patient and does not take adequate account of the physician's role in contributing to noncompliance.

In addition to assuring the appropriate diagnosis and treatment of the patient, the physician has responsibilities in the physician-patient relationship that bear directly on patient compliance. Patient compliance is best achieved in a physician-patient relationship of mutual understanding and cooperation. Authoritarian physicians competing for power and control over patients directly undermine the mutual understanding and consent that is vital to a successful patient-doctor relationship. Authoritarian physicians and passive patients who see themselves as "following doctor's orders" without an adequate understanding of the goals and purposes of their own medical therapy set the stage for noncompliance. The successful physician-patient relationship has the patient actively involved in his or her care, with both physician and patient having a mutual understanding of the goals of care. Therefore, when confronted with a noncompliant patient, the physician first must be sure a paternalistic or authoritarian attitude has not contributed to a passive and noncompliant patient.

NONCOMPLIANCE: ITS FORMS AND QUANTITATIVE ASPECTS

The busy clinician, even if familiar with the problem of noncompliance, often is not aware of its myriad forms and of how common the problem is (Table 54–1). A number of careful studies have provided solid quantitative data regarding the magnitude of the problem of noncompliance. Some patients manifest noncompliance by delaying to obtain appropriate medical care, while others fail to appear for scheduled appointments. The patient may either not keep scheduled appointments with his or her own physician or not follow through on referrals recommended by the primary physician. Medical appointments initiated by physicians for preventive care are kept only about one-half the time, while medical appointments initiated by patients are kept about 75 percent of the time. Patients comply about 75 percent of the time with a regimen of 2 weeks or less of medication prescribed for an illness such as a urinary tract infection, pneumonia, or streptococcal sore throat.[3,4] Patients who receive short courses of medication or immunization for preventive care successfully complete the entire course of treatment only 60 percent of the time. Compliance with long-term medication regimens for either prevention or cure is about 50 percent, regardless of the condition under treatment or the population studied. Patients' compliance with dietary regimens (e.g., weight reduction, low cholesterol diet, hemodialysis diets) varies from 30 to 70 percent, while patients' cooperation with preventive health regimens, such as seatbelt use and smoking cessation, varies from 15 to 30 percent in numerous studies.[5] Given the results of all these studies, understanding and increasing patient compliance is clearly an important aspect of *every* patient's care.

FACTORS AFFECTING MEDICAL COMPLIANCE

Studies of factors that affect medical compliance have focused on the kind of illness, severity, complexity of the drug regimen, and appointment keeping. Most studies demonstrate little or no correlation between most diseases and compliance. However, patients with major psychiatric illness or dementia have been demonstrated to have poorer medical compliance with prescribed regimens than patients who do not suffer these illness.[6] In most cases, disease

TABLE 54–1 Forms of Medical Noncompliance

Appointment Noncompliance

  Not keeping a scheduled appointment for preventive care (e.g., visit for Pap smear, breast examination, immunization, periodic health examination)

  Not keeping a scheduled appointment for treatment diagnosis (e.g., referral to specialist for evaluation, follow-up visit for management of hypertension or diabetes)

  Delay in seeking appropriate medical care

Medication Noncompliance

  Failure to complete treatment course for short-term acute illness (e.g., streptococcal pharyngitis, urinary tract infection)

  Failure to maintain treatment regimen for long-term prevention (e.g., antihypertensive drugs)

  Failure to maintain treatment regimen for long-term treatment (e.g., diabetic, cardiac, or antituberculous treatment)

Noncompliance with Dietary and Preventive Measures

  Failure to adhere to recommended diet (e.g., ADA diet, weight loss, low sodium diet)

  Nonadherence to preventive measures (e.g., smoking cessation, safety measures such as seat belt use)

severity also has no relation to patient compliance with medical regimens. For most diseases, an increase in the severity of symptoms does not increase compliance. Significantly, however, as patients' levels of disability increase from chronic diseases, their compliance with medical regimens does increase.[7] For example, renal transplant recipients follow their complex drug regimens in over 90 percent of instances. It is unclear whether the increased compliance in these conditions is related to increased medical supervision for extremely ill patients or whether the patient simply has a greater motivation to comply with medical regimen. Ironically, patients who initially comply with medical regimens and who experience rapid clinical improvement early in the course of treatment subsequently have lower compliance rates completing the regimen.

Several interesting findings appear when the characteristics of drug medication regimens are analyzed for their relation to patient compliance. Obviously, medications that are given by injection or by infusion require direct medical supervision, and therefore compliance rates are higher. Unfortunately, many medications used in the long-term treatment of chronic illness are not amenable to parenteral administration. Compliance with different types of oral medications is extraordinarily variable. Patients tend to have higher compliance rates for cardiac drugs, antihypertensive agents, and diabetic drugs than they do for drugs administered for symptomatic improvement, such as antihistamines, analgesics, and antacids.[8,9] The longer a drug is prescribed, the lower the compliance rate. Clearly established also is that the greater the number of medications prescribed and the more frequently patients are required to take medications the less likely they are to comply.[10] Curiously, patients who are asked to take higher doses of individual medications seem to be more compliant with the regimen.

The impact of significant side effects of drugs on medical compliance is unclear. Some patients persist in taking medications despite serious side effects, while others may cease taking medication even in the absence of significant side effects. The cost of medication can be a significant barrier to patient compliance, especially in patients who take multiple medications over long periods of time. Obviously, patients who lack the financial resources or the medical insurance coverage to afford expensive medications are much less likely to comply with the prescribed regimen.

Several factors affect patients' behaviors with regard to keeping scheduled appointments and following through on referrals made by their primary physician. Patients referred to other clinicians for consultation or treatment are much less likely to follow through on the referral if a long period of time (more than 2 weeks) elapses between the time the appointment is made and the actual referral appointment. Patients referred from screening programs are much less likely to attend a follow-up appointment than those who are either self-referred or referred from specific physicians. In addition, patients referred from one physician to another are much more likely to attend the referral appointment if they have been referred to a specific physician, rather than to a general group practice or clinic setting. In office practice, patients are more likely to attend a scheduled appointment if they are given a specific appointment time and if they know that they will see a specific physician. Patients who have been kept waiting longer than 15 to 30 minutes at previous appointments are less likely to attend their next scheduled office visit.[11]

DETECTING MEDICAL NONCOMPLIANCE

Physicians are poor predictors of whether their patients will follow a prescribed medication regimen or will appear for scheduled office visits. In this section, we discuss some of the ways physicians can more readily detect noncompliance in the office setting (Table 54–2). The detection of patients who do not comply with scheduled return visits or referrals is relatively easy, provided that the physician has a practical and convenient means of recording office visits, cancellations, and "no shows", as well as a way of tracking patients who have been referred to other physicians for consultation.

On the other hand, the detection of patients who are noncompliant with medication regimens is more difficult. Many physicians use the presence of the desired outcome (e.g., lowered blood pressure in hypertensive patients) as evidence that the patient has been compliant with a prescribed regimen. Unfortunately, the relationship between therapeutic outcome and compliance is often confounded by other factors that are not related to compliance. For example, the hypertensive patient's blood pressure may return towards normal as a result of the physician's reassurance or of the interaction of multiple medications, rather than from compliance with a particular medication. Some

TABLE 54–2 Methods of Detecting Medical Noncompliance

Appointment Noncompliance
    Record cancellations and "no shows" in the office
    Keep a "tickle file" of patients scheduled for visits for preventive care
    Keep a record of patients referred for consultations with other physicians

Medication Noncompliance
    Take a detailed medication history at each visit and ask about patient's
        adherence
    Review medication diaries
    Medication monitoring (pill counts)
    Measure drug and drug metabolite levels where possible

patients who are noncompliant readily report their failure to follow a medical regimen, and there is some evidence to suggest that those patients who do admit to noncompliance are more amenable to strategies to improve their compliance. Another technique for assessing medication compliance is by means of pill counting. Pill counts at regular intervals and the provision of regular pill dispensers to patients may help to improve compliance. Physicians who initiate pill counts with patients should do so in a nonjudgmental and supportive environment and should be aware that pill counts may overestimate pill use. Compliance with common medications measured by pill count may be confounded by the use of these medications by other family members and by patients who knowingly discard medication prior to pill counts in order to appear compliant. One can also determine if the patient has had a prescription filled, but obviously there is no guarantee that the patient has taken the medication, even if the prescription has been filled.

More direct measures of assessing medication compliance include measurements of drug or drug metabolite levels in blood and urine. The unavailability of accurate, inexpensive, and readily available drug and metabolite assays for all the medications commonly used limits this technique. The clinician must also have an adequate appreciation of the pharmacokinetics of the medications being taken by the patient as well as of biologic variation among patients. Failure to appreciate these aspects of direct measurement of drug and metabolite levels in blood and urine may lead the physician to conclude falsely that a patient is noncompliant with the medical regimen.

TECHNIQUES FOR IMPROVING PATIENT COMPLIANCE

Several techniques have been identified for improving patients' compliance. In patients being treated acutely for a self-limited illness, the importance of explicit verbal instructions to the patient, accompanied by detailed written instructions, cannot be overemphasized. The physician should make every effort to determine if the regimen prescribed is consistent with the patient's work, homelife, and daily rituals. For example, patients for whom drugs are prescribed three times a day with meals may be noncompliant if the patient is accustomed to eating only two meals a day. Short course medications (10 days or less) that can be administered parenterally may be preferable to oral medications. Special packaging or oral medications (pill packs) that remind the patient of the dosing regimen and the duration of administration can be extremely helpful in facilitating patient compliance. Written instructions should be accompanied by date reminders or pill calendars that instruct patients in drug administration. Telephone follow-up by office personnel, by allied health professionals, or by the physician also facilitate patient compliance with short-term medication regimens.

Compliance with long-term medical regimens for chronic illnesses is more difficult to achieve. An effective means of assuring higher patient compliance in these cases is to increase the frequency of office visits, home visits, or telephone monitoring. Patient education regarding the name, the dosing regimen, and the purpose of medications may be helpful in encouraging patients to comply with their medical regimen, but this by no means guarantees compliance. As noted earlier, drug levels of medications amenable to measurement by laboratory tests, such as digoxin and cardiac antiarrhythmics, can be followed as a good indicator of patient compliance. Unfortunately, few of the medications commonly used in practice for the treatment of chronic conditions or long-term prevention are available in parenteral forms amenable to use in office practice on a routine basis. Ongoing areas of research in biomedical engineering may provide for long-term administration of drugs by subcutaneous depot; currently, however, these techniques are only experimental. Transcutaneous administration of medications (e.g., long-acting nitrates) also may increase patient compliance, but no solid data to substantiate this possibility yet exist. The use of pill-dispensing packages or packs has limited usefulness in the treatment of long-term chronic illness, but such pill packs may become more widely available in the future. The critical ingredient in assuring patient compliance remains ongoing physician supervision.

Many physicians in office practice commonly assume that patients who initially are compliant with medical regimens will continue to be compliant. Evidence shows that patients on long-term medication regimens become less compliant as time goes on. Therefore, an important part of every office visit is reevaluation of the patient's compliance with already instituted medical regimens. The patient should be instructed to bring all medications at each office visit. A brief review of factors that may precipitate noncompliance should be included as part of each visit. First, a careful history should be taken to determine if side effects from the medical regimen have developed; physicians must carefully question patients about the development of medication side effects that might otherwise not have been noted by the patient (e.g., new onset of sleep disturbances or sedation). The physician should inquire whether family members are supportive of the patient's continuation of the medical regimen, and should be aware of the possibility that any disruption in the patient's social, working, or family life may contribute to noncompliance. Increasing depression in patients requiring chronic medical regimens may contribute to lack of adherence to the regimen. The physician must consider whether the increasingly noncompliant patient may have lost faith in the physician. Finally, in patients with multiple chronic illnesses, with terminal illness, or with complaints that do not yield easily to medical explanation, the physician must be aware of any overt or subconscious message that the patient feels the physician has given up on alleviating the suffering, symptoms, and cause of the patient's illness.

The easiest way to begin helping patients who are noncompliant is to increase the frequency of supervision. Office visits to either the physician or allied health personnel can be increased; these visits need not and should not be long, but should provide the patient with an opportunity to review their medication regimen and to ask questions about any problems with the regimen or side effects they are experiencing. Sometimes, regular telephone contact with patients can alleviate their anxiety and improve medical compliance. Another successful method is to institute goals to achieve between visits and to have the patient identify factors that interfere with compliance. At the next office visit, the physician and the patient can mutually solve problems to improve compliance. Other helpful strategies include the modification of a patient's regimen to a less frequent dosing schedule, a decrease in the total number of pills taken, and the tailoring of the medication regimen to the work, dietary, and sleeping habits of the patient.

Patients living either alone or in unsupportive, disruptive social situations may require the assistance of other health professionals to achieve compliance. The physician should refer such patients to social service agencies, visiting nurse associations, and other home care agencies to assist in both assessing and ensuring compliance with medical regimens. Allied office personnel such as nurse practitioners, physician assistants, and office medical technicians often can be helpful to support patients in the continuation of their prescribed medical regimen. In patients with known or suspected psychiatric disease, with depression, or with organic brain syndrome with increasing dementia, the physician may require evaluation and assistance from mental health professionals as well as from social service agencies to ensure adequate patient supervision. In the case of patients with tuberculosis and some sexually transmitted diseases, the physician may seek the assistance of public health agencies to achieve compliance. Many industries now have available occupational health programs that may reinforce and encourage patients through the workplace to comply with therapeutic and preventive medical regimens.

Several techniques are available to increase patient compliance with attending scheduled office visits and following through on referrals. As noted previously, a short time between the initiation of a referral and the actual appointment date is the greatest inducement to patient compliance in accepting referrals. Other effective techniques include writing letters to the patient and following up with telephone calls, as well as facilitating the patient's arrival at unfamiliar destinations. In addition to efficient and timely sheduling of office visits, both mail and telephone reminders have been shown to be effective in improving patient attendance at scheduled office visits. It should be noted that patients are more apt to attend an office visit that they themselves scheduled. Appointments initiated by the physician for preventive checkups or follow-up visits are much more frequently complied with if the patient receives an additional mail or telephone reminder. Mailed reminders have shown no distinct advantage over telephone reminders; whichever technique appears most practical and cost effective within the context of an individual physician's office practice is advisable. We believe that attention to the details and techniques we have discussed will improve the patient-doctor relationship overall and will enhance adherence to a prescribed medical regimen.

References

1. Haynes RB, Taylor DW, Sackett DL, eds. Compliance in health care. Baltimore: The Johns Hopkins University Press, 1979:1.
2. Shiel RC, Baker JA. Resolving noncompliance in patient care. J Manipulative Physiol Ther 1983; 6(1):37-40.
3. Bergman AB, Werner RJ. Failure of children to receive penicillin by mouth. N Engl J Med 1963; 268:1334-1338.
4. Mushlin AI, Appel FA. Diagnosing patient non-compliance. Arch Int Med 1977; 137:318-321.
5. Sackett DL, Snow JC. The magnitude of compliance and noncompliance. In: Haynes RB, Taylor DW, Sackett DL, eds. Compliance in health care. Baltimore: The Johns Hopkins University Press, 1979:11.
6. Blackwell B. Treatment compliance. In: Grast JH, Jefferson JW, Spitzer RL, eds. Treatment of mental disorders. Oxford: Oxford University Press, 1982.
7. Donabedian A, Rosenfeld LS. Follow-up study of chronically ill patients discharged from the hospital. J Chronic Dis 1964; 17:847-862.
8. Hemmuniki E, Heskkila J. Elderly peoples' compliance with prescriptions and quality of medication. Scand J Soc Med 1975; 3:87-92.
9. Hulka BS, Kupper LL, Cassel JC, Efird R, Burdette J. Medication use and misuse: physician-patient discrepancies. J Chronic Dis 1975; 28:7-21.
10. Hulka BS, Cassel JC, Kupper LL. Communication, compliance and concordance between physicians and patients with prescribed medications. Am J Public Health 1976; 66:847-853.
11. Haynes RB. Determinants of compliance: the disease and the mechanics of treatment. In: Haynes RB, Taylor DW, Sackett DL, eds. Compliance in health care. Baltimore: The Johns Hopkins University Press, 1979:49.

INDEX

Lotensin®
benazepril hydrochloride

Tablets

Prescribing Information

> **Use in Pregnancy**
> When used in pregnancy during the second and third trimesters, ACE inhibitors can cause injury and even death to the developing fetus. When pregnancy is detected, Lotensin should be discontinued as soon as possible. See WARNINGS, Fetal/Neonatal Morbidity and Mortality.

DESCRIPTION

Benazepril hydrochloride is a white to off-white crystalline powder, soluble (>100 mg/mL) in water, in ethanol, and in methanol. Benazepril's chemical name is 3-[[1-(ethoxy-carbonyl)-3-phenyl-(1S)-propyl]amino]-2,3,4,5-tetrahydro-2-oxo-1H-1-(3 S)-benzazepine-1-acetic acid monohydrochloride; its structural formula is:

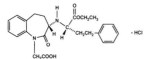

Its empirical formula is $C_{24}H_{28}N_2O_5 \bullet HCl$, and its molecular weight is 460.96.

Benazeprilat, the active metabolite of benazepril, is a non-sulfhydryl angiotensin-converting enzyme inhibitor. Benazepril is converted to benazeprilat by hepatic cleavage of the ester group.

Lotensin is supplied as tablets containing 5 mg,10 mg, 20 mg, and 40 mg of benazepril for oral administration. The inactive ingredients are cellulose compounds, colloidal silicon dioxide, crospovidone, hydrogenated castor oil (5-mg, 10-mg, and 20-mg tablets), iron oxides, lactose, magnesium stearate (40-mg tablets), polysorbate 80, propylene glycol (5-mg and 40-mg tablets), starch, talc, and titanium dioxide.

CLINICAL PHARMACOLOGY
Mechanism of Action

Benazepril and benazeprilat inhibit angiotensin-converting enzyme (ACE) in human subjects and animals. ACE is a peptidyl dipeptidase that catalyzes the conversion of angiotensin I to the vasoconstrictor substance, angiotensin II. Angiotensin II also stimulates aldosterone secretion by the adrenal cortex.

Inhibition of ACE results in decreased plasma angiotensin II, which leads to decreased vasopressor activity and to decreased aldosterone secretion. The latter decrease may result in a small increase of serum potassium. Hypertensive patients treated with Lotensin alone for up to 52 weeks had elevations of serum potassium of up to 0.2 mEq/L. Similar patients treated with Lotensin and hydrochlorothiazide for up to 24 weeks had no consistent changes in their serum potassium (see PRECAUTIONS).

Removal of angiotensin II negative feedback on renin secretion leads to increased plasma renin activity. In animal studies, benazepril had no inhibitory effect on the vasopressor response to angiotensin II and did not interfere with the hemodynamic effects of the autonomic neurotransmitters acetylcholine, epinephrine, and norepinephrine.

ACE is identical to kininase, an enzyme that degrades bradykinin. Whether increased levels of bradykinin, a potent vasodepressor peptide, play a role in the therapeutic effects of Lotensin remains to be elucidated.

While the mechanism through which benazepril lowers blood pressure is believed to be primarily suppression of the renin-angiotensin-aldosterone system, benazepril has an antihypertensive effect even in patients with low-renin hypertension. In particular, Lotensin was antihypertensive in all races studied, although it was somewhat less effective in blacks than in nonblacks.

Pharmacokinetics and Metabolism

Following oral administration of Lotensin, peak plasma concentrations of benazepril are reached within 0.5-1.0 hours. The extent of absorption is at least 37% as determined by urinary recovery and is not significantly influenced by the presence of food in the GI tract.

Cleavage of the ester group (primarily in the liver) converts benazepril to its active metabolite, benazeprilat. Peak plasma concentrations of benazeprilat are reached 1-2 hours after drug intake in the fasting state and 2-4 hours after drug intake in the nonfasting state. The serum protein binding of benazepril is about 96.7% and that of benazeprilat about 95.3%, as measured by equilibrium dialysis; on the basis of in vitro studies, the degree of protein binding should be unaffected by age, hepatic dysfunction, or concentration (over the concentration range of 0.24-23.6 μmol/L).

Benazepril is almost completely metabolized to benazeprilat, which has much greater ACE inhibitory activity than benazepril, and to the glucuronide conjugates of benazepril and benazeprilat. Only trace amounts of an administered dose of Lotensin can be recovered in the urine as unchanged benazepril, while about 20% of the dose is excreted as benazepril, 4% as benazepril glucuronide, and 8% as benazeprilat glucuronide.

The kinetics of benazepril are approximately dose-proportional within the dosage range of 10-80 mg.

The effective half-life of accumulation of benazeprilat following multiple dosing of benazepril hydrochloride is 10-11 hours. Thus, steady-state concentrations of benazeprilat should be reached after 2 or 3 doses of benazepril hydrochloride given once daily.

The kinetics did not change, and there was no significant accumulation during chronic administration (28 days) of once-daily doses between 5 mg and 20 mg. Accumulation ratios based on AUC and urinary recovery of benazeprilat were 1.19 and 1.27, respectively.

When dialysis was started two hours after ingestion of 10 mg of benazepril, approximately 6% of benazeprilat was removed in 4 hours of dialysis. The parent compound, benazepril, was not detected in the dialysate.

The disposition of benazepril and benazeprilat in patients with mild-to-moderate renal insufficiency (creatinine clearance >30 mL/min) is similar to that in patients with normal renal function. In patients with creatinine clearance ≤30 mL/min, peak benazeprilat levels and the initial (alpha phase) half-life increase, and time to steady-state may be delayed (see DOSAGE AND ADMINISTRATION).

Benazepril and benazeprilat are cleared predominantly by renal excretion in healthy subjects with normal renal function. Nonrenal (i.e., biliary) excretion accounts for approximately 11-12% of benazeprilat excretion in healthy subjects. In patients with renal failure, biliary clearance may compensate to an extent for deficient renal clearance.

In patients with hepatic dysfunction due to cirrhosis, levels of benazeprilat are essentially unaltered. The pharmacokinetics of benazepril and benazeprilat do not appear to be influenced by age.

In studies in rats given[14]C-benazepril, benazepril and its metabolites crossed the blood-brain barrier only to an extremely low extent. Multiple doses of benazepril did not result in accumulation in any tissue except the lung, where, as with other ACE inhibitors in similar studies, there was a slight increase in concentration due to slow elimination in that organ.

Some placental passage occurred when the drug was administered to pregnant rats.

Pharmacodynamics

Single and multiple doses of 10 mg or more of Lotensin cause inhibition of plasma ACE activity by at least 80-90% for at least 24 hours after dosing. Pressor responses to exogenous angiotensin I were inhibited by 60-90% (up to 4 hours post-dose) at the 10 mg dose.

Administration of Lotensin to patients with mild-to-moderate hypertension results in a reduction of both supine and standing blood pressure to about the same extent with no compensatory tachycardia. Symptomatic postural hypotension is infrequent, although it can occur in patients who are salt- and/or volume-depleted (see **WARNINGS**).

In single-dose studies, Lotensin lowered blood pressure within 1 hour, with peak reductions achieved 2-4 hours after dosing. The antihypertensive effect of a single dose persisted for 24 hours. In multiple dose studies, once-daily doses of 20-80 mg decreased seated pressure (systolic/diastolic) 24 hours after dosing by about 6 -12 /4-7 mmHg. The trough values represent reductions of about 50% of that seen at peak.

Four dose-response studies using once-daily dosing were conducted in 470 mild-to-moderate hypertensive patients not using diuretics. The minimal effective once-daily dose of Lotensin was 10 mg; but further falls in blood pressure, especially at morning trough, were seen with higher doses in the studied dosing range (10-80 mg). In studies comparing the same daily dose of Lotensin given as a single morning dose or as a twice-daily dose, blood pressure reductions at the time of morning trough blood levels were greater with the divided regimen.

During chronic therapy, the maximum reduction in blood pressure with any dose is generally achieved after 1-2 weeks. The antihypertensive effects of Lotensin have continued during therapy for at least two years. Abrupt withdrawal of Lotensin has not been associated with a rapid increase in blood pressure.

In patients with mild-to-moderate hypertension, Lotensin 10-20 mg was similar in effectiveness to captopril, hydrochlorothiazide, nifedipine SR, and propranolol.

The antihypertensive effects of Lotensin were not appreciably different in patients receiving high- or low-sodium diets.

In hemodynamic studies in dogs, blood pressure reduction was accompanied by a reduction in peripheral arterial resistance, with an increase in cardiac output and renal blood flow and little or no change in heart rate. In normal human volunteers, single doses of benazepril caused an increase in renal blood flow but had no effect on glomerular filtration rate.

Use of Lotensin in combination with thiazide diuretics gives a blood-pressure-lowering effect greater than that seen with either agent alone. By blocking the renin-angiotensin-aldosterone axis, administration of Lotensin tends to reduce the potassium loss associated with the diuretic.

INDICATIONS AND USAGE

Lotensin is indicated for the treatment of hypertension. It may be used alone or in combination with thiazide diuretics.

In using Lotensin, consideration should be given to the fact that another angiotensin-converting enzyme inhibitor, captopril, has caused agranulocytosis, particularly in patients with renal impairment or collagen-vascular disease. Available data are insufficient to show that Lotensin does not have a similar risk (see **WARNINGS**).

CONTRAINDICATIONS

Lotensin is contraindicated in patients who are hypersensitive to this product or to any other ACE inhibitor.

WARNINGS

Angioedema

Angioedema of the face, extremities, lips, tongue, glottis, and larynx has been reported in patients treated with angiotensin-converting enzyme inhibitors. In U.S. clinical trials, symptoms consistent with angioedema were seen in none of the subjects who received placebo and in about 0.5% of the subjects who received Lotensin. Angioedema associated with laryngeal edema can be fatal. If laryngeal stridor or angioedema of the face, tongue, or glottis occurs, treatment with Lotensin should be discontinued and appropriate therapy instituted immediately. **Where there is involvement of the tongue, glottis, or larynx, likely to cause airway obstruction, appropriate therapy, e.g., subcutaneous epinephrine injection 1:1000 (0.3 mL to 0.5 mL) should be promptly administered (see ADVERSE REACTIONS).**

Hypotension

Lotensin can cause symptomatic hypotension. Like other ACE inhibitors, benazepril has been only rarely associated with hypotension in uncomplicated hypertensive patients. Symptomatic hypotension is most likely to occur in patients who have been volume- and/or salt-depleted as a result of prolonged diuretic therapy, dietary salt restriction, dialysis, diarrhea, or vomiting. Volume- and/or salt-depletion should be corrected before initiating therapy with Lotensin.

In patients with congestive heart failure, with or without associated renal insufficiency, ACE inhibitor therapy may cause excessive hypotension, which may be associated with oliguria or azotemia and, rarely, with acute renal failure and death. In such patients, Lotensin therapy should be started under close medical supervision; they should be followed closely for the first 2 weeks of treatment and whenever the dose of benazepril or diuretic is increased.

If hypotension occurs, the patient should be placed in a supine position, and, if necessary, treated with intravenous infusion of physiological saline. Lotensin treatment usually can be continued following restoration of blood pressure and volume.

Neutropenia/Agranulocytosis

Another angiotensin-converting enzyme inhibitor, captopril, has been shown to cause agranulocytosis and bone marrow depression, rarely in uncomplicated patients, but more frequently in patients with renal impairment, especially if they also have a collagen-vascular disease such as systemic lupus erythematosus or scleroderma. Available data from clinical trials of benazepril are insufficient to show that benazepril does not cause agranulocytosis at similar rates. Monitoring of white blood cell counts should be considered in patients with collagen-vascular disease, especially if the disease is associated with impaired renal function.

Fetal/Neonatal Morbidity and Mortality

ACE inhibitors can cause fetal and neonatal morbidity and death when administered to pregnant women. Several dozen cases have been reported in the world literature. When pregnancy is detected, ACE inhibitors should be discontinued as soon as possible.

The use of ACE inhibitors during the second and third trimesters of pregnancy has been associated with fetal and neonatal injury, including hypotension, neonatal skull hypoplasia, anuria, reversible or irreversible renal failure, and death. Oligohydramnios has also been reported, presumably resulting from decreased fetal renal function; oligohydramnios in this setting has been associated with fetal limb contractures, craniofacial deformation, and hypoplastic lung development. Prematurity, intrauterine growth retardation, and patent ductus arteriosus have also been reported, although it is not clear whether these occurrences were due to the ACE inhibitor exposure.

These adverse effects do not appear to have resulted from intrauterine ACE inhibitor exposure that has been limited to the first trimester. Mothers whose embryos and fetuses are exposed to ACE inhibitors only during the first trimester should be so informed. Nonetheless, when patients become pregnant, physicians should make every effort to discontinue the use of benazepril as soon as possible.

Rarely (probably less often than once in every thousand pregnancies), no alternative to ACE inhibitors will be found. In these rare cases, the mothers should be apprised of the potential hazards to their fetuses, and serial ultrasound examinations should be performed to assess the intraamniotic environment.

If oligohydramnios is observed, benazepril should be discontinued unless it is considered life-saving for the mother. Contraction stress testing (CST), a nonstress test (NST), or biophysical profiling (BPP) may be appropriate, depending upon the week of pregnancy. Patients and physicians should be aware, however, that oligohydramnios may not appear until after the fetus has sustained irreversible injury.

Infants with histories of *in utero* exposure to ACE inhibitors should be closely observed for hypotension, oliguria, and hyperkalemia. If oliguria occurs, attention should be directed toward support of blood pressure and renal perfusion. Exchange transfusion or dialysis may be required as means of reversing hypotension and/or substituting for disordered renal function. Benazepril, which crosses the placenta, can theoretically be removed from the neonatal circulation by these means; there are occasional reports of benefit from these maneuvers with another ACE inhibitor, but experience is limited.

No teratogenic effects of Lotensin were seen in studies of pregnant rats, mice, and rabbits. On a mg/m² basis, the doses used in these studies were 60 times (in rats), 9 times (in mice), and more than 0.8 times (in rabbits) the maximum recommended human dose (assuming a 50 kg woman). On a mg/kg basis these multiples are 300 times (in rats), 90 times (in mice) and more than 3 times (in rabbits) the maximum recommended human dose.

PRECAUTIONS
General
Impaired Renal Function: As a consequence of inhibiting the renin-angiotensin-aldosterone system, changes in renal function may be anticipated in susceptible individuals. In patients with severe congestive heart failure whose renal function may depend on the activity of the renin-angiotensin-aldosterone system, treatment with angiotensin-converting enzyme inhibitors, including Lotensin, may be associated with oliguria and/or progressive azotemia and (rarely) with acute renal failure and/or death. In a small study of hypertensive patients with renal artery stenosis in a solitary kidney or bilateral renal artery stenosis, treatment with Lotensin was associated with increases in blood urea nitrogen and serum creatinine; these increases were reversible upon discontinuation of Lotensin or diuretic therapy, or both. When such patients are treated with ACE inhibitors, renal function should be monitored during the first few weeks of therapy. Some hypertensive patients with no apparent preexisting renal vascular disease have developed increases in blood urea nitrogen and serum creatinine, usually minor and transient, especially when Lotensin has been given concomitantly with a diuretic. This is more likely to occur in patients with preexisting renal impairment. Dosage reduction of Lotensin and/or discontinuation of the diuretic may be required. **Evaluation of the hypertensive patient should always include assessment of renal function (see DOSAGE AND ADMINISTRATION).**

Hyperkalemia: In clinical trials, hyperkalemia (serum potassium at least 0.5 mEq/L greater than the upper limit of normal) occurred in approximately 1% of hypertensive patients receiving Lotensin. In most cases, these were isolated values which resolved despite continued therapy. Risk factors for the development of hyperkalemia include renal insufficiency, diabetes mellitus, and the concomitant use of potassium-sparing diuretics, potassium supplements, and/or potassium-containing salt substitutes, which should be used cautiously, if at all, with Lotensin (see **Drug Interactions**).

Cough: Cough has been reported with the use of ACE inhibitors. Characteristically, the cough is nonproductive, persistent, and resolves after discontinuation of therapy. ACE inhibitor-induced cough should be considered as part of the differential diagnosis of cough.

Impaired Liver Function: In patients with hepatic dysfunction due to cirrhosis, levels of benazeprilat are essentially unaltered.

Surgery/Anesthesia: In patients undergoing surgery or during anesthesia with agents that produce hypotension, benazepril will block the angiotensin II formation that could otherwise occur secondary to compensatory renin release. Hypotension that occurs as a result of this mechanism can be corrected by volume expansion.
Information for Patients
Pregnancy: Female patients of childbearing age should be told about the consequences of second- and third-trimester exposure to ACE inhibitors, and they should also be told that these consequences do not appear to have resulted from intrauterine ACE inhibitor exposure that has been limited to the first trimester. These patients should be asked to report pregnancies to their physicians as soon as possible.

Angioedema: Angioedema, including laryngeal edema, can occur with treatment with ACE inhibitors, especially following the first dose. Patients should be so advised and told to report immediately any signs or symptoms suggesting angioedema (swelling of face, eyes, lips, or tongue, or difficulty in breathing) and to take no more drug until they have consulted with the prescribing physician.

Symptomatic Hypotension: Patients should be cautioned that lightheadedness can occur, especially during the first days of therapy, and it should be reported to the prescribing physician. Patients should be told that if syncope occurs, Lotensin should be discontinued until the prescribing physician has been consulted.

All patients should be cautioned that inadequate fluid intake or excessive perspiration, diarrhea, or vomiting can lead to an excessive fall in blood pressure, with the same consequences of lightheadedness and possible syncope.

Hyperkalemia: Patients should be told not to use potassium supplements or salt substitutes containing potassium without consulting the prescribing physician.

Neutropenia: Patients should be told to promptly report any indication of infection (e.g., sore throat, fever), which could be a sign of neutropenia.
Drug Interactions
Diuretics: Patients on diuretics, especially those in whom diuretic therapy was recently instituted, may occasionally experience an excessive reduction of blood pressure after initiation of therapy with Lotensin. The possibility of hypotensive effects with Lotensin can be minimized by either discontinuing the diuretic or increasing the salt intake prior to initiation of treatment with Lotensin. If this is not possible, the starting dose should be reduced (see **DOSAGE AND ADMINISTRATION**).

Potassium Supplements and Potassium-Sparing Diuretics: Lotensin can attenuate potassium loss caused by thiazide diuretics. Potassium-sparing diuretics (spironolactone, amiloride, triamterene, and others) or potassium supplements can increase the risk of hyperkalemia. Therefore, if concomitant use of such agents is indicated, they should be given with caution, and the patient's serum potassium should be monitored frequently.

Oral Anticoagulants: Interaction studies with warfarin and acenocoumarol failed to identify any clinically important effects on the serum concentrations or clinical effects of these anticoagulants.

Lithium: Increased serum lithium levels and symptoms of lithium toxicity have been reported in patients receiving ACE inhibitors during therapy with lithium. These drugs should be coadministered with caution, and frequent monitoring of serum lithium levels is recommended. If a diuretic is also used, the risk of lithium toxicity may be increased.

Other: No clinically important pharmacokinetic interactions occurred when Lotensin was administered concomitantly with hydrochlorothiazide, chlorthalidone, furosemide, digoxin, propranolol, atenolol, naproxen, or cimetidine.

Lotensin has been used concomitantly with beta-adrenergic-blocking agents, calcium-channel-blocking agents, diuretics, digoxin, and hydralazine, without evidence of clinically important adverse interactions. Benazepril, like other ACE inhibitors, has had less than additive effects with beta-adrenergic blockers, presumably because both drugs lower blood pressure by inhibiting parts of the renin-angiotensin system.

Carcinogenesis, Mutagenesis, Impairment of Fertility
No evidence of carcinogenicity was found when benazepril was administered to rats and mice for up to two years at doses of up to 150 mg/kg/day. When compared on the basis of body weights, this dose is 110 times the maximum recommended human dose. When compared on the basis of body surface areas, this dose is 18 and 9 times (rats and mice, respectively) the maximum recommended human dose (calculations assume a patient weight of 60 kg). No mutagenic activity was detected in the Ames test in bacteria (with or without metabolic activation), in an in vitro test for forward mutations in cultured mammalian cells, or in a nucleus anomaly test. In doses of 50-500 mg/kg/day (6-60 times the maximum recommended human dose based on mg/m² comparison and 37-375 times the maximum recommended human dose based on a mg/kg comparison), Lotensin had no adverse effect on the reproductive performance of male and female rats.

Pregnancy Categories C (first trimester) and D (second and third trimesters)
See **WARNINGS**, Fetal/Neonatal Morbidity and Mortality.

Nursing Mothers
Minimal amounts of unchanged benazepril and of benazeprilat are excreted into the breast milk of lactating women treated with benazepril. A newborn child ingesting entirely breast milk would receive less than 0.1% of the mg/kg maternal dose of benazepril and benazeprilat.

Geriatric Use
Of the total number of patients who received benazepril in U.S. clinical studies of Lotensin, 18% were 65 or older while 2% were 75 or older. No overall differences in effectiveness or safety were observed between these patients and younger patients, and other reported clinical experience has not identified differences in responses between the elderly and younger patients, but greater sensitivity of some older individuals cannot be ruled out.

Pediatric Use
Safety and effectiveness in children have not been established.

ADVERSE REACTIONS
Lotensin has been evaluated for safety in over 6000 patients with hypertension; over 700 of these patients were treated for at least one year. The overall incidence of reported adverse events was comparable in Lotensin and placebo patients.

The reported side effects were generally mild and transient, and there was no relation between side effects and age, duration of therapy, or total dosage within the range of 2 to 80 mg. Discontinuation of therapy because of a side effect was required in approximately 5% of U.S. patients treated with Lotensin and in 3% of patients treated with placebo.

The most common reasons for discontinuation were headache (0.6%) and cough (0.5%). (See **PRECAUTIONS**, Cough).

The side effects considered possibly or probably related to study drug that occurred in U.S. placebo-controlled trials in more than 1% of patients treated with Lotensin are shown below.

PATIENTS IN U.S. PLACEBO-CONTROLLED STUDIES

	LOTENSIN (N = 964)		PLACEBO (N = 496)	
	N	%	N	%
Headache	60	6.2	21	4.2
Dizziness	35	3.6	12	2.4
Fatigue	23	2.4	11	2.2
Somnolence	15	1.6	2	0.4
Postural Dizziness	14	1.5	1	0.2
Nausea	13	1.3	5	1.0
Cough	12	1.2	5	1.0

Other adverse experiences reported in controlled clinical trials (in less than 1% of benazepril patients), and rarer events seen in postmarketing experience, include the following (in some, a causal relationship to drug use is uncertain):

Cardiovascular: Symptomatic hypotension was seen in 0.3% of patients, postural hypotension in 0.4%, and syncope in 0.1%; these reactions led to discontinuation of therapy in 4 patients who had received benazepril monotherapy and in 9 patients who had received benazepril with hydrochlorothiazide (see **PRECAUTIONS** and **WARNINGS**). Other reports included angina pectoris, palpitations, and peripheral edema.

Renal: Of hypertensive patients with no apparent preexisting renal disease, about 2% have sustained increases in serum creatinine to at least 150% of their baseline values while receiving Lotensin, but most of these increases have disappeared despite continuing treatment. A much smaller fraction of these patients (less than 0.1%) developed simultaneous (usually transient) increases in blood urea nitrogen and serum creatinine.

Fetal/Neonatal Morbidity and Mortality: See WARN-INGS, Fetal/Neonatal Morbidity and Mortality.

Angioedema: Angioedema has been reported in patients receiving ACE inhibitors. During clinical trials in hypertensive patients with benazepril, 0.5% of patients experienced edema of the lips or face without other manifestations of angioedema. Angioedema associated with laryngeal edema and/or shock may be fatal. If angioedema of the face, extremities, lips, tongue, or glottis and/or larynx occurs, treatment with Lotensin should be discontinued and appropriate therapy instituted immediately (see **WARNINGS**).

Gastrointestinal: Constipation, gastritis, vomiting, and melena.

Dermatologic: Apparent hypersensitivity reactions (manifested by dermatitis, pruritus, or rash) and flushing.

Neurologic and Psychiatric: Anxiety, decreased libido, hypertonia, insomnia, nervousness, and paresthesia.

Other: Arthralgia, arthritis, asthenia, asthma, bronchitis, dyspnea, impotence, infection, myalgia, sinusitis, sweating, and urinary tract infection.

Clinical Laboratory Test Findings
Creatinine and Blood Urea Nitrogen: Of hypertensive patients with no apparent preexisting renal disease, about 2% have sustained increases in serum creatinine to at least 150% of their baseline values while receiving Lotensin, but most of these increases have disappeared despite continu-

Lotensin® benazepril hydrochloride

ing treatment. A much smaller fraction of these patients (less than 0.1%) developed simultaneous (usually transient) increases in blood urea nitrogen and serum creatinine. None of these increases required discontinuation of treatment. Increases in these laboratory values are more likely to occur in patients with renal insufficiency or those pretreated with a diuretic and, based on experience with other ACE inhibitors, would be expected to be especially likely in patients with renal artery stenosis (see **PRECAUTIONS**, General).

Potassium: Since benazepril decreases aldosterone secretion, elevation of serum potassium can occur. Potassium supplements and potassium-sparing diuretics should be given with caution, and the patient's serum potassium should be monitored frequently (see **PRECAUTIONS**).

Hemoglobin: Decreases in hemoglobin (a low value and a decrease of 5 g/dL) were rare, occurring in only 1 of 2014 patients receiving Lotensin alone and in 1 of 1357 patients receiving Lotensin plus a diuretic. No U.S. patients discontinued treatment because of decreases in hemoglobin.

Other (causal relationships unknown): Clinically important changes in standard laboratory tests were rarely associated with Lotensin administration. Elevations of liver enzymes, serum bilirubin, uric acid, and blood glucose have been reported, as have scattered incidents of hyponatremia, electrocardiographic changes, leukopenia, eosinophilia, and proteinuria. In U.S. trials, less than 0.5% of patients discontinued treatment because of laboratory abnormalities.

OVERDOSAGE

Single oral doses of 3 g/kg benazepril were associated with significant lethality in mice. Rats however, tolerated single oral doses of up to 6 g/kg. Reduced activity was seen at 1 g/kg in mice and at 5 g/kg in rats. Human overdoses of benazepril have not been reported, but the most common manifestation of human benazepril overdosage is likely to be hypotension.

Laboratory determinations of serum levels of benazepril and its metabolites are not widely available, and such determinations have, in any event, no established role in the management of benazepril overdose.

No data are available to suggest physiological maneuvers (e.g., maneuvers to change the pH of the urine) that might accelerate elimination of benazepril and its metabolites. Benazeprilat can be removed from the body by dialysis, but this intervention should rarely, if ever, be required.

Angiotensin II could presumably serve as a specific antagonist-antidote in the setting of benazepril overdose, but angiotensin II is essentially unavailable outside of scattered research facilities. Because the hypotensive effect of benazepril is achieved through vasodilation and effective hypovolemia, it is reasonable to treat benazepril overdose by infusion of normal saline solution.

DOSAGE AND ADMINISTRATION

The recommended initial dose for patients not receiving a diuretic is 10 mg once-a-day. The usual maintenance dosage range is 20-40 mg per day administered as a single dose or in two equally divided doses. A dose of 80 mg gives an increased response, but experience with this dose is limited. The divided regimen was more effective in controlling trough (pre-dosing) blood pressure than the same dose given as a once-daily regimen. Dosage adjustment should be based on measurement of peak (2-6 hours after dosing) and trough responses. If a once-daily regimen does not give adequate trough response an increase in dosage or divided administration should be considered. If blood pressure is not controlled with Lotensin alone, a diuretic can be added.

Total daily doses above 80 mg have not been evaluated.

Concomitant administration of Lotensin with potassium supplements, potassium salt substitutes, or potassium-sparing diuretics can lead to increases of serum potassium

(see **PRECAUTIONS**).

In patients who are currently being treated with a diuretic, symptomatic hypotension occasionally can occur following the initial dose of Lotensin. To reduce the likelihood of hypotension, the diuretic should, if possible, be discontinued two to three days prior to beginning therapy with Lotensin (see **WARNINGS**). Then, if blood pressure is not controlled with Lotensin alone, diuretic therapy should be resumed.

If the diuretic cannot be discontinued, an initial dose of 5 mg Lotensin should be used to avoid excessive hypotension.

Dosage Adjustment in Renal Impairment

For patients with a creatinine clearance <30 mL/min/1.73 m^2 (serum creatinine >3 mg/dL), the recommended initial dose is 5 mg Lotensin once daily. Dosage may be titrated upward until blood pressure is controlled or to a maximum total daily dose of 40 mg.

HOW SUPPLIED

Lotensin is available in tablets of 5 mg, 10 mg, 20 mg, and 40 mg, packaged with a desiccant in bottles of 100 tablets. Lotensin is also supplied in blister packages (1 tablet/blister), in Accu-Pak® Unit Dose boxes containing 10 strips of 10 blisters each.

Each tablet is imprinted with LOTENSIN on one side and the tablet strength ("5", "10", "20", or "40") on the other. Samples, when available, are identified by the word *SAMPLE* on each tablet.

The National Drug Codes for the various packages are:

Dose	Tablet Color	Bottle of 100	Accu-Pak®
5 mg	light yellow	NDC 0083-0059-30	NDC 0083-0059-32
10 mg	dark yellow	NDC 0083-0063-30	NDC 0083-0063-32
20 mg	tan	NDC 0083-0079-30	NDC 0083-0079-32
40 mg	dark rose	NDC 0083-0094-30	NDC 0083-0094-32

Storage: Do not store above 86° F (30° C). Protect from moisture.

Dispense in tight container (USP).

Printed in U.S.A.   C92-18 (Rev. 3/92)

C I B A

Dist. by :
CIBA Pharmaceutical Company
Division of CIBA-GEIGY Corporation
Summit, New Jersey 07901

ISBN 1-55664-076-5